Medical Management of Kidney and Electrolyte Disorders

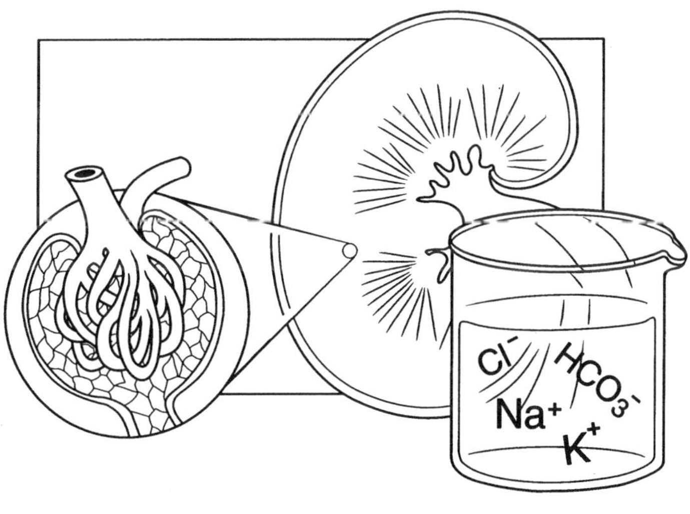

Clinical Guides to Medical Management

Consulting Editor

Burton E. Sobel, M.D.
Medical Center Hospital of Vermont
University of Vermont
Burlington, Vermont

Medical Management of Heart Disease, edited by Burton E. Sobel

Medical Management of Rheumatic Musculoskeletal and Connective Tissue Diseases, edited by Jan Dequeker, Gabriel Panayi, Theodore Pincus, and Rodney Grahame

Medical Management of Atherosclerosis, edited by John LaRosa

Medical Management of Liver Disease, edited by Edward L. Krawitt

Medical Management of Pulmonary Diseases, edited by Gerald S. Davis; Associate Editors: Theodore W. Marcy and Elizabeth A. Seward

Medical Management of Diabetes Mellitus, edited by Jack L. Leahy, Nathaniel G. Clark, and William T. Cefalu

Medical Management of Kidney and Electrolyte Disorders, edited by F. John Gennari

Additional Titles in Preparation

Medical Management of Kidney and Electrolyte Disorders

edited by

F. John Gennari

University of Vermont
Burlington, Vermont

MARCEL DEKKER

DEKKER

MARCEL DEKKER, INC. NEW YORK • BASEL

To my parents, who taught me from the start to think outside the envelope and gave me the gifts of love, discipline, energy, and intellectual curiosity that have enriched my life and work.

ISBN: 0-8247-8869-9

This book is printed on acid-free paper.

Headquarters
Marcel Dekker, Inc.
270 Madison Avenue, New York, NY 10016
tel: 212-696-9000; fax: 212-685-4540

Eastern Hemisphere Distribution
Marcel Dekker AG
Hutgasse 4, Postfach 812, CH-4001 Basel, Switzerland
tel: 41-61-261-8482; fax: 41-61-261-8896

World Wide Web
http://www.dekker.com

The publisher offers discounts on this book when ordered in bulk quantities. For more information, write to Special Sales/Professional Marketing at the headquarters address above.

Current printing (last digit):
10 9 8 7 6 5 4 3 2 1

PRINTED IN THE UNITED STATES OF AMERICA

Foreword

The Medical Management series was developed to provide practitioners, whether they be generalists or specialists, with current and comprehensive information pertinent to the care of their patients. The material is presented in a format consistent with the nature of clinical experience and epistemology. Thus, cardinal signs and symptoms rather than diagnostic labels are points of departure.

This component of the series, edited by Dr. F. John Gennari, addresses kidney and electrolyte disorders. It does so elegantly, thoroughly, thoughtfully, and practically.

Renal disease knows no definitive specialty borders. Whether it presents as eclampsia requiring an obstetrician's wisdom, glomerulonephritis challenging the pediatrician, drug induced interstitial nephritis challenging the internist's acumen, or hypertensive or diabetic nephropathy identified and treated by a conscientious cardiologist, renal disease must be recognized and aggressively managed by each patient's personal physician. Generally, in internal medicine and family practice as well as in emergency medicine, all too often the first recognition of kidney disease is end-stage renal disease following an indolent, subtle course concealed as a result of patient denial or inadequately aggressive diagnostic evaluation.

Medical Management of Kidney and Electrolyte Disorders identifies and highlights symptoms of renal and electrolyte disorders in Part I with four chapters written by internationally respected authorities. Clinical presentation and laboratory evaluation are the subjects of Part II comprising ten chapters by authorities who cover a broad spectrum ranging from the nephrotic syndrome and hematuria to derangements in tonicity, potassium, calcium, phosphorus, and magnesium balance and metabolism. The bulk of the book, Part III, comprises 18 chapters. They address management of renal disease and electrolyte disorders. The presentations cover acute and chronic renal failure; hypertensive and diabetic nephropathy; glomerular, tubular, and interstitial disorders; drug- and toxin-induced nephropathy; kidney stones and infections; obstructive nephropathy and inherited renal diseases; kidney disease in special settings such as pregnancy and hypertension; management of recipients of kidney transplants; treatment of acid-base, tonicity, and electrolyte disorders; and modification of drug dosage in patients with renal insufficiency.

As is the case for the preceding components of the Medical Management series, the focus of this book is on authoritative guidance rather than encyclopedic review. Each chapter is designed to serve as a clinician's "consultant" to aid in the interpretation and development of inferences derived from recognition of cardinal signs and symptoms of disease. The material should facilitate the concerned clinician's consideration of pathophysiological mechanisms underlying disease and their diagnostic and therapeutic implications instead of reinforcing reliance on algorithms and recipes.

Dr. Gennari has assembled a truly outstanding group of authorities from his own institution and throughout the United States. Their contributions provide definitive delineation of kidney and electrolyte disorders and their management that should serve the reader well. Because of its breadth and scope, the book should be useful to generalists and specialists; students, house staff, and fellows; attendings in academic medical centers; practitioners in rural and urban settings; and hospital-, office-, and emergency room–based physicians. It is hoped that this contribution to the Medical Management series will complement its well-received previous publications addressing medical management of atherosclerosis, heart disease, diabetes mellitus, pulmonary disease, liver disease, and dramatic musculoskeletal and connective tissue diseases.

Burton E. Sobel, M.D.

Preface

Kidney diseases, and disorders of fluid and electrolyte balance, can sometimes be a source of confusion for physicians who interact with these important clinical problems only intermittently. This book was conceived to remove that confusion, by providing a comprehensive and concise source of information for the practitioner. To accomplish this goal, experts in specific areas of nephrology have contributed their knowledge. Their contributions include information about pathophysiology, clinical presentation, diagnosis, and treatment, presented in a succinct and readable manner. Although many authors contributed, the book has been carefully edited for consistency of style and approach, and the information has been filtered by a single editor to ensure its accessibility for the reader. It was written with the primary care physician in mind, but should also be a useful reference text for emergency room physicians, hospitalists, intensive care physicians, and all physicians with an interest in this area.

The book is organized into three parts to allow physicians to enter the subject from a variety of perspectives. The first four chapters approach the subject from the viewpoint of patients' symptoms, allowing readers to determine whether their patient's complaint can be accounted for by renal or electrolyte disorders. The subsequent ten chapters approach the topic from the perspective of physical and laboratory findings, defining the characteristic syndromes with which patients present and taking the reader through the key laboratory findings that are the hallmarks of these disorders. The third and largest portion of the book covers the subject from the perspective of specific diseases, and focuses on diagnosis and management. These chapters enable the physician with a question about a specific disease to obtain information about its presentation, diagnosis, and management. A centerpiece of this section of the book is a comprehensive chapter that covers the diagnosis and management of glomerular diseases in a concise and readily accessible manner. In addition, the key topics of the management of chronic renal insufficiency and diabetic nephropathy are reviewed in this section of the book, with particular attention to strategies designed to slow progression to end-stage renal disease. The last chapter of the book covers the important topic of drug dosage modification in patients with renal disease.

This book is intended to provide comprehensive information about all the disorders that comprise the subspecialty of nephrology, but a special highlight is its coverage of electrolyte disorders, an area of particular interest to the editor. The chapters covering these disorders, four of which were written by the editor, are interspersed among all three parts of the book. The first part contains a chapter that covers the symptoms of electrolyte disorders, a unique contribution. In the second part, the pathophysiology, clinical presentation, and tools for diagnosis of these disorders are covered. The specific treatments for electrolyte disorders are presented separately in the third part of the book, allowing the clinician with specific questions about treatment to find the answers quickly.

This book will benefit practitioners of medicine who must manage the increasing population of patients with renal and electrolyte disorders as our population ages. By providing pragmatic and accessible information, it should help to dissolve confusion and provide a rational approach to these disorders.

F. John Gennari, M.D.

Contents

Foreword Burton E. Sobel *iii*
Preface *v*
Contributors *xi*

Part I: Symptoms of Renal and Electrolyte Disorders

1. Oligurìa and Polyuria 1
Gertrude S. Lefavour

2. Edema 19
Rainer Lang

3. Uremia 39
Jeffrey A. Kraut

4. Symptoms of Electrolyte Disorders 57
Deborah B. Adey

Part II: Clinical Presentation and Laboratory Evaluation of Renal Diseases and Electrolyte Disorders

5. Interpretation of Blood Urea Nitrogen (BUN) and Creatinine 75
Gregorio T. Obrador and Andrew S. Levey

6. Asymptomatic Hematuria/Proteinuria 95
Wolfgang J. Weise

7. The Nephrotic Syndrome 113
Ruth C. Campbell and Gerald C. Groggel

8. The Nephritic Syndrome 129
Ann Guillot

9. Secondary Hypertension 137
Jeffrey M. Rimmer

10. Urinary Tract Infection: Physical and Laboratory Findings 157
Mary B. Ramundo, W. Kemper Alston, and Christopher J. Grace

11. Diagnosis of Acid-Base Disorders 169
F. John Gennari

12. Diagnosis of Tonicity Disorders 191
Alan S. Segal

13. Diagnosis of Disorders of Potassium Balance 217
James A. Strom, John T. Harrington, and Geetha Narayan

14. Diagnosis of Disorders of Calcium, Phosphorus, and Magnesium Metabolism 237
F. John Gennari

Part III: Management of Renal Diseases and Electrolyte Disorders

15. Acute Renal Failure 251
Matthew G. Chaffin and Jonathan Himmelfarb

16. Chronic Renal Insufficiency 269
Robert N. Santella

17. Hypertension in Patients with Renal Disease 293
Stephen C. Textor

18. Diabetic Nephropathy 309
Gerald C. Groggel

19. Primary and Secondary Glomerular Diseases 321
Laura M. Dember

20. Drug- and Toxin-Induced Renal Injury 367
William M. Bennett

21. Management of Kidney Stones 393
Melanie P. Derman and David A. Bushinsky

22. Treatment of Urinary Tract Infections 409
Christopher J. Grace, W. Kemper Alston, and Mary B. Ramundo

23. Obstructive Nephropathy 425
E. Darracott Vaughan Jr., Frederick A. Gulmi, and Diane Felsen

24. Inherited Renal Diseases 447
William D. Kaehny

25. Hypertension and Kidney Disease in Pregnancy 465
Susan Hou and Claudia Peano

26. Management of Cardiovascular Complications in Patients with Chronic Renal Insufficiency 489
Deepak Malhotra and William L. Henrich

27. Medical Management of Renal Transplant Patients 499
John D. Scandling

28. Treatment of Acid-Base Disorders 521
F. John Gennari

29. Treatment of Hypertonicity and Hypotonicity 535
Alan S. Segal

30. Treatment of Hypokalemia and Hyperkalemia 549
Geetha Narayan, John T. Harrington, and James A. Strom

31. Treatment of Calcium, Phosphorus, and Magnesium Disorders 565
F. John Gennari

32. Drug Dosing in Renal Insufficiency 575
Carl J. Possidente

Index *589*

Contributors

Deborah B. Adey, M.D. Assistant Clinical Professor, Division of Nephrology, Department of Medicine, University of California, San Francisco, California

W. Kemper Alston, M.D. Associate Professor, Infectious Diseases Unit, Department of Medicine, Fletcher Allen Health Care, University of Vermont, Burlington, Vermont

William M. Bennett, M.D. Medical Director, Solid Organ and Cellular Transplantation Unit, Department of Medicine, Legacy Good Samaritan Hospital, Portland, Oregon

David A. Bushinsky, M.D. Professor of Medicine, and Chief, Nephrology Unit, University of Rochester Medical Center, Rochester, New York

Ruth C. Campbell, M.D. Fellow, Division of Nephrology, Department of Medicine, University of Alabama, Birmingham, Alabama

Matthew G. Chaffin, M.D. Androscoggin Clinical Associates, Lewiston, Maine

Laura M. Dember, M.D. Assistant Professor, Renal Section, Department of Medicine, Boston University School of Medicine, Boston, Massachusetts

Melanie P. Derman, M.D. Nephrology Department, Beth Israel Deaconess, Boston, Massachusetts

Diane Felsen, Ph.D. Associate Research Professor of Pharmacology, Department of Urology, Weill Medical College of Cornell University, New York, New York

F. John Gennari, M.D. Professor of Medicine and Director, Nephrology Unit, Department of Medicine, University of Vermont, Burlington, Vermont

Christopher J. Grace, M.D. Associate Professor, Infectious Diseases Unit, Department of Medicine, Fletcher Allen Health Care, University of Vermont, Burlington, Vermont

Gerald C. Groggel, M.D. Associate Professor, Department of Internal Medicine, University of Nebraska Medical Center, Omaha, Nebraska

Ann Guillot, M.D. Professor, Department of Pediatrics, University of Vermont, Burlington, Vermont

Frederick A. Gulmi, M.D. Attending Urology Physician, Department of Urology, Brookdale University Hospital and Medical Center, and Assistant Professor, Department of Urology, Health Sciences Center at Brooklyn, State University of New York, Brooklyn, New York

John T. Harrington, M.D. Dean and Professor, Tufts University School of Medicine, Boston, Massachusetts

William L. Henrich, M.D. Chairman, Department of Medicine, University of Maryland School of Medicine, Baltimore, Maryland

Jonathan Himmelfarb, M.D. Director, Division of Nephrology and Renal Transplantation, Department of Medicine, Maine Medical Center, Portland, Maine

Susan Hou, M.D. Professor, Loyola University Medical Center, Maywood, Illinois

William D. Kaehny, M.D. Professor, Renal Diseases and Hypertension, University of Colorado School of Medicine, and VA Medical Center, Denver, Colorado

Jeffrey A. Kraut, M.D. Chief, Dialysis Unit, VA Greater Los Angeles Health Care System, and Professor of Medicine, UCLA School of Medicine, Los Angeles, California

Rainer Lang, M.D. Attending Nephrologist, Klinikum Nürnberg, University Erlangen-Nürnberg, Nürnberg, Germany

Gertrude S. Lefavour, M.D. Associate Professor, Nephrology Unit, Department of Medicine, University of Medicine and Dentistry of New Jersey (UMDNJ)–Robert Wood Johnson Medical School, New Brunswick, New Jersey

Andrew S. Levey, M.D. Chief, Division of Nephrology, New England Medical Center, and Professor, Tufts University School of Medicine, Boston, Massachusetts

Deepak Malhotra, M.D., Ph.D. Division of Nephrology, Department of Medicine, Medical College of Ohio, Toledo, Ohio

Geetha Narayan, M.D. Associate Director, Division of Nephrology, St. Elizabeth's Medical Center, and Assistant Professor, Tufts University School of Medicine, Boston, Massachusetts

Gregorio T. Obrador, M.D., M.P.H. Associate Dean for Academic Affairs, Panamerican University School of Medicine, Mexico City, Mexico

Claudio Peano Rush-Presbyterian-St. Luke's Medical Center, Chicago, Illinois

Carl J. Possidente, Pharm.D. Pharmacist Clinician, Department of Pharmacotherapy, Fletcher Allen Health Care, University of Vermont, Burlington, Vermont

Mary B. Ramundo, M.D. Assistant Professor, Infectious Diseases Unit, Department of Medicine, Fletcher Allen Health Care, University of Vermont, Burlington, Vermont

Jeffrey M. Rimmer, M.D. Professor, Nephrology Unit, Department of Medicine, University of Vermont, Burlington, Vermont

Robert N. Santella, M.D., F.A.C.P. Assistant Professor, Department of Internal Medicine, University of South Dakota School of Medicine, Sioux Falls, South Dakota

John D. Scandling, M.D. Professor and Medical Director, Renal Transplantation, Department of Medicine, Stanford University, Stanford, California

Alan S. Segal, M.D. Assistant Professor, Departments of Medicine, Molecular Physiology and Biophysics, and Pharmacology, University of Vermont, Burlington, Vermont

James A. Strom, M.D. Chief of Nephrology, St. Elizabeth's Medical Center, and Associate Professor, Tufts University School of Medicine, Boston, Massachusetts

Stephen C. Textor, M.D. Professor, Mayo Medical School, and Divisions of Hypertension and Nephrology, Mayo Clinic, Rochester, Minnesota

E. Darracott Vaughan Jr., M.D. Chairman, Department of Urology, Weill Medical College of Cornell University, New York, New York

Wolfgang J. Weise, M.D., F.A.C.P. Assistant Professor, Nephrology Unit, Department of Medicine, University of Vermont, Burlington, Vermont

1
Oliguria and Polyuria

Gertrude S. Lefavour
University of Medicine and Dentistry of New Jersey–Robert Wood Johnson Medical School, New Brunswick, New Jersey

I. INTRODUCTION

Of the symptoms and signs associated with renal disease, changes in the volume of urine produced may either be unnoticed or be misinterpreted by the patient. In many instances, however, such changes can provide useful clues to the nature of the underlying disorder as well as being important in management. The reason for poor patient reporting in this regard reflects the great diversity in urine output under normal conditions. Daily urine output can vary from as little as 500 mL of maximally concentrated urine (close to 1200 mOsm/kg H_2O) to as much as 12–15 L of very dilute urine (approximately 50 mOsm/kg H_2O), depending on the need for water balance at any given time. This normal range in urine volume, regulated to maintain water balance, together with the equally precise regulation of volume status, allows most of us to vary intake of water and solutes without giving any thought to limits or to the volume of urine produced.

This chapter is directed at introducing the clinician to disorders of urinary volume —oliguria, polyuria, and anuria. Although the precise volumes that define these three abnormalities are somewhat arbitrary, the most commonly agreed-on values are as follows. Oliguria is defined as a urine volume of less than 400–500 mL/24 hours (<20 mL/hr). Polyuria is defined as a urine volume of greater than 3 L/24 hr (>2 mL/min). Anuria is literally the absence of urine but is defined in the clinical setting as less than 50–100 mL/day. In addition to these three categories of abnormal volume, the chapter will address the symptoms of nocturia, the passage of abnormal amounts of urine in the night, and frequency, a symptomatic increase in the frequency of voiding.

II. ANURIA

Anuria is the condition in which urine output is minimal (50–100 mL/24 hr). It is extremely important to separate anuria from oliguria because the former often indicates the presence of a reversible condition if intervention is undertaken expeditiously. Thus anuria is a medical emergency, not only for salvage of renal function if the cause is correctable, but also to prevent complications of severe

Table 1 Causes of Anuria and Oliguria

- Anuria
  - Bilateral obstruction of urinary tract[a]
  - Bilateral obstruction of renal arteries or veins[a]
  - Cortical necrosis
  - Rapidly progressive glomerulonephritis
  - Shock (particularly in elderly)
  - Pelvic injury, surgical ligation (inadvertent) of ureters
  - Shock wave lithotripsy
  - Following immunoglobulin, thrombolytic or antithrombotic therapy
- Oliguria
  - Prerenal
    - Hemodynamic instability—hemorrhage, burns, GI losses, extravascular sequestration
    - Hypotension, shock
    - Congestive heart failure
    - Sepsis
    - Hepatorenal syndrome
    - Medications—ACE inhibitors, angiotensin II receptor blockers, NSAIDs
  - Intrarenal
    - Ischemic tubular necrosis—hypoperfusion, postoperatively, burns, hemorrhage, pancreatitis, sepsis, trauma, obstetric complications
    - Nephrotoxic tubular necrosis—aminoglycoside antibiotics, radiocontrast, amphotericin, chemotherapeutic agents, myoglobinuria, solvents, heavy metals
    - Glomerular, vascular—acute glomerulonephritis, malignant hypertension, vasculitis, hemolytic uremic syndrome, cholesterol emboli, cortical necrosis
    - Acute interstitial nephritis
  - Postrenal
    - Intratubular obstruction by crystals
    - Intrinsic or extrinsic obstruction of renal pelvis, ureters, urethra by stones, clots, tumor, infection, fibrosis
    - Neurogenic bladder

[a] Or unilateral obstruction of solitary functioning kidney.

renal failure. Surprisingly, some patients may fail to notice or report even complete cessation of urine output until more than a day has elapsed. The disorder quickly produces other symptoms, however, and patients usually come to medical attention in a timely fashion.

Anuria is most commonly associated with bilateral urinary tract obstruction or obstruction of a solitary kidney. An additional useful clue to obstruction is urine output fluctuating between anuria and oliguria or even polyuria. The second most common cause of anuria is acute complete obstruction of the renal arteries or veins (or obstruction of a single vessel if a solitary functioning kidney). Other causes of anuria include diffuse cortical necrosis, rapidly progressive glomerulonephritis, shock (particularly in the elderly), pelvic injury, inadvertent surgical ligation of the ureters, shock wave lithotripsy, or following immunoglobulin, thrombolytic, or antithrombotic therapy (Table 1).

The initial evaluation of a patient with anuria should include the placement of a bladder catheter and renal ultrasound to assess whether obstruction is present (see Chapters 15 and 23 for more details of workup and differential diagnosis). A period of time should elapse after placing a urinary catheter to ascertain that urine is not being produced. If there is no evidence of obstruction, one must cast a wider diagnostic net quickly with particular consideration of arterial occlusion in the patient with a high risk for this problem.

III. OLIGURIA

Oliguria (<400–500 mL urine/day) can be defined physiologically as the production of inadequate amounts of urine to excrete the daily solute and/or water load, leading to accumulation of salt and water as well as nitrogenous wastes and to the eventual development of symptomatic uremia. An individual ingesting a typical North American diet must excrete about 600 mOsmoles (about half of which is salt and half urea) to maintain solute and nitrogen balance. Even if the urine is maximally concentrated (1000–1200 mOsm/kg H_2O), this solute load requires the excretion of at least 500 mL of urine per day. In fact, one rarely can stay in solute balance with a urine output of less than 600–700 mL/day.

Oliguria is almost always associated with acute renal failure, i.e., a large and abrupt drop in glomerular filtration rate (GFR). In chronic renal insufficiency, urine volume is usually maintained at normal or even increased volumes, due to adaptive changes in the remaining nephrons and a loss of concentrating ability (see later). Although an asymptomatic elevation in blood urea nitrogen (BUN) and creatinine is the most common sign of acute renal failure (ARF), oliguria may be the initial clue to the presence of a renal problem. A useful approach to the patient with oliguria is to divide the causes into three general categories:

prerenal, intrarenal, and postrenal. Although oliguria is commonly observed in each of these general categories, urine flow is not always decreased in acute renal failure. Acute renal failure is covered in more detail in Chapter 15 and obstruction in Chapter 23.

A. Prerenal

The major abnormality in prerenal acute renal failure is a decrease in renal blood flow (RBF), due either to decreased renal perfusion pressure or to increased renal vascular resistance (or both), producing oliguria by both decreasing GFR and increasing tubular reabsorption of salt and water. With prompt recognition and treatment of the underlying hemodynamic problem, urine output (and renal function) will usually return to normal. However, if left unrecognized and untreated, intrarenal damage can occur (see below). Any cause of hemodynamic instability can lead to oliguria, including hemorrhage, burns, gastrointestinal fluid losses, or extravascular sequestration of fluid. Hypotension from any cause can cause oliguria. In patients without hypotension, decreased renal perfusion can lead to oliguric states in patients with severe congestive heart failure, sepsis, or hepatorenal syndrome (see Table 1 and Chapter 15).

Two classes of medication—angiotensin-converting enzyme (ACE) inhibitors (and their close cousin, angiotensin receptor blockers) and prostaglandin inhibitors (nonsteroidal anti-inflammatory drugs, or NSAIDs)—deserve special emphasis because of their common use and propensity to reduce glomerular filtration by altering intrarenal hemodynamics. In patients with congestive heart failure, severe liver disease, or underlying chronic renal insufficiency, these drugs may cause prerenal oliguria. Patients with bilateral renal artery stenosis or significant volume depletion are also at increased risk. The elderly (>65 years) are particularly susceptible to developing prerenal oliguria either through medication use or because of dehydration (or volume depletion) from disease or inadequate intake. In addition, these same patients have an increased susceptibility to drug-induced nephrotoxic injury and obstructive uropathy.

Important information is frequently available from both the history and physical examination to help in the diagnosis of a prerenal cause for oliguria. Careful attention should be paid to medication use, excessive fluid loss, possible inadequate intake, history of heart disease, or advanced liver disease. On physical examination, attention should be focused on extracellular fluid volume status. Because tubular function is intact in prerenal azotemia, the urine should be concentrated and have a low sodium concentration ($[Na^+] < 20$ mEq/L) and the fractional excretion of sodium (FE_{Na}) should be less than 1% (see Chapter 15). In addition, the urinary sediment should not contain notable abnormalities. It should be emphasized, however, that none of these findings is diagnostic, and the diagnosis of prerenal versus an intrarenal cause of acute renal failure can sometimes be extremely difficult.

B. Intrarenal

Damage to any of the major structures of the kidney (i.e., glomeruli, tubules, or interstitium) can cause oliguric acute renal failure. By far the most common of these injuries, accounting for over 90% of intrarenal causes of oliguria, is acute tubular necrosis (ATN). Acute renal failure caused by ischemic or nephrotoxic insults is associated with focal necrosis of the tubular epithelium, hence the term ATN. Ischemic etiologies are most common and represent a continuum of the causes of prerenal azotemia (i.e., hypoperfusion from any cause), including post-operative vasoconstriction, hemorrhage, pancreatitis, burns, sepsis, trauma, or obstetric complications. Drugs such as aminoglycoside antibiotics, radiocontrast dyes, amphotericin, or antineoplastic agents are the next most common. Other nephrotoxic etiologies include pigments such as myoglobinuria, solvents such as carbon tetrachloride, bichloride of mercury, or ethylene glycol, or heavy metals such as mercury, platinum, lead, or cadmium (see Chapter 20).

In the history, information should be sought regarding hypotension, recent exposure to nephrotoxins, or risk factors for myoglobinuria. As in the case of prerenal acute renal failure, the physical examination should focus attention on extracellular fluid volume, possible limb ischemia, or evidence of prolonged lying in one position. There are no pathognomonic laboratory findings that can separate intrarenal from prerenal acute renal failure. Because tubular damage is present, however, urine [Na^+] is usually higher than in prerenal oliguria, and the FE_{Na} is typically $> 2\%$. In addition, the urinary sediment often reflects the tubular damage by manifesting the presence of pigmented granular casts or renal tubular epithelial cells.

Acute interstitial nephritis (AIN) is a much rarer cause of oliguria. When present, it is most commonly associated with hypersensitivity reactions to drugs, particularly antibiotics, diuretics, and NSAIDs. Important information from the history and physical examination includes a history of drug exposure, infection, or hematuria and the finding of a rash or fever. The laboratory findings suggestive of allergic interstitial nephritis include minimal proteinuria (<1 g/day), eosinophilia, eosinophiluria, hematuria, pyuria, and casts containing white cells. The interstitial nephritis caused by NSAIDs is an exception, commonly manifested by heavy proteinuria (>3 g/day), and rarely associated with fever, eosinophilia, or oliguria. Recovery from any drug-induced interstitial nephritis usually occurs with discontinuation of the offending agent, although complete recovery may take months.

Glomerular and vascular etiologies such as acute glomerulonephritis, malignant hypertension, vasculitis, hemolytic uremic syndrome, cholesterol emboli, and cortical necrosis are rarer causes than tubular or interstitial injury. Severe oliguria or even anuria is a common presentation in rapidly progressive glomerulonephritis (RPGN) and is an important predictor of poor recovery of renal function. For each of these diseases distinctive physical findings and laboratory results can lead one to the appropriate diagnosis (see Chapters 8 and 19). In most instances, the urinalysis is suggestive of glomerular disease (proteinuria, hematuria, red cell casts). Prompt diagnosis is important in many of these disorders to avoid permanent loss of renal function.

C. Postrenal

Anything that produces obstruction to both kidneys (or obstruction of a solitary kidney) can produce oliguria, although anuria or anuria alternating with oliguria or polyuria is particularly suggestive of obstruction. Intratubular obstruction by crystals such as uric acid (urate nephropathy or as part of the tumor lysis syndrome) or induced by drugs such as acyclovir, sulfadiazine, and recently indinavir is a form of obstruction (intratubular). Obstruction can involve the pelvis of the kidney or ureters (stones, clot, tumor, or infection) or the lower tract (bladder outlet obstruction, neurogenic bladder) and can be extrinsic or intrinsic.

When considering a diagnosis of obstruction, one should question the patient about a history of kidney stones, recurrent urinary tract infection, retroperitoneal or pelvic disease, or neurological disease and inquire about lower urinary tract symptoms such as frequency, urgency, dysuria, or dribbling. Physical findings suggestive of obstruction include a palpable bladder, prostate enlargement, or pelvic pathology. Typically the urine sediment is unremarkable, and the FE_{Na} is $>1\%$. The placement of a urinary catheter may be curative (at least temporarily) in the case of lower tract obstruction. A prompt diagnosis is important since obstructive causes of oliguria can usually be relieved and renal function preserved (see Chapter 23).

IV. POLYURIA

In contrast to anuria and oliguria, polyuria does not necessarily represent a pathological process. An increase in urine volume can be an appropriate response to an increase in fluid intake. The first step in the management of a complaint of polyuria is to determine whether any pathological process is present. As discussed further below, this can sometimes be a vexing diagnostic problem. The amount of fluid ingested is determined by demographic and cultural factors as well as by psychosocial factors, and by abnormalities in hormonal, neurological and hemodynamic stimuli. Polyuria may merely be the manifestation of a self-driven increase in fluid intake or be due to medical advice (up to 4 L/day intake recommended in some patients with cystine stones). Polydipsia is frequently associated with polyuria and may be either the cause or the result of the increase in urine volume.

A. Frequency and Nocturia

Before undertaking a discussion of polyuria, it is important to distinguish it from frequency and nocturia. Frequency is the voiding of small amounts of urine at frequent intervals. Frequency is most often caused by bladder irritation (e.g., cystitis) or by decreased bladder capacity or impaired bladder emptying. Patients who report frequency should not have an abnormally large urine output. Nocturia is the passage of excessive urine in the night. Patients with nocturia usually have decreased urine volume during the day, so that total urine output is not excessive. However, as discussed below, nocturia can also be a symptom of polyuria. Nocturia is most commonly associated with edema-forming states, e.g., congestive heart failure or nephrotic syndrome, and is due to dependent edema fluid reentering the circulation when the patient lies down to sleep at night. In addition it is a common feature of chronic renal insufficiency because the patient is unable concentrate the urine at night (see later).

B. Physiology of Urine Concentration and Dilution

Over half the glomerular filtrate produced daily is reabsorbed in the proximal tubule, a site at which no change in urine tonicity occurs. The primary site that enables both dilution and concentration of the urine is the thick ascending limb of Henle's loop, where sodium is reabsorbed virtually without water, via a specific furosemide-sensitive membrane transporter (the $Na^+/K^+/2Cl^-$ cotransporter). This transporter reduces the osmolality of the tubular fluid entering the distal nephron to approximately 100 mOsmol/kg and delivers solute in excess of water to the descending vasa recta, increasing the tonicity of the medullary interstitium. This single event is multiplied by the countercurrent events that occur in the loop of Henle and adjacent vasa recta, leading to an increase in tonicity at the tip of the renal papilla to as high as 1200 mOsmol/kg under optimal conditions. The high tonicity of the renal papilla is due not only to NaCl accumulation, but also to urea that is added to the countercurrent system in the medullary collecting ducts. Although generated by solute transport and countercurrent multiplication, papillary hypertonicity is maintained by limiting blood flow to the papilla. Any factor that either impedes solute transport or increases papillary blood flow rate will impair the ability to concentrate the urine.

The high papillary osmolality provides the driving force for urine concentration, but the degree to which the urine is concentrated is regulated by adjustments in collecting duct water permeability. Antidiuretic hormone (arginine vasopressin or ADH), secreted by the posterior pituitary gland, binds to a unique receptor (V2 receptor) on the basolateral membrane of the collecting duct epithelial cell and initiates a cellular signaling pathway that adjusts water permeability by inserting water channels in the membrane adjacent to the urine space. In the absence of ADH, collecting duct water permeability is extremely low and the urine remains dilute despite papillary interstitial hypertonicity. Moreover, as the urine traverses the collecting tubule in the absence of ADH, solute absorption continues and urine osmolality falls from 100 mOsmol/kg in the early distal tubule to its minimum value of 50 mOsmol/kg.

ADH secretion is regulated by osmoreceptors located in the hypothalamus that respond to very small changes in plasma osmolality (1–2%). Thirst is also stimulated by increases in plasma osmolality. In addition to osmoreceptors, ADH secretion is stimulated by changes in extracellular volume, so that a 10–20% reduction in ECF volume will also stimulate ADH release, regardless of plasma osmolality. Conversely, ECF volume expansion will blunt the secretion of ADH even when plasma osmolality rises.

C. Pathophysiology of Polyuria

From the above information, it is apparent that the ability to concentrate the urine will be impaired if (1) ADH is not present, (2) the collecting duct is unresponsive to ADH, or (3) medullary tonicity is reduced.

V. CAUSES OF POLYURIA

It is useful to approach a search for the cause of polyuria in your patient by separating the causes into two broad groups: water diuresis and solute diuresis. The former is due to abnormal water excretion, whereas the latter is due to abnormal solute excretion. Water diuresis is either driven by high levels of water intake or is the result of one of the three defects outlined above. Solute diuresis is driven by the need to excrete large amounts of solute in the urine (either through high intake or generation of solute) and is always the result of a loss of medullary hypertonicity due to a solute-induced increase in medullary blood flow.

A simple examination of the urine is usually all that is necessary to determine which of these two categories is responsible for the polyuria. In water diuresis, the urine is usually dilute [specific gravity (S.G.) < 1.010, or osmolality $<$ 250 mOsm/kg H_2O], solute excretion is not excessive, and there is no glycosuria. In solute diuresis, the urine is usually equal to or slightly more concentrated than the plasma (S.G. $= 1.010–1.015$, osmolality $= 300–500$ mOsm/kg H_2O) and a solute (e.g., glucose, sodium, or urea) is present in abnormally large amounts.

Osmolar and free water clearances are theoretical constructs that have little clinical utility and are largely of historical interest. They were developed and used in early studies designed to define the factors responsible for the renal control of solute and water balance. Osmolar clearance (C_{osm}) is defined as the volume of urine (per unit time) required to excrete urine solute at the osmolality of plasma. Free water clearance is defined as the difference between urine volume and C_{osm}. If urine volume was greater than C_{osm}, then free water clearance had a positive value, whereas if C_{osm} was greater than urine volume, free water clearance was said to be negative. These clearances are now rarely measured and they contain incorrect assumptions, particularly regarding the lumping together of urea and electrolyte excretion. The only legacy of this approach is the persistent use of the term ''free water'' rather than ''water'' when discussing replacement fluids (see Table 2).

A. Water Diuresis

Water diuresis, characterized by the excretion of large volumes of dilute urine, is divided into two broad categories: diabetes insipidus (DI), in which increased excretion is primary, and disorders of thirst in which the polyuria is secondary to increased intake of large quantities of fluid (see Table 3). DI itself is divided into central diabetes insipidus (central DI), the result of inadequate production or excessive breakdown of ADH, and nephrogenic diabetes insipidus (nephrogenic DI), due to unresponsiveness of the kidney to ADH.

1. Central Diabetes Insipidus

Central DI is characterized by the passage of large quantities of very dilute urine and is almost always accompanied by increased thirst and nocturia (see Table

Table 2 Commonly Used Formulas

Term	Name	Calculation	Units
C_{osm}	Osmolal clearance	$(U_{osm}) \times V/P_{osm}$	mL/min
C_{H2O}	Free water clearance	$V - C_{osm}$	mL/min
$C_{osm(E)}$	Electrolyte osmolal clearance	$(U_{[Na]} + U_{[K]}) \times V/P_{[Na]}$	mL/min
FE_{Na}	Fractional excretion of sodium	$\frac{(U_{Na}/P_{Na})}{(U_{Cr}/P_{Cr})} \times 100$	%
U_{TS}	Urinary total solute	$(U_{osm}) \times$ total volume (TV)	mOsmol
U_E	Urinary electrolyte solute	$2 \times (U_{[Na]} + U_{[K]}) \times TV$	mOsmol
U_{NE}	Urinary nonelectrolyte solute	$U_{TS} - U_E$	mOsmol
UAG	Urinary anion gap	$(U_{[Na]} + U_{[K]}) - U_{[Cl]}$	mEq

V = Urine volume in mL/min; TV = Urine volume in L/day.

Table 3 Causes of Water Diuresis

Central diabetes insipidus (CDI)
Idiopathic
Trauma, surgery, burns
Hypoxic encephalopathy or severe ischemia
Primary, secondary malignancies—lung, breast, leukemia, lymphoma
Infiltrative disease—Langerhans cell histiocytosis, eosinophilic granuloma, Sarcoidosis
Infection
Familial
Nephrogenic diabetes insipidus (NDI)
Amyloidosis, Sjögren's syndrome
Chronic tubulointerstitial renal disease
Hypokalemia
Drugs—lithium, demeclocycline, cidofovir, foscarnet, methoxyflurane, amphotericin B, aminoglycosides, cisplatin, rifampin
Hypercalcemia
Hereditary—X-linked recessive, autosomal recessive
Sickle cell disease or trait
Obstruction
Recovery from ATN
Postrenal transplantation
Pregnancy-related DI
Preexisting DI (central or nephrogenic)
Occurring during pregnancy—vasopressin responsive, vasopressin-resistant, vasopressin dDAVP–sensitive, vasopressin—dDAVP–resistant, postpartum in Sheehan's syndrome
Excessive water intake
Compulsive water drinking (psychogenic polydipsia)
Thirst center defect, infiltrative disease, trauma

3). In the absence of restricted access to water, serum [Na^+] and osmolality are usually normal or high normal but not markedly elevated. The most common cause of central DI is damage to the neurohypophysis either from surgery or trauma. After such damage, a triphasic response is frequently seen. Initially, a diuretic phase occurs due to ADH deficiency lasting 1–6 days. This is followed by a period of antidiuresis (approximately 5 days) due to release of stored ADH from the damaged neurons. Finally, permanent DI develops if damage is sufficient. Other causes (listed in Table 3) include primary and metastatic tumors, infiltrative and infectious etiologies, and familial, although up to half of cases are idiopathic. Sporadic as well as autosomal dominant inherited forms of central DI present in childhood.

A second cause of ADH deficiency is the result of accelerated metabolism of this hormone. During pregnancy ADH is degraded rapidly due to release of vasopressinase from the placenta. Although this increase in ADH breakdown is not a significant problem in normal women, those with subclinical impairment in ADH production or who have well-controlled central DI frequently become symptomatic during pregnancy. Since the synthetic analog desamino-D-AVP (dDAVP) is resistant to inactivation by vasopressinase, it is usually effective in gestational DI. There are reports of transient vasopressin-responsive, as well as vasopressin-resistant–dDAVP-sensitive, and vasopressin and dDAVP-resistant disease, all resolving after delivery. The coexistence of central DI with Sheehan's syndrome has also been reported as well as transient DI and fatty liver of pregnancy.

2. Nephrogenic Diabetes Insipidus

Nephrogenic DI, resulting from unresponsiveness or resistance of the collecting tubules to ADH, occurs rarely as either an X-linked or autosomal recessive familial disease. These familial disorders have been shown to be due to specific mutations in the gene encoding the V2 receptor or, more rarely, the gene encoding the water channel itself. Nephrogenic DI is much more commonly due to one of a wide variety of acquired disease states or drug-induced disorders of urine concentration (see Table 3). The most striking of these occurs with the drug lithium. This agent blocks the intracellular signal of ADH, leading to symptomatic polyuria despite adequate ADH secretion in approximately 20% of the people taking this drug. The defect is reversible if the drug is discontinued after a short course of therapy but may become permanent after prolonged use. Hypercalcemia also interferes with the cellular effects of ADH and causes a reversible water diuresis.

Most of the other causes of nephrogenic DI are due to a loss of medullary hypertonicity. Furosemide and other loop diuretics completely ablate papillary hypertonicity and lead to the production of isotonic urine. Early on in the course of renal insufficiency, urinary concentrating ability is lost due to disruption of the countercurrent process. In the elderly, urinary concentrating ability is diminished as well, presumably due to the loss of functioning nephrons. Impairment of urinary concentrating capacity due to medullary washout is sometimes termed "partial nephrogenic DI" because the urine is not more dilute than plasma and, as a result, symptomatic polyuria is not usually a problem.

3. Polydipsia

Disorders of thirst regulation cause primary polydipsia, leading secondarily to symptomatic polyuria. This disorder occurs most commonly in patients with psychiatric disease, particularly those with schizophrenia. Compulsive water drinking, up to 8–12 L/day, can occur in these patients with resultant polyuria. The cause is unknown and may be multifactorial. The drugs used to treat schizophrenia have anticholinergic effects, causing a dry mouth, and these may contribute to increased fluid intake. Such patients can frequently be distinguished from those with central DI by a more gradual onset of polyuria, a wider diurnal variation in urine volume (patients with central or nephrogenic DI have constant urine output, thus significant nocturia). As in central DI the urine is very dilute, but individuals with primary polydipsia may have a low serum sodium concentration. As a result of prolonged intake of excess water and production of dilute urine, maximum urinary osmolality is impaired by downregulation of ADH secretion as well as partial washout of the medullary interstitial gradient. Primary polydipsia occurs much more rarely due to abnormalities in the thirst center in the hypothalamus.

B. Solute Diuresis

A solute diuresis inhibits the concentrating capacity of the kidney, causing urine osmolality to be between 300 and 500 mOsm/kg, even in the presence of high concentrations of ADH (see Table 4). The reduction in concentrating capacity is the result of a reduction in papillary solute content (''medullary washout''), in turn caused by an increase in papillary blood flow and, in some instances, by impairment of Na^+ reabsorption in the loop of Henle. The most common cause of polyuria due to solute diuresis is uncontrolled diabetes mellitus. Hyperglycemia causes renal vasodilation and increases papillary blood flow, reducing total papillary solute content. In addition, the filtration of glucose in amounts that

Table 4 Causes of Solute Diuresis

Electrolyte
Volume expansion from saline loading
Sodium wasting—cystic disease, Bartter's syndrome, adrenal insufficiency, cerebral salt wasting
Diuretic administration
Bicarbonate loading, carbonic anhydrase administration
Nonelectrolyte
Glucose—poorly controlled diabetes mellitus, DI patients treated with large volumes of dextrose in water
Urea—hypercatabolic states, high protein feedings, relief of urinary tract obstruction, recovery from ATN
Mannitol
Glycerol
Radiocontrast
Mixed diuresis (solute and water)

exceed the kidney's ability to reabsorb this solute leads to impairment of sodium reabsorption in the loop of Henle, further impairing urinary concentrating ability. A solute diuresis can also occur if excess sodium chloride is ingested or administered. The latter is the reason that ingesting seawater will hasten dehydration by impairing urinary concentrating ability as compared to not drinking anything.

Given these two common causes of polyuria, one should always test the urine in a polyuric patient for the presence of glucose as well as measuring urinary sodium excretion. Glycosuria in the absence of hyperglycemia can be an incidental finding in some forms of renal disease. This so-called renal glycosuria is never sufficient to cause polyuria. Only when the glycosuria is secondary to hyperglycemia does the characteristic polyuria occur. The finding of a random urine $[Na^+]$ greater than 50–70 mEq/L in a polyuric patient is supportive of Na^+-induced solute diuresis. If this test is equivocal, one can measure total urinary solute excretion: the urine osmolality multiplied by the total (24-hr) volume. The contribution of electrolytes is determined by $2 \times (U_{[Na]} + U_{[K]}) \times$ 24-hour volume (or $2 \times U_{[Cl]}$ if urine chloride concentration is greater than $U_{[Na]} + U_{[K]}$). The total urinary solute minus the electrolyte contribution is then equal to the amount of nonelectrolyte solute (see Table 2).

An electrolyte solute excretion rate of >600 mOsm in 24 hours is abnormally high (see Table 2). This is usually the result of excessive salt ingestion or volume expansion with parenteral saline administration. However, a high urinary electrolyte excretion rate can also be due to increased NaCl losses from renal salt wasting syndromes such as medullary cystic disease, Bartter's syndrome, adrenal insufficiency, surreptitious diuretic abuse, or cerebral salt wasting (see Chapter 12). In these settings failure to concentrate the urine is probably due to factors other than the solute in the urine. The urinary anion gap, usually used in the assessment of hyperchloremic metabolic acidosis and determined by $(U_{[Na]} + U_{[K]}) - U_{[Cl]}$, if highly positive, implies significant excretion of an anion other than chloride, e.g., bicarbonate as in bicarbonate loading or carbonic anhydrase inhibitor administration. On occasion ketoanions can contribute significantly to the polyuria as in diabetic, starvation, or alcoholic ketoacidosis, or there may be a high excretion of anionic drugs such as salicylates.

When high rates of nonelectrolyte solute are present in the urine, the total solute excretion will be high (>1000 mOsmol/day), and half or more will be accounted for by nonelectrolyte excretion. Examples of nonelectrolyte causes of solute diuresis are mannitol, glycerol, and radiocontrast administration. Excessive rates of urea excretion may be seen in several settings, i.e., following relief of urinary tract obstruction or during the recovery phase of ATN (see above), or associated with high protein intake either enterally or parenterally, or in highly catabolic states. Whether urea per se is the cause of solute diuresis in these settings is unclear because many other solutes are also being excreted and urea infusions usually do not cause polyuria. In certain polyuric states, excretion of both water and solute is increased. Such patients may excrete a dilute urine (U_{osm} = 150–300 mOsm/kg), but when measured, solute excretion is >900–1000 mOsm per day. This situation occurs most commonly when physicians administer excess water and solute and the kidneys are responding appropriately by excreting the excess.

VI. DIAGNOSIS

The initial step in evaluating a patient who complains of polyuria is to confirm the diagnosis by measuring urine volume. The measurement need not be extremely accurate. If the urine volume is greater than 3 L/day, the diagnosis is established. The next step is to determine the cause. For this purpose, helpful clues are often present in the history. For instance, an abrupt onset of marked polyuria, particularly with recent cranial surgery, shock, ischemia, or trauma, suggests central DI. Patients with central DI have a predilection for iced or very cold water, for some unknown reason. Underlying malignancy (hypercalcemia), prolonged lithium use, or a history of disorders associated with chronic hypokalemia would be consistent with nephrogenic DI. Minimal nocturia is suggestive of primary polydipsia. A family history is suggestive of inherited forms of DI. The recent administration of mannitol, radiocontrast, or excessive saline, the finding of persistently elevated blood glucose or high protein feedings suggests a solute diuresis. Physical examination should focus on whether the patient is volume expanded.

Laboratory studies should include determinations of serum electrolytes, BUN, creatinine, glucose, and calcium. Urine specific gravity and dipstick glucose measurements will quickly assess whether glycosuria is present and whether the diuresis if associated with a dilute urine (<1.010). The latter assessment can be confirmed by measurement of urine osmolality. Further laboratory assessment will depend on whether the cause is still unclear. As discussed above, one can analyze the amount and nature of the solute excreted in the urine when necessary to separate water diuresis from solute diuresis and to define the nature of the excess solute responsible for the polyuria.

VII. DETERMINATION OF THE CAUSE OF WATER DIURESIS

The cause of a water diuresis (central or nephrogenic DI, primary polydipsia) must be determined for proper treatment (see Table 5). In many instances, the diagnosis will be obvious and testing beyond that outlined above is not necessary. For example, if the patient already manifests hypertonic dehydration with a urine osmolality of <150 mOsm/kg H_2O or a specific gravity of <1.003, then the

Table 5 Etiology of Water Diuresis

	Central DI	Nephrogenic DI	1° Polydipsia
Onset	Abrupt	Variable	Gradual
Urine volume	Large	Moderate	Variable
Nocturia	Severe	Moderate	May be absent
History of psychiatric disease	No	No	Frequent
Serum osmolality	High normal	High normal	Low, low normal
Serum sodium	High normal	High normal	Low, low normal

diagnosis is DI rather than primary polydipsia. If patients with DI have access to water and are able to respond to their thirst, however, they will not be dehydrated but will complain of excess thirst. In such instances, a provocative test is needed to separate DI from primary polydipsia. Unfortunately, the provocative test is water deprivation, which can be dangerous for the patient with severe central or nephrogenic DI. Nonetheless, a correctly done water deprivation test (see below) can in most instances separate DI from primary polydipsia and can separate nephrogenic from central DI. The major diagnostic problem is defining partial defects in ADH secretion and separating them from primary polydipsia.

Water restriction testing must be done under careful supervision because severe dehydration and hypertonicity can develop rapidly in some patients. Testing can be done in the outpatient setting, but the patient should be allowed ad-lib fluid intake until 2 hours before the start of the test. Baseline measurements of weight, serum and urine osmolalities, and serum sodium are obtained, and then all fluids are withheld. Hourly determinations of body weight and urine osmolality with serum measurements of sodium and osmolality are made every 2 hours until 3% of body weight is lost or urine osmolality fails to increase by >30 mOsm/kg H_2O over 2–3 hours despite rising serum osmolality or serum osmolality of >295. Five units of aqueous vasopressin is then given subcutaneously (or 10 μg of dDAVP by nasal insufflation) with measurements of urine osmolality after 30, 60, and 120 minutes. Although the results take longer to get back, serum ADH levels should also be obtained at baseline and after dehydration (but before vasporessin administration) to assist in the interpretation of the test.

The normal response to fluid restriction is a two- to fourfold rise in U_{osm} without further change after AVP because endogenous hormone effects are maximal when serum osmolality reaches 295–300 mOsm/kg. In complete DI, U_{osm} remains low and increases by at least 50% (usually 100–800%) following vasopressin administration. Endogenous ADH levels should also be low. In partial central DI, U_{osm} usually rises to >300 with fluid restriction, and there is a subnormal response to AVP (10–50%). If either partial or complete central DI is suggested by this functional test, magnetic resonance imaging of the brain is recommended to identify any brainstem lesions.

In nephrogenic DI a submaximal increase (up to 45%) in U_{osm} is observed during restriction without further change from administered AVP, and the urine remains hypotonic. Polydipsic patients will increase urine osmolality to 500 or greater with fluid restriction but demonstrate no further change with AVP. This subnormal response is due to medullary washout or downregulation of ADH release from prolonged polydipsia and polyuria. Occasionally the distinction between partial CDI and polydipsia is difficult even with measurement of ADH levels. Referral to a nephrologist or endocrinologist is appropriate in some cases to determine the specific diagnosis.

VIII. TREATMENT OF POLYURIA

Once a diagnosis has been established, a treatment plan to control polyuria can be formulated. In the case of diabetes insipidus, if thirst mechanisms are intact and no acute illness is present, the patient will usually be in normal water balance and have a normal serum sodium concentration. If not, then water deficits should be corrected (see Chapter 29). For the stable patient with central DI, the aim of therapy is to provide adequate hormone replacement therapy to decrease nocturia and allow adequate sleep. The synthetic analog of ADH, dDAVP, is usually given once or twice a day to achieve this goal. Care must be taken to avoid overdosage, which will result in hyponatremia. In patients with partial deficiencies in ADH secretion, agents such as chlorpropramide, clofibrate, and carbamazepine have been used with variable success to augment the effects of ADH on the kidney or to stimulate its secretion.

In patients with nephrogenic DI, the polyuria is obviously unresponsive to hormone replacement therapy or to drugs that augment the effects of ADH. The first step in treatment is to correct the underlying cause, if possible (e.g., hypercalcemia) or to discontinue the offending drug (e.g., lithium). When this is not possible or if DI is permanent (e.g., from longstanding lithium use), the use of thiazide diuretics together with salt restriction to cause mild volume depletion can reduce urine volume significantly. Amiloride is the preferred diuretic in lithium-induced nephrogenic DI because it helps block lithium uptake by the distal nephron. Nonsteroidal anti-inflammatory agents such as indomethacin or tolmetin can further reduce urine volume by causing a reduction in GFR in diuretic-treated patients. In addition, the use of a low-protein, low-sodium diet to decrease urinary solute can significantly reduce daily urine volume.

Primary polydipsia is often the most difficult problem to manage. Patient education is the mainstay of therapy. Avoidance, if possible, of drugs causing dry mouth, restriction of fluid, and frequent weighing to detect rapid weight gains and therefore potential hyponatremia all have a role.

The treatment of a solute diuresis should be directed at addressing the underlying cause. Appropriate control of blood glucose will reduce urine volume in diabetes-induced polyuria. Removal or reduction of the offending solute will correct the problem when other solutes are responsible.

SUGGESTED READINGS

Bendz H, Aurell M, Balldin J, Mathe AA, Sjodin I. Kidney damage in long-term lithium patients: a cross-sectional study of patients with 15 years or more on lithium. Nephrol Dial Transplant 1994; 9:1250–1254.

Berl T, Schrier RW. Disorders of water metabolism. In: Schrier RW, ed. Renal and Electrolyte Disorders. 4th ed. Boston: Little, Brown and Company, 1992:1–88.

Durr JA. Diabetes insipidus in pregnancy. Am J Kidney Dis 1987; 9:276–283.

Gennari FJ, Kassirer JP. Osmotic diuresis. N Engl J Med 1974; 291:714–720.

Goldman MB, Robertson GL, Luchins DJ, Hedeker D. The influence of polydipsia on water excretion in hyponatremic, polydipsic, schizophrenic patients. J Clin Endocrinol Metab 1996; 81:1465–1470.

Harris HW Jr, Zeidel ML. Cell biology of vasopressin. In: Brenner BM, ed. Brenner & Rector's The Kidney. 5th ed. Philadelphia: W. B. Saunders Company, 1996:516–531.

Kamel KS, Ethier JH, Richardson RMA, Bear RA, Halperin ML. Urine electrolytes and osmolality: when and how to use them. Am J Nephrol 1990; 10:89–102.

Klahr S, Miller SB. Acute oliguria. N Engl J Med 1998; 338:671–675.

Knepper MA, Rector FC Jr. Urine concentration and dilution. In: Brenner BM, ed. Brenner & Rector's The Kidney. 5th ed. Philadelphia: W. B. Saunders Company, 1996: 532–570.

Ledingham JGG, Crowe MJ, Forsling ML, Phillips PA, Rolls BJ. Effects of aging on vasopressin secretion, water excretion, and thirst in man. Kid Int 1987; 32(suppl 21):S90–S92.

Mindell JA, Chertow GM. A practical approach to acute renal failure. Med Clin North Am 1997; 81:731–748.

Morrison G, Singer I. Hyperosmolal states. In: Narins RG, ed. Maxwell & Kleeman's Clinical Disorders of Fluid and Electrolyte Metabolism. 5th ed. New York: McGraw-Hill, Inc. 1994:617–658.

Narins RG, Riley LJ Jr. Polyuria: simple and mixed disorders. Am J Kidney Dis 1991; 17:237–241.

Navarro JF, Quereda C, Quereda C, Gallego N, Antela A, Mora C, Ortuno J. Nephrogenic diabetes insipidus and renal tubular acidosis secondary to foscarnet therapy. Am J Kidney Dis 1996; 27:431–434.

Oster JR, Singer I, Thatte L, Grant-Taylor I, Diego JM. The polyuria of solute diuresis. Arch Intern Med 1997; 157:721–729.

Palevsky PM. Hypernatremia. In: Greenberg A, ed. Primer on Kidney Diseases. 2nd ed. San Diego: Academic Press, 1998:64–70

Robertson GL. Diabetes insipidus. Endocrin Metab Clin North Am 1995; 24:549–572.

Robertson GL, Berl T. Pathophysiology of water metabolism. In: Brenner BM, ed. Brenner & Rector's The Kidney. 5th ed. Philadelphia: W. B. Saunders Company, 1996: 873–928.

Rose BD, ed. UpToDate. Vol. 6, No. 1.

Sato N, Ishizaka H, Yagi H, Matsumoto M. Posterior lobe of the pituitary in diabetes insipidus: dynamic MR imaging. Radiology 1993; 186:357–360.

Toto RD. Approach to the patient with acute renal failure. In: Greenberg A, ed. Primer on Kidney Diseases. 2nd ed. San Diego; Academic Press, 1998:253–259.

Zeudek ML. Recent advances in water transport. Sem in Nephrol 1998; 18:167–177.

Zerbe RL, Robertson GL. A comparison of plasma vasopressin measurements with a standard indirect test in the differential diagnosis of polyuria. N Engl J Med 1981; 305: 1539–1546.

2 Edema

Rainer Lang
University Erlangen-Nürnberg, Nürnberg, Germany

I. INTRODUCTION

Humans can eat as little or as much salt as they like and drink just a few sips or more than two gallons of liquid a day and still be able to maintain a relatively constant blood volume. The kidneys promptly excrete any unneeded water and salt or minimize the loss of salt and water as needed. Adequate blood volume is the prerequisite of adequate tissue perfusion, and adequate perfusion is required for normal cell and organ function—fundamental for life. Because of its importance, it is not surprising that blood volume is highly regulated.

There are some disorders, however, in which tissue perfusion is challenged, the most common of which is heart failure. In this situation the body tries to increase vascular volume to restore tissue perfusion. Yet some if not most of what was meant to fill the vascular bed leaves the vessels and accumulates in the interstitium. As a result, edema, one of the telltale signs of congestive heart failure, develops. Edema is a visible or palpable expansion of the interstitial fluid volume. It often appears first in the extremities but may also be present in other locations such as the lungs or in the abdominal cavity. Edema occurs in the nephrotic syndrome, renal insufficiency, congestive heart failure, liver cirrhosis, and in several other conditions, as will be discussed later. Edema can also form locally when venous or lymphatic obstruction or local tissue damage occurs. Most commonly, however, edema is a generalized condition with symmetrical involvement, as in the disorders mentioned above.

General edema is invariably associated with renal Na^+ retention, which may be the primary event, as in acute glomerulonephritis, or the response to another disorder, as in congestive heart failure. Regardless of the cause, general edema can only form if Na^+ intake exceeds Na^+ excretion. This chapter will focus on the causes, symptoms, and management of generalized edema.

II. PATHOPHYSIOLOGY

A. Volume Regulation

The fluid contained in the vascular and interstitial compartments together make up the extracellular fluid (ECF) volume. ECF volume accounts for only about 20% of body weight but harbors nearly three quarters of total body Na^+. Because Na^+ and its accompanying anions make up most (>90%) of the total solute contained in the ECF and because the solute concentration (osmolality) of the body fluids is also regulated (see later), the absolute amount of Na^+ in the body determines the size of the ECF volume. Thus, regulation of Na^+ balance by the kidneys also controls ECF volume and indirectly determines vascular volume as well. Vascular volume is maintained within narrow limits despite considerable fluctuations in daily fluid and Na^+ intake. In fact, a 2–3% reduction in vascular volume results in virtual elimination of Na^+ from the urine even before changes in cardiovascular parameters are detectable.

Whenever volume homeostasis is challenged, hemodynamic responses are activated within minutes and result in changes in heart rate, peripheral resistance, and venous capacitance (Table 1). Within a few hours Na^+ and water balance is adjusted by changes in the excretion of Na^+ and water by the kidneys and by

Table 1 Integrated Response to Hypovolemia

	Hemodynamic changes	Na^+ and water balance
Onset	Minutes	Hours
Response	↑ Cardiac contractility	Thirst
	↑ Heart rate	Renal sodium and water retention
	↑ Peripheral resistance	
	↑ Venous constriction	
Stimulated	Catecholamines	Catecholamines
	Angiotensin II	Angiotensin II
	ADH	ADH
	Endothelin	Aldosterone
	Prostaglandin H_2	
	Thromboxane A_2	
Suppressed	Prostaglandin E_2	Prostaglandin E_2
	Atrial natriuretic peptide	Atrial natriuretic peptide
	Nitric oxide	Nitric oxide

behavioral signals to the brain (e.g., increasing or decreasing thirst). Additionally, fluid can be shifted between the vascular and interstitial compartment across the capillary membranes either to help restore vascular volume in the face of volume depletion or to decrease vascular volume if it is abnormally increased. Thus the interstitium functions as a volume buffer for the vascular compartment.

B. Effective Vascular Volume

Pressures in the venous and arterial systems are continuously monitored by specialized baroreceptor sensing cells, and these cells can initiate effector responses to stabilize vascular volume when these pressures change. Baroreceptors in the pulmonary veins and the atria sense the filling of the low-pressure regions of the circulation. Arterial baroreceptors located in the carotid sinus, the aortic arch, and the juxtaglomerular apparatus sense arterial filling pressures. These latter sensors are the guardians of what is termed ''effective vascular volume.'' Because the arterial circulation is such a small fluid compartment ($<2\%$ of total body water), small changes of its volume can have substantial effects and are therefore vigorously compensated for, whereas similar changes in the venous compartment are better tolerated.

In hypovolemia, baroreceptor activation sets off a cascade of responses that result in increased levels of angiotensin II, aldosterone, catecholamines, endothelin, antidiuretic hormone (ADH), prostaglandins, and other hormones. Not surprisingly, virtually all of these hormones have the ability to directly or indirectly alter total peripheral and renal vascular resistance and to decrease renal Na^+ excretion. ADH has the additional property of facilitating water reabsorption in the collecting duct, which is why dilutional hyponatremia is a common finding in severe heart failure or advanced cirrhosis, and sometimes in nephrotic syndrome, conditions where the arterial baroreceptors sense hypovolemia.

In response to overfilling of the vasculature (hypervolemia), hormones that cause vasodilation and/or natriuresis are released. These include atrial natriuretic peptide (ANP), prostaglandin E_2, and nitric oxide (NO).

From the foregoing, it is apparent that ECF volume regulation is a multifactorial process. The redundancy of the regulatory system not only makes it resilient and flexible, but also assures its continuing operation if one or more regulatory responses are impaired. The system becomes much less flexible when cardiac or renal function is impaired.

C. Starling Forces

The physiological factors involved in the balance between vascular and interstitial fluid distribution are called Starling forces. These include capillary and interstitial hydrostatic and oncotic pressures and the permeability of the capillary wall that separates the vascular from the interstitial space.

Arterial, venous, and lymphatic pressures influence capillary and interstitial hydrostatic pressures. Capillary hydrostatic pressure in addition is locally regulated by pre- and postcapillary sphincters. The oncotic pressures of plasma and interstitial fluid counterbalance the driving force of the associated hydrostatic pressures. Vascular permeability does not change in most settings where edema formation occurs, unless there is associated microvascular injury. The sum of all these transcapillary pressures is termed the net transcapillary pressure, which describes the net driving force for transcapillary fluid movement. Local protective mechanisms allow flexibility to buffer changes in the net transcapillary pressure. For example, when fluid shifts from the capillary lumen into the interstitium, it increases the interstitial hydrostatic pressure, dilutes interstitial proteins, and reduces interstitial oncotic pressure. The higher interstitial hydrostatic pressure in turn augments lymphatic flow, which washes out protein and thus further reduces interstitial oncotic pressure. In moderate hypoalbuminemia, interstitial and plasma albumin concentrations tend to equilibrate, minimizing the oncotic imbalance. Edema formation reflects exhaustion of these local protective mechanisms.

III. STATES OF VOLUME DYSREGULATION

Although the first clinical impression of a patient with edema suggests fluid volume overload, the problem is somewhat more complex. For example, in certain settings the effective vascular volume may still be seriously reduced despite considerable interstitial volume expansion (edema). Patients with edema have excess Na^+ and water in their body, but this excess isotonic fluid is often distributed inappropriately in the ECF compartment. We cannot measure effective vascular volume directly, but it can be estimated from hormone levels, renal or cardiac responses, and of course with clinical experience. Renal sodium excretion varies directly with the effective vascular volume, and it is important to understand this concept for edema therapy.

A. Congestive Heart Failure

Congestive heart failure is the prototypical example for a condition of low effective vascular volume. Forward failure from decreased cardiac output results in low pressures at the baroreceptors. They in turn induce a cascade of events that ultimately increases plasma (and interstitial) volume by compensatory renal Na^+ retention. This response is homeostatic in the sense that some of the retained Na^+ and water contributes to vascular volume, which in turn increases cardiac filling pressures, cardiac output, and systemic pressure. Although some of the extra volume stays within the vascular compartment, the remainder enters the interstitium and eventually appears clinically as edema. Because arterial filling pressures are the most tightly regulated, the response to what the arterial baroreceptors sense overrides signals from the low-pressure system and Na^+, and water retention usually continues despite the release of ANP from the dilating atria. If these responses are able to restore effective vascular volume to normal, then renal Na^+ excretion will again match intake and a new steady-state of balance will be achieved. In high-output cardiac failure, such as occurs in thyrotoxicosis, the effective vascular volume is reduced primarily due to peripheral vasodilation. The kidneys respond with Na^+ retention just as outlined above for low-output failure.

In mild heart failure this adaptive response improves myocardial performance. However, with progression of cardiac disease and worsening failure, renal Na^+ and water retention does not restore effective vascular volume to normal, and with continued Na^+ and water intake, edema worsens. Furthermore, diastolic filling pressures and volumes increase, which makes stroke work less efficient. The high peripheral vascular resistance with or without accompanying high blood pressure fed by the continued release of vasoconstrictor hormones (see earlier) may embarrass cardiac function further as well. ANP levels are elevated in parallel with the severity of the disease, and the hormone has a role in renal and peripheral vasodilation with hemodynamic improvement. Its natriuretic effect, however, is blunted, possibly because of reduced sodium delivery to its site of action in the collecting duct. Angiotensin-converting enzyme (ACE) inhibitors as well as angiotensin receptor (AT1) blockers restore the diuretic response to exogenous ANP in animals with severe congestive heart failure presumably by increasing distal Na^+ delivery.

B. Renal Insufficiency

The damaged kidney is remarkable in its ability to continue to maintain Na^+ balance. To achieve this balance when the glomerular filtration rate (GFR) (and the filtered load of Na^+) is reduced requires downregulation of tubular Na^+ reabsorption in the remaining nephrons in order to match Na^+ excretion with intake. Unfortunately, the natriuretic response to acute Na^+ intake becomes more and more delayed as GFR falls. As a result, ECF volume expansion ensues and this change increases systemic blood pressure. For reasons that are unclear, the renin-angiotensin-aldosterone system and sympathetic nervous activity are not appropriately suppressed for the degree of plasma volume expansion in patients with chronic renal insufficiency. Additionally, accumulation of oxygen free radicals suppresses NO synthesis, thus impairing another vasodilatory and natriuretic pathway. Eventually, sufficient Na^+ retention occurs to produce clinical edema. Given the diet ingested by most of our patients, it is not surprising that hypertension and edema are characteristic features of advanced renal insufficiency. It should be noted, however, that the ability to conserve Na^+ is also impaired, presumably due to the downregulation of tubular Na^+ reabsorption, so that volume depletion can occur with severe dietary Na^+ restriction or overdiuresis.

Edema is a typical feature of *acute poststreptococcal glomerulonephritis*, occurring in about 85% of cases (see Chapters 8 and 19). GFR is almost always reduced in acute disease, and urine output falls to frankly oliguric levels (see Chapter 1 for definitions) in about half of the patients. Avid renal Na^+ retention causes acute volume expansion with hypertension, heart failure, and edema. Proteinuria is usually not in the nephrotic range and is not likely to contribute to edema formation. *Rapidly progressive glomerulonephritis* is not typically associated with severe edema formation despite similar reductions in GFR and mild to moderate proteinuria. Why Na^+ retention is less pronounced is not known.

Edema formation is extremely common in patients with *diabetic nephropathy* due to the additive effects of renal insufficiency, hypoalbuminemia, increased capillary permeability, and autonomic neuropathy. This spectrum of disturbances plus the comorbidities that are almost always present once diabetic nephropathy develops poses a real medical challenge.

C. Nephrotic Syndrome with Normal Renal Function

Nephrotic syndrome is characterized by proteinuria, hypoalbuminemia, and edema formation due to Na^+ retention (see Chapter 7). Despite the sometimes huge increase in ECF volume caused by Na^+ and water retention in this disorder, it is not clear whether the effective vascular plasma volume is increased, normal, or decreased. Two views of the pathophysiology of the edema in the nephrotic syndrome have experimental support. The first or classic view is that the edema is due to the decrease in plasma oncotic pressure, per se, with a resultant decrease in effective vascular volume triggering renal Na^+ retention. This is the ''underfill'' view of nephrotic edema. The second view is that a primary renal insult leads both to proteinuria and Na^+ retention. According to this view, the effective vascular volume is increased or ''overfilled'' and edema is due to the resultant imbalance in Starling forces. Differentiating between hypovolemic and hypervolemic nephrotic syndrome has clinical and therapeutic implications. In the former scenario, aggressive diuresis could lead to hypotension and vascular collapse; in the latter scenario, diuresis can be pursued with impunity. However, it is often difficult to make a distinction between these two views because of the difficulties in assessing plasma volume, and research studies have shown conflicting results. Clinically, nephrotic syndrome with low effective vascular volume should be suspected in patients with postural hypotension, a normal GFR, a serum albumin <2 g/dL, and/or minimal change disease (see Chapter 7).

D. Cirrhosis of the Liver

Cirrhosis stimulates renal Na^+ and water retention early in its course. This change in renal Na^+ handling eventually leads to ascites formation as liver disease progresses. With near end-stage liver disease, GFR also declines and renal failure may develop. However, changes in renal function appear to be functional in nature in many cases. The most dramatic demonstration of the functional nature of these changes is that kidneys transplanted from patients with cirrhosis into patients with normal liver function have worked normally with respect both to filtration rate and Na^+ balance.

Patients with cirrhosis frequently have an elevated cardiac output, but they behave as if they were volume depleted, as evidenced by avid Na^+ retention, progressive activation of the renin-angiotensin-aldosterone system, stimulation of the sympathetic nervous system (e.g., norepinephrine), and ADH secretion. This disparity is caused by vasodilation, mainly in the splanchnic region, and by multiple arteriovenous fistulas, some of which are visible as spider nevi. These abnormalities lead to a relative underfilling of the arterial circulation. Arterial baroreceptors sense low pressures and induce a hyperdynamic circulatory response and Na^+ and water retention (Table 1).

E. Other Causes of Edema

Idiopathic edema is a disorder that most commonly affects menstruating women who appear otherwise healthy. The edema may initially be present only premenstrually, when plasma volume is increased, but it eventually persists throughout the menstrual cycle. These patients appear to have an abnormal response to assuming upright posture, characterized by excessive pooling of volume in the lower extremities. Hypovolemia from loss of fluid into the interstitium triggers renal Na^+ retention and a weight gain of several kilograms during daytime. A variety of clinical studies have demonstrated minor abnormalities in capillary permeability and hormonal regulation of electrolyte balance in women with this disorder, but no conclusive pathophysiology has been elucidated. As a result, idiopathic edema has been dismissed by some as being paradoxically induced by the chronic diuretic use. According to this view, Na^+-retaining mechanisms are normally activated in response to diuretic-induced hypovolemia. When the patient attempts to discontinue the diuretics, a rapid "rebound" edema follows, which implies to the patient and the physician that continued diuretic therapy is indeed indicated. Rebound weight gain is a normal response to diuretic discontinuation, however, and it may be exaggerated by chronic potassium depletion. Post-diuretic edema after long-term diuretic therapy can be avoided if diuretics are tapered over at least 2 weeks and potassium losses are adequately replaced. Diuretic dependence probably plays a role in the majority, but not all, cases of idiopathic edema.

Up to 80% of *pregnancies* are associated with edema that worsens with gestation time. The edema of pregnancy is associated with peripheral venous and arterial vasodilation and a new low-resistance shunt, the placenta. The renin-angiotensin-aldosterone system and other volume regulatory systems are activated to restore the effective plasma volume and compensate for the enlarged vascular bed. Taken together, these mechanisms result in increased heart rate and stroke volume in the presence of low blood pressure. Towards the end of the pregnancy edema formation is enhanced by increased capillary hydrostatic pressure in the lower extremities that is only partially compensated for by decreased interstitial oncotic pressure. Diuretics have no place in the management of this physiological form of edema.

Edema formation in *preeclampsia* has a different pathophysiology (see Chapter 25). It originates as a result of the release of factors from the ischemic placenta that impair normal endothelial integrity and cause fluid loss into the interstitium. Edema formation is facilitated by the concomitant presence of hypertension, proteinuria, and hypoalbuminemia. Edema alone does not make the diagnosis of preeclampsia; hypertension and proteinuria are essential components. The presence of edema is actually associated with a better outcome than the nonedematous variant of preeclampsia.

Some degree of *capillary leak* may contribute to edema formation in patients with diabetes. There are also cases of episodic capillary leak syndromes, in most of which a monoclonal gammopathy was eventually diagnosed. A variety of cytokines have been shown to induce capillary leak, among which are interleukins 1, 2, and 4, tumor necrosis factor, and bradykinin. There is no evidence that similar alterations in capillary membranes play a significant role for edema formation in congestive heart failure or renal disease.

Drugs, particularly potent vasodilators, can induce edema. This is especially true for calcium channel blockers, which can abolish autoregulation of the precapillary sphincters and thus expose the capillary bed to higher hydrostatic pressures. All vasodilators induce some degree of renal Na^+ retention and can cause edema by this mechanism, including calcium channel blockers, minoxidil, hydralazine, clonidine, and α_1 blockers such as terazosin. Fludrocortisone, estrogens, and nonsteroidal anti-inflammatory drugs (NSAIDs) directly stimulate renal Na^+ reabsorption. The pathogenesis of postdiuretic edema was discussed above.

IV. CLINICAL PRESENTATION AND EVALUATION

Bilateral leg edema is more likely to be caused by a systemic disorder than by local factors. In one review of a group of patients in whom venous insufficiency was felt to be the primary cause in the majority, careful diagnostic evaluation revealed that only 22% had venous insufficiency alone. In the others, 33% had cardiac disease, 42% had pulmonary hypertension with or without additional cardiac disease, and 18% had renal disease; drugs may have contributed in 16%, and no cause was identifiable in 27%. Thus, although venous insufficiency is much more common than congestive heart failure or kidney disease (25–30% vs. $<1\%$ in the general population), bilateral leg edema should raise the clinical suspicion and initiate a search for a systemic cause. In such a patient, the physician should always initiate a workup to establish the cause before beginning diuretic treatment.

A. History

In most patients, obtaining a history and symptoms of congestive heart failure or hepatic cirrhosis is straightforward. In some patients with these diseases and in many patients with renal disease, however, there may be no symptoms other than edema. In the patient with renal disease, a history of noting foamy urine (from its protein content) or periorbital swelling in the morning can occasionally be elicited. Abrupt occurrence of bilateral leg edema may be caused by the acute onset of the nephrotic syndrome or after excessive salt intake in a previous compensated state of heart failure or renal insufficiency. A diagnosis of deep vein thrombosis or even bilateral iliac thrombosis is much less likely but may be considered.

B. Differential Diagnosis

Chronic venous insufficiency is typically associated with brawny induration or venous stasis ulcers. These signs may be absent in unilateral venous edema of recent onset. The first and most persistent symptom of lymphedema is a puffiness of the dorsum of the foot that does not disappear even with bed rest. Primary lymphedema is caused by an inherited defect in the lymphatic system with hypoplasia or varicose dilatation that affects women 10 times more commonly than men. Symptoms sometimes do not become apparent until after the age of 35 years. Acquired lymphedema can be secondary to lymphatic obstruction from carcinoma, infection, radiation, or retroperitoneal fibrosis.

If idiopathic edema is suspected, a history of diuretic or laxative abuse as well as anorectic behavior should be sought. Increased hydrostatic pressure over a long working day produces a small degree of lower leg edema in almost everyone and is not a sign of disease. Weight gains of 1–3 pounds are common. This swelling promptly resolves overnight and should not be medically treated.

So-called lipedema is not true edema and does not pit on pressure. It results from subcutaneous accumulation of fatty tissue in the legs and always spares the feet. It affects women almost exclusively and may be familial. In myxedema, mucopolysaccharides are deposited in subcutaneous, submucosal, and subendothelial spaces, and these substances bind water and Na^+ and impair lymphatic clearance. Mental disturbances, hypothermia, and changes in the skin as well as other typical symptoms of hypothyroidism are almost always present.

Drugs, namely vasodilators, diuretics, laxatives, and nonsteroidal analgesics, may provide clues for drug-induced edema. Questions about salt intake are often more educational than helpful, since most patients are unaware of the salt content of their diet. Family history can be helpful in the diagnosis of hereditary kidney, heart, or liver diseases.

C. Physical Examination

Clinically detectable edema does not occur until ECF volume has increased by at least 2–3 liters. It is found primarily in the dependent areas of the body in a symmetrical distribution—in the lower extremities in ambulatory patients or over the sacrum and along proximal thighs in a bedridden patient. It is likely to redistribute to other areas of the body with changes in posture, a feature that differentiates it from local edema. Periorbital edema occurs in supine patients with severe nephrotic syndrome where the low periorbital interstitial hydrostatic pressure does not effectively compensate for the decreased plasma oncotic pressure.

Central venous pressure is elevated in right-sided heart failure and less often in renal insufficiency. It is normal or may even be decreased in patients with cirrhosis. Patients with ascites and associated jugular vein distention should always be evaluated for possible right-sided heart failure. Ascites is associated with all causes of general edema but is most commonly found in cirrhosis and right-sided heart failure. Pulmonary edema is a typical feature of left-sided heart failure (due either to systolic or diastolic dysfunction), but it can also occur in patients with renal insufficiency and normal left ventricular function after excessive Na^+ intake and retention. Pulmonary edema does not occur in the nephrotic syndrome if GFR is normal or near normal or in hepatic cirrhosis. The presence or absence of hypertension, postural hypotension and tachycardia, peripheral vascular filling and cyanosis, and the moisture of mucus membranes gives clues to estimate the status of effective vascular volume.

D. Laboratory Evaluation

Renal disease can be evaluated easily in the office by urine dipstick testing. The absence of protein or blood on urine dipstick makes intrinsic renal disease highly unlikely. If proteinuria (1+ or greater) is present on dipstick testing, it should be quantitated in a spot urine sample or a 24-hour collection (see Chapters 6 and 7). In a spot urine sample, the measured protein concentration divided by the measured creatinine concentration provides a reasonable estimate of proteinuria (in g/day). Examination of the urine sediment in patients with hematuria and proteinuria is essential to further characterize the nature of the renal disease (see Chapter 6).

With the exception of the nephrotic syndrome, a normal serum creatinine value essentially excludes renal disease as a cause of the edema. Measurement of creatinine or iothalamate clearance is rarely necessary or indicated (see Chapter 5). In severe heart failure or liver cirrhosis, the kidneys react appropriately to the prerenal condition, and creatinine values may fluctuate from day to day reflecting changes in effective vascular volume.

Measurement of urine Na^+ concentration in a random sample is rarely helpful in establishing the cause of edema. In general, urine Na^+ concentration should be inappropriately low in all edema states. In acute disease, Na^+ excretion may indeed serve as an indicator of the renal response to what is being sensed by the arterial baroreceptors. Because of the confounding effect of concomitant blood pressure medication and/or diuretics or the inability to adequately concentrate or dilute the urine in chronic renal insufficiency, however, interpretation of the test results is often difficult. In patients with cirrhosis receiving diuretic therapy, urine Na^+ concentrations may be helpful in guiding treatment. Values below 10 mEq/L can indicate too vigorous volume removal with an increased risk of developing hepatorenal syndrome. Measurement of Na^+ concentration in a 24-hour urine collection allows the physician to assess dietary Na^+ intake and base dietary advice on the finding, because in the steady state, Na^+ excretion is virtually equal to Na^+ intake.

A low serum Na^+ concentration is a sign of the severity of congestive heart failure or liver cirrhosis and indicates a poor prognosis, particularly when present in the absence of diuretic therapy. This dilutional hyponatremia reflects inadequate water excretion due to continuous ADH release. It provides no information regarding Na^+ balance (see Chapter 12).

Serum albumin concentration is typically low in the nephrotic syndrome and can fall to levels as low as 1 g/dL in severe disease. However, hypoalbuminemia is not specific to the nephrotic syndrome; it can occur in malnourished or very ill patients and is a feature of advanced cirrhosis as well.

Measurement of volume regulatory hormones such as renin, aldosterone, norepinephrine, ADH, or ANP is generally not useful in the clinical setting. Results may well be in the normal range in the compensated state or may not be interpretable unless Na^+ and water balance, posture and influences of concomitant medications are carefully controlled for. Primary hyperaldosteronism does not cause clinically detectable edema.

Liver and thyroid function tests are helpful in confirming the clinical suspicion of cirrhosis or hypothyroidism with myxedema. Imaging studies such as chest x-ray and echocardiogram may confirm a clinical diagnosis of congestive heart failure or pulmonary hypertension. Venous insufficiency or deep vein thrombosis can best be studied with Duplex ultrasound. CT of the abdomen is useful in the evaluation of lymphedema and has replaced lymphangiography.

V. TREATMENT

The key therapeutic principle in treating generalized edema is to reverse the underlying cause if possible. If this goal cannot be accomplished, the next goal should be an attempt to restore the effective vascular volume towards normal. The specific approach depends on the abnormality causing the edema. In congestive heart failure, steps to improve cardiac function should be initiated. In the nephrotic syndrome, maneuvers to reduce proteinuria should be instituted. In hepatic cirrhosis maneuvers to reduce splanchnic and peripheral vasodilation should be considered. The third goal of therapy should be to reduce dietary Na^+ intake. In the absence of continually adding more Na^+ to the body than can be excreted, edema cannot worsen regardless of the cause. When the patient is properly educated and motivated, edema can often be controlled simply by reducing Na^+ intake. Unfortunately, in most cases diuretics are necessary to alleviate the symptoms of the edematous patient.

A. Diuretics

Diuretics are potent disrupters of volume regulation, which makes them valuable for the treatment of edema. With the exception of the carbonic anhydrase inhibitors, all clinically useful diuretics interfere with Na^+ reabsorption by blocking specific transport mechanisms. They are grouped into classes according to their site of action along the nephron (Table 2). Most of the side effects are class specific and can be explained by the physiological role of the transporter that is inhibited.

Loop diuretics are potent natriuretic agents (see Table 2). They have a rapid onset and short duration of action. The peak natriuresis occurs within 2 hours if taken by mouth, and the duration of effect lasts only 4–8 hours. The effectiveness of these agents is limited by the adaptive response of the kidney to the reduction in effective vascular volume induced by their administration. This adaptive response, mediated by angiotensin II as well as α-adrenergic stimulation, increases Na^+ reabsorption in the proximal tubule and in the collecting duct. The limitation in the diuretic effectiveness of these agents, not unexpectedly, is most evident in patients with edema states characterized by low effective vascular volumes, such as congestive heart failure and cirrhosis. Loop diuretics are very effective in patients with ECF volume overload due to impaired renal function.

Table 2 Diuretics

Type	Na^+ transporter inhibited	Maximal effect on Na^+ excretion
Loop diuretics: Furosemide, bumetanide, piretanide, torasemide, ethacrynic acid	$Na^+ - K^+$-$2Cl^-$ transporter in the loop of Henle	Up to 25% of filtered Na^+
Thiazides: Hydrochlorothiazide, chlorthalidone, indapamide, metolazone	Na^+-Cl^- cotransporter in distal tubule	3–5% of filtered Na^+
K^+-sparing diuretics: Amiloride, triamterene, spironolactone	Epithelial Na^+channel in the collecting duct	1–2% of filtered Na^+
Carbonic anhydrase inhibitors: Acetazolamide, methazolamide	Na^+/H^+ exchanger, H^+-ATPase in proximal tubule and loop of Henle	Minimal due to distal compensation

Loop diuretics typically produce metabolic alkalosis and hypokalemia by increasing Na^+ delivery to the collecting duct where its reabsorption promotes H^+ and K^+ excretion and can cause significant magnesium loss by mechanisms not clearly defined. Loop diuretics are ototoxic when peak blood levels exceed 50–100 mg/L. Such blood levels may be achieved by rapid bolus intravenous administration. Unlike most other drugs, the dosage of the loop diuretics should be increased in renal insufficiency to as high as 160 mg twice daily of furosemide as needed to obtain a diuretic response.

Thiazides are less potent but nonetheless effective diuretic agents. They have a gradual onset and more prolonged duration of action than the loop diuretics. The peak natriuresis after a single oral dose occurs within 3–6 hours, and the duration of action is 6–48 hours, depending on the particular thiazide used. The natriuretic response decreases markedly with impaired renal function (GFR < 30 mL/min, creatinine > 3 mg/dL). Metolazone may be more effective than other thiazides in patients with impaired renal function because it accumulates and provides higher concentrations at its site of action in the kidney.

Thiazides can produce significant hypokalemia and metabolic alkalosis along with magnesium loss, by the same mechanisms as outlined above for the loop diuretics. In contrast to the loop diuretics, however, the thiazides decrease renal calcium excretion and can rarely cause mild hypercalcemia. The thiazides impair renal diluting capacity, but not the ability to concentrate the urine. As a result hyponatremia, sometimes severe, can occur. Loop diuretics and thiazides are chemically related and can impair glucose tolerance, lipid metabolism, and uric acid excretion.

Potassium-sparing diuretics are the least potent of the clinically useful diuretics. Their main asset, inhibition of K^+ excretion, is also their potentially major liability. They should not be used in situations of impaired K^+ excretion, such as renal insufficiency, hyperkalemic renal tubular acidosis, and only very cautiously if at all in combination with inhibitors of the renin-angiotensin-aldosterone system. Amiloride and triamterene block the collecting duct Na^+ channel, preventing Na^+ reabsorption at this site and thereby reducing the driving force for K^+ secretion. Because such a small portion of filtered Na^+ is reabsorbed in the collecting duct, these drugs are not effective by themselves in the treatment of edema. Instead, they are typically used in combination with loop diuretics or thiazides to minimize K^+ losses. Triamterene is potentially nephrotoxic and can induce stone formation. Spironolactone is a competitive inhibitor of aldosterone and effectively blocks the action of this hormone by preventing its binding to the mineralocorticoid receptor in the collecting duct. Because of its antialdosterone effect, this drug is uniquely useful in disorders in which edema is related to high aldosterone levels. Its use is limited by its antiandrogenic side effects such as gynecomastia.

Azetazolamide is a potent inhibitor of H^+-linked Na^+ reabsorption, primarily in the proximal tubule through its effect on the enzyme carbonic anhydrase. The diuretic effect of acetazolamide, however, is normally small and short-lived due to adaptive increases in Na^+ reabsorption along the nephron at sites that are independent of H^+ secretion (e.g., in the loop of Henle, distal tubule, and collecting duct). In addition, acetazolamide causes metabolic acidosis through the loss of bicarbonate in the urine and hypokalemia by stimulating K^+ secretion in the collecting duct. Its use is currently limited to patients with metabolic alkalosis or chronic respiratory acidosis.

B. Mechanism of Edema Mobilization

Diuretics acutely reduce vascular volume. This reduction lowers venous and capillary hydrostatic pressures and increases plasma oncotic pressure, both of which promote the movement of fluid from the interstitium to the blood compartment. Overzealous diuresis depletes vascular and ECF volume, decreases cardiac output, and impairs renal function. The first dose of a loop diuretic or thiazide usually produces a prompt diuresis. Continued treatment, however, establishes a new equilibrium within a few days, in which Na^+ excretion no longer exceeds intake. This braking phenomenon limits weight loss to 1–2 kg in the nonedematous patient. When a short-acting diuretic is used in a person ingesting enough Na^+, the drug-induced Na^+ loss is followed by the retention of an equivalent amount of Na^+ during the remainder of the day, resulting in no weight loss at all. On a sufficiently restricted diet, however, the acute natriuresis exceeds Na^+ intake and a negative sodium balance can be achieved. With prolonged use, loop diuretics may lose efficacy due to upregulation of Na^+ transport in the distal tubule and collecting duct.

C. Edema Therapy—General Guidelines

Regardless of its etiology, treatment of mild edema should start with dietary Na^+ restriction. The patient should be instructed that just discontinuing added salt at the table is not sufficient. Ideally, dietary Na^+ should be reduced to about 100 mEq/day, a diet in which foods should be chosen that do not contain salt. Further restriction to a minimum of 50 mEq/day may be necessary in some patients with refractory edema. The patient should also be educated that the "salt substitute" or "diet salt" available in the supermarket is simply KCl. The use of KCl as a salt substitute should be discouraged in any patient with renal insufficiency or who is taking a K^+-sparing diuretic, because of the risk of life-threatening hyperkalemia.

Bed rest reduces hydrostatic pressure in the lower extremities and minimizes activation of the renin-angiotensin-aldosterone and sympathetic nervous systems during therapy. Bed rest has been shown to be helpful in the treatment of the edema caused by heart failure or liver cirrhosis, improving the response to diuretics. Prolonged bed rest, however, is not recommended because of its deleterious effects on muscle and bone.

If renal function is normal and the edema is mild, a thiazide is a useful first choice for a diuretic agent. In most patients with edema, however, loop diuretics should be used from the start, because they are the most potent and the response is most predictable. The initial goal is to find the effective single dose. One can start with 40 mg of furosemide and then double the dose until adequate diuresis ensues (manifested by weight loss of 0.5–1 kg) or a maximum dose of 160–200 mg is reached. Because of variability in the absorption of an oral dose, intravenous furosemide is often more effective at a lower dose. The maximum intravenous dose recommended by many is 200 mg. When an effective dose is reached, it can be repeated twice daily if need be. In the acute setting an intravenous loop diuretic can be given as a bolus (e.g., 40 mg of furosemide in patients with normal renal function or up to 200 mg in renal insufficiency) or as continuous infusion (e.g., 0.25–1.0 mg/kg/hr of furosemide).

The most important education for patients taking diuretics is to have them understand the relationship between changes in weight and edema. They should weigh themselves on a regular basis and record the data, so that decisions about adjusting the diuretic dose can easily be made. They can also be trained to assess their lower extremity edema on a regular basis. Because salt intake varies from day to day, even with the most rigid diet, frequent variations in diuretic dose may be necessary as well. The patients can make these adjustments themselves if they do the appropriate monitoring at home.

1. Acute Pulmonary Edema

Acute left ventricular dysfunction with pulmonary edema is the only life-threatening form of edema and requires immediate specific therapy of the underlying myocardial ischemia, arrhythmia, or hypertension. Intravenous furosemide (40 mg) reduces left ventricular filling pressures within 15 minutes due to an increase in venous capacity and reduction in peripheral resistance. Similar effects can be produced with nitrates, hydralazine, and positive inotropic agents. Diuresis ensues after 30–60 minutes of an intravenous loop diuretic and decreases preload and end-diastolic pressure by reducing plasma volume. Because they reduce preload, diuretics run the risk of reducing cardiac output in some patients and causing compensatory vasoconstriction. Thus, they should only be used with other agents that act more directly on the heart. Acute pulmonary edema can also be the result of volume excess in a patient with renal failure. Though a high dose of intravenous furosemide should be tried in this situation, removal of fluid by dialysis may be necessary if little or no response occurs to the diuretic.

2. Chronic Congestive Heart Failure

Diuretic therapy for congestive heart failure is a double-edged sword. On the one hand, the negative Na^+ balance induced by diuretics and dietary Na^+ restriction improves cardiac dilatation and pulmonary and peripheral edema. On the other hand, fluid removal diminishes effective vascular volume and reduces cardiac filling pressures, causing a reduction in cardiac output and contractility. On balance, most patients with congestive heart failure benefit from diuretic therapy with less pulmonary congestion and increased exercise tolerance, even in the presence of lower cardiac output. Eventually, however, the failing heart is unable to sustain adequate output unless filling pressures are high. In this setting diuretics worsen the situation. A telltale sign of this problem is a rise in serum creatinine and BUN when the patient is placed on a diuretic.

ACE inhibitors improve natriuresis and induce hemodynamic and neurohormonal changes that lead to a reduction of both preload and after load. These agents are well documented to reduce morbidity and mortality in patients with congestive heart failure. Spironolactone has also been shown to have a beneficial effect in clinical trials. Diuretics have only very limited usefulness in isolated right-sided heart failure, because cardiac output is so dependent on high filling pressures.

3. Cirrhosis of the Liver

Medical treatment of cirrhotic ascites is essentially supportive, dictated by the patient's discomfort, impaired cardiovascular or respiratory function, and potential for infection. Only 10% of patients respond to dietary Na^+ restriction and bed rest alone. When the edema requires treatment, spironolactone is the recommended first agent. This increases the proportion of responding patients to 65%. The addition of a loop diuretic may produce clinical improvement in an additional 20%. Spironolactone therapy usually starts at a dose of 50–100 mg/day, although doses of up to 600 mg have been used safely and effectively. If maximal doses of spironolactone do not cause an adequate diuresis, a loop diuretic can be given and spironolactone continued.

In cirrhotic patients with ascites and no peripheral edema, the reabsorptive capacity of the peritoneal capillaries and lymphatics is limited to about 300–900 mL/day. Diuretic therapy should be monitored to avoid daily weight loss beyond this limit to avoid prerenal azotemia or vascular collapse. When peripheral edema is also present, more vigorous diuresis is safe. Severe ascites may require large volume paracentesis to alleviate symptoms from abdominal pressure. Paracentesis appears to be safer than diuretic therapy with respect to encephalopathy and renal and electrolyte disturbances, particularly when albumin replacement is given concomitantly. Overdiuresis of ascites and peripheral edema in patients with cirrhosis inevitably causes a rise in serum creatinine. When this occurs diuretics should be discontinued, and it may even be necessary to infuse isotonic saline to restore effective vascular volume to normal.

4. Nephrotic Syndrome

Treatment of edema in patients with the nephrotic syndrome should be regarded solely as supportive therapy, and institution of diuretic therapy should be based on clinical judgement (see Chapter 7). As with all causes of edema, the initial approach to the edema of the nephrotic syndrome should be to restrict dietary Na^+ intake. This approach is the safest intervention, but unless the patient is extremely motivated, it is not usually successful in preventing progressively worsening edema. Unfortunately, patients with the nephrotic syndrome are often resistant to diuretic therapy in the usual dosage. There are multiple reasons for this resistance. Furosemide is highly protein bound and hypoalbuminemia increases its volume of distribution, which lowers its plasma concentration and slows renal elimination. Proteinuria also reduces the concentration of unbound drug in the tubular lumen, the only site from which it is active. When urinary albumin concentrations exceed 4 g/L, two to three times the normal dose is needed to deliver adequate amounts of unbound, active drug to the loop of Henle. Finally, there is a high degree of renal Na^+ avidity, presumably due to increased numbers and activity of Na^+ transporters, increasing the dosage requirement of the inhibitor.

If a high dose of a loop diuretic is not successful in controlling the edema, additional blockade of Na^+ reabsorption sites with a thiazide diuretic potentiates the diuretic effect. A danger in some patients with the nephrotic syndrome is the development of orthostatic hypotension with aggressive diuresis. Patients who are hypertensive are likely to be plasma volume expanded, and edema mobilization should not be associated with adverse symptoms. In patients with severe hypoalbuminemia and normal renal function, however, effective vascular volume may be significantly decreased (see earlier). Diuretic therapy in this situation is likely to worsen symptoms of vascular volume depletion despite the continued presence of edema. If treatment of edema is deemed necessary in such patients, diuretics should be used cautiously, with care taken to reduce weight very gradually (<1 kg/day).

5. Chronic Renal Insufficiency

Expansion of vascular volume due to inadequate Na^+ excretion contributes to the development both of hypertension and edema in renal insufficiency. Thus, dietary Na^+ restriction should be the mainstay of therapy. Nonetheless, diuretics are an important adjunct to therapy in patients who are unable to control edema with dietary changes, particularly because they reduce blood pressure as they reduce ECF volume. In patients with renal insufficiency, loop diuretics are the agents of choice because of the variability in response to thiazides and the risk of hyperkalemia with the K^+-sparing diuretics. Higher doses of loop diuretics are needed to achieve a response in these patients because less of the drug reaches the site in the kidney where it is active. In addition, the filtered load of Na^+ is reduced when the GFR is decreased and there is less flexibility in tubular reabsorption, all of which limits the effectiveness of any diuretic regimen. Combination therapy of a loop diuretic with metazolone can enhance the natriuretic effect at relatively low doses. Eventually, filtration is reduced to so great an extent that all diuretics become ineffective, and then dialysis therapy is necessary to remove excess fluid.

D. Refractory Edema

Diuretics occasionally fail to ameliorate edema even at high doses. The initial approach to this problem is to find out if the diuretic works at all, provided that the patient takes it. Thus the first question to ask the patient is whether or not urine output increases within 2 or 3 hours after taking the diuretic. Patients usually have no problem in determining if a diuretic is effective, because significant diuresis disrupts daytime activities or sleep.

1. Adequate Diuresis but Edema Does Not Change

By far the most common cause of this problem is excessive dietary Na^+ intake. The patient and his or her family should be quizzed carefully about diet, and they should be reeducated about the importance of dietary Na^+ restriction. To drive home the point, one can measure urinary Na^+ excretion in a 24-hour sample at a time when weight is constant. In this setting Na^+ excretion should be virtually the same as intake. Subsequently, a rigorous dietary assessment and counseling may be necessary to eliminate hidden sources of salt from the diet. The patient's medication list and use of over-the-counter drugs (e.g., NSAIDs) should also be reviewed to identify drugs that impair Na^+ excretion. One should also reexamine the diagnosis. For example, the patient with bilateral leg edema from venous stasis may show a good initial response to diuretics. However, the kidneys will soon compensate for the iatrogenic reduction in effective plasma volume. The edema will not be fully mobilized until the underlying problem of increased venous hydrostatic pressure is solved or the patient becomes symptomatic from hypovolemia.

2. Diuretic Produces No Increase in Urine Output Even At Maximal Dose

There are two major causes for this problem. The first is that intestinal absorption of the drug is impaired. Such impairment can occur in severe edema states and has been ascribed to the presence of edema in the bowel wall. The second is that the renal response to the drug is impaired for one of the following reasons: (1) in renal failure the drug may not reach its site of action in the tubular lumen in sufficiently high concentration, (2) in proteinuric states, the luminal drug is bound to filtered albumin and is thus ineffective, (3) compensatory increase in Na^+ reabsorption at other sites in the nephron diminishes the diuretic effect of the drug, or (4) the diuretic-induced decrease in effective vascular volume reduces GFR and the filtered load of Na^+.

If poor intestinal reabsorption is the problem, intravenous therapy is the solution. If the renal response is impaired because of upregulation of Na^+ transport at other sites in the nephron, combining diuretics that work at different sites in the nephron can address this problem. In edematous patients with normal renal function, any combination of a loop diuretic with a thiazide or spironolactone is reasonable, with the choice depending mainly on the anticipated side effects or the underlying pathophysiology (see earlier). Even acetazolamide combined with a loop diuretic may work. In patients with renal insufficiency, spironolactone should not be used, and metolazone is the recommended thiazide to use in combination with a loop diuretic. Metolazone appears to have an additional effect on proximal Na^+ reabsorption at a relatively low dose. However, its absorption from the intestine is poor and sometimes erratic, and there may be several days of lag time before its effect is apparent. It has an extremely prolonged serum half-life in renal insufficiency, and diuresis may continue for days after the drug is discontinued.

In cirrhosis loop diuretics have been successfully combined with spironolactone and/or metolazone. In heart failure the use of spironolactone in combination with furosemide has the additional advantage of blocking pro-arrhythmogenic aldosterone effects that are not prevented by ACE inhibitors alone. The combination of acetazolamide with furosemide is less effective but may have a role in congestive heart failure with diuretic-induced alkalosis.

Diuretics are potent tools in clinical medicine. Poor diuretic response does not necessarily result from using the wrong diuretic or the wrong combination thereof, but may just indicate severe volume contraction. Repeated reassessment of the effective vascular volume and awareness of the complications of diuretic therapy are essential for their successful use.

SUGGESTED READINGS

Andreoli TE. Edematous states: an overview. Kidney Int Suppl 1997; 59:S2–10.

Blankfield RP, Finkelhor RS, Alexander JJ, et al. Etiology and diagnosis of bilateral leg edema in primary care. Am J Med 1998; 105:192–197.

Brater DC. Diuretic therapy. N Engl J Med 1998; 339:387–395.

Brater DC, Anderson SA, Brown-Cartwright D. Response to furosemide in chronic renal insufficiency: rationale for limited doses. Clin Pharmacol Ther 1986; 40:134–139.

Dikshit K, Vyden JK, Forrester JS, Chatterjee K, Prakash R, Swan HJ. Renal and extrarenal hemodynamic effects of furosemide in congestive heart failure after acute myocardial infarction. N Engl J Med 1973; 288:1087–1090.

Ellison DH. The physiologic basis of diuretic synergism: its role in treating diuretic resistance. Ann Intern Med 1991; 114:886–894.

Gines P, Arroyo V, Quintero E, et al. Comparison of paracentesis and diuretics in the treatment of cirrhotics with tense ascites. Results of a randomized study. Gastroenterology 1987; 93:234–241.

Orth SR, Ritz E. The nephrotic syndrome. N Engl J Med 1998; 338:1202–1211.

Oster JR, Epstein M, Smoller S. Combined therapy with thiazide-type and loop diuretic agents for resistant sodium retention. Ann Intern Med 1983; 99:405–406.

Pockros PJ, Reynolds TB. Rapid diuresis in patients with ascites from chronic liver disease: the importance of peripheral edema. Gastroenterology 1986; 90:1827–1833.

Schrier RW, Fassett RG. A critique of the overfill hypothesis of sodium and water retention in the nephrotic syndrome. Kidney Int 1998; 53:1111–1117.

Schrier RW. Pathogenesis of sodium and water retention in high-output and low-output cardiac failure, nephrotic syndrome, cirrhosis, and pregnancy (1) [erratum in N Engl J Med 1989; 320:676]. N Engl J Med 1988; 319:1065–1072.

Schrier RW. Pathogenesis of sodium and water retention in high-output and low-output cardiac failure, nephrotic syndrome, cirrhosis, and pregnancy (2) [erratum in N Engl J Med 1989; 320:676]. N Engl J Med 1988; 319:1127–1134.

Taylor SH. Refocus on diuretics in the treatment of heart failure. Eur Heart J 1995; 16(suppl F):7–15.

Wilcox CS. Diuretics. In: Brenner BM, ed. Brenner and Rector's The Kidney, 5th ed. Philadelphia: W.B. Saunders, 1996:2299–2330.

3
Uremia

Jeffrey A. Kraut
VA Greater Los Angeles Health Care System and UCLA School of Medicine, Los Angeles, California

I. INTRODUCTION

The term uremia, literally "urine in the blood," is used to describe the symptoms associated with far advanced renal disease. As implied by its literal meaning, uremic symptoms were thought to arise solely from the retention of intoxicating agents in the body as a result of decreased excretion by the kidney. However, in addition to its role in the excretion of potentially toxic substances, the kidney regulates fluid, electrolyte, and acid-base balance, secretes the key regulatory hormones renin, vitamin D, and erythropoietin, and metabolizes many hormones. Not surprisingly, the symptoms of uremia result from derangements in all of these functions of the kidney. As outlined in Table 1, the symptoms of uremia encompass virtually all the major organ systems in the body.

In the following discussion, the signs and symptoms arising in the course of renal failure are arranged according to the organ system primarily affected. However, it should be clear from the discussion that many of the symptoms are due to abnormalities in more than one organ system. In each of the organ systems discussed below, the typical time in the course of renal disease that each of the symptoms appear is reviewed, as is any distinctions in symptomatology between acute and chronic renal insufficiency. For ease of access, these aspects are also summarized at the end of the chapter and in Tables 2 and 3. Factors that have been implicated in the pathogenesis of uremic symptoms are summarized in Table 4.

Table 1 Signs and Symptoms of Uremia

Organ system	Signs and symptoms
Musculoskeletal	
Renal osteodystrophy	Bone pain, fractures, tendon rupture
Myopathy	Muscle weakness, pain
Neurological	Confusion, stupor, coma, paresthesias, dysesthesias
Cardiopulmonary	Hypertension, cardiomyopathy, chest pain, friction rub, shortness of breath, murmurs, peripheral edema
Gastrointestinal	Abdominal pain, early satiety, bleeding, diarrhea, anorexia, nausea, vomiting
Dermatological	Pruritus, calcium deposits
Endocrine	Infertility, decreased basal metabolism, carbohydrate intolerance
Hematological	Purpura, easy bruisability, anemia, prolonged bleeding, decreased lymphocyte function, decreased neutrophil function
Urogenital	Nocturia, polyuria, dysmenorrhea, amenorrhea, impotence, loss of libido

II. SIGNS AND SYMPTOMS OF RENAL FAILURE

A. Skin

Pruritus is a common symptom in patients with far advanced chronic renal insufficiency, and this problem persists in many patients receiving dialysis therapy. The pruritus is diffuse and often unrelenting, causing some patients to scratch incessantly and to produce multiple excoriations. Typically, the itchiness does not respond well to antihistamines or skin lotions. The pathogenesis of this abnormality is multifactorial, but the major factor appears to be disordered calcium homeostasis. As hyperparathyroidism develops (see Chapters 14 and 16), the ionic concentrations of calcium and phosphorus in the extracellular compartment rise to levels at which precipitation of calcium phosphate occurs. A characteristic site for this precipitation is in the subcutaneous tissue, producing an inflammatory response in the skin and the symptom of pruritus. Unless hyperparathyroidism is far advanced, the subcutaneous calcifications are not visible on x-ray. In far advanced cases, the calcium deposits can become large enough to cause skin breakdown and then are seen on physical exam. Uncontrolled hyperparathyroidism should be suspected if the calcium-phosphorus product (serum calcium in mg/dL × serum phosphorus in mg/dL) is greater than 70. Usually the serum parathyroid hormone (PTH) level is also markedly increased, and elevations in PTH secretion have been implicated even in the absence of a high calcium-phos-

Table 2 Relationship Between Onset of Signs and Symptoms of Uremia and GFR

GFR = 40–80 mL/min; serum creatinine = 1.5–2.5 mg/dL (mild renal insufficiency)
- Hypertension
- Increase in PTH (variable)
- Vitamin D deficiency

GFR = 15–40 mL/min; serum creatinine = 2.5–5.0 mg/dL (moderate renal insufficiency)
- Hyperphosphatemia
- Hypocalcemia
- Renal osteodystrophy
- Anemia
- Anorexia

GFR < 15 mL/min; serum creatinine > 5.0 mg/dL (severe renal insufficiency)
- Left ventricular hypertrophy
- Cardiomyopathy
- Valvular calcifications[a]
- Congestive heart failure
- Pericarditis[b]
- Anorexia
- Nausea and vomiting
- Mental confusion
- Purpura
- Rectal bleeding and diarrhea

[a] Most frequent in dialysis patients on dialysis for several years.
[b] Uncommon except with marked elevation of BUN levels.

Table 3 Comparison of Most Frequent Signs and Symptoms in Acute Versus Chronic Renal Failure

Sign or symptom	Acute renal failure	Chronic renal failure
Anemia	Common, except in very acute setting	Common
Hyperkalemia	Common	Common
Acidosis	Common	Common
CNS changes	More prominent	Common
Peripheral neuropathy	Does not occur	Common
Pruritus	Rare	Common
Bone pain and bone disease	Does not occur	Common
Anorexia, nausea, vomiting	More prominent	Common
Cardiomyopathy	Rare	Common

Table 4 Factors Implicating in the Pathogenesis of Uremic Symptoms

Retained end products of metabolism
Urea
Creatinine
Guanidinosuccinic acid
Methylguanidine
Methylamines
''Middle molecules'' (300–3000 daltons)
Parathyroid hormone
Metabolic acidosis
Anemia

phorus product. When these abnormalities are present, control of serum calcium and phosphorus levels and suppression of PTH secretion usually lead to resolution or marked improvement in symptoms, unless the process is far advanced. In some patients without advanced skin involvement, however, pruritus continues unabated despite control of serum calcium, phosphorus, and PTH. It has been postulated that, in these patients, pruritus is actually one of the clinical manifestation of peripheral neuropathy. When adequate control of calcium, phosphorus, and PTH fails to ameliorate the pruritus, ultraviolet treatments are sometimes effective in reducing symptomatology.

In addition to pruritus, dryness and scaling of the skin, altered pigmentation, and reduced sweating are observed in a large number of patients with chronic renal failure. Moreover, when uremia is severe (BUN $>$ 150–200 mg/dL), a whitish deposit on the skin can appear (uremic frost). This deposit appears to be due to precipitation of ammonia.

B. Musculoskeletal System

Musculoskeletal symptoms are frequently observed in patients with advanced chronic renal insufficiency, but are extremely uncommon in individuals with acute renal failure. As with many of the symptoms associated with renal failure, this difference indicates that a prolonged (months to years) exposure to renal failure is required to bring about the pathological changes responsible for the signs and symptoms of musculoskeletal disorders.

1. Myopathy

Muscle weakness is frequently observed in patients with chronic renal failure. The weakness is usually confined to the proximal musculature and evolves slowly over months to years. Patients initially have difficulty arising from a seated position. A waddling gait can develop eventually. In some patients, the myopathy can become severe enough to limit ambulation, leading to confinement to a wheelchair. Upper extremity weakness can progress to the point where patients become unable to hold their arms above their head to comb their hair. In most instances, these more advanced symptoms occur after the patient has reached end-stage renal disease and has been receiving dialysis therapy.

The cause of the muscle weakness is unclear. Plasma levels of muscle enzymes are usually normal, and electromyographic abnormalities are absent or nonspecific. Muscle biopsy shows mild nonspecific myopathic alterations on light microscopy and severe degenerative changes on electron microscopy. The muscle weakness is associated with increased PTH levels, phosphate depletion, low vitamin D levels, and excess aluminum accumulation, and all of these factors have been implicated in the pathogenesis of this disorder. Suppression of elevated PTH levels, supplementation with vitamin D, and removal of aluminum have indeed led to improvement both in the clinical and pathological findings. Other suggested but unproven contributory factors include carnitine deficiency and iron overload.

A much earlier symptom is muscle cramping, usually in the lower extremities, which typically occurs at rest rather than with exercise. The patient usually complains of this problem developing at night after retiring. Whether this latter symptom is an early manifestation of neuropathy or myopathy is unclear. In some patients, the symptom is relieved by quinine or clonazepam.

2. Bone Disease

Bone pain is a symptom that develops in some patients late in the course of chronic renal failure. It typically involves the long bones and vertebrae and can be extremely disabling. The pain is usually vague in nature and deep-seated, often located in the low back, hips, knees, or legs. As expected, the pain is exacerbated by weight bearing or exercise and frequently varies in intensity. Physical findings are usually scant: occasionally, pressure produces localized tenderness of the chest wall or pelvis, but more often the physical examination is negative. If bone disease is severe, loss of height due to vertebral compression fractures, fracture of long bones, or deformities particularly of the hands and clavicles can be seen. In children, growth can be stunted.

These signs and symptoms are the result of pathological changes in bone that accompany chronic renal insufficiency, termed renal osteodystrophy, and include osteitis fibrosa cystica, osteomalacia, and adynamic bone disease (see Chapter 16). Although more than one of these abnormalities can occur simultaneously, osteomalacia is the most common pathological disorder noted in patients with bone pain or bone fractures. Pathological changes in bone can be observed even in patients with mild renal insufficiency, but they are most prominent in patients with far advanced or end-stage renal disease. Over 80% of patients have abnormalities on bone biopsy immediately prior to the initiation of dialysis, a time when glomerular filtration rate is usually less than 10 mL/min.

The pathogenesis of the various types of bone disease is multifactorial (see Chapter 16). Although osteitis fibrosa cystica is predominately due to the effects of excess PTH secretion and a decrease in 1,25-dihydroxycholecalciferol (the active form of vitamin D, calcitriol) secretion by the kidney, this disorder may be exacerbated by the metabolic acidosis that commonly accompanies chronic renal insufficiency. Metabolic acidosis appears to worsen bone disease either by directly stimulating osteoclast action or by augmenting the effects of PTH on bone. The severity of the bone lesions in patients with secondary hyperparathyroidism appears to be directly correlated with the level of PTH and the duration of the renal failure. Bone disease is more severe if PTH levels are substantially elevated, i.e., >400 pg/mL (more than 20- to 30-fold the normal value) and the renal disease has been present for a prolonged period of time. PTH levels can be normal or low in patients with osteomalacia or adynamic bone disease. Metabolic acidosis, diabetes mellitus, excess aluminum, and suppression of parathyroid hormone secretion by excessive calcitriol administration are some of the factors implicated in producing osteomalacia.

Bone pain can also be due to bone cysts produced by amyloid deposits. Patients with longstanding renal failure accumulate β_2-microglobulin, which can result in amyloid production and deposition. When bone pain is the result of these amyloid deposits, there is usually evidence of amyloid deposition in other parts of the body. The most common site is in the carpal tunnel, and patients present with carpal tunnel syndrome (see below).

The specific cause of the bone pain in a given patient may be difficult to discern. X-ray findings are commonly absent or nonspecific. In patients with bone symptoms, attention should be directed at calcium and phosphorus homeostasis. Control of hyperparathyroidism, osteomalacia, or adynamic bone disease may ameliorate the symptoms.

3. Spontaneous Tendon Rupture

Rupture of various tendons can occur in patients with longstanding chronic renal failure with minimal stress. Tendon rupture is seen most frequently in the quadriceps, triceps, or extensor tendons of the fingers. When present, tendon rupture can produce excruciating pain and often leads to extensive deformities of and inability to move the affected extremity. Abnormalities of collagen underlie the weakening of individual tendons. Metabolic acidosis and hyperparathyroidism are probably the two primary contributory factors.

4. Arthritis

Arthritic symptoms including pain and stiffness of large joints are noted in a small group of patients with chronic renal failure. Physical examination can reveal erythema and swelling. Joint inflammation can be due to deposition of calcium pyrophosphate or calcium apatite, and in these cases synovial biopsy reveals either calcium pyrophosphate or apatite crystal deposition, respectively. Erosive arthritis and joint effusions can also be the consequence of amyloidosis due to β_2-microglobulin deposition.

5. Ischemic Vascular Disease

In a small number of patients, digital ischemia leading to Raynaud's phenomenon and/or gangrene of the digits is observed. Symptoms of pain, numbness, or tingling of the hands and feet might be present upon exposure to cold or, if ischemia is severe enough, even in the absence of cold exposure. The digital ischemia is the result of metastatic calcifications in blood vessels and/or excess PTH levels and has been termed "calciphylaxis." In some instances, suppression of PTH secretion has led to marked amelioration of the symptoms. However, the response to the reduction of PTH levels will depend upon the extent of the metastatic calcifications, and in many cases reduction in PTH levels has little impact.

C. Ocular System

The most prominent symptom involving the eyes is pain, tenderness, and erythema of the conjunctivae, the "red eye syndrome." Examination of the eye reveals conjunctival inflammation. Corneal calcification can also be observed, producing band keratopathy and decreased visual acuity. The corneal calcification and red eye syndrome are due to metastatic deposition of calcium phosphate salts, occurring in uncontrolled hyperparathyroidism (see earlier).

D. Cardiovascular System

1. Pericarditis

Traditionally, pericarditis has been listed as the primary cardiovascular abnormality occurring in uremia. However, pericarditis is now rare in patients with either acute or chronic renal failure, probably because dialysis therapy is initiated earlier in the course of the disease and because closer attention is paid to the adequacy of therapy (see Chapter 26). Much more common now is cardiomyopathy (see below). Nonetheless, when pericarditis develops, signs and symptoms can vary from persistent chest pain to unexplained hypotension. Because it is potentially life-threatening, the diagnosis should be considered in any patient with advanced renal insufficiency or end-stage renal disease and appropriate testing undertaken. The treatment for this disorder is intensive hemodialysis.

2. Cardiomyopathy

The declining incidence of pericarditis has been more than counterbalanced by a rising incidence of symptomatic congestive heart failure. Abnormal cardiac function, including left ventricular hypertrophy, dilated cardiomyopathy, ischemic cardiac disease, and mitral and aortic valvular dysfunction, occurs in 30–70% of patients either at the time of initiation of dialysis or after they have been maintained on dialysis for a variable period of time (see Chapter 26). Symptoms and signs of cardiac disease such as palpitations, shortness of breath, chest pain, peripheral edema, ascites, pulmonary edema, and pleural effusion can be very prominent. Most importantly, cardiac disease is the most common underlying cause of death in patients with end-stage renal failure.

The pathogenesis of the cardiac disease is multifactorial. Anemia, elevated PTH levels, hypertension, metastatic calcifications, and abnormal homocysteine levels have all been implicated as pathogenic factors in the genesis of these cardiac abnormalities. Although the term "uremic cardiomyopathy" has sometimes been used to define the heart failure seen in patients with end-stage renal disease, traditional toxins such as urea nitrogen, creatinine, and aliphatic amines probably play little role in the pathogenesis of this disorder.

3. Hypertension

As discussed in detail in Chapters 9, 16, and 17, hypertension is almost universally present in patients with advanced chronic renal insufficiency. The hypertension is due primarily to sodium retention by the diseased kidneys, but abnormalities in the renin-angiotensin system, catecholamine secretion, and other volume and vasoconstrictive regulatory hormones also contribute. As in patients with normal renal function, hypertension is rarely associated with any symptoms. When severe, it can present with headaches and visual disturbances. Even when no symptoms are present, however, this disorder should be treated aggressively, because it contributes to cardiac morbidity (see above), increases the risk of stroke, and accelerates the progression to end-stage renal disease (see Chapter 16).

E. Nervous System

Uremia is associated with both central nervous system abnormalities and with peripheral neuropathy. Disturbances of the central nervous system are prominent in acute renal failure, first appearing in the majority of patients when the BUN and creatinine rise above 120–130 mg/dL and 8–9 mg/dL, respectively. Subtle alterations in mental status occur first and can progress to disorientation and confusion. Torpor and signs of toxic psychosis can occur. Cranial nerve abnormalities such as nystagmus and facial asymmetries can occur. Dysarthria, diffuse weakness, and fasciculations are other abnormalities noted. On physical examination, reflexes are often increased. The EEG is usually grossly abnormal, displaying slow delta waves. These EEG alterations are not improved immediately despite aggressive dialysis therapy, but return to normal with recovery of renal function.

Involvement of the central nervous system is also a predictable consequence of chronic renal failure, first appearing with moderate to severe renal impairment. In the early stages, the patient might become disinterested in the environment and display difficulty concentrating and a reduced ability for abstract thinking. Drowsiness, lethargy, and apathy develop, and patients may note difficulty sleeping. Psychiatric disturbances including delusions, depression, mania, euphoria, and occasionally paranoid tendencies are noted. There can be signs of neuromuscular irritability. Fibrillary muscle twitching is present early, followed by involvement of larger muscle groups. Deep tendon reflexes are often exaggerated. As renal failure becomes more severe, tremors, hiccups, decreased coordination, asterixis, and diffuse myoclonus can develop. Mental status changes evolve into stupor and coma. Convulsions are rare in patients with uncomplicated renal failure but are not infrequent when renal failure and hypertensive encephalopathy coexist.

The relationship between the degree of chronic renal failure and the extent of neurological disturbances is unclear. However, it is safe to say that clinically significant neurological disturbances usually do not occur until the glomerular filtration rate falls below 15–20 mL/min. Severe neurological sequelae, including changes in consciousness and coma, are not observed until the BUN is greater than 150–200 mg/dL.

The pathogenesis of these central nervous system abnormalities is not completely defined but appears to be multifactorial in origin. Brain metabolism and oxygen utilization are depressed. The reduction in metabolism is due to both impaired neurotransmission and inhibition of Na^+/K^+ ATPase and other enzyme activity. Amino acids and metabolic end products 300–3000 daltons in size (''middle molecules'') (see Table 4) and certain hormones produced in excess such as PTH have been implicated as possible uremic toxins.

Peripheral neuropathy is uncommon in patients with acute renal failure but is extremely common in patients with chronic renal failure. Peripheral nerve damage was first noted in patients with chronic renal failure over 100 years ago, but it was not recognized as an important problem until the early 1960s when chronic dialysis therapy first became available, presumably because patients died quickly of their renal failure before that time. The exact prevalence of neuropathy is not clear, but it has been estimated that 65% (range 10–83%) of patients with chronic renal failure have some evidence of neuropathy at the time of initiation of chronic dialysis (GFR < 10 mL/min). However, clinically significant neuropathy is rare in nondiabetic patients until the glomerular filtration rate falls below 12 mL/min. The failure to define the prevalence of neuropathy more precisely is probably related to discordance between the symptoms and objective physical findings or abnormalities noted on nerve conduction studies. Abnormal nerve conduction is often present in the absence of either symptoms or abnormalities on physical examination.

The peripheral neuropathy noted in patients with chronic renal failure is essentially indistinguishable from that noted with alcoholism or diabetes mellitus. Uremic neuropathy is a distal symmetrical, mixed polyneuropathy. Both motor and sensory nerves are affected, but the sensory nerves are characteristically more severely involved. The lower extremities are more commonly affected than the upper extremities. A mononeuropathy has also been described that involves the median nerve, producing wasting, motor loss, and sensory symptoms of the hands. This carpal tunnel syndrome is most common in dialysis patients and is related to deposition of amyloid material in this area (see earlier). Its occurrence is related to the duration of chronic renal failure, increasing after 10 years on dialysis.

Peripheral neuropathy can also present as a restless leg syndrome (akathesia) that is comprised of two components: a sensory component characterized by paresthesias, described as an achy or crawling feeling in the lower extremities, and a motor component, usually described as an inability to sit still. These symptoms are more prominent in the distal portion of the extremities and are worse at night. Alternatively, patients can experience burning, constriction, swelling, and tenderness predominately of the distal extremities (burning foot syndrome).

By the time patients complain of paresthesias, clinical evidence of peripheral neuropathy is usually present. The severity and progression of neuropathy is variable, but in general it changes only slowly over months to years. In rare cases it progresses rapidly. Depressed or abolished ankle reflexes and reduced vibratory perception are the initial physical findings. Atrophy and weakness of distal leg muscles can develop with foot drop, but prominent motor weakness is uncommon. Autonomic neuropathy, although most prominent in diabetic patients with renal failure, can also be seen in patients with other causes of renal failure. This can contribute to sexual dysfunction noted in some patients (see below).

Pathologically, uremic neuropathy is characterized by demyelination and structural impairment of axons. The pathogenesis of the neuropathy is multifactorial. Uremic toxins in the middle-molecule range (300–3000 daltons), including substances such as methylguanidine and myoinositol (Table 4), have been implicated in inhibiting enzymes such as transketolase and Na^+/K^+ ATPase. A contributing role for these substances is supported by the observation that the neuropathy is often less severe in patients maintained on chronic peritoneal dialysis, a form of treatment in which these substances are removed more effectively, than in patients receiving hemodialysis. Elevated PTH levels has also been suggested as a contributory factor to neuropathy by raising intracellular calcium levels of peripheral nerves. Indeed, parathyroidectomy prevents the slowing of nerve conduction noted in uremic dogs. However, nerve-conduction velocity is not improved by parathyroidectomy in humans, and therefore the precise role of PTH remains unclear.

F. Gastrointestinal System

Gastrointestinal symptoms are often among the most prominent abnormalities that bring the patient with chronic renal insufficiency to the attention of a physician.

1. Anorexia

As renal failure progresses and GFR falls below 15–25% of normal, a subtle loss of appetite commonly develops. Nutritional analysis indicates that in patients with advanced chronic renal insufficiency, spontaneous protein intake drops to as low as 0.5 g/kg body weight (as compared to the usual North American intake of greater than 1 g/kg body weight). The decrease in protein and overall calories can lead to significant weight loss, mimicking the findings in patients with an occult malignancy. However, anorexia is not inevitable, and some patients with marked renal insufficiency have no weight loss or loss of appetite. When present, anorexia evolves in a typical way. The individual describes normal hunger up to the point of actually seeing or smelling the food, but then becomes nauseated. Many patients, however, merely describe a general loss of appetite. Early satiety with abdominal bloating is occasionally noted in end-stage renal failure patients receiving dialysis therapy. When studied, these individuals have impaired gastric emptying. These symptoms are relieved by metoclopramide, a stimulator of gastric nerves, and presumably are due to uremic autonomic neuropathy.

2. Nausea and Vomiting

When the GFR falls below 10–15 mL/min, nausea and vomiting can develop. These symptoms often develop in the setting of an intercurrent illness such as an upper respiratory illness or diarrhea. Both the loss of appetite and the nausea and vomiting have been attributed to retained toxins, as they commonly abate when the GFR is acutely increased with ECF volume expansion or after the initiation of protein restriction or dialysis therapy. In addition, these symptoms can persist in patients with end-stage renal disease who are not receiving adequate dialysis therapy. The retained toxins responsible for these symptoms are undefined. Recent studies have implicated the metabolic acidosis that regularly attends the course of chronic renal failure in contributing importantly both to the reduction in appetite and the weight loss.

Significant pathological changes can be seen in the gastrointestinal tract that probably contribute, in part, to the gastrointestinal symptoms. Endoscopic signs of gastroduodenal mucosal inflammation with petechiae and erosions are seen in almost 50% of patients with severe renal failure, whether or not they are on dialysis. Recent studies have documented that *Helicobacter pylori* is seen in 68% of the uremic subjects with gastritis, and this pathogen may contribute to the relatively high prevalence of gastritis in uremic patients.

3. Diarrhea

When severe azotemia is present (BUN > 150–200 mg/dL), a profuse bloody diarrhea may develop. Pathological examination of the GI tract in these patients reveals the presence of multiple ulcers in association with hemorrhagic lesions. Pseudomembranes are also common. The lesions have been attributed to the effects of high levels of ammonia resulting from the breakdown of urea in the gut. Gastrointestinal bleeding in the absence of diarrhea can also be seen. Another potential cause is amyloid infiltration of any portion of GI tract leading to small and large intestinal bleeding or bowel infarction. If the latter is present, symptoms will also include abdominal pain.

G. Urogenital System

Alterations in the pattern of urination can be particularly disturbing for patients with renal disease. A decrease in urination can be one of the first abnormalities noted by patients with acute, but not chronic, renal failure. In the latter disorder, in fact, nocturia and polyuria, resulting from an impairment in renal concentrating ability, are more characteristic. These symptoms appear early in the course of renal insufficiency, generally occurring when GFR falls to less than 40 mL/min. Only when renal insufficiency is far advanced (GFR < 5 mL/min) does urine output fall to noticeably low levels. The shift in the diurnal pattern of urination can mimic other disorders, including partial obstruction and diabetes mellitus, and lead the physician away from the proper diagnosis. Gross hematuria and "foaminess" of the urine are other symptoms of either acute or chronic renal disease that can alarm the patient. The latter is due to heavy proteinuria, a concomitant finding in many forms of renal disease (see Chapters 6 and 7).

Both men and women with renal insufficiency often develop sexual problems, including decreased libido, impotence, and infertility. These problems are multifactorial in origin, relating to fatigue from anemia (see below), depression, associated illnesses, and alternations in reproductive hormone secretion. Secretion of testosterone is commonly decreased in men, and the pituitary hormones regulating the menstrual cycle in women are usually disordered, causing amenorrhea.

H. Hematological System

1. Anemia

Anemia is a common feature of both acute and chronic renal failure. Although patients with uncomplicated acute renal failure (e.g., radiocontrast dye induced) typically have hematocrit levels in the normal range, anemia can develop quickly if the acute renal failure persists for longer than a few days or can be present at the onset if complicating illnesses are present. Most, but not all, patients with chronic renal insufficiency develop anemia when the GFR falls below 25–30% of normal. Although there is a strong correlation between the degree of anemia and the severity of chronic renal insufficiency, the relationship is quite variable. Some patients have symptomatic anemia with creatinine levels as low as 2 mg/dL, and others maintain a near normal hematocrit with creatinine levels as high as 6–8 mg/dL. Anemia contributes not only to symptoms of weakness, fatigue, and shortness of breath, but also to the pathogenesis of the cardiomyopathy noted with chronic renal failure (see earlier). The anemia is due primarily to decreased red cell production as a consequence of erythropoietin deficiency (see Chapter 16).

2. Abnormal Bleeding Tendency

Patients with either acute or chronic renal failure develop a bleeding diathesis, due primarily to abnormal platelet function. The bleeding tendency is characterized by minor purpuric lesions, nosebleeds, gastrointestinal bleeding, and bleeding from invasive procedure sites. In uremic patients, the abnormality can be detected by measuring the bleeding time, which is typically prolonged. The bleeding diathesis is rapidly corrected by dialysis, in most instances. In patients not receiving dialysis, administration of desmopressin (DDAVP) will transiently correct the disorder.

3. White Blood Cell Function

Depressed lymphocyte function and altered chemotaxis contribute to the susceptibility to infection in patients with chronic renal failure. In addition, this defect in function decreases the likelihood of developing immunity after vaccination and may lead to false-negative results in skin testing for tuberculosis. Although these abnormalities are improved by dialysis therapy, lymphocyte and neutrophil function remain below normal.

III. TIME COURSE OF APPEARANCE OF SYMPTOMS

Table 2 summarizes the relationships between renal function and the development of associated laboratory abnormalities, signs, and symptoms in patients with renal disease. As is apparent from the table, chronic renal insufficiency is almost always a symptomless disease until far advanced. Early in the course of the disease, the only clue that renal function is disturbed is the development of hypertension, and this finding is only present in 30–50% of patients with mild renal insufficiency. Vitamin D deficiency occurs early but is only evident if the level in the blood is measured. Only when GFR falls to less than 25–35% of normal do symptoms begin to appear, and the early symptoms are probably due in large part to the development of anemia. When GFR falls to less than 15% of normal, more general signs and symptoms occur and the typical associated problems of renal failure develop. Two points should be emphasized about these signs and symptoms. First, their development is extremely variable from patient to patient. Second, none of the signs and symptoms are not pathognomonic for renal disease. They are, in fact, quite nonspecific, with the exception of renal osteodystrophy. When patients come to you with any of these symptoms, a serum creatinine should be part of the workup, and this simple test can easily determine whether renal insufficiency is present. Even when renal insufficiency is present, one must consider other diagnoses that might coexist and contribute to the patient's symptoms. This is particularly true with the finding of anemia.

IV. SYMPTOMS IN ACUTE VERSUS CHRONIC RENAL FAILURE

Table 3 summarizes the differences in the symptoms found in acute and chronic renal failure. As can be seen, the major differences are in the presence of peripheral neuropathy, pruritus, bone disease, and cardiac failure. In patients with uncomplicated acute renal failure (e.g., induced by a drug or toxin), none of the above signs and symptoms should be present. By contrast, the central nervous system findings and the gastrointestinal symptoms are more prominent when the BUN and creatinine rise rapidly to high levels. Many patients with acute renal failure have other diseases, and therefore none of the above distinctions is very specific. Differentiating acute from chronic renal failure rests largely on historical creatinine measurements. In their absence, it is often difficult to distinguish the two diagnoses. If the patient recovers renal function rapidly, then the diagnosis of acute renal failure is confirmed.

V. EFFECT OF DIALYSIS ON THE UREMIC SYNDROME

Table 5 depicts the expected effect of dialysis on the most prominent signs and symptoms noted in the patient with renal failure. As can be seen, dialysis is extremely effective in ameliorating the central nervous system abnormalities noted with renal failure. Effective dialysis can also prevent significant progression of peripheral neuropathy, but usually it does not reverse existing nerve damage. Dialysis reverses the signs and symptoms of pericarditis, but it has little impact on either the accelerated atherosclerosis or the cardiomyopathy commonly observed in the patient with chronic renal failure. In patients with anorexia and

Table 5 Effect of Dialysis on the Signs and Symptoms of Uremia

Sign or symptoms	Effect of dialysis
CNS	
Drowsiness	Marked improvement
Decreased attentiveness	
Impaired memory	
Confusion, stupor, coma	
Peripheral neuropathy	
Dysesthesias	Stabilizes but does not reverse
Restless leg syndrome	
Decreased sensation	
Decreased motor function	
Cardiovascular	
Pericarditis	Marked improvement
Cardiomyopathy	Little effect
Gastrointestinal	
Anorexia, nausea, vomiting	Marked improvement
Enterocolitis	Marked improvement
Peptic ulcer disease	Improved
Dermatological	
Pruritus	Improved?
Hyperpigmentation	
Hematological	
Anemia	Improved
Platelet dysfunction	Improved
Impaired neutrophil and lymphocyte function	Improved

nausea, or with uremic enterocolitis, dialysis therapy usually produces a rapid improvement in symptoms. The anemia of renal failure is improved by dialysis but not corrected, as are the abnormalities in platelet, lymphocyte, and neutrophil function. Finally, dialysis has a variable effect on the dermatological and endocrinological abnormalities of renal failure.

REFERENCES

Cohen G, Haag-Weber M, Horl WH. Immune dysfunction in uremia. Kidney Int 1997; 62:S79–S82.

DeMarchi S, Cecchin E, Villalta D, et al. Relief of pruritus and decreases in plasma histamine concentrations during erythropoetin therapy in patients with uremia. N Engl J Med 1992; 326:969–974.

Fargnoli D. Symbolic equations and impotence in uremia. Contrib Nephrol 1990; 77:56–64.

Franklin SS. Uremia: newer concepts in pathogenesis and treatment. Med Clin North Am 1970; 54:411–430.

Fraser CL, Arieff AI. Nervous system complications in uremia. Ann Intern Med 1988; 109:143–153.

Graham KA, Goodship THJ, Bushinsky DA, Gennari FJ, Walls J, Pickering W, et al. Does metabolic acidosis have clinically important consequences in dialysis patients? Sem Dial 1998; 11:14–24.

Guarnieri G, Toigo G, Fiotti N, et al. Mechanisms of malnutrition in uremia. Kidney Int 1997; 62:S41–S44.

Haag-Weber M, Hori WH. Dysfunction of polymorphonuclear leukocytes in uremia. Sem Nephrol 1996; 16:192–201.

Hakim RM, Lazarus JM. Initiation of dialysis. J Am Soc Nephrol 1995; 6:1319–1328.

Jubelirer SJ. Hemostatic abnormalities in renal disease. Am J Kid Dis 1985; 5:219–225.

Kang JY. The gastrointestinal tract in uremia. Digest Dis Sci 1993; 38:257–268.

Massry SG, Smogorzewski M. The heart in uremia. Sem Nephrol 1996; 16:214–221.

Merrill JP, Hampers CL. Uremia. N Engl J Med 1970; 282:1014–1021.

Merrill JP, Hampers CL. Uremia. N Engl J Med 1970; 282:953–961.

Mitch WE. Mechanisms causing loss of lean body mass in uremia. Adv Nephrol 1997; 26:133–142.

O'Keeffe ST. Restless leg syndrome. A review. Arch Int Med 1996; 156:243–248.

Parfrey PS. Cardiac and cerebrovascular disease in chronic uremia. Am J Kidney Dis 1993; 21:77–80.

Parfrey PS, Harnett JD, Foley RN. Heart failure and ischemic heart disease in chronic uremia. Curr Opinion Nephrol Hypertension 1995; 4:105–110.

Prezant DJ. Effect of uremia and its treatment on pulmonary function. Lung 1990; 168: 1–14.

Sagripanti A, Barsotti G. Bleeding and thrombosis in chronic uremia. Nephron 1997; 75: 125–139.

Teschan PE. Uremia: an overview. Sem Nephrol 1994; 14:199–204.

Tolkoff-Rubin NE, Rubin RH. Uremia and host defenses. N Engl J Med 1990; 322:770–772.

Venkatesan J, Henrich WL. Cardiac disease in chronic uremia:management. Adv Renal Replacement Ther 1997; 4:249–266.

Wesely SA, Liebowitz B, Katims JJ. Neuropathy of uremia: evaluation by nerve conduction velocity versus neurospecific current perception threshold. Nephron 1989; 52: 317–322.

4
Symptoms of Electrolyte Disorders

Deborah B. Adey
University of California, San Francisco, California

I. INTRODUCTION

Electrolyte and acid-base disorders are often associated with characteristic symptoms, but they can also be asymptomatic, or cause only nonspecific symptoms, particularly when the disturbance is mild. Recognition of both specific and nonspecific symptoms is important because it allows the physician to uncover these disorders in a timely fashion and to intervene before life-threatening complications develop. In this chapter, the pathophysiology of each of the major electrolyte and acid-base disturbances is summarized briefly, and then the commonly encountered symptoms are reviewed. The symptoms are summarized for each of the electrolyte disorders in Tables 1–4. For a more complete description of the pathophysiology, diagnosis, and management of these disorders, the reader is referred to the chapters specifically dealing with each of these disorders.

II. TONICITY DISORDERS: HYPO- AND HYPERNATREMIA

Abnormalities in serum Na^+ concentration are among the most common electrolyte disturbances encountered, and they reflect, in most instances, abnormalities in serum tonicity (see Chapter 12). Sodium is the predominant extracellular solute, and therefore its concentration is closely correlated with serum osmolality, which is normally maintained in the relatively narrow range of 285–295 mOsmol/kg H_2O. Serum osmolality, and therefore Na^+ concentration ($[Na^+]$), is maintained by a feedback mechanism involving antidiuretic hormone (ADH) and thirst, which interact to regulate water balance. ADH acts in the kidney to facilitate water reabsorption in the distal nephron, and thirst stimulates the ingestion of water. In addition to sensing and responding to changes in tonicity, this regulatory system responds to changes in vascular volume through baroreceptors in the carotid arteries, aortic arch, right atrium, and kidney. Thus, a reduction in vascular volume stimulates both thirst and the release of ADH even when the body fluids are hypotonic, and vascular volume expansion blunts both these signals even when tonicity is increased. The normal regulation of serum tonicity and its disorders are discussed in Chapter 12. The present chapter reviews the symptoms associated with hypotonicity, i.e., abnormal water retention, and hypertonicity, i.e., abnormal water losses. The former problem is identified clinically by the presence of hyponatremia and the latter by the presence of hypernatremia.

A. Hyponatremia

Hyponatremia, defined as a serum sodium concentration of less than 135 mEq/L, is caused in most instances by abnormal retention of water, resulting in hypotonicity of the body fluids (see Chapter 12 for exceptions). Strikingly, the most common causes of hyponatremia are not the result of impaired osmoreceptor function or abnormalities in ADH secretion, but are due to factors operating on Na^+ and water reabsorption in the kidney. The most common cause is the use of diuretics. Thiazide diuretics have a greater propensity for causing hyponatremia than do the loop diuretics. Other common causes of altered water metabolism include renal failure, liver failure, and heart failure. The syndrome of inappropriate ADH release (SIADH) is an entity that is often considered as the etiology of hyponatremia, but it is actually quite uncommon. SIADH is a condition in which vasopressin release continues despite serum hypoosmolality and vascular volume expansion. There are several known and postulated causes for SIADH, including certain tumors, infections, and intracranial lesions. A reset osmostat is a variant of SIADH in which patients are able to excrete a water load, but do so at a lower osmolality than normal. This condition can be seen in the elderly, in the setting of alcoholism, tuberculosis, and malnutrition. It is a normal feature of pregnancy. Because the hyponatremia induced by a reset osmostat is mild, it is only rarely symptomatic.

The symptomatic manifestations of hyponatremia are dependent on both the severity of hypotonicity and the rapidity with which it develops (Table 1). Most symptoms are a result of the decrease in intracellular tonicity in the central nervous system (CNS) induced by water retention. A reduction in extracellular osmolality shifts water into cells, causing cell swelling and, in the case of the CNS, cerebral edema. The initial symptoms are headache, nervousness, and agitation, sometimes associated with vomiting. If acute hyponatremia is severe (serum $[Na^+] < 120$ mEq/L), symptoms may progress rapidly to disorientation, stupor, seizures, or coma. If severe cerebral edema occurs, transtentorial herniation may occur, resulting in respiratory arrest and death.

Table 1 Symptoms of Tonicity Disorders: Hypo/Hypernatremia

	General	Neuromuscular	Mental status	Cardiopulmonary
Acute hyponatremia				
Mild/Moderate ($[Na^+] < 125$ mEq/L)	Can be asymptomatic			
Severe ($[Na^+] < 125$ mEq/L)	Vomiting Malaise	Headache Stupor Seizures	Disorientation Agitation Coma	None
Chronic hyponatremia	Usually asymptomatic until very severe ($[Na^+] < 115$ mEq/L)			
Hypernatremia	Irritability	Hyperreflexia Focal neurological Findings if subdural hemorrhage	Lethargy Somnolence	None

Fortunately, protective mechanisms ameliorate cell swelling in the CNS in states of sustained hypotonicity. Initially as the brain tissue swells there is an efflux of fluid into the brain interstitium and drainage into the cerebral spinal fluid. Intracellular adaptation to hypotonicity occurs over a period of hours to 2–3 days. Initially potassium, the predominant intracellular cation, is extruded, decreasing intracellular osmotic pressure. Subsequently, organic osmolytes, including taurine, phosphocreatine, myoinositol, glutamine, and glutamate are removed from the cells by metabolic processes. These metabolic events further decrease intracellular osmolality and limit water entry into the cells. As a result of these protective responses, the symptoms described above are markedly diminished when hyponatremia develops more slowly and is sustained. Symptoms of chronic hyponatremia usually develop only when the serum [Na^+] falls below 115 mEq/L or if the patient has an underlying neurological condition. Patients with less severe sustained hyponatremia are usually asymptomatic.

Because of the cellular adaptations described above, severe cellular damage, termed central pontine myelinolysis or osmotic demyelinating syndrome, can occur when serum [Na^+] is corrected too rapidly, particularly after a prolonged period of exposure to hyponatremia. The etiology is unclear but is felt to be a result of brain dehydration and shrinking of the axons away from the myelin sheath. This disorder should be suspected when a patient's neurological status improves initially and then deteriorates during treatment, or 2–6 days after the correction of hyponatremia. Symptoms are often vague, most typically manifested by psuedobulbar palsy, mutism, swallowing dysfunction, and quadriparesis. Despite the nomenclature, the lesions observed by magnetic resonance imaging can be extra-pontine. See Chapter 29 for guidelines in treating hyponatremia to avoid this complication.

B. Hypernatremia

Hypernatremia, defined as a serum [Na^+] greater than 145 mEq/L, is a state of water deficiency (see Chapter 12). This condition occurs most commonly in those who are unable to obtain water under their own volition—the very young and the very old. Thirst is a powerful defense against hypernatremia, and diminished thirst leaves one susceptible to hypersomolar states. Primary hypodipsia results from destruction of the thirst centers in the hypothalamus from such etiologies as malignancies, trauma, granulomatous disease, or vascular disease. More common, however, is a situation of diminished fluid intake combined with decreased renal concentrating ability or increased insensible losses. In a hospital setting, a patient may become hypernatremic as a result of hyperalimentation causing osmotically induced diarrhea or causing impairment of renal concentrating ability due to osmotic diuresis from hyperglycemia or high urea production. Sustained inappropriate fluid replacement in the setting of ongoing hypotonic fluid losses can also result in hypernatremia. Less commonly, hypernatremia is due primarily to diabetes insipidus, that is, a failure in ADH secretion or a failure in its effectiveness in the kidney. Central diabetes insipidus is caused by decreased or absent production/secretion of vasopressin, and nephrogenic diabetes insipidus is caused by inherited abnormalities in the vasopressin receptor or by certain drugs (e.g., lithium).

As noted above, intense thirst is the major symptom in otherwise normal individuals who experience even a slight increase in serum [Na^+]. In patients with impaired thirst or who cannot signal their thirst to others, hypernatremia produces symptoms caused by cellular dehydration in the central nervous system. They include generalized irritability, confusion, and lethargy that can progress to coma, hyperreflexia, and spasticity (Table 1). In states of water deficit, water shifts from the intracellular compartment to the ECF compartment, resulting in cell shrinkage. In the CNS, cell shrinkage causes the brain parenchyma to shrink away from the pia and dural covering, producing traction on the dural veins and sinuses and a potential for intracranial hemorrhage. If hemorrhage occurs, symptoms will be referable to the focal nature of the intracranial bleed.

In a similar fashion to the response to hypotonicity, cellular defense mechanisms protect against cell shrinkage in hypertonic states. These defenses include electrolyte entry and the production of new intracellular osmolytes by metabolic processes to limit water exodus. Despite these defenses, with the exception of primary hypodipsia, an extremely rare condition, most patients develop symptoms of confusion and lethargy when the serum [Na^+] is greater than 155 mEq/L, although patients are often symptomatic at serum sodium levels well below 155 mEq/L.

III. DISORDERS OF POTASSIUM BALANCE: HYPO- AND HYPERKALEMIA

Disorders of potassium balance (hypokalemia and hyperkalemia) are extremely common and are often symptomatic. As discussed in Chapter 13, potassium is maintained in the intracellular compartment by the continual expenditure of energy through the activity of the Na^+/K^+ ATPase pump. The continual action of the Na^+/K^+ ATPase pump establishes the resting membrane potential that is critical for cardiac and muscle cell function. Regulatory processes maintain serum [K^+] between 3.6 and 4.5 mEq/L, a value less than 1/30 of the intracellular concentration.

Potassium intake varies widely. Diets high in fruits and vegetables contain large amounts of potassium, whereas some diets (e.g., tea and toast) contain very little potassium. Ingested potassium is absorbed and rapidly transferred to the intracellular compartment, a process facilitated through stimulation of the Na^+/

K^+ ATPase pump by insulin and β-adrenergic catecholamines. Excretion of K^+ occurs predominantly via the kidneys (80%), with 15% excreted via the gastrointestinal tract, and 5% excreted via sweat. Aldosterone plays a dominant role in potassium balance by regulating K^+ secretion by the renal tubules.

A. Hypokalemia

Hypokalemia (serum $[K^+] < 3.6$ mEq/L) can be due either to depletion of body K^+ stores or to a shift of K^+ into cells (see Chapter 13). Most commonly hypokalemia is a manifestation of K^+ depletion caused by diuretic use or diarrhea. Because potassium is contained in most foods, decreased intake is not a common cause for a low serum $[K^+]$ but may be a contributing factor in the presence of other circumstances. Uncontrolled diabetes can cause hypokalemia because of K^+ losses in the urine induced by glycosuria. In this setting, the hypokalemia may be masked by insulin deficiency because this hormone is key for K^+ entry into cells. With insulin treatment, the hypokalemia rapidly emerges. β-Adrenergic catecholamine release also stimulates K^+ entry into cells and can result in hypokalemia in the absence of K^+ depletion. Trauma victims are found to be mildly or moderately hypokalemic within an hour of presentation likely as a result of catecholamine release, but return to normal values within 24 hours.

Hereditary or congenital causes of hypokalemia are rare but should be considered in the child or young adult or when other possibilities have been exhausted. Familial hypokalemic periodic paralysis is a rare cause of transient hypokalemia that can be precipitated by a high-carbohydrate diet or strenuous exercise.

Hypokalemia hyperpolarizes muscle cell membranes, making them more refractory to developing an action potential. The symptoms of hypokalemia are predominantly related to this effect. Mild hypokalemia (serum $[K^+]$ 3.0–3.5 mEq/L) is often asymptomatic. If symptoms develop, they are quite nonspecific and include fatigue, muscle weakness, and constipation due to smooth muscle dysfunction (Table 2). Moderately severe hypokalemia (2.0–3.0 mEq/L) may result in more severe constipation, muscle weakness, or rhabdomyolysis. If serum $[K^+]$ falls to less than 2.0 mEq/L, muscle paralysis can ensue leading eventually to respiratory failure. Strikingly, hypokalemia has very little effect on cardiac signal conduction in the absence of underlying heart disease. In patients with normal cardiac function, even severe hypokalemia (serum $[K^+] < 2.0$ mEq/L) only rarely causes cardiac arrhythmias. By contrast, patients with underling cardiac disease, especially if treated with digoxin, can develop life-threatening arrhythmias with only mild hypokalemia. Hypokalemia produces characteristic changes in the electrocardiogram, although these do not correlate well with serum $[K^+]$. The ECG findings in patients with hypokalemia include U waves and S-T segment flattening. In patients with ischemic heart disease, reentrant cardiac arrhythmias may occur and can result in cardiac arrest. Hypokalemia can also

Table 2 Symptoms of Hypo/Hyperkalemia

	General	Neuromuscular	Mental status	Cardiopulmonary
Hypokalemia				
Mild ($[K^+] > 3.0$ mEq/L)	Often asymptomatic Fatigue Constipation	None	None	Cardiac arrhythmias[a]
Moderate ($[K^+]$ 2.5–3.0 mEq/L)	Fatigue Constipation	Muscle weakness	None	Cardiac arrhythmias[a]
Severe ($[K^+] < 2.5$ mEq/L)	Fatigue Constipation	Rhabdomyolysis Ascending paralysis	None	Cardiac arrhythmias[a]
Hyperkalemia				
Mild/Moderate ($[K^+] < 6.5$ mEq/L)	------------ Asymptomatic	------------	None	Sudden life-threatening cardiac arrhythmias
Severe ($[K^+] > 6.5$ mEq/L)	Weakness	Muscle weakness Falling down Ascending paralysis	None	Sudden life-threatening cardiac arrhythmias

[a] Only in patients with ischemic heart disease or taking digoxin.

result in disturbances in renal function. Abnormalities in both urinary concentrating and diluting capabilities have been documented in chronic hypokalemia, as has a decrease in creatinine clearance.

B. Hyperkalemia

Hyperkalemia (serum $[K^+] > 5.0$ mEq/L) is less common than hypokalemia, with the exception of patients with renal insufficiency (see Chapter 13). Renal excretion of excess K^+ is the main regulator of body K^+ stores. In acute renal failure, potassium levels can rise rapidly. In chronic renal insufficiency, K^+ secretion into the colon is adaptively increased, facilitating K^+ excretion in the stool. In addition, renal K^+ excretion is well maintained in the absence of excessive K^+ intake. Nonetheless, mild to moderate hyperkalemia (serum $[K^+]$ 5–5.5 mEq/L) is a common feature of renal insufficiency. In the absence of renal insufficiency, drug-induced hyperkalemia, increased release of potassium from cells, aldosterone deficiency, or resistance to aldosterone need to be considered (see Chapter 13).

Mild hyperkalemia (serum $[K^+]$ 5.0-6.0 mEq/L) is rarely symptomatic, but moderate (6.0–6.5 mEq/L) and severe (>6.5 mEq/L) hyperkalemia can cause sudden and serious cardiac arrhythmias (Table 2). Patients can present with chest pain resembling a myocardial infarction or with a cardiac arrest. The electrocardiographic changes are characteristic. In patients with mild to moderate hyperkalemia, peaked T waves (>5 mm) may be seen but are not uniformly present. With more severe hyperkalemia, the QRS complex widens and first-degree A-V block can develop. Eventually the QRS complex deteriorates into a sinusoidal pattern and cardiac arrest occurs. These events usually occur only when the serum $[K^+]$ is greater than 7.0 mEq/L but can rarely occur with less severe hyperkalemia. With potassium levels > 9.0 mEq/L, patients may experience atrioventricular dissociation, ventricular tachycardia, or ventricular fibrillation. Occasionally patients will present first with the other major symptom associated with hyperkalemia, muscle weakness. Muscle weakness is usually seen when the serum $[K^+]$ is greater than 7.0 mEq/L and can progress to an ascending paralysis with paresthesias of the hands or feet, similar to that seen in hypokalemia.

IV. DISORDERS OF CALCIUM AND PHOSPHORUS HOMEOSTASIS

Parathyroid hormone (PTH) and vitamin D are the principal mediators of both calcium and phosphorus balance (see Chapter 14). PTH maintains ionized calcium concentration in the extracellular compartment within a narrow range, 1.1–1.3 mmol/L (8.8–10.4 mg/dL for serum calcium concentration if albumin concentration is normal). PTH promotes the release of calcium from bone and stimulates its reabsorption by the kidney. PTH also causes phosphate release from bone but prevents its accumulation in the ECF by promoting phosphate excretion by the kidney. PTH also increases production of the active form of vitamin D, calcitriol, a hormone that promotes calcium absorption from the gut and also inhibits the secretion of PTH. Dysregulation of calcium and phosphorus balance can result from abnormalities in PTH release or its effectiveness or from abnormalities in calcitriol production or secretion. In addition, calcium and phosphorus balance can be disordered by abnormalities in the release of calcium from bones or in the renal tubular transport of these ions that are independent of PTH and calcitriol (see Chapter 14).

A. Hypocalcemia

Hypocalcemia is most commonly observed in patients with low serum albumin concentration, necessitating either calculation or measurement of the ionized [Ca^{2+}] to determine whether calcium homeostasis is disrupted (see Chapter 14). A low ionized [Ca^{2+}] (< 1.1 mmol/L) can develop when there is a failure of PTH synthesis or action, inadequate calcitriol, or excess calcium loss from either the gastrointestinal tract or kidney. With the exception of chronic renal insufficiency, deficiency in calcitriol is an uncommon cause of hypocalcemia in the United States, given the fortification of milk with vitamin D. Strict vegetarians can be at risk for vitamin D deficiency, as can people in certain cultures that require strict adherence to a dress code that allows minimal skin exposure to sunlight. Severe liver disease results in inadequate synthesis of vitamin D as well as decreased albumin synthesis. Gastrointestinal losses of calcium can develop in severe diarrhea or other malabsorption syndromes.

Mild hypocalcemia (ionized [Ca^{2+}] 1.0–1.1 mmol/L, or serum calcium 8–9 mg/dL in a patient with a normal serum albumin concentration) is often asymptomatic. More severe hypocalcemia causes a wide variety of symptoms, presumably all related to impaired nerve and muscle function (Table 3). Patients may present with depression, psychosis, or emotional lability. They may complain of paresthesias (circumoral and acral), muscle cramps, weakness, or fatigue. Severe cases can manifest laryngeal stridor or seizures. Cardiovascular effects of hypocalcemia include inhibition of cardiac contractility, bradycardia, and hypotension, due to both these cardiac effects and peripheral vasodilation.

B. Hypercalcemia

Hypercalcemia, defined as a serum [Ca^{2+}] > 10.5 mg/dL or, more specifically, a serum ionized [Ca^{2+}] > 1.3 mmol/L, is a common clinical finding. When severe (serum [calcium] > 13 mg/dL), it can present as a medical emergency with con-

Table 3 Symptoms of Disorders of Calcium, Magnesium, and Phosphorus Concentration

	General	Neuromuscular	Mental status	Cardiopulmonary
Hypocalcemia	Weakness Fatigue	Paresthesias Muscle cramps Seizures[a]	Apathy	Tachyarrhythmias[a]
Hypercalcemia	Anorexia Nausea, vomiting Constipation Polyuria	Muscle weakness	Depression[a] Psychosis[a] Obtundation[a]	Bradycardia[a] Vasodilation[a]
Hypomagnesemia	Anorexia Weakness Malaise	Carpopedal spasm Seizures[a]	Apathy	Tachyarrhythmias
Hypermagnesemia	Weakness	Paralysis[a]	Lethargy Somnolence	Hypotension[a] Bradycardia[a] Cardiac arrest[a]
Hypophosphatemia	Weakness Hemolytic anemia[a]	Multiple effects[a] including ataxia Cranial nerve palsies Paresis Rhabdomyolysis Myopathies, myalgias (see text)	Irritability	Respiratory arrest[a]
Hyperphosphatemia	Pruritus	Symptoms of hypocalcemia	None	None

[a] when severe

fusion and acute renal failure. Hypercalcemia is most often the result of increased bone resorption, due to abnormal PTH release or from a PTH-related peptide produced by certain tumors or to direct stimulation of osteoclast activity by other tumors (e.g., multiple myeloma). It can rarely occur as a result of vitamin D intoxication or immobilization (see Chapter 14).

Historically, hypercalcemia has been associated with the symptom complex described by the well-known medical adage, "stones, bones, psychic moans, and abdominal groans." Though patients rarely present with all these symptoms, this adage still provides a framework to evaluate the symptoms of hypercalcemia. Symptoms are primarily related to the CNS and gastrointestinal tract and can include depression, mild mental status changes to frank psychosis, or obtundation (Table 3). Gastrointestinal effects can include anorexia, nausea, vomiting, and constipation, especially in patients with chronic hypercalcemia. Hypercalcemia interferes with renal concentrating ability both by a direct effect in the collecting duct and by causing renal arteriolar vasoconstriction. This defect in renal concentrating ability in turn can lead to volume depletion and worsening of the hypercalcemia. Calcium can precipitate with the kidney and exacerbate the decline in glomerular filtration rate. Chronic hypercalcemia can result in nephrolithiasis, nephrocalcinosis, or interstitial nephritis.

C. Hypophosphatemia

Hypophosphatemia is defined as a serum phosphorus concentration of < 2.5 mg/dL, but serious consequences rarely develop unless the phosphorus falls below 1.0 mg/dL. Hypophosphatemia develops either from renal or gastrointestinal losses. Renal losses occur in hyperparathyroidism, after renal transplantation, in Fanconi's syndrome, and in the diuretic phase of recovery form acute tubular necrosis. Inadequate intake or inadequate absorption from the gastrointestinal tract can also lead to hypophosphatemia. Phosphate binders (calcium carbonate, magnesium salts, aluminum salts) used to treat peptic ulcer disease, laxatives, and oral iron all impair phosphate absorption from the gut. Inadequate intake of phosphorus occurs with eating disorders such as anorexia nervosa, alcoholism, or in anatomical disruption of the gastrointestinal tract produced by gastrectomy, Crohn's disease, gastrointestinal bypass, or gluten enteropathies.

Hypophosphatemia can also be seen with intracellular shifts in phosphorus. Hospitalized patients receiving parenteral or enteral nutrition after prolonged malnutrition can exhibit hypophosphatemia with the "refeeding syndrome." This is felt to be secondary to enhanced phosphorylation of carbohydrates and utilization of ATP. The "hungry bone syndrome" can be seen after parathyroidectomy and result in severe hypocalcemia and hypophosphatemia as bone remineralization occurs. Other transcellular shifts include rapid uptake by actively replicating cells, after strenuous exercise, or in alcohol withdrawal.

Mild hypophosphatemia is of little consequence and is an asymptomatic condition. However, as phosphorus levels approach 1.0 mg/dL, more serious adverse effects are likely to develop due to depletion of intracellular adenosine triphosphate (ATP). Neuromuscular effects are most common and range from mild anxiety and irritability to more severe effects of dysarthrias, dysphagias, ballismus, anisocoria, nystagmus, ataxia, or respiratory arrest (Table 3). Other neurological sequelae may include paresthesias, cranial nerve palsies, and paresis. Rhabdomyolysis is a well-recognized complication of severe hypophosphatemia, but myopathy and myalgias may be the presenting symptoms. Patients may complain of bone pain, anorexia, or generalized weakness. When hypophosphatemia is extremely severe (phosphorus < 0.5 mg/dL), a hemolytic anemia can develop.

D. Hyperphosphatemia

Hyperphosphatemia is defined as a serum phosphorus of >4.5 mg/dL. The most common cause is renal insufficiency or failure, either acute or chronic. Hyperphosphatemia is an almost universal problem in patients with end-stage renal disease who are ingesting an adequate diet; its management is discussed in Chapter 16. In the absence of renal failure, hyperphosphatemia is a rare occurrence.

Mild hyperphosphatemia is asymptomatic. More severe hyperphosphatemia is associated with hypocalcemia and metastatic calcification. The consequent hypocalcemia is directly responsible for many of the symptoms associated with hyperphosphatemia. Symptoms range from mild neuromuscular irritability with carpopedal spasm and paresthesias to seizures and severe hypotension. Metastatic calcification is commonly seen in the end-stage renal disease patient. Sites of calcification include lung, gastric mucosa, kidney and cornea, as well as arterial and arteriolar vessel walls. Deposition of calcium phosphate in arteriolar walls can affect the smooth muscles of the vessel walls and interfere with normal hemostasis. The most common symptom of hyperphosphatemia, however, is pruritis (Table 3). This symptom can be a particularly vexing problem in patients with chronic renal insufficiency or with end-stage renal disease who have the combination of sustained hyperphosphatemia and autonomous hyperparathyroidism. As a result they do not become hypocalcemic as phosphate concentration rises, promoting the deposition of calcium phosphate in the skin. This symptom is manifest by extensive excoriations in the arms and legs.

V. DISORDERS OF MAGNESIUM BALANCE: HYPO- AND HYPERMAGNESEMIA

Magnesium is the fourth most prevalent cation in the body and plays a key role in metabolic processes and enzymatic actions, neuromuscular transmission, as well as cardiovascular tone (see Chapter 14). The body maintains a precise balance of magnesium, as it does for sodium, potassium, and calcium, but how this is achieved is not completely understood. The kidney adjusts magnesium excretion in response to changes in dietary intake. The gastrointestinal tract also plays an important role in the maintenance of magnesium balance. Approximately 30–40% of dietary magnesium is absorbed in the gastrointestinal tract, specifically the jejunum and ileum, and the amount absorbed is also regulated, although to a lesser degree than is the renal excretion of this ion.

A. Hypomagnesemia

Hypomagnesemia (serum [Mg^{2+}] < 1.5 mEq/L) is probably the most underdiagnosed electrolyte disorder. Because only a small fraction of magnesium in the body is in the extracellular compartment, deficiency in this ion may not be detected until total body [Mg^{2+}] is significantly reduced. The most common causes of magnesium deficiency are gastrointestinal losses and diuretic use. Acute or chronic diarrhea can result in profound loss of magnesium, and malabsorptive states can permit saponification and chelation of magnesium salts in the gut, impairing absorption of this ion.

The symptoms of hypomagnesemia are nonspecific and often occur in association with disordered levels of other cations (Table 3). Symptoms that can be attributed specifically to hypomagnesemia include carpopedal spasm with Chvostek and Trousseau signs, lethargy, weakness, anorexia, nausea, apathy, and seizures. Cardiac tachyarrhythmias have also been noted.

B. Hypermagnesemia

Hypermagnesemia (serum [Mg^{2+}] > 2.5 mEq/L) is a rare problem and only occurs in the settings of either excessive magnesium administration or renal insufficiency. Magnesium sulfate is given to women in preterm labor to stop uterine contractions. In this setting the target for the magnesium level is just into the toxic range (4–6 mEq/L). The most common form of magnesium administration, laxative use, does not produce hypermagnesemia in the absence of renal insufficiency. In a similar fashion, magnesium-containing antacids are not a problem, except in patients with renal insufficiency. In this group of patients, chronic ingestion of such antacids may lead to toxic magnesium levels and should be avoided.

The symptoms of hypermagnesemia are related to magnesium's role in neuromuscular conduction. At mild toxicity, as is often seen in women being treated for preterm labor, symptoms are lethargy, drowsiness, and diminished deep-tendon reflexes (Table 3). As the toxicity increases, new symptoms appear including somnolence, paralysis, and bradycardia. The latter may progress to complete heart block and eventually to cardiac arrest.

VI. DISORDERS OF ACID-BASE EQUILIBRIUM

Acid-base disorders are common, especially in hospitalized patients, and are characterized by abnormalities in blood pH, PCO_2, and serum $[HCO_3^-]$. The pH of the body fluids is normally tightly regulated and maintained in a narrow range (7.38–7.42) by the interplay of pulmonary and renal control mechanisms, the former regulating PCO_2 and the latter regulating serum $[HCO_3^-]$. Acid-base disorders occur when these regulatory mechanisms are disrupted and are divided into four major categories: metabolic acidosis, respiratory acidosis, metabolic alkalosis, and respiratory alkalosis (see Chapter 11).

A. Metabolic Acidosis

Metabolic acidosis results from either addition of excess acid to the body (endogenous production or exogenous ingestion) or loss of HCO_3^- from the body (either in the urine or stool) (see Chapter 11). In either case, the manifestation of metabolic acidosis is a primary reduction in serum $[HCO_3^-]$, usually to less than 20 mEq/L, leading to a reduction in blood pH. The reduction in pH engendered by the fall in serum $[HCO_3^-]$ initiates an adaptive hyperventilatory response that lowers PCO_2, minimizing the fall in pH that would otherwise occur. The most common causes of metabolic acidosis are due to runaway endogenous acid production (as occurs in diabetic ketoacidosis) or to alkali loss with severe diarrhea (e.g., cholera).

The symptoms of acidemia are largely determined by the etiology of the acidosis. The most characteristic and general symptom of metabolic acidosis is Kussmaul respiration (Table 4). The patient with Kussmaul breathing complains of breathlessness, due to the ventilatory adaptive response to a fall in serum $[HCO_3^-]$. This cause of breathlessness is readily diagnosed by measurement of arterial blood gases. This symptom, however, only occurs with severe acute metabolic acidosis. With milder degrees of metabolic acidosis, the hyperventilation is asymptomatic, particularly when the acidosis is sustained. Mild to moderate chronic metabolic acidosis (e.g., renal tubular acidosis) (see Chapter 11) is usually an asymptomatic condition. If symptoms develop they are most commonly related to other electrolyte disorders that are a component of the acidosis (e.g., hypokalemia in some forms of renal tubular acidosis). In a similar fashion, the symptomatic manifestations of more severe and acute metabolic acidosis are reflective of the etiology underlying the illness and are difficult to attribute to acidemia, per se. For example, most of the symptoms of diabetic ketoacidosis are attributable to the hyperosmolality, volume depletion, and hyperglycemia that occur in this disorder. Severe acidosis ($pH < 7.20$) has a negative inotropic effect on the heart and may be a contributing factor in symptoms of heart failure.

Table 4 Symptoms of Acid-Base Disorders

	Specific for acidosis/ alkalosis	Others
Metabolic acidosis		
Acute	Shortness of breath (Kussmaul ventilation) Malaise	Symptoms due to associated findings (e.g., hypo- or hyperkalemia, hypertonicity)
Chronic	Usually asymptomatic	
Respiratory acidosis		
Acute	Shortness of breath, lethargy, somnolence	Symptoms due to hypoxemia
Chronic	Often asymptomatic when mild Shortness of breath, lethargy, somnolence	
Metabolic alkalosis		
$[HCO_3^-] < 40$ mEq/L	Asymptomatic	Symptoms due to hypokalemia
$[HCO_3^-] > 40$ mEq/L	Delirium, stupor Seizures Cardiac arrhythmias	Symptoms due to hypokalemia and hypoxemia
Respiratory alkalosis		
Acute	Circumoral and acral paresthesias Clouded sensorium	Symptoms due to hypocalcemia, hypophosphatemia
Chronic	Asymptomatic	

B. Respiratory Acidosis

Respiratory acidosis is the result of CO_2 retention and is manifested by an increase in PCO_2, usually to a level greater than 45 mmHg. As its name implies, respiratory acidosis is caused by respiratory failure. An immediate rise in the partial pressure of CO_2 results when ventilation ceases or is inadequate. In states of ventilatory insufficiency a new equilibrium develops in which PCO_2 is higher than normal, the level dependent on the degree of ventilatory insufficiency. Because CO_2 is in equilibrium with the weak acid H_2CO_3, the pH of the blood falls resulting in acidemia. The adaptive response to hypercapnia is an increase in serum $[HCO_3^-]$ that occurs through changes in renal acid excretion and HCO_3^- reabsorption.

Respiratory acidosis presents with a spectrum of manifestations that range from nearly asymptomatic in a well-compensated chronic respiratory acidosis, to lethargy, confusion, and coma with acute exacerbations of respiratory failure (Table 4). Acute respiratory acidosis is more commonly associated with symptoms of shortness of breath, particularly when it occurs with congestive heart failure, severe pneumonia, or during an asthma attack.

C. Metabolic Alkalosis

Metabolic alkalosis is caused by a primary increase in serum [HCO_3^-] to levels greater than 30 mEq/L and is most commonly caused by the selective loss of chloride from the body fluids. Such losses can occur with vomiting, nasogastric drainage, or diuretic administration. Much more rarely it is induced by abnormal mineralocorticoid production or by tubular transport abnormalities (see Chapter 11). The increase in serum [HCO_3^-] increases blood pH, eliciting a compensatory hypoventilatory response to increase PCO_2.

Unless severe (serum [HCO_3^-] > 40 mEq/L), metabolic alkalosis is usually an asymptomatic condition (Table 4). When symptoms do appear, they are most likely related to the associated hypokalemia (see above). When metabolic alkalosis is severe, delirium, seizures, and stupor may develop. These symptoms are probably multifactorial in origin, involving factors such as hypokalemia, a decrease in ionized calcium, and hypoxemia due to the compensatory hypoventilation that accompanies metabolic alkalosis. Myocardial irritability is enhanced in the presence of moderate to severe metabolic alkalosis, potentiating supraventricular, and ventricular arrhythmias. The arrhythmias may be refractory to treatment until the pH is reduced.

D. Respiratory Alkalosis

Respiratory alkalosis is caused by a primary reduction in PCO_2 to levels less than 36 mmHg and is caused by hyperventilation. Hyperventilation can occur secondary to hypoxemia or it can be induced independent of hypoxemia, a condition termed primary hyperventilation. Primary hyperventilation occurs in a wide variety of clinical settings, including cerebral injury, progesterone excess, salicylate intoxication, liver failure, pulmonary emboli, and the anxiety hyperventilation syndrome. The adaptive response to respiratory alkalosis is a reduction in serum [HCO_3^-], accomplished by a change in renal acid excretion and HCO_3 reabsorption.

Patients with acute respiratory alkalosis develop characteristic symptoms, including circumoral and acral paresthesias (Table 4). These symptoms are related to increased binding of calcium to albumin and are similar to those described above for hypocalcemia. Chronic respiratory alkalosis is always an asymptomatic condition.

SELECTED READINGS

Tonicity Disorders: Hypo/Hypernatremia

Arieff AI, Llach F, Massry S. Neurologic manifestations and morbidity of hyponatremia: correlation with brain water and electrolytes. Medicine 1976; 55:121–129.

Bartter FC, Schwartz WB. The syndrome of inappropriate secretion of antidiuretic hormone. Am J Med. 1967; 42:790–806.

Devita MV, Michelis MF. Perturbations in sodium balance: hyponatremia and hypernatremia. Clin Lab Med 1993; 13:135–148.

Fried LF, Palevsky PM. Hyponatremia and hypernatremia. Med Clin North Am 1997; 81: 585–609.

Snyder NA, Feigel DW, Arieff AI. Hypernatremia in elderly patients. Ann Int Med 1987; 107:309–319.

Stern RH, Cappucio JD, Silver SM, Cohen EP. Neurologic sequelae after treatment of severe hyponatremia: a multicenter perspective. J Am Soc Nephrol 1994; 4:1522–1530.

Disorders of Potassium Homeostasis

Mandal AK. Hypokalemia and Hyperkalemia. Med Clin North Am 1997; 81:611–639.

Latta K, Hisano S, Chan JCM. Perturbations in potassium balance. Clin Lab Med 1993; 13:149–159.

Defronzo RA, Bia M, Smith D. Clinical disorders of hyperkalemia. Ann Rev Med 1982; 33:521–554.

Disorders of Calcium, Phosphorus, and Magnesium Metabolism

Nussbaum SR. Pathophysiology and Management of Severe Hypercalcemia. Endocrin Metab Clin North Am 1993; 22:343 362.

Bourke E, Delaney V. Assessment of hypocalcemia and hypercalcemia. Clin Lab Med 1993; 13:157–181.

Weisinger JR, Bellorin-Font E. Magnesium and phosphorus. Lancet 1998; 352:391–396.

Acid/Base Disturbances

Riley LJ, Ilson BE, Narins RG. Acute metabolic acid-base disorders. Crit Care Clin 1987; 5:699–722.

Rimmer JM, Gennari, FJ. Metabolic alkalosis. J Intensive Care Med 1987; 2:137–150.

5

Interpretation of Blood Urea Nitrogen (BUN) and Creatinine

Gregorio T. Obrador
Panamerican University School of Medicine, Mexico City, Mexico

Andrew S. Levey
New England Medical Center and Tufts University School of Medicine, Boston, Massachusetts

Although the kidney carries out a wide variety of tasks, glomerular filtration rate (GFR) is considered the best index of overall renal function in both health and disease. The serum concentrations of creatinine (S_{cr}) and urea nitrogen (historically referred as blood urea nitrogen, BUN) are commonly used in clinical practice because they provide a good estimate of GFR and are widely available and inexpensive. However, several renal and extrarenal factors can importantly influence the serum concentrations of these substances. An understanding of such factors is therefore critical for proper interpretation of S_{cr} and BUN.

In this chapter we review the aspects of the excretion, metabolism, and measurement of creatinine and urea that are essential for proper interpretation of the S_{cr} and BUN. The principles covered are applied to clinical situations that are frequently encountered in the primary care setting.

I. GLOMERULAR FILTRATION RATE

The level of GFR is the best index of overall renal function for several reasons: it is a direct measure of the rate of filtration; it is reduced prior to the onset of symptoms of renal failure; impairment in GFR correlates with the severity of some of the structural abnormalities observed in chronic renal diseases; and signs and symptoms of uremia occur when GFR falls below 5–10 mL/min. However, it is not an ideal index. GFR is difficult to measure, and the measurement is not sensitive for detecting early damage to the kidney. In addition, the GFR can be affected by factors other than structural damage. These issues are discussed below.

A. Normal Range of GFR

Because GFR varies directly with renal size, which in turns varies with body size, GFR is conventionally factored by body surface area. In normal individuals, GFR is approximately 125 mL/min/1.73 m^2 or 180 L/day/1.73 m^2. The value of 1.73 m^2 reflects the average value for young men and women. Despite adjustment for body surface area, the normal GFR for women is approximately 8% lower than that for men. GFR also declines with age. In men, the normal GFR declines approximately 10 mL/min/1.73 m^2 for every decade of life after 40 years. Hence, the normal GFR in an 80-year-old man is approximately 80 mL/min/1.73 m^2. Cross-sectional studies in normal women indicate that the decrement in GFR with age is roughly similar.

B. Determinants of GFR

Glomerular filtration is a passive process of ultrafiltration of plasma across the semipermeable glomerular capillary wall. The GFR we measure is the sum of the filtration rates of each of the approximately 2 million nephrons:

$$\text{GFR} = \text{N} \times \text{SNGFR} \tag{1}$$

where N is the number of nephrons and SNGFR is single nephron GFR. The determinants of SNGFR are expressed in the equation:

$$\text{SNGFR} = K_f \times P_{UF} = A \times P \times (\Delta P - \Delta\pi) \tag{2}$$

where K_f is the glomerular ultrafiltration coefficient, the product of glomerular capillary surface area (A) and its hydraulic permeability (P), and P_{UF} is the net ultrafiltration pressure, the difference between the mean transcapillary hydrostatic (ΔP) and oncotic ($\Delta\pi$) pressure gradients. Although not explicit in this equation, SNGFR varies directly with the renal plasma flow because of the relationship between renal plasma flow and both ΔP and $\Delta\pi$.

It is not possible to measure SNGFR or its determinants in humans. However, these factors have been quantitated both in normal animals and in animals with experimentally induced renal diseases and reduced nephron mass. In animals with a reduction in functioning nephrons, glomerular capillary hypertension (increased ΔP) and glomerular hypertrophy (increased A) are observed in the remaining nephrons. These changes both increase single nephron GFR, thereby sustaining overall GFR at a level higher than would be expected from the decline in the number of nephrons. Indeed, despite a two-thirds reduction in nephron mass, GFR is only reduced by approximately 30% because of the increase in

Table 1 Conditions Other Than Renal Disease That Affect GFR

Pregnancy
Alterations in renal perfusion
Marked excess or deficit of extracellular fluid volume
Nonsteroidal anti-inflammatory drugs
Acute protein load and habitual protein intake
Blood glucose control (in diabetics)
Level of arterial blood pressure and class of antihypertensive agents

Source: Levey AS. Clinical evaluation of renal function. In: Greenberg A, ed. Primer of Kidney Diseases. San Diego: Academic Press, 1994, pp 20–26.

SNGFR in the remaining nephrons. Consequently, the GFR may not accurately reflect the physical extent of renal injury in a variety of renal diseases. Moreover, GFR is affected by conditions other than renal disease, such as changes in extracellular volume or renal perfusion (Table 1). These conditions alter GFR by changing SNGFR rather than reflecting changes in the number of nephrons and can occur both in healthy individuals and in patients with renal disease.

C. Measurement of GFR from Renal Clearance

Because GFR cannot be measured directly, it is assessed by renal clearance. Renal clearance, measured in units of mL/min (or L/day), is a theoretical concept defined as the volume of plasma from which a substance is completely removed during a particular time period. The measurement of renal clearance is based on the premise that the amount of a substance cleared from the plasma by the kidney during a particular time interval must be equal to its excretion into the urine:

$$P_x C_x = U_x V \tag{3}$$

where P_x is the average plasma or serum concentration of substance x, C_x is the plasma clearance of substance x, U_x is the urinary concentration of substance x, and V is the urine flow rate. Therefore, by knowing the urine and plasma concentrations of a substance and the urine flow rate, one can rearrange Eq. (3) to calculate the clearance (C_x):

$$C_x = U_x V / P_x \tag{4}$$

If substance x is freely filtered across the glomerular capillary wall and excreted only by glomerular filtration, its rate of glomerular filtration is equal to its rate of urinary excretion:

$$\text{GFR} \times P_x = U_x V \tag{5}$$

where the term GFR $\times$ P_x is the filtered load of x. By substitution into Eq. (4):

$$GFR = C_x \tag{6}$$

Hence, substance x would be defined as an "ideal filtration marker" if its renal clearance could be used to assess GFR.

The term U_xV is the sum of the rates of excretion of substance x by glomerular filtration (GFR $\times$ P_x), tubular secretion (TS_x) and tubular reabsorption (TR_x):

$$U_xV = GFR \times P_x + TS_x - TR_x \tag{7}$$

If substance x also undergoes tubular reabsorption or secretion, then urinary excretion does not equal the filtered load and clearance does not equal GFR. Therefore, the value for the renal clearance of x depends not only on the level of renal function, but also on the mechanism of renal excretion. The clearance of x would exceed GFR for substances that are filtered and secreted and would be less than GFR for substances that are filtered and reabsorbed.

D. Measurement of GFR from Renal Clearance of Exogenous Markers

Inulin, a 5200 dalton polymer of fructose, is an ideal filtration marker because it is freely filtered at the glomerulus and is not reabsorbed, secreted, or metabolized by the renal tubules. It is not bound to plasma proteins and is nontoxic and physiologically inert. For these reasons its renal clearance is regarded as the "gold standard" for the measurement of GFR. However, measurement of inulin clearance requires a continuous intravenous infusion as well as a carefully timed urine collection. Hence, this method is not easily adapted to clinical practice and remains largely a research tool. To simplify the assessment of GFR, investigators have studied other clearance methods, using bolus injection techniques and alternative filtration markers, such as $[^{125}I]$iothalamate and $[^{99m}Tc]$DTPA. Simultaneous measurements of renal clearance of these markers by alternative methods, and of inulin, by classic techniques, reveal similar although not identical results. These alternative methods for measuring GFR have become popular in clinical research in recent years but have not yet been adopted in practice.

E. Measurement of GFR from Renal Clearance of Endogenous Markers

Creatinine (molecular mass, 113 daltons) fulfills most, but not all, of the requirements for an ideal filtration marker. It is not protein bound and is freely filtered; it is not metabolized and is physiologically inert. However, in individuals with normal renal function, tubular secretion accounts for 5–10% of excreted creatinine. In patients with reduced GFR, the fraction of excreted creatinine that enters the tubule by secretion is increased and may account for up to 60% of the creatinine in the urine. Consequently, the level of creatinine clearance can substantially exceed GFR. Moreover, there is considerable variation in tubular secretion of creatinine among individuals and over time in the same individual. Despite these limitations, creatinine clearance is commonly used to estimate GFR because it is easier to measure and less expensive than direct measurements using radioisotopic methods. Most commonly, creatinine clearance is calculated from a 24-hour urine collection for creatinine and a single measurement of serum creatinine.

Urea (molecular mass, 60 daltons) can also be used as a filtration marker, but it is even less reliable than creatinine. The reason is that urea is not only filtered by the glomerulus but is also reabsorbed by the tubules (see later). As a result, urea clearance underestimates GFR. By coincidence, when the GFR is <20 mL/min/1.73 m^2, the proportion of the filtered load of urea that is reabsorbed approximates the proportion of excreted creatinine that is secreted. Consequently, in patients with advanced chronic renal disease, the average of the values for creatinine and urea clearance may provide a close approximation to the GFR.

F. Estimation of GFR from Serum Solute Concentration

To understand the relationship between GFR and the concentration of an individual solute (e.g., creatinine) in the serum, the concept of steady state of solute balance is critical. A steady state with regard to substance x is achieved when its rate of generation in body fluids (from either endogenous production or exogenous intake) is constant and equal to its rate of disappearance from body fluids (from either excretion or metabolism). In these circumstances, the serum concentration of x is constant. In the steady state, if substance x is excreted only in the urine, its generation and urinary excretion are equal, as depicted in the equation:

$$G_x = U_xV \tag{8}$$

where G_x is the generation rate of x. An important corollary is that, in the steady state, the rate of generation of solutes excreted in the urine can be assessed from their rate of urinary excretion. For an ideal filtration marker, the steady-state serum concentration is determined by the GFR and by its rate of generation and urinary excretion:

$$S_x = G_x/\text{GFR} = U_xV/\text{GFR} \tag{9}$$

Thus, for any given G_x, S_x is inversely related to GFR, and GFR can be assessed from the level of S_x.

II. SERUM CREATININE AS AN INDEX OF GFR

The use of serum creatinine as an index of GFR is based on two assumptions: (1) creatinine is an ideal filtration marker whose clearance (C_{cr}) equals GFR, and (2) creatinine balance is in a steady state, with creatinine generation rate (G_{cr}) being equal to renal excretion rate ($U_{cr}V$). Under these conditions, the serum level (S_{cr}) would be inversely related to GFR:

$$S_{cr} = G_{cr}/GFR = U_{cr}V/GFR \tag{10}$$

In reality, neither assumption is entirely correct. Tubular secretion, generation, and extrarenal elimination of creatinine may vary among individuals and over time in an individual. This variation can affect S_{cr} even if GFR remains constant. Consequently, in some circumstances serious errors can result from the estimation of GFR from serum creatinine. A summary of factors and clinical conditions that influence S_{cr} is presented in Table 2. With proper understanding of these concepts and limitations, S_{cr} provides a useful index of GFR for clinical decision making in most circumstances.

A. Renal Handling of Creatinine

In normal individuals, the magnitude of the GFR in relation to creatinine production rate is sufficient to maintain a low S_{cr}. The normal value for S_{cr} is approximately 0.8–1.2 mg/dL (71–106 μmol/L) with slightly lower values in women than in men. Figure 1 shows the expected changes in creatinine excretion, balance, and S_{cr} following a 50% decrement in GFR in a hypothetical setting in which the generation of creatinine is unchanged and creatinine excretion is accomplished only by glomerular filtration. A new steady state is reached when the S_{cr} rises sufficiently so that the filtered load of creatinine, and hence its urinary excretion, again equals its generation. In the new steady state, the 50% reduction in GFR results in a reciprocal doubling in S_{cr}. Although the assumptions upon which this analysis is based are not quite accurate (see earlier), in the steady state, changes in GFR are reflected by reciprocal changes in S_{cr}.

Because of the inverse relationship between S_{cr} and GFR, a large change in GFR is required to raise S_{cr} from the normal to the elevated range. However, once S_{cr} is elevated, even small changes in GFR raise it substantially more. In the hypothetical example shown in Figure 1, an increase in S_{cr} from 1.0 to 2.0 mg/dL represents a fall in GFR from 120 to 60 mL/min. By contrast, a rise in S_{cr} from 6.0 to 12.0 mg/dL reflects a reduction in GFR from 20 to 10 mL/min. Thus, a small elevation of S_{cr} above the normal range represents a major loss in GFR, and subsequent increments reflect progressively smaller decrements in GFR. Expression of the S_{cr} as its reciprocal ($1/S_{cr}$) allows the magnitude of decline in GFR to be more clearly appreciated, and this representation is used in some

Table 2 Factors and Clinical Conditions That Influence Serum Creatinine

Factor/Clinical condition	Effect on S_{cr}	Comment
Creatinine generation		
Reduced muscle mass	Decrease	Common in children, women, older and malnourished patients
Gain in muscle mass	Increase	Increased generation due to release of creatinine from muscle
Vigorous prolonged exercise	Increase	Increased generation due to release of creatinine from muscle
Rhabdomyolysis	Increase	Increased generation due to release of creatinine from muscle
Ingestion of cooked meat	Increase	Transient increase in creatinine generation; however, the increase in S_{cr} may be blunted by transient increase in GFR
Creatinine measurement		
Imprecision in the low range	Variable	Most of the commonly used creatinine assays are imprecise in the low range
Positive interferences	Increase	Glucose, uric acid, ascorbate, acetoacetate, pyruvate, other ketoacids, protein
Negative interferences	Decrease	Bilirubin or other substances present in the serum of jaundiced patients
Therapy with cephalosporins and flucytosine	Increase	Interference with the picric acid and iminohydrolase assays for creatinine, respectively
Renal function		
Decreased GFR	Increase	Physiological conditions and drugs (see Table 1), acute and chronic renal failure (see below)
Inhibition of tubular secretion	Increase	Blocking of tubular secretion of creatinine by cimetidine and trimethropin
Acute renal failure	Increased	Elevation of the serum creatinine to a level consistent with severity of renal failure may take several days
Chronic renal failure	Increased	Reduced renal creatinine excretion; however, the increase in P_{cr} may be blunted by increased renal tubular secretion and extrarenal elimination, as well as reduced creatinine generation due to loss of muscle mass and protein restriction

S_{cr} = Serum creatinine.

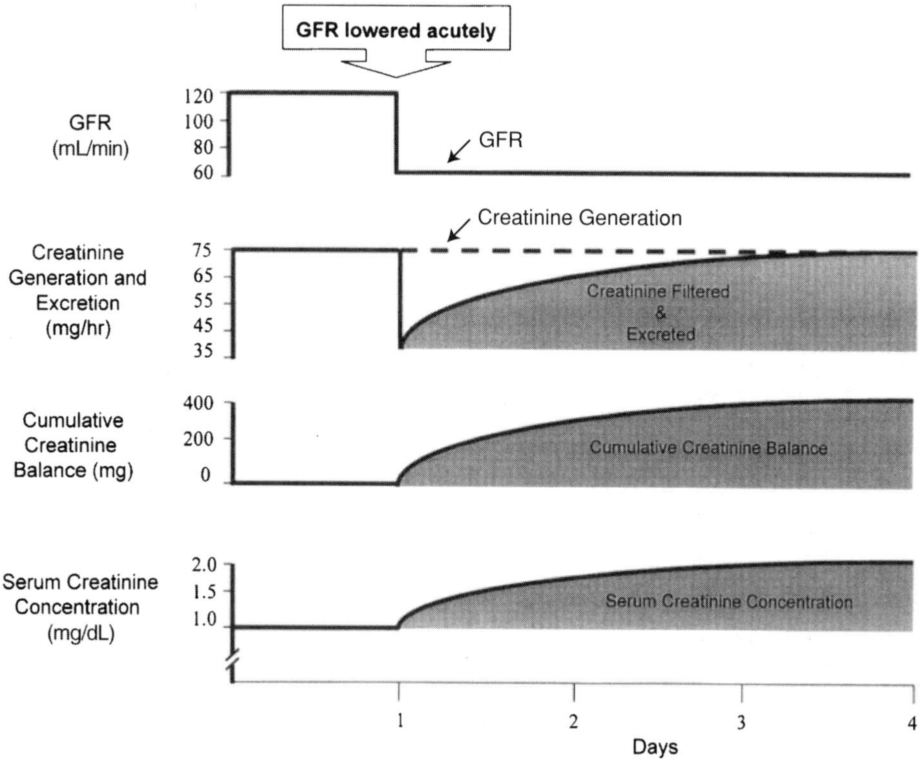

Figure 1 Effect of a sudden decrease in GFR on creatinine excretion, production, balance and serum creatinine concentration. (Modified with permission from Kassirer JP. N Engl J Med 1971; 285:385–389.)

clinical studies to depict progression of renal disease. In clinical practice, however, the rate of rise in serum creatinine is used to assess progression of renal insufficiency.

As discussed earlier, C_{cr} may not accurately reflect GFR in renal insufficiency because a greater proportion of creatinine is excreted by tubular secretion when GFR declines (Fig. 2, left panel). In patients with advanced chronic renal insufficiency, tubular secretion accounts for as much as 60% of creatinine excretion. Consequently, as GFR declines the rise in S_{cr} is less than would be expected if creatinine were excreted solely by filtration. As a result, the increase in S_{cr} underestimates the magnitude of the reduction in GFR. At the extreme, serum creatinine may remain normal despite a reduction in GFR to as low as 20 mL/

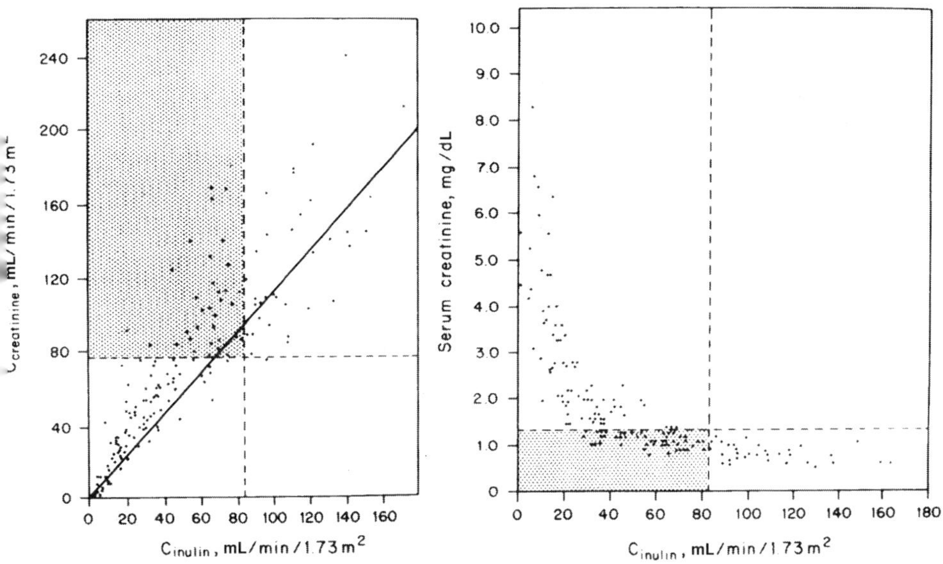

Figure 2 Relationship of creatinine clearance (left) and serum creatinine (right) to GFR (inulin clearance) in patients with renal disease. Horizontal lines indicate lower limit of normal for creatinine clearance (left) and upper limit of normal for serum creatinine (right). Vertical lines indicate lower limit of normal for GFR. Diagonal line (left) is the line of identity. Shaded areas indicate the proportion of patients in whom the level of creatinine clearance or serum creatinine is normal despite reduced GFR. (Reprinted with permission from Shemesh O. Kidney Int 1985; 28:830–838, and Levey AS, Annu Rev Med 1988; 39:465–490.)

min/1.73 m^2 (Fig. 2, right panel). As a general guideline, any elevation of the steady-state S_{cr} above the normal range indicates a substantial reduction in GFR.

B. Creatinine Metabolism

1. Creatinine Generation

Creatinine is a stable end product of metabolism, formed by the nonenzymatic dehydration of creatine in muscle. Creatine is synthesized primarily in the liver, enters the circulation, and is actively taken up by muscle cells, which contain approximately 98% of the total body pool. In muscle cells, excess creatine is metabolized, and the creatinine produced by this conversion leaves the intracellular compartment and is excreted by the kidney. Dietary creatine contained in meat is another source of creatinine and may account for 30% of daily creatinine generation. Cooking meat converts a variable fraction of creatine into creatinine, which is then absorbed and also enters the creatinine pool. Overall, creatinine generation parallels total muscle mass and, to a lesser extent, meat intake.

2. Extrarenal Creatinine Elimination

Creatinine is eliminated almost entirely by renal excretion; insignificant amounts are excreted in feces and sweat. In patients with renal disease, the renal excretion of creatinine is lower than in normal individuals. This reduction is due at least in part to enhanced creatinine elimination by extrarenal routes, probably because of degradation by intestinal microorganisms. Indeed, extrarenal elimination may account for as much as 68% of the total creatinine excretion in advanced renal insufficiency. Therefore, urinary creatinine excretion is reduced in chronic renal disease.

C. Measurement of Serum Creatinine

The alkaline picrate reaction, described by Jaffé in 1886, remains the dominant assay for measurement of creatinine in clinical laboratories today. Under alkaline conditions, creatinine reacts directly with picrate ion to form an equimolar complex whose red-orange color is easily detected and quantified. The advantages of methods using the Jaffé reaction are their simplicity and their wide clinical acceptance. The disadvantage is that as much as 20% of the color reaction in serum or plasma arises from substances other than creatinine. In an attempt to measure ''true creatinine,'' methods that separate creatinine from these noncreatinine chromogens have been developed. The most commonly used is the kinetic alkaline picrate method, which takes advantage of the differential rate of color development for noncreatinine chromogens versus that for creatinine. However, although these methods significantly reduce positive interferences from noncreatinine chromogens, they do not completely eliminate the problem. As a result, total chromogen and not ''true creatinine'' is the value used in clinical practice.

D. Estimation of Creatinine Clearance and GFR from Serum Creatinine

In 1976, Cockcroft and Gault derived a formula, which now bears their name, to estimate C_{cr} from steady-state S_{cr}. The formula is particularly simple to use and accounts for differences in creatinine generation due to the effects of body weight, age, and gender on body muscle mass:

$$C_{cr} = \frac{(140 - \text{age}) \times \text{weight}}{S_{cr} \times 72} \tag{10}$$

In this formula, C_{cr} is in mL/min, age is in years, weight is in kg, and S_{cr} is in mg/dL. The value for C_{cr} calculated from this formula should be multiplied by 0.85 in women because a lower fraction of the body weight is composed of muscle. Also, in patients with marked obesity or ascites, lean or ideal body mass should be used for the calculation. This formula provides a good estimate of C_{cr}, but it consistently overestimates GFR in patients with renal disease.

Recently, an equation to predict GFR, rather than C_{cr}, was developed using data from the Modification of Diet in Renal Disease (MDRD) Study. This equation uses simple demographic and laboratory information, including the S_{cr}, and predicts GFR adjusted for body surface area:

$$\text{GFR}/1.73\ \text{m}^2 = 170 \times [S_{cr}]^{-.999} \times [\text{Age}]^{-.176} \times [0.762 \text{ if female}] \times [1.180 \text{ if black}] \times [\text{BUN}]^{-.170} \times [\text{Alb}]^{+.318} \quad (11)$$

In this formula, GFR is in mL/min/1.73 m^2 of body surface area, S_{cr} is in mg/dL, age is in years, BUN is in mg/dL, and serum albumin (Alb) is in g/dL. The advantages of this equation are (1) it predicts GFR rather than C_{cr}; (2) it predicts GFR over the full range of values; (3) it is more accurate and precise than other equations, including the Cockcroft-Gault equation; and (4) collection of a timed urine sample and measurement of height and weight are not required. However, this equation has not been validated in children ($<$18 years), the elderly ($>$70 years), type I and type II diabetics taking insulin, pregnant women, those with serious comorbid conditions, or renal transplant recipients. Nonetheless, computing and reporting GFR predicted from S_{cr} could be implemented in clinical laboratories by routinely requesting basic patient demographic and laboratory data. As described below, we recommend routinely using the MDRD Study prediction equation or the Cockcroft-Gault equation to predict GFR or creatinine clearance from S_{cr} in patients with chronic renal disease.

III. EFFECTS OF COMMON CLINICAL CONDITIONS ON SERUM CREATININE

A. Variation in Muscle Mass, Malnutrition, Muscle Disorders, and Diet

The steady state can be disturbed by changes in creatinine production as well as in GFR. Since creatinine generation parallels muscle mass, individuals with lower muscle mass such as women, children, the elderly, those who are malnourished, and patients with muscle wasting disorders will have lower baseline S_{cr}. As a consequence, S_{cr} may remain within normal limits despite a substantial reduction in GFR. Dietary meat intake also contributes to creatinine generation, and patients who restrict their meat intake may also have low S_{cr}.

Conversely, if creatinine generation is acutely increased, as may occur in severe rhabdomyolysis, the S_{cr} can increase out of proportion to changes in GFR. Also, cooked meat and its broth contain enough creatinine to transiently increase the S_{cr} by as much as 1.0 mg/dL, even though GFR remains normal. Measurement of S_{cr} after ingestion of meat may reveal an elevated level and suggest a reduction on GFR. If this is suspected, measurement of S_{cr} in the fasting state will eliminate the elevation due to creatinine ingestion.

B. Drug-Induced Inhibition of Creatinine Secretion

Some medications, such as cimetidine and trimethoprim, competitively inhibit the organic base secretory pump in the proximal tubule responsible for creatinine secretion. This results in a transient decrease in creatinine excretion and an increase in the S_{cr} to a new steady-state level. The elevation in S_{cr} is usually less than 0.5 mg/dL in patients with normal GFR. The elevation is greater in patients with reduced GFR because a greater proportion of renal creatinine excretion is due to secretion. Ranitidine, another organic base, has little effect on S_{cr}, in part because of the much smaller doses used.

C. Measurement Errors

Although the methods currently used to measure creatinine are more precise than the original Jaffé reaction method, two problems remain. First, most methods are imprecise in the lower range. Indeed, analytical variability may account for 80–90% of day-to-day variability in S_{cr} results in an individual. Hence, it can be difficult to determine whether changes in the serum level within the normal range represent analytical variability or changes in GFR, particularly among individuals with low muscle mass such as women and children.

The second problem is that various substances can interfere with the serum assays, leading to spurious elevations in the serum level (Table 2). Glucose, uric acid, ascorbate, acetoacetate, pyruvate, other ketoacids, and protein can cause positive interferences with the alkaline picrate reaction. Although overestimation from these noncreatinine chromogens does not usually impact on clinical decision making, the measured S_{cr} may increase by 0.5–2 mg/dL or more in patients with ketoacidosis. This effect is rapidly reversed with correction of the ketoacidosis.

Cephalosporins can also cause spurious elevations of the S_{cr}. After intravenous administration of cefoxitin, S_{cr} may be falsely elevated by as much as 2.8 mg/dL at the time of the peak concentration of the drug in serum. Other cephalosporins known to contribute to the colorimetric reaction include cephalothin, cefazolin, and cefamandole. Another positive interference occurs with the antifungal flucytosine and an enzymatic method that uses the enzyme iminohydrolase (Ektachem method; Eastman Kodak Co., Rochester, NY). Flucytosine may increase the S_{cr} concentration by as much as 6 mg/dL, which may lead to emergency consultation for "acute renal failure."

Finally, negative interferences with the creatinine assays can also occur. Although the mechanism is not completely understood, high concentrations of bilirubin or other compounds in the serum of jaundiced patients can interfere with the alkaline picrate reaction resulting in a lower S_{cr}.

D. Acute Renal Insufficiency

In acute renal insufficiency, the steady state is lost as a result of rapid deterioration in renal function, and thus the S_{cr} no longer follows a reciprocal relationship with GFR. Instead, a more complex relationship is observed (Fig. 3). As GFR falls abruptly, S_{cr} rises only slowly. Indeed, if the renal excretion of creatinine is near zero, the rate of rise of S_{cr} will parallel the rate of creatinine generation. In acute renal failure, GFR is typically less than 10 mL/min/1.73 m^2, and the serum creatinine rises by 0.5–2.5 mg/dL per day. In the recovery phase, improvement in S_{cr} lags behind the improvement in GFR. Thus, S_{cr} remains elevated after GFR begins to improve, slowing falling over a period of 3–5 days or longer. Only when GFR stabilizes will a new steady state emerge, with S_{cr} again reflecting GFR.

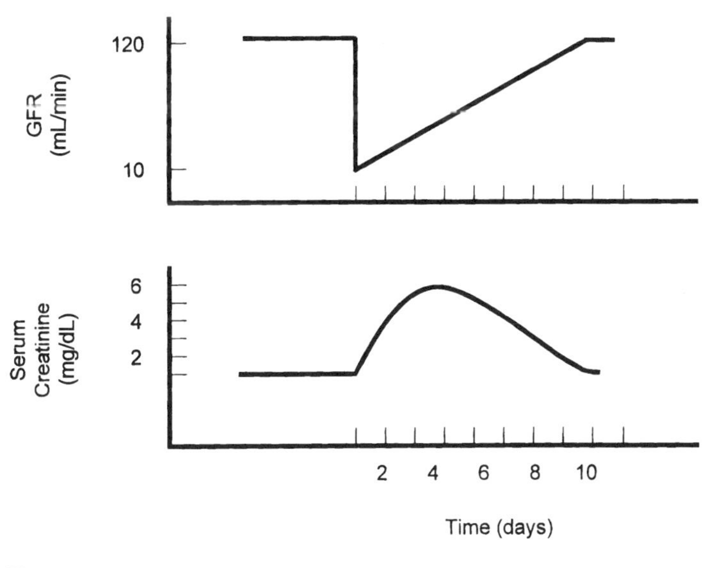

Figure 3 Hypothetical changes in (top) glomerular filtration rate (GFR) and (bottom) serum creatinine in acute renal failure. (Modified with permission from Moran SM, Myers BD. Kidney Int 1985; 27:928–937.)

1. Drug Dosing in Acute Renal Insufficiency

Given the non–steady-state relationship between S_{cr} and GFR in acute renal insufficiency, one should be wary of drug-dosing nomograms that relate drug dosage to S_{cr}. These nomograms are based on the assumption that the S_{cr} is a steady-state value, and their use may lead to errors in dosing if renal function is changing. For example, if GFR suddenly declines from 125 to 10 mL/min, S_{cr} on day 1 may still be normal since there will not have been enough time for creatinine to accumulate in the plasma. On day 2, S_{cr} may increase to 2 mg/dL. Only after several days does the S_{cr} rise to a level consistent with the reduced GFR. If, based on the assumption that a S_{cr} of 2 mg/dL on day 2 reflects a 50% loss in GFR, the above patient were given half the dose of a medication that is entirely excreted by the kidney (e.g., an aminoglycoside), toxic levels will occur.

2. Dialysis Considerations in Acute Renal Failure

Another application of these concepts is that dialysis may be necessary before S_{cr} reaches a steady-state value typically associated with severe renal insufficiency. For example, a patient who develops anuric acute renal failure will have an initial S_{cr} that is only slightly above the baseline, despite a GFR that is effectively equal to zero. Only after sufficient time has elapsed will S_{cr} increase to a value usually associated with severe renal insufficiency. However, dialysis may be required for fluid overload, hyperkalemia, or acidosis even though S_{cr} is not yet elevated to a high level.

E. Chronic Renal Insufficiency

Although it is an insensitive marker of renal insufficiency, a persistently elevated serum creatinine is often the first indication that chronic renal disease is present. A serum creatinine greater than 1.5 mg/dL in men and greater than 1.2 mg/dL in women generally reflects a substantial decrease in GFR and should prompt an investigation to determine whether renal insufficiency is due to a functional change (Table 1) or to structural renal disease. After exclusion of functional causes, assessment of the urine sediment, protein excretion, and, in most instances, a renal ultrasound should be undertaken to determine the cause of renal disease. Because of the utility of early interventions to slow the progression of chronic renal disease, the primary care physician should either initiate these actions on their own (see Chapter 16) or refer patients to nephrologists as soon as the diagnosis of chronic renal disease is established.

Serum creatinine is the standard tool used in clinical practice to monitor the rate of progression of chronic renal disease and the effects of intervention to slow progression. However, as described earlier, the rise in serum creatinine with progressive decline in GFR may be masked by increases in renal tubular secretion and extrarenal elimination of creatinine. In addition, meat intake is often restricted, and malnutrition and muscle wasting are common, thus decreasing creatinine generation. Overall, the combination of these factors makes it difficult to assess the level of GFR or changes in GFR from the level of S_{cr} or changes in S_{cr} in patients with chronic renal disease. To overcome these difficulties, we recommend routinely estimating GFR or creatinine clearance using the S_{cr} and the MDRD Study equation or the Cockcroft-Gault equation.

1. Monitoring the Rate of Progression of Chronic Renal Disease

Patients with chronic renal disease generally have a very slow decline in GFR (2–10 mL/min per year), corresponding to a very slow increase in S_{cr} (0.1 mg/dL per month until very late in their course). A faster decline in GFR indicates the presence of a rapidly destructive process. Such patients should be referred in a timely fashion to a nephrologist for a full workup of the cause and initiation of appropriate therapy when indicated. Delay in referral can lead to irreversible damage with many forms of rapidly progressive renal insufficiency.

2. Initiation of Dialysis and Transplantation for End-Stage Renal Disease

The average value for predicted GFR at the initiation of dialysis for end-stage renal disease in the United States is approximately 7 mL/min/1.73 m^2, although there is a wide range. The high morbidity and mortality of patients with end-stage renal disease has led some to speculate that this value is too low. The average value for serum creatinine is approximately 8 mg/dL, with lower mean values in the elderly, women, whites, smaller individuals, and diabetics. The range of serum creatinine values is also wide, with almost 25% of patients having values less than or equal to 5.0 mg/dL. Reliance on serum creatinine, rather than predicted GFR or creatinine clearance, to assess the level of function may lead to overestimation of the level of renal function and subsequent delay in referral and initiation of dialysis and transplantation. Such delays can contribute to morbidity and mortality for patients with chronic renal disease. In general, referral to a nephrologist for consideration for dialysis and renal transplantation should occur at levels of GFR high enough to allow time for preparation for these therapies (20–25 mL/min/1.73 m^2).

IV. BUN AS AN INDEX OF GFR

Like creatinine, urea is freely filtered by the glomerulus, and thus its clearance is affected by GFR. The normal range for steady-state BUN levels is 10–15 mg/

dL, a value 10–15 times the S_{cr}. However, the BUN provides a less precise estimate of the GFR than S_{cr} for two main reasons: (1) urea generation is primarily determined by protein intake and is more variable than creatinine generation, and (2) renal tubular reabsorption of urea varies with level of hydration and renal perfusion. Therefore, the level of BUN should not be interpreted as an index of GFR. In fact, the BUN should not be evaluated without a concurrent S_{cr}. When evaluated in relation to S_{cr} (BUN/S_{cr} ratio) the BUN can provide clues to the level of protein intake, the presence of a catabolic state, and changes in renal perfusion or hydration. In this section, we discuss pertinent information regarding renal urea handling and metabolism of urea, measurement of BUN, and interpretation of the BUN/S_{cr} ratio. A summary of factors and clinical conditions that influence BUN is presented in Table 3.

A. Renal Handling of Urea

Urea is freely filtered by the glomerulus and follows a complex pattern along the nephron, with reabsorption in the proximal tubule, secretion in the loop of Henle, and a second wave of reabsorption in the collecting tubule. This complex pattern allows for urea recycling in the medullary interstitium, an important component of the urinary concentrating mechanism. The final wave of reabsorption in the collecting duct determines urea clearance and is directly related to salt and water reabsorption at this site in the nephron. When collecting duct salt and water reabsorption are increased, urea reabsorption also increases, reducing its clearance, and when collecting duct salt and water reabsorption are blunted, urea reabsorption is blunted as well, increasing its clearance. In states of antidiuresis, urea clearance falls to as low as 35–40% of GFR (net urea reabsorption of 60–65%), and in diuretic states it rises to as high as 80–100% of GFR. This variation in urea clearance relative to GFR (and C_{cr}) causes the BUN to rise proportionately more than S_{cr} in antidiuretic states and to result in a lower BUN in diuretic states. This variable relationship is a clinically useful tool, defined as the BUN/S_{cr} ratio, and is used to assess the causes of a reduction in GFR. The normal range of values for this ratio is 10–15.

B. Urea Metabolism

Urea is an end product of protein catabolism. In an individual in a steady state of nitrogen balance, urea generation and excretion by the kidney is equivalent to dietary protein intake. Urea is synthesized in the liver by deamination of amino acids not used for protein synthesis. Dietary protein intake is normally the main determinant of urea generation. Because of the close association between urea production and protein intake, measurement of urinary urea nitrogen excretion is used as an indicator of protein intake in the steady state. Each gram of urea

Table 3 Factors and Clinical Conditions That Influence BUN

Factor/Clinical condition	Effect on BUN	Comment
Urea generation		
Increased dietary protein	Increase	Increased urea generation
Increased tissue breakdown	Increase	Increased urea generation
Impaired protein synthesis	Increase	Increased urea generation
Restriction of dietary protein	Decrease	Reduced urea generation
Malnutrition	Decrease	Reduced urea generation
Liver dysfunction	Variable	Decreased GFR, increased urea reabsorption, decreased urea generation
Hydration		
Overhydration (hypotonic fluid administration, syndrome of inappropriate ADH secretion)	Decrease	Reduced urea reabsorption
Dehydration (water deprivation, diabetes insipidus)	Increase	Increased urea reabsorption
Renal perfusion		
Increased renal perfusion (volume expansion, pregnancy)	Decrease	Increased GFR, reduced urea reabsorption
Reduced renal perfusion (volume depletion, congestive heart failure)	Increase	Reduced GFR, increased urea reabsorption, increased urea generation
Renal function		
Decreased GFR	Increase	Physiological conditions and drugs (see Table 1), acute and chronic renal failure

Source: Levey AS. Clinical evaluation of renal function. In: Greenberg A, ed Primer of Kidney Diseases. San Diego: Academic Press, 1994, pp 20–26.

excreted is equivalent to 6.25 g of protein ingested. Variations in protein intake have little effect on the BUN in individuals with normal renal function, but in the setting of chronic renal insufficiency, when adjustments in urea clearance are limited, the BUN level and BUN/S_{cr} ratio reflect the level of protein intake. When urea clearance is limited in states in which endogenous protein breakdown is increased, such as trauma, gastrointestinal bleeding, catabolic states (e.g., congestive heart failure, sepsis, or administration of corticosteroids), the BUN/S_{cr} will be high. Rarely, toxins that impair protein synthesis, such as tetracycline, can also increase the BUN/S_{cr} ratio. The most common presentation of a very high BUN/S_{cr} ratio (>40 : 1) is in patients with severe congestive heart failure. Conversely, a low BUN and low ratio of BUN/S_{cr} will be observed in patients with reduced urea generation due to liver dysfunction, malnutrition, or dietary protein restriction.

C. Urea Measurement

Several methods for measuring urea nitrogen in blood, including direct and indirect methods, are commercially available. Most of these methods depend on the increase in conductivity of a sample following treatment with urease. The coefficient of variation of the methods commonly used for measuring BUN is approximately 5%. Relatively few drugs or compounds interfere with measurement of urea nitrogen.

D. Interpretation of the BUN/S_{cr} Ratio in Acute Renal Failure

Analysis of the BUN/S_{cr} ratio is sometimes helpful in uncovering the cause of acute renal failure, but it is not specific. In conditions associated with reduced renal perfusion (''prerenal conditions''), GFR is reduced and urea reabsorption is increased. Therefore, urea clearance is reduced more than creatinine clearance. In addition, in most prerenal settings, urea production is also increased. As a result both of increased production and decreased excretion, BUN increases faster than the S_{cr} leading to an increased BUN/S_{cr} ratio. A ratio of >20 is typical for prerenal conditions. It should be emphasized, of course, that a high ratio may also be seen in patients with structural renal damage associated with increased urea reabsorption (such as the early phase of acute glomerulonephritis or obstruction of the urinary tract) or with increased urea generation (such as high protein intake, gastrointestinal bleeding, or therapy with corticosteroids).

A normal BUN/S_{cr} ratio is typically seen in acute tubular necrosis. However, prerenal conditions should not be excluded by a normal ratio because diminished urea production (such as a low protein intake or liver disease) may blunt the expected rise in BUN despite enhanced tubular reabsorption.

V. SUMMARY

Despite its limitations, the serum creatinine concentration (S_{cr}) is the most useful marker we have of GFR in clinical practice. To maximize its utility, the S_{cr} must be interpreted in light of concepts of renal physiology, creatinine metabolism, analytical chemistry, and detailed clinical information. Equations to predict GFR or creatinine clearance are especially important in estimating the level of renal function from S_{cr} and in the management of chronic renal disease. Because of the variability in urea generation and reabsorption, the BUN is a much less reliable reflection of the GFR. In fact, the BUN is of little use except when examined in relation to the S_{cr}. The BUN/S_{cr} ratio can be a useful guide to the status of protein intake, hydration, and renal perfusion and is sometimes useful in the differential diagnosis of acute renal failure.

REFERENCES

Cockcoft DW, Gault MH. Prediction of creatinine clearance from serum creatinine. Nephron 1976; 16:31–41.

Kassirer JP. Clinical evaluation of kidney function: glomerular function. N Engl J Med 1971; 285:385–389.

King AJ, Levey AS. Dietary protein and renal function. J Am Soc Nephrol 1993; 3:1723–1737.

Levey AS. Nephrology forum: measurement of renal function in chronic renal disease. Kidney Int 1990; 38:167–184.

Levey AS. Assessing the effectiveness of therapy to prevent the progression of renal disease. Am J Kidney Dis 1993; 22:207–214.

Levey AS. Clinical evaluation of renal function. In: Greenberg A, ed. Primer on Kidney Diseases. San Diego, CA: Academic Press, 1994, pp 20–26.

Levey AS, Bosch JP, Breyer JA, Greene T, Rogers N, Roth D, for the Modification of Diet in Renal Disease (MDRD) Study Group. A more accurate method to estimate glomerular filtration rate from serum creatinine: a new prediction equation derived from the Modification of Diet in Renal Disease Study. Ann Intern Med 1999; 130: 461–470.

Luke RG. Uremia and the BUN. N Engl J Med 1981; 305:1213–1215.

Moran SM, Myers BD. Course of acute renal failure studied by a model of creatinine kinetics. Kidney Int 1985; 27:928–937.

Perrone RD, Madias NE, Levey AS. Serum creatinine as an index of renal function: new insights into old concepts. Clin Chem 1992; 38:1933–1953.

Rose BD. Clinical assessment of renal function. In: Rose BD, ed. Pathophysiology of Renal Disease. New York: McGraw-Hill, 1987:1–39.

Shemesh O, Golbetz H, Kriss JP, Myers BD. Limitations of creatinine as a filtration marker in glomerulopathic patients. Kidney Int 1985; 28:830–838.

Walser M. Progression of chronic renal failure in man. Kidney Int 1990; 37:1195–1210.

Yager HM, Harrington JT. Evaluation of serum electrolytes, creatinine, and blood urea nitrogen. In: Jacobson HR, Striker GE, Klahr S, eds. The Principles and Practice of Nephrology. St. Louis: Mosby, 1995.

6
Asymptomatic Hematuria/ Proteinuria

Wolfgang J. Weise
University of Vermont, Burlington, Vermont

I. INTRODUCTION

Hematuria and proteinuria are the most common abnormalities detected on routine urinalysis in patients who have few or no symptoms of underlying intrinsic renal or urological disease. In this setting it is important for the primary care physician to differentiate between relatively benign and common causes of hematuria/proteinuria and more serious but less common causes that require referral to a urologist or nephrologist. Appropriate evaluation of these abnormalities can identify patients with serious illness expeditiously and avoid exposure of others to unnecessary testing and anxiety.

This chapter will review the approach to the patient with asymptomatic hematuria/proteinuria in the primary care setting and provide guidelines for referring patients to the appropriate specialist. The combined finding of abnormal hematuria and proteinuria is a major feature of the nephritic syndrome, and the approach to the diagnosis and management of that disorder is discussed in more detail in Chapter 8. The approach to the diagnosis and management of nephrotic-range (>3.5 g/24 h) proteinuria is discussed further in Chapter 7.

II. HEMATURIA

Hematuria that is not explained by an obvious underlying condition is relatively common. Hematuria may be grossly visible (gross hematuria) or microscopic. It is, however, important to remember that the degree of hematuria bears no relation to the underlying cause and that any degree of hematuria, transient or persistent, should be considered a sign of serious disease until proven otherwise. Developing a rational strategy for evaluation of hematuria is problematic because erythrocytes can be present in the urine of healthy individuals and the number of erythrocytes that defines an abnormality is controversial.

A. Defining Abnormal Hematuria

Different studies have defined an ''abnormal'' number of erythrocytes from as low as one to as many as 30 erythrocytes per high power field. The lower the cut-off value of erythrocytes chosen, the more false-positive test results; the higher the cut-off, the more likely the test will miss significant abnormalities. At the same time, these studies have reported microhematuria in 4–7% of ''normal'' controls. These data imply absence of urological or intrinsic renal disease, but not all controls underwent complete diagnostic testing, making the significance of these findings uncertain. Different definitions of what constitutes an abnormal number of erythrocytes also explain the relatively wide range of patients reported with asymptomatic microscopic hematuria. Its prevalence is estimated at between 5% and 13% of the general population. For the purposes of this review, microscopic hematuria is defined as three or more red cells per high-power field on microscopic urine analysis (see below), a definition that is widely used.

B. Detection of Hematuria

1. Microscopic Urine Analysis

The gold standard for detecting red cells in the urine is microscopic examination of the urine sediment. The number of erythrocytes per high-power field depends on preparation technique. Unfortunately there is no universally accepted method for preparing the urine sediment. The most widely used technique is to centrifuge 10–12 mL of urine at 2000–2500 rpm for 5 minutes and then pour off the supernatant, leaving approximately 0.25–0.5 mL in the tube. After resuspension, one drop is placed on a slide with a cover slip and the number of red cells counted in 5–10 high-power fields. Although phase contrast microscopy allows better visualization of all cellular elements of the urine sediment, standard light microscopy is used in most laboratories.

2. Urine Dipstick Analysis

A more convenient test that is commonly used as the initial screen for hematuria is the dipstick for hemoglobin. In this test, cellulose strips dipped into a urine specimen record the ability of hemoglobin to catalyze the reaction between hydrogen peroxide and a chromagen. The resulting reaction causes the chromagen to turn green, and the degree of color change is directly related to the amount of hemoglobin present. The dipstick for hemoglobin can detect the hemoglobin released from as few as 1 or 2 erythrocytes per high-power field. In patients with microscopic hematuria (i.e., 3 or more red blood cells per high-power field), the test is negative in 16% of patients, is trace positive in approximately 39%, and is positive in about 45%. False-negative results can be seen in the presence of reducing agents such as vitamin C. In patients without microscopic hematuria, the test is negative in 85%, trace positive in 14%, and negative in 1%. False-positive tests almost always suggest the presence of myoglobin or free hemoglobin, findings that should be further investigated.

C. Diagnosis of the Source of the Hematuria

Intrinsic lesions of the genitourinary tract involving the kidneys, ureters, bladder, prostate, or urethra can all produce hematuria. The distribution of these lesions associated with asymptomatic microscopic hematuria in the general clinical population is outlined in Table 1. The initial step in the evaluation of microscopic hematuria does not require referral to a subspecialist (nephrologist or urologist) but rather consists of a thorough medical history, including a review of medications and an inquiry for specific conditions. The first step in this process is to consider the possibility that the hematuria is drug-induced.

Table 1 Distribution of Urological Findings in Asymptomatic Patients with Microhematuria

Categories of urological disease	% (range)
Serious	2.3 (0–5.3)
Uroepithelial neoplasia	0.1 (0–1.2)
Ureteral calculus	0.9 (0–2.2)
Prostatic cancer	0.5 (0–4.1)
Renal neoplasia	0.4 (0–1.1)
Other	0.3 (0–1.8)
Moderately serious	18.2
Renal calculi	3.3
Urinary tract infection	0.5
Nephrosis and/or renal insufficiency	14.4
Minor	50.5

Source: Modified from Mohr DN, et al. Asymptomatic microhematuria and urologic disease: a population-based study. JAMA 1986; 256:224–229.

1. Drug-Induced Hematuria

Drugs implicated in causing hematuria include nonsteroidal anti-inflammatory drugs (NSAIDs), which can cause both interstitial nephritis and papillary necrosis (see Chapter 20). Other drugs commonly associated with interstitial nephritis are antibiotics, including the penicillins, cephalosporins, quinolones, rifampin, and trimethoprim-sulfamethoxazole. Papillary necrosis should be considered in patients with diabetes mellitus, patients with a history of analgesic abuse, and African American patients with sickle-cell trait or disease. Cyclophosphamide and ifosfamide can cause a hemorrhagic chemical cystitis, a complication avoided by pretreatment water loading. A newer protease inhibitor, indinavir, for the treatment of HIV infection has also been associated with hematuria. The underlying mechanism is thought to be crystalluria and urolithiasis, and again hematuria and acute renal failure can be prevented by generous oral fluid intake. Use of anticoagulants increases the occurrence of microscopic hematuria by either spontaneous bleeding or induction of bleeding from an occult lesion. Significant urological causes have been reported in up to 45% of such patients.

2. Transient vs Persistent Hematuria

Once a drug-induced cause has been excluded, the evaluation should focus on whether the history or physical examination suggests a specific cause and, related to this question, whether the hematuria is transient or persistent. Transient microscopic hematuria is a common finding in young adults. Up to 40% of these individuals are found to have hematuria on at least one occasion and 16% on two or more occasions. Fever, infection, exercise, and trauma are the most common causes of transient hematuria, and close follow-up without further evaluation is probably the best approach in young adults. The situation is different in older adults (>50 years) who have a higher incidence of urological malignancies and in whom even transient hematuria increases this risk significantly. In such patients, a complete urological evaluation should be undertaken (see later).

Vigorous exercise, trauma, and sports-related injury are well-established causes of hematuria. Up to 18% of marathon runners have hematuria that usually resolves within 48–72 hours. Concurrent pyuria and bacteruria associated with hematuria suggest urinary tract infection. In such individuals, the hematuria will disappear after treatment of the cystitis. In women, cyclic hematuria that is usually present during or shortly after menstruation suggests endometriosis of the urinary tract. Contamination of urine during menses is also a possible cause of hematuria and can be ruled out by repeating the urinalysis after cessation of menstruation.

Persistent hematuria suggests other causes. Hematuria detected in hospital or nursing home patients is frequently related to the presence of indwelling catheters. A positive family history of renal disease or hematuria points towards inherited intrinsic renal diseases (e.g., polycystic kidney disease, Alport's syndrome, and benign familial hematuria) as the underlying cause of the hematuria. Patients with persistent hematuria as the only manifestation of glomerular disease and adults with isolated hematuria who had negative radiographic and cystoscopic evaluations are likely to have normal renal tissue on biopsy or one of following disorders:

1. IgA-nephropathy, often characterized by gross hematuria after upper respiratory tract infections and a negative family history
2. Alport's syndrome or other forms of hereditary nephritis, in which gross hematuria is uncommon and family history is usually positive for hematuria and renal failure
3. Benign familial hematuria, characterized by thin glomerular basement membranes on renal biopsy and a positive family history of hematuria but not renal failure

All these patients should be referred to a nephrologist for evaluation and decision regarding the need for renal biopsy and for assistance in management. Although a biopsy will define the specific pathology responsible for the hematuria in most instances, it is rarely undertaken in patients with isolated hematuria (with the exception of defining a lesion for genetic counseling) because the prognosis is excellent in most of these disorders. Follow-up studies of asymptomatic hematuria have shown that none of the patients develop renal failure. When biopsied, patients who are found to have normal renal tissue have a high incidence of urolithiasis (25%) and should have urological follow-up.

When asymptomatic patients present with both hematuria and proteinuria, by contrast, they have an almost 15% chance of developing chronic renal failure. Because treatment can modify the course of some of the diseases causing this presentation, a more aggressive diagnostic approach is justified. Most nephrologists will consider renal biopsy if there is evidence of progressive renal failure, increasing proteinuria, or elevated blood pressure in addition to hematuria.

3. Glomerular Versus Nonglomerular Sources of Hematuria

As part of the initial evaluation, one should also determine, if possible, whether the hematuria is of glomerular or nonglomerular origin. The problem with making this distinction is the difficulty in detecting the pathognomonic changes on urinalysis. In many cases a nephrologist is required to make this assessment. The finding of dysmorphic erythrocytes and, in particular, the presence of red cell casts in a patient with microscopic hematuria strongly suggests that glomerular disease is the cause of the hematuria (see Chapter 8). If one can make this diagnosis, visualization of the lower urinary tract is usually unnecessary (see later). Red cell casts are virtually pathognomonic for glomerular hematuria, although their absence by no means excludes glomerular bleeding. Urine protein excretion exceeding 500 mg per day in the absence of gross hematuria is also strongly suggestive of a glomerular lesion. Erythrocyte morphology is less helpful in distinguishing between glomerular and nonglomerular bleeding. With bleeding from the lower urinary tract, the erythrocytes are usually round and uniform, but when the bleeding is from the kidney and particularly when it is glomerular in origin, the erythrocytes may have dysmorphic features (irregular outer membrane). The exact predictive value of erythrocyte morphology in the diagnosis of hematuria is not known because most examiners have limited experience assessing red cell morphology. This test is probably most helpful when all of the red cells are either normal or clearly dysmorphic. Acanthocytes, which are ring-formed dysmorphic erythrocytes with one or more membrane protrusions of variable size and shape, may be more specific and are best detected by phase contrast microscopy. A study from a referral center reports a sensitivity of 52% and specificity of 98% for glomerular disease when 5% or more of the erythrocytes are comprised of acanthocytes. The diagnostic yield of this test in a primary care setting is not known, but it is likely to be less accurate.

4. Decision to Proceed with Imaging Studies

The unequivocal finding of red cell casts is such a strong indicator of glomerular disease that further diagnostic studies to exclude lower urinary tract bleeding are usually unnecessary. In the absence of this finding, and particularly when there is no associated proteinuria, the age of the patient is the most important factor to consider in deciding whether to initiate further evaluation. Studies both in the urological referral setting and in the population at large have found that serious urological lesions are almost exclusively limited to patients older than 50 years. Serious lesions are defined as conditions leading to increased morbidity or mortality and whose natural history can be influenced by early detection and therapy. Bladder neoplasms and ureteral stones account for most of these lesions. About 13% of all elderly patients with microscopic hematuria referred to a urologist are found to have a urological neoplasm compared to 1% of the cases in general practice, but malignancies rarely occur in patients under the age of 50 years. The risk of bladder cancer is increased twofold in cigarette smokers and in dye and chemical workers who have been exposed to aromatic amines. Patients with a history of analgesic abuse also have a high risk of developing transitional cell cancer, and the risk persists even after discontinuation of analgesics and the development of end-stage renal disease.

The likelihood of finding serious urologic lesions in patients with asymptomatic hematuria who are younger than 50 years, have no known risk factors, and have a normal physical examination and normal basic laboratory tests is probably less than 1%. In taking a cautious approach, I recommend that any

Table 2 Initial Diagnostic Evaluation of Asymptomatic Patients with Microhematuria

Urine sediment
Urine cytology
Serum creatinine
Intravenous pyelography (IVP)
Cystoscopy

patient with a higher pretest probability be referred for urological evaluation. Commonly performed tests are outlined in Table 2.

D. Diagnostic Tests

There is no optimal diagnostic strategy for assessing the source of asymptomatic hematuria. It has been difficult to assess the utility of specific tests for two reasons:

1. Patients referred for urological evaluation are likely to have more severe disease than the population not referred to a specialist, leading to a falsely high sensitivity of the various diagnostic tests for detection of serious lesions.
2. Patients without hematuria usually do not undergo diagnostic evaluation, and it is therefore not possible to estimate to what degree microscopic hematuria and serious urological lesions are actually related. This problem is termed the so-called workup bias in all the published studies.

1. Renal Imaging

As an initial imaging study, most physicians will order an intravenous pyelogram (IVP) or a renal ultrasound looking for silent stones, renal masses, or polycystic kidney disease. An IVP may also detect medullary sponge kidney in a young patient, a condition that may not be seen by ultrasonography. Advanced bladder cancer can produce filling defects on IVP, making it a reasonable first choice in elderly patients. In the patients with a contraindication to IVP (dye allergy), ultrasound should be used instead. Although this test is safer and less expensive, it has not been shown to be sufficiently efficacious to replace the IVP as the first line renal imaging study. Computer tomography (CT) and magnetic resonance imaging (MRI) are usually not required as part of the initial evaluation, but they may be considered if there is concern about a renal lesion. The diagnostic accuracy of these two imaging studies in detecting a renal mass is as good if not better than the IVP.

2. Cystoscopy

Cystoscopy is considered the gold standard for clinically detectable lesions of the lower urinary tract because it allows visualization of the ureteral orifices, bladder, and the urethra. The indications for cystoscopy are not completely defined. Of patients with documented tumors of the bladder, less than one half have abnormalities identified by IVP. In general, cystoscopy is recommended in patients with defined risk factors, exposure to certain dyes, heavy smoking, and analgesic abuse and in men over the age of 50 years. The distribution of lesions identified among these patients evaluated for microscopic hematuria is shown in Table 3. The diagnostic yield of cystoscopy is very low in men under the age of 40 years and in low-risk women.

3. Urine Cytology

A freshly voided morning urine specimen is usually recommended for cytological examination. The specimen is fixed with alcohol and the cells stained by appropriate staining methods. As with other tests in this section, the operating characteristics of urine cytology and the evaluation of microscopic hematuria have not been precisely determined. Among patients with suspected or established urological malignancy, the sensitivity and specificity is reported to be as high as 80% and 90%, respectively. False-positive results are most commonly seen in patients with stones and chronic infection and those who have undergone chemotherapy or radiation therapy of the bladder. Low-grade bladder cancer accounts for most of the false-negative results. Newer urine-based markers (NMP22, DTA, FDP)

Table 3 Lower Urinary Tract Lesions Identified by Cystoscopy in Asymptomatic Patients with Microscopic Hematuria Referred for Urological Evaluation

Lesion	% average of several studies
Urethral lesions	20
Benign prostatic hypertrophy	15
Prostate cancer	1
Bladder cancer	7
Cystitis	3
Miscellaneous	6

appear to be more sensitive than urine cytology and therefore more accurate in detecting low-grade bladder cancer.

4. Other Diagnostic Tests

In evaluating young patients with microscopic hematuria, a plain radiograph of the abdomen (KUB) may be helpful since the prevalence of silent renal calculi in this patient population is sufficiently high. Other procedures include biopsy of the prostate or kidney when clinically indicated. The combination of normal findings on IVP, cystoscopy, and urine cytology is usually sufficient to exclude urinary malignancy. Not more than 1% of older patients with initial negative evaluation will develop a urological neoplasm on reevaluation after up to 5 years.

E. Unexplained Hematuria

Patients with persistent isolated hematuria and complete negative urological evaluations are likely to have mild glomerular disease (as discussed above) or a predisposition for stone formation. Idiopathic hypercalciuria and hyperuricosuria have been reported in up to one third of children or young adults with apparently isolated hematuria. In both disorders, family history is often positive for renal stone disease and these patients are at increased risk for symptomatic urolithiasis. Treatment with a thiazide diuretic for hypercalciuria or allopurinol for hyperuricosuria usually eliminates hematuria. No cause of hematuria is found in at least 10% of patients despite extensive investigation.

F. Summary

Our ability to recommend strategies for evaluating microscopic hematuria is clearly limited by some of the problems discussed in this chapter. There are still controversies and uncertainty regarding the definition of hematuria, operating characteristics of specific tests, and the benefit of early detection and treatment of lesions identified in asymptomatic patients.

With this limited evidence in mind, the following definitions and strategies are recommended:

1. Abnormal hematuria is defined as three or more erythrocytes per high-power field or a positive dipstick for hemoglobin.
2. Additional urinary abnormalities such as proteinuria and erythrocyte casts or elevated serum creatinine and blood pressure suggest glomerular disease. These patients should be referred to a nephrologist for evaluation.
3. In patients younger than 50 years without risk factors for cancer, hypercalciuria and hyperuricosuria should first be excluded. An IVP can be

justified to exclude medullary sponge kidney or silent stones. If the result of the IVP is normal, clinical follow-up is advised.

4. Patients who have any risk factor for cancer or are older than 50 years should undergo a urological evaluation, including IVP or renal ultrasound, cystoscopy, and urine cytology.

III. PROTEINURIA

Proteinuria is a common finding in clinical practice. The reported incidence of proteinuria discovered on routine urinalysis ranges from less than 1% to about 9%. As with hematuria, the finding of proteinuria may represent a serious underlying disorder or it may reflect a benign condition with a favorable prognosis. Chapter 7 reviews the pathophysiology of abnormal renal protein handling and the approach to the patient with heavy proteinuria, and Chapter 8 reviews the combined finding of proteinuria and hematuria. In this chapter the approach to evaluating isolated mild to moderate proteinuria is discussed. This condition typically occurs in asymptomatic patients in whom proteinuria is detected incidentally by dipstick during routine urinalysis. The different diagnostic categories of isolated proteinuria are outlined in Table 4. By definition, these patients do not have abnormal hematuria or cellular casts; the urinary sediment is normal. Quantitative measurement of urinary protein can be used to assist in the diagnosis of renal disease and to assess progression and response to therapy. However, it is also commonly used as a screening test for populations at risk for renal damage, particularly diabetic and hypertensive patients. This application of the laboratory assessment of proteinuria is discussed in detail in Chapters 17 and 18.

Table 4 Diagnostic Categories of Isolated Proteinuria

Types of proteinuria
Glomerular
Tubular
Overflow
Quantity of proteinuria
Nonnephrotic range (<3.5 g/day)
Nephrotic range (≥3.5 g/day)
Conditions under which protein is excreted
Transient or intermittent
Orthostatic
Persistent

A. Pathophysiology of Proteinuria

The glomerulus consists of capillaries that are permeable to fluid and small solutes but provide an effective filtration barrier for plasma macromolecules such as protein. The glomerular basement membrane and the epithelial cell foot processes form this barrier, impeding filtration of protein primarily on the basis of molecular weight and charge (size and charge selectivity). Under normal physiological conditions, the urine protein excretion is limited to less than 150 mg/day. Moreover, only about 20–40% of the excreted protein is albumin. The remainder is a mixture of low molecular weight globulin fragments and Tamm-Horsfall glycoprotein, the latter secreted by renal tubular epithelial cells. Most of the filtered albumin is reabsorbed by the proximal tubule. The urinary albumin excretion rate in healthy individuals is <30 mg/day.

B. Types of Proteinuria

1. Glomerular Proteinuria

Glomerular proteinuria is caused by increased glomerular permeability to plasma proteins and may vary in amount from minimal to nephrotic range (>3.5 g/day/1.73 m^2). The primary protein lost through the glomerulus is albumin, and the urine dipstick test detects only this protein. The proteinuria of diabetic nephropathy and other glomerular diseases, as well as benign causes of proteinuria such as exercise-induced or orthostatic proteinuria, fall into this category.

2. Tubular Proteinuria

Tubular proteinuria, a much rarer problem, is caused by impaired tubular reabsorption of the lower molecular weight proteins normally filtered by the glomerulus. This defect is usually the result of tubular interstitial disease. Typically the proteins excreted are low molecular weight proteins such as β_2-microglobulin and immunoglobulin light chains. In the early stages of tubular proteinuria, the dipstick test may be negative because this method does not detect these proteins. Progressive tubular interstitial disease, however, is associated with nephron loss and results in the secondary glomerular damage and loss of albumin in the urine. The resulting proteinuria usually measures less than 2 g/day.

3. Overflow Proteinuria

Overflow proteinuria is caused by overproduction of a low molecular weight protein that overwhelms the normal proximal tubular reabsorptive capacity. This type of proteinuria is almost always associated with immune globulin light chains produced by an underlying multiple myeloma or monoclonal gammopathy of uncertain significance.

Table 5 Common Causes of Different Types of Proteinuria

Glomerular Proteinuria
Primary glomerular disease
Minimal change disease
Focal segmental glomerulosclerosis
Membranous nephropathy
Membranoproliferative glomerulonephritis
Glomerular disease associated with systemic disease
Diabetes mellitus
Collagen vascular disorders (e.g., lupus nephritis)
Amyloidosis
Infection (e.g., HIV, hepatitis B and C, endocarditis)
Glomerular disease associated with drugs
Nonsteroidal anti-inflammatory drugs
Gold
Penicillamine
Tubular proteinuria
Hypertensive nephrosclerosis
Tubularinterstitial disease due to
Analgesic abuse
Heavy metals
Lithium
Overflow proteinuria
Paraproteinemias
Multiple myeloma
Light chain disease
Amyloidosis

There is tremendous overlap among the causes of proteinuria, but most cases of persistent proteinuria seen in primary care are due to glomerular proteinuria. Common causes of the various types of proteinuria are outlined in Table 5.

C. Detection and Measurement of Proteinuria

1. Dipstick Measurement

Proteinuria is usually detected by dipstick analysis, a semiquantitative method to estimate the protein concentration in urine. The colorimetric reaction of an indicator dye correlates directly with the concentration of protein in the urine. The dipstick positive results are usually recorded between trace (10–20 mg/dL) and 3+ (>500 mg/dL). It should be emphasized that the dipstick measures urine protein concentration, not total amount. Thus, for example, a patient excreting a dilute urine may have a negative dipstick test despite excreting an abnormal amount of protein, because the concentration is low. By contrast, the dipstick may be positive in highly concentrated urine, even though protein excretion is not abnormally increased. False-positive results can occur in markedly alkaline urine (because the protein indicator is affected by pH) and in patients presenting with gross hematuria (see Sec. II).

2. Laboratory Measurement

When a urine sample is sent to the laboratory for a quantitative protein measurement, the sulfosalicylic acid test (SSA) is the most common method used for analysis. This test is based on the denaturation and precipitation of protein by the acid. The amount of protein present is estimated by the degree of turbidity, and proteins other than albumin are detected. This feature makes the SSA test helpful when multiple myeloma is suspected in older patients. A positive SSA test with a simultaneously obtained negative or slightly positive dipstick suggests the presence of proteins other than albumin in the urine. A positive result for free monoclonal light chains confirms the diagnosis of multiple myeloma or monoclonal gammopathy of uncertain significance.

3. Microalbuminuria Measurement

This test is discussed in detail in Chapter 18, but it should be emphasized that it differs from the technique used to measure total urinary protein. The analysis for microalbuminuria uses an antibody to human albumin and therefore only detects albumin. It should only be obtained when the dipstick test is negative because it is used to detect very small, but abnormal, amounts of albumin in the urine.

D. Evaluation of Isolated Proteinuria

The approach to the patient with isolated proteinuria begins with a complete medical history and physical examination to uncover systemic diseases in which proteinuria commonly occurs. These diseases include diabetes mellitus, hypertension, or collagen vascular disease. Regardless of whether a systemic disease is identified, two additional questions need to be answered: (1) How much protein is being excreted? and (2) Under what conditions is the protein excreted? A third and related question of what protein is excreted has already been discussed in Section III.B.

1. Quantity of Proteinuria

A quantitative measurement of urine protein excretion should be undertaken in all patients with proteinuria. This can be accomplished by a 24-hour urine collection or, more conveniently, by measuring the protein and creatinine concentrations in a random urine sample and then calculating the protein-to-creatinine ratio (mg/mg). This ratio correlates closely with daily urine protein excretion in g/ 1.73 m^2 of body surface area.

The quantity of protein excreted is important for both management and prognosis. Most patients with benign forms of proteinuria excrete less than 2 g/ day. In primary glomerular diseases (e.g., focal segmental glomerulosclerosis, membranous nephropathy) the degree of proteinuria correlates closely with the risk of progressive renal failure. Prognosis is often poor in patients with nephrotic range proteinuria while patients with mild proteinuria generally do not progress and rarely need therapy with immunosuppressive agents.

2. Conditions Under Which Protein is Excreted

(a) Transient Proteinuria. Many patients with isolated mild proteinuria have a transient pattern of pattern of protein excretion. In normal individuals, proteinuria will be found in 4% of men and 7% of women on a single examination, with spontaneous and complete resolution on subsequent examinations. High fever, strenuous exercise, exposure to cold, emotional stress, and congestive heart failure are common precipitating events for this type of proteinuria. The transient increase in protein excretion may be mediated by angiotensin II or norepinephrine-induced changes in glomerular permeability. After resolution of the invoking event, urine protein excretion returns to normal. Progressive renal disease has not been reported in these patients, and no further evaluation and follow-up is necessary.

(b) Idiopathic Transient Proteinuria. Idiopathic transient proteinuria is defined as proteinuria found during routine urinalysis in apparently healthy individuals and absent with subsequent urine specimens. This presentation is common in children and young adults, some of whom may have occasional positive results for proteinuria if urine samples are repeatedly tested on follow-up. There is no increased morbidity or mortality associated with this condition.

(c) Orthostatic Proteinuria. This pattern of proteinuria occurs most commonly in children and young adults and is characterized by increased protein excretion in the upright position but normal protein excretion when the patient is supine. Almost one in five young men with proteinuria on urinalysis have this pattern of protein excretion. The underlying mechanism is not fully understood, but neurohumoral activation and altered glomerular permeability have been invoked. To make the diagnosis of orthostatic proteinuria, it is necessary to collect

a split urine sample over a 24-hour period. The patient is instructed to collect a 16-hour upright collection, usually between 7 a.m. and 11 p.m.; a separate overnight 8-hour collection is obtained between 11 p.m. and 7 a.m. The diagnosis of orthostatic proteinuria is confirmed when the overnight protein excretion is normal (<50 mg/8 h) and not just less than when in the upright position as is seen in many patients with glomerular diseases. The total amount of protein excreted is usually less than 1 gram per day, but nephrotic range proteinuria has rarely been reported. Orthostatic proteinuria is a benign condition. Kidney biopsy, when done, shows either normal renal tissue or mild mesangial proliferation. Renal function remains normal after as long as 50 years, and most patients are in remission after more than 10 years of follow-up.

(d) Persistent Proteinuria. Detecting a persistent pattern of proteinuria should raise the greatest concern of physicians evaluating a patient with isolated proteinuria. The reasons for this concern are twofold. First, persistent proteinuria usually reflects some significant underlying renal or systemic disease, and second, this pattern is associated with a higher mortality rate than transient or orthostatic proteinuria due to the increased risk of progressive renal disease.

Renal biopsy studies in patients with persistent low-grade proteinuria (usually <1 g/day) show normal renal tissue or mild mesangial changes in approximately three out of four patients. Glomerular lesions are seen in about 20%. The most common of these are focal segmental glomerulosclerosis, IgA nephropathy, and membranous nephropathy. In general, a greater proportion of patients will have glomerular disease when urine protein excretion is above 1 g/day.

Because isolated low-grade proteinuria is sometimes seen with urinary obstruction, polycystic kidney disease or reflux nephropathy, all patients should undergo renal ultrasound examination to exclude these conditions. Baseline laboratory tests should include an estimation of glomerular filtration rate (GFR) by measuring serum creatinine concentration or creatinine clearance. Serological studies such as serum complement levels (C3, C4), antinuclear antibodies (ANA), antistreptolysin titer (ASO), and antineutrophil cytoplasmic antibodies (ANCA) are not helpful in asymptomatic patients and should only be obtained when specific diseases are clinically suspected (e.g., collagen vascular disease, systemic vasculitis). For optimal care, the patient should be referred to a nephrologist in order to evaluate whether further workup is needed and to provide assistance in management.

E. Prognosis and Recommended Interventions

The prognosis for patients with persistent proteinuria is directly related to the degree of proteinuria. Patients with nonnephrotic range proteinuria (<3.5 g/day), with normal renal function, and absence of systemic disease usually have a benign course; end-stage renal disease is uncommon even after 20 years of follow-up. Patients with nephrotic range proteinuria have the highest risk for developing end-stage renal disease, and that risk is further increased by the presence of a systemic disease and impaired renal function at the time of diagnosis. These patients should clearly be referred to a nephrologist for renal biopsy and further management (see Chapter 7).

In patients with diabetic nephropathy and many nondiabetic chronic nephropathies, dietary protein restriction and antihypertensive therapy are effective treatments that retard renal disease progression (see Chapter 16). In general, lowering systemic blood pressure will decrease proteinuria. This antiproteinuric effect is more prominent with angiotensin-converting enzyme (ACE) inhibitors and the nondihydrophyridine calcium-channel blockers (i.e., verapamil and diltiazem). Whenever proteinuria is reduced (independent of mechanism and drug used), renal function is protected from declining over time. As a result, reduction of urine protein excretion to levels of <1 g/day and optimal blood pressure control (<135/85 mmHg) should be the ultimate goal of all physicians caring for patients with progressive proteinuric renal diseases.

F. Summary

The following recommendations should be considered as general guidelines for evaluation of the patient with isolated asymptomatic proteinuria and with normal renal function:

1. A positive result on dipstick should be at least repeated twice. Negative results on follow-up testing indicate a transient proteinuria, and no follow-up is needed.
2. When the dipstick is repeatedly positive, quantitative measurement of urine protein excretion (24-hour urine collection or protein/creatinine ratio calculated from measurements in a random urine sample) should be undertaken. Patients with proteinuria of <1 g/day (or with a protein/creatinine ratio <1.0) should be followed up yearly. The risk for progression is low.
3. In young patients (<30 years) with proteinuria, orthostatic proteinuria should be ruled out with appropriate urine collection. If the abnormal proteinuria is confined to the upright posture, yearly follow-up is sufficient because the risk for progression is low.
4. In patients with persistent proteinuria, structural renal disease should be evaluated by renal ultrasound. Further steps may include urological evaluation (urinary obstruction) or yearly follow-up (polycystic kidney disease, reflux nephropathy) with close monitoring of proteinuria, blood pressure, and renal function.

5. Patients with proteinuria of uncertain etiology, particularly with nephrotic range proteinuria, should be referred to a nephrologist for further evaluation (e.g., renal biopsy) and management.

Two points should be emphasized with regard to these recommendations. The first is that they do not apply to the patient who has abnormal hematuria in association with the proteinuria. Such patients need early referral to a nephrologist for further diagnostic workup and management (see Chapter 8). The second is that they do not apply to the patient with an abnormal or rising serum creatinine concentration. Again these patients should be referred to a nephrologist (see Chapter 16).

SUGGESTED READINGS

Abuelo JG. Proteinuria: Diagnostic principles and procedures. Ann Int Med 1983; 98: 186–191.

Andres A, Praga M, Bello I, Diaz-Rolón JA, Gutierrez-Millet V, Morales JM, Rodicio JL. Hematuria due to hypercalciuria and hyperuricosuria in adult patients. Kidney Int 1989; 36:96–99.

Carson CC III, Segura JW, Greene LF. Clinical importance of microhematuria. JAMA 1979; 241:149–150.

Fogazzi GB, Fenili D. Urinalysis and microscopy. In: Oxford Textbook of Clinical Nephrology. 2d ed. New York: Oxford University Press, 1998:21–38.

Golin AL, Howard RS. Asymptomatic microscopic hematuria. J Urol 1980; 124:389–391.

Greene LF, O'Shaughnessy EJ Jr, Hendricks ED. Study of five hundred patients with asymptomatic microhematuria. JAMA 1956; 161:610–613.

Kanwar YS, Liu ZZ, Kashihara N, Wallner EI. Current status of the structural and functional basis of glomerular filtration and proteinuria. Semin Nephrol 1991; 11:390–413.

Köhler H, Wandel E, Brunck B. Acanthocyturia—a characteristic marker for glomerular bleeding. Kidney Int 1991; 40:115–120.

Mohr DN, Offord KP, Owen RA, Melton LJ III. Asymptomatic microhematuria and urologic disease. A population-based study. JAMA 1986; 256:224–229.

Nieuwhof C, Doorenbos C, Grave W, de Heer F, de Leeuw P, Zeppenfeldt E, van Breda Vriesman PJC. A prospective study of the natural history of idiopathic non-proteinuric hematuria. Kidney Int 1996; 49:222–225.

Remuzzi G, Bertani T. Pathophysiology of progressive nephropathies. N Engl J Med 1998; 339:1448–1456.

Reuben DB, Wachtel TJ, Brown PC, Driscoll JL. Transient proteinuria in emergency medical admissions. N Engl J Med 1982; 306:1031–1033.

Robinson RR. Isolated proteinuria in asymptomatic patients. Kidney Int 1980; 18:395–406.

Rytand DA, Spreiter S. Prognosis in postural (orthostatic) proteinuria. Forty to fifty-year follow-up of six patients after diagnosis by Thomas Addis. N Engl J Med 1981; 305:618–621.

Topham PS, Harper SJ, Furness PN, Harris KPG, Walls J, Feehally J. Glomerular disease as a cause of isolated microscopic haematuria. Q J Med 1994; 87:329–335.

Van Savage JG, Fried FA. Anticoagulant associated hematuria: a prospective study. J Urol 1995; 153:1594–1596.

7
The Nephrotic Syndrome

Ruth C. Campbell
University of Alabama, Birmingham, Alabama

Gerald C. Groggel
University of Nebraska Medical Center, Omaha, Nebraska

I. INTRODUCTION

The nephrotic syndrome is a clinical entity characterized by proteinuria, hypoalbuminemia, edema, hyperlipidemia, and lipiduria. It is not the result of one pathological process; rather, it occurs in many disease states and is the common end result of a number of different types of glomerular insults. The causes of the nephrotic syndrome are divided into primary (i.e., an isolated glomerular disease) and secondary (associated with a systemic disease). The primary causes are defined by their pathological histology (Table 1). The most common secondary causes of nephrotic syndrome are diabetes mellitus, systemic lupus erythematosus, and amyloidosis (Table 2). The approach to the patient with the nephrotic syndrome is threefold: (1) to identify the underlying pathologic process, (2) to minimize or reverse renal impairment, and (3) to treat the extrarenal complications.

II. PATHOPHYSIOLOGY

The hallmark of the nephrotic syndrome is proteinuria. The major component of the proteinuria is albumin, comprising over 80–90%, followed by IgG. Albumin is a medium weight (60 kDa), negatively charged protein that is virtually excluded from the urine in the healthy kidney. The albumin contained in the blood that passes through the kidney is kept from the urinary space by the three layers of

Table 1 Primary Causes of the Nephrotic Syndrome

Minimal change disease (16%)[a]
Mesangial proliferative glomerulonephritis (12%)
IgM nephropathy
IgA nephropathy
Focal segmental glomerulosclerosis (32%)
Membranous nephropathy (34%)
Membranoproliferative glomerulonephritis (5%)

[a] Numbers in parentheses indicate the approximate percentage of adults with isolated (primary) nephrotic syndrome who have each diagnosis.

the glomerular capillary wall, which act as a filter. These layers are the fenestrated capillary endothelial cell, the glomerular basement membrane, and the slit diaphragms of the epithelial cell foot processes (see Fig. 1). In addition to putting a size restraint on the filtration of larger molecules, these layers also present a charge barrier. The components of the capillary wall are negatively charged, and the negative charge acts as a barrier to filtration of smaller negatively charged proteins such as albumin. Any injury to the glomerulus that affects either the pore size or the charge of the filter will allow more protein into the urinary space.

Normally, the small amount of protein that passes the glomerular basement membrane is reabsorbed and metabolized to its component amino acids in the proximal tubule. If enough protein leaks into the glomerular filtrate, however,

Table 2 Secondary Causes[a] of the Nephrotic Syndrome

Diabetes mellitus
Systemic lupus erythematous
Amyloidosis
Drugs
Vasculitis
Neoplasms
Infections—bacterial, viral protozoal, parasitic
HIV-associated nephropathy
Preeclampsia
Chronic renal allograft rejection
Alport's syndrome
Obesity
Renal artery stenosis

[a] Listed in decreasing order of importance.

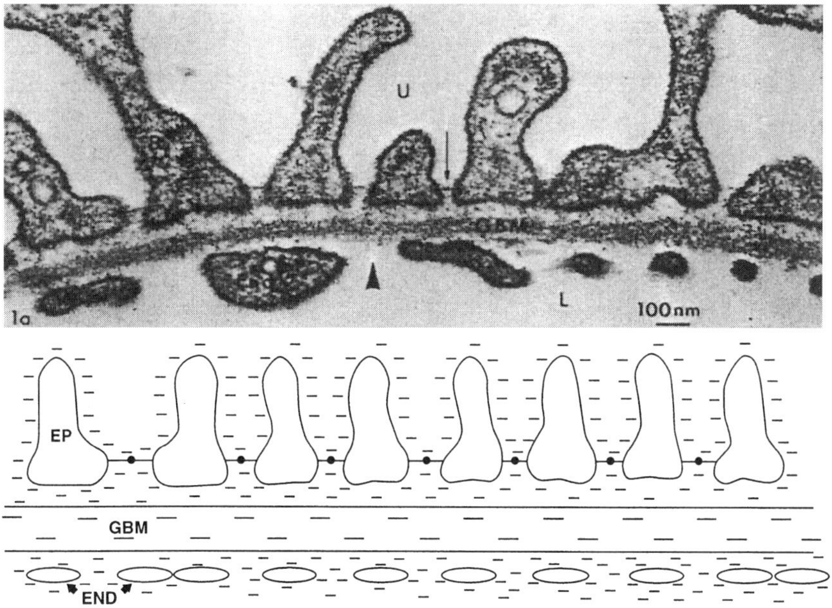

Figure 1 Electron micrograph of the glomerular filtration barrier including endothelial cells (END), glomerular basement membrane (GBM), and epithelial cells (EP). At bottom is a schematic of this barrier with the anionic charges represented. U is urinary space. (From Venkatachalam et al., 1978.)

the ability of the proximal tubule to reabsorb it is overwhelmed and the protein is lost in the urine. Both reabsorption and catabolism of filtered protein are increased in the nephrotic syndrome. The total amount of lost protein, therefore, is the amount that is excreted plus the amount reabsorbed and catabolized.

The body's response to the increased loss of albumin due to renal excretion and catabolism is to increase hepatic synthesis of this protein. However, in nephrotic patients, the increase in hepatic synthesis does not keep pace with the renal losses. This disequilibrium is not because urinary losses are too massive for the liver to match. The hepatic response to hypoalbuminemia is suboptimal in nephrotic patients, and this impairment results in hypoalbuminemia. The reason for the impaired synthesis of albumin is not known.

Once the nephrotic syndrome develops, the large amount of protein crossing the glomerular basement membrane may, by itself, cause further injury to the glomeruli and tubules, independent of the initial insult. An important goal of therapy, thus, is to minimize the proteinuria, a therapeutic goal that will reduce the hypoalbuminemia and may also decrease the risk of further renal damage (see sec. VIII). Control of the proteinuria and improvement in serum albumin levels will also lead to a reduction in edema and will decrease the extrarenal complications such as hyperlipidemia and hypercoagulability (see later).

III. EVALUATION AND DIAGNOSIS

The nephrotic syndrome has a wide range of clinical presentations. It should be considered in patients with proteinuria detected on screening exam, in patients with underlying illnesses that predispose to renal complications such as diabetes, in patients with worsening renal function, in patients with hypoalbuminemia, and in patients who present with edema, transudative pleural effusions, or ascites.

Nephrotic syndrome is diagnosed by the combined presence of greater than 3.5 g of protein in the urine per 24 hours (per 1.73 m^2 of body surface area), hypoalbuminemia, and edema. Patients with greater that 3.5 g of proteinuria/ 24 hours, but without hypoalbuminemia or edema, are referred to as having

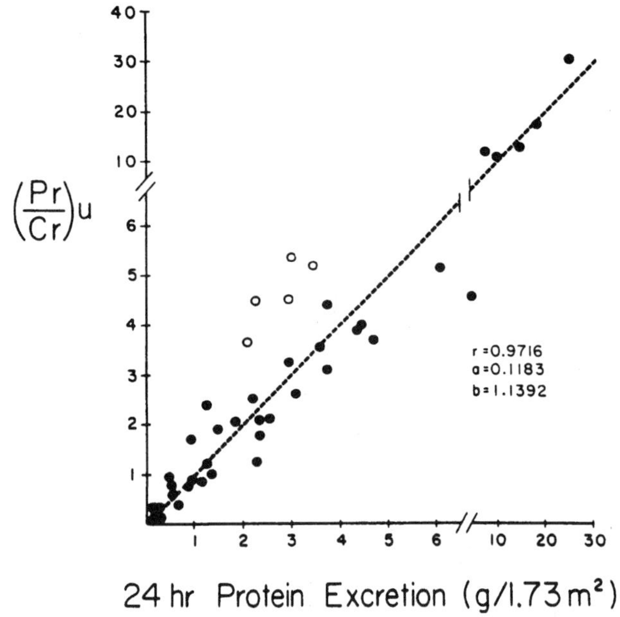

Figure 2 Ratio of urinary protein to creatinine concentration (Pr/Cr) in a random, single voided specimen expressed as a function of 24-hour protein excretion. (From Ginsberg et al., 1983.)

"nephrotic-range" proteinuria. The defining quantity of proteinuria of 3.5 g is clearly arbitrary. Some patients with severe hypoalbuminemia (<2 g/dL) may have only 2–3 g of proteinuria and still have a clinical course consistent with the nephrotic syndrome.

A. Measurement of Urinary Protein Excretion

Urinary protein excretion has traditionally been assessed in a 24-hour urine collection. A well-timed collection, however, is difficult for patients to complete at home and can lead to inaccurate information. An easier and better method is to obtain a random urine specimen and to measure both urinary protein and creatinine concentrations. The protein/creatinine concentration ratio in such a random sample correlates very well with the value measured in a 24-hour specimen (see Fig. 2). When calculating the ratio, the concentrations of protein and creatinine must be in the same units. The urine specimen should be collected during the day and should not be from an early morning void. The value of the ratio corresponds approximately to grams per 24 hours so that a ratio of greater than 3.5 represents nephrotic-range proteinuria. The normal ratio should be less than 0.2. This method assumes a 24-hour creatinine excretion of only 1 g and therefore may underestimate the degree of proteinuria in a male patient with a large muscle mass and therefore a higher rate of creatinine excretion. The method also assumes a stable glomerular filtration rate (GFR) and so should only be used for patients with stable renal function.

B. Further Workup

Once the nephrotic syndrome is diagnosed, a search for the underlying cause should be undertaken. Many renal and systemic disorders can affect the glomeruli and cause nephrotic-range proteinuria (see Table 1 and 2). Of the systemic causes, diabetes is by far the most common and, in fact, is probably the most common cause of the nephrotic syndrome in the United States. Other systemic causes are much rarer. The most common primary glomerular disorder in the adult is membranous nephropathy, followed by focal segmental glomerulosclerosis and minimal change disease.

1. History, Physical Examination, and Initial Laboratory Evaluation

The first step in identifying the cause is a thorough history and physical examination, with particular attention to the presence of systemic disease and use of drugs that might cause the nephrotic syndrome (Table 3; see later). Initial laboratory tests should include serum creatinine and electrolytes, calcium, phosphorus, lipid

Table 3 Drugs Associated with the Nephrotic Syndrome

Well-established relationship
Nonsteroidal anti-inflammatory drugs
Gold
Probenecid
Organic mercurials
Penicillamine
Interferon α
Intravenous heroin use
Rare reported cases
Captopril
Lithium
Mesantoin
Trimethadone
Paradione
Phenindione
Tolbutamide
Chlorpropamide
Clonidine

profile, total serum protein and albumin, hepatitis screen, complement studies, antinuclear antibodies (ANA), antineutrophil cytoplasmic antibodies (ANCA), and CBC. The latter screening tests are recommended because the nephrotic syndrome occurs in patients with hepatitis and with systemic vasculitis as well as with systemic lupus erythematosis. Diabetes mellitus should always be screened for with a glycosylated hemoglobin. Patients over the age of 40 years should be evaluated for multiple myeloma with serum and urine protein electrophoresis and immunofixation. HIV testing should be considered in the initial evaluation as well.

In addition to the blood work, all patients should have a urinalysis with microscopic exam. The urine sediment typically contains oval fat bodies, which are fat-laden epithelial cells, and fatty casts. When examined under polarized light, the lipid droplets in the cells and casts show the characteristic Maltese cross pattern (doubly refractile fat bodies). Patients with the nephrotic syndrome can also have white cells, red cells, and cellular casts in their urine sediment, depending on the specific cause. None of these findings are pathognomonic for a specific disease, however, and a renal biopsy is needed for the precise diagnosis.

2. Renal Biopsy

Except for a minority of patients, diagnosing the cause of the nephrotic syndrome requires a renal biopsy. All adults and children over the age of 12 with the nephrotic syndrome need to be considered for renal biopsy, and younger children should always be evaluated by a nephrologist. Patients with diabetes mellitus who present with the nephrotic syndrome are not routinely biopsied but should also be referred to a nephrologist for evaluation and recommendations for treatment. Patients with type 1 diabetes for longer than 10 years with associated retinopathy and no history, physical examination findings, or laboratory results suggestive of another cause or with type 2 diabetes with no findings suggestive of another cause do not need a biopsy because of the high probability that diabetic nephropathy is the cause (see Chapter 18 for more detailed recommendations). A diabetic patient without retinopathy (particularly type 1) or who has rapidly deteriorating renal function may have another cause for the nephrotic syndrome, and biopsy should be considered.

Identification of the specific etiology of the nephrotic syndrome in a particular patient is necessary for making decisions about disease-specific therapy and also can provide prognostic information. Additional laboratory tests may be ordered based on the pathology seen on the biopsy. The list of causes is quite extensive (Tables 1 and 2), and further testing should be based on the biopsy results.

IV. PROGNOSIS

The prognosis for renal function in patients with the nephrotic syndrome depends on the underlying pathology. Some postinfectious injuries remit spontaneously. Minimal change disease can remit spontaneously or with corticosteroid treatment and, in children and young adults, has a very good prognosis. Some disorders, such as focal segmental glomerulosclerosis, progress more commonly to end-stage renal disease. Treatment of specific disorders is presented in Chapter 19. In general, treatment usually involves corticosteroids and often cytotoxic drugs as well. Treatment decisions should be made in conjunction with a nephrologist. It is worth emphasizing that with many glomerular diseases that cause the nephrotic syndrome early treatment may be the best hope for preserving renal function, so timely identification of the pathology is important.

V. ASSOCIATED DISEASES

The renal pathology can also alert the clinician to the presence of other, unsuspected illnesses. Membranous nephropathy, for example, is associated with malignancy. Patients with membranous nephropathy should have a thorough history and physical to screen for malignancy, have a chest x-ray, and be up to date on cancer screening exams (e.g., mammogram, papanicolaou (PAP) smear, sigmoidoscopy, prostate specific antigen (PSA) with digital exam). If the history or physical is suggestive of malignancy, a more extensive workup should be undertaken. Malignancy can also develop after the presentation of membranous nephropathy, so patients with membranous nephropathy and an initial negative evaluation should be followed carefully. If an underlying malignancy is present, successful treatment of the tumor is associated with remission of the nephrotic syndrome. Minimal change disease is also associated with malignancy, particularly lymphoma and Hodgkin's disease.

Therapy for the secondary causes of the nephrotic syndrome is also based on the underlying illness. Good glycemic control for diabetics should be a goal, although glycemic control is better proven to prevent diabetic nephropathy than to reverse it. The therapy for lupus nephritis is highly dependent on the biopsy results and can be controversial. It usually includes cytotoxic agents, and again, treatment decisions should be made in conjunction with a nephrologist.

VI. DRUGS ASSOCIATED WITH THE NEPHROTIC SYNDROME

A wide variety of drugs have been reported to cause the nephrotic syndrome, but the relationship is tenuous for many of these reports (Table 3). The drugs for which a cause-and-effect relationship has been established include gold, probenecid, organic mercurials, penicillamine, interferon α, and the nonsteroidal anti-inflammatory drugs (NSAIDs). In rare instances captopril, lithium, and certain anticonvulsant drugs (mesantoin, trimethadone, and paradione) appear to cause the nephrotic syndrome. In addition to these prescribed drugs, intravenous heroin and cocaine use are well documented to be associated with the development of focal glomerulosclerosis and the nephrotic syndrome (see Chapter 20).

The most common cause, by far, of drug-induced nephrotic syndrome is NSAIDs. These drugs cause minimal change disease coupled with a characteristic interstitial nephritis (see Chapter 20). The nephrotic syndrome begins after several months on the drug (although the duration of exposure needed is quite variable). In all instances, discontinuation of the offending drug is indicated. With NSAIDs, this action almost always leads to remission of the nephrotic syndrome within 1 month.

VII. COMPLICATIONS

Nephrotic syndrome is defined by its major complications: edema, hypoalbuminemia, and hyperlipidemia. In addition, patients with nephrotic syndrome are at increased risk for infection and have a hypercoagulable state. Nephrotic patients may also have endocrine abnormalities due to loss of hormones and binding proteins in the urine. Loss of renal function is a major complication. Renal function may deteriorate gradually because of chronic proteinuria or because of progression of the underlying renal disease. Nephrotic patients may also develop acute renal failure due to overdiureses or intrarenal edema. Each of these problems and their management is discussed below.

A. Edema

Edema is one of the defining characteristics of the nephrotic syndrome, but, surprisingly, the pathophysiology of this problem and its relationship to hypoalbuminemia remain incompletely understood. The traditional view that the edema is due to decreased oncotic pressure caused by hypoalbuminemia may not apply in many patients with the nephrotic syndrome. This view, now termed the ''underfill model,'' is based on the supposition that decreased oncotic pressure in the intravascular space, due to hypoalbuminemia, leads to a loss of fluid into the interstitial space, particularly in areas where vascular hydrostatic pressure is increased. Hence edema is seen in the lower extremities in the evening and around the face and eyes early in the day. According to this model, patients with nephrotic syndrome should have a decreased intravascular volume, which in turn stimulates Na^+ retention by the kidney by activation of the renin/angiotensin/aldosterone system. If true, this model has implications for therapy. Treatment of edema may further embarrass the vascular compartment, causing symptoms from severe vasoconstriction.

Evaluation of vascular volume and the renin/angiotensin/aldosterone system in patients with nephrotic syndrome, however, have not supported this simple construction. One group of patients who may have a significant ''underfill'' component to their edema are those with severe hypoalbuminemia (serum albumin levels <2 g/dL). These patients have shown evidence of decreased intravascular volume more consistently.

The lack of experimental support for the underfill model has led researchers to look for other possible explanations for the edema. This search has resulted in a second model, edema due to primary retention of Na^+ by the kidney, leading to vascular ''overfill'' and edema formation due to increased hydrostatic pressure coupled with hypoalbuminemia. According to this model, renal injury from the disease that causes the proteinuria also impairs the normal renal response to extracellular fluid (ECF) volume expansion, resulting in Na^+ retention. This event is independent of the hypoalbuminemia, but, in the presence of a low albumin, the Na^+ retention is manifest primarily by edema rather than hypertension. There is considerable experimental evidence to support this pathophysiology in most adults with the nephrotic syndrome. The specific cause of the Na^+ retention is not defined completely, but current work points to an apparent resistance to atrial natruretic peptide (ANP) in the collecting duct in patients with nephrotic syndrome. In normal individuals, ingestion of salt is followed by expansion of ECF volume, which in turn causes the secretion of ANP in response to activation of right atrial stretch receptors. The secreted ANP promotes Na^+ excretion by inhibiting collecting duct Na^+ reabsorption. In patients with nephrotic syndrome, ANP is released and complexes with its receptor in the collecting duct normally, but the intracellular message is inappropriately degraded. This leads to a blunted response to ANP and consequent Na^+ retention. The same pathophysiology is seen in the more inflammatory forms of glomerular disease (i.e., glomerulonephritis and the nephritic syndrome) (see Chapters 8 and 19). The implications of the ''overfill'' and ''underfill'' models of edema for therapy are discussed below and in Chapter 2.

B. Hyperlipidemia

Hyperlipidemia is almost invariably present in patients with the nephrotic syndrome. Typically, total cholesterol, very-low-density lipoproteins (VLDL), and low-density lipoproteins (LDL) are all elevated. Changes in triglycerides and high-density lipoproteins (HDL) levels are variable. The hyperlipidemia is due to both increased synthesis and decreased degradation. Hypoalbuminemia is a stimulus for increased hepatic synthesis of cholesterol and infusion of albumin decreases cholesterol synthesis. It is unclear, however, whether the increase in cholesterol synthesis is entirely due to decreased serum albumin concentration.

In addition to increased synthesis, catabolism of lipids in nephrotic patients is abnormal. Lipoprotein lipase (LPL), the enzyme that breaks down triglycerides in chylomicrons and VLDL particles, has impaired activity. HDL may be normal or low in nephrotic syndrome. Low levels may contribute to impaired catabolism of LDL and VLDL. HDL function may be impaired either because of losses in the urine of HDL itself or because of loss into the urine of some necessary, but undefined, cofactors.

The significance of the hyperlipidemia as a risk factor for cardiovascular disease in patients with nephrotic syndrome is unclear; few studies have assessed this problem. One retrospective study did find an increase in the incidence of myocardial infarction. The risk of the hyperlipidemia probably needs to be viewed in the context of other risk factors and the duration of the proteinuria. For patients with long-standing nephrotic syndrome, the associated hyperlipidemia is likely to be a risk factor for atherosclerosis and should be treated (see further below).

C. Hypercoagulability

Patients with the nephrotic syndrome suffer from hypercoagulability to a variable extent. The cause of the clotting tendency is unclear, but it appears to be multifactorial. One factor is the underlying disease. For example, patients with membranous nephropathy have a higher incidence of deep venous thrombosis than patients with minimal change disease. The loss of clotting cascade proteins (antithrombin III in particular) in the urine may be a contributing factor, but urinary levels of antithrombin III in patients with nephrotic syndrome are not uniformly elevated. Other clotting abnormalities include elevated fibrinogen levels and platelet hyperaggregability, but it has been difficult to use these levels as predictors of thrombosis. One hypothesis is that endothelial cell damage occurs in some patients with the nephrotic syndrome as well as changes in the clotting cascade. This combination of abnormalities would certainly predispose to thrombus formation, but the hypothesis is unproven as yet.

D. Renal Vein Thrombosis

Of particular concern in patients with the nephrotic syndrome is renal vein thrombosis. The incidence of this complication is unclear, but it appears to occur most commonly in patients with membranous nephropathy (with a widely varying incidence, 5–50%, in published reports). It is less common in other types of nephrotic syndrome. Patients with serum albumin levels of <2 g/dL are at greater risk. Renal vein thrombosis can present with flank pain, hematuria, and worsening renal failure but much more commonly produces no symptoms. In the asymptomatic patient, its only manifestation may be a sudden deterioration in renal function. In some instances the first manifestation is a symptomatic pulmonary embolus. In patients with a clinical presentation consistent with pulmonary embolus and negative Doppler studies of the legs, renal vein thrombosis should be considered.

E. Infection

Patients with the nephrotic syndrome have increased susceptibility to infection for many reasons. Hypogammaglobulinemia may result from the loss of IgG in the urine. Complement factors are also lost in the urine. Cell-mediated immunity appears to be depressed. These factors combine to increase the risk of infection, and, in fact, sepsis was a common cause of death in nephrotic patients before the advent of corticosteroid therapy. Patients with the nephrotic syndrome are particularly susceptible to infections at sites of edema, for example, cellulitis of the lower extremities or spontaneous bacterial peritonitis. Patients with sustained nephrotic syndrome should receive pneumococcal vaccine, although the antibody response is poor. Immunoglobulin therapy may be a consideration for patients with severe hypogammaglobulinemia. There are no guidelines for its use in nephrotic patients.

F. Endocrine Abnormalities

Abnormalities of calcium and vitamin D metabolism are present in patients with the nephrotic syndrome. Vitamin D binding protein is lost in the urine, leading to reduced vitamin D levels. A reduction in vitamin D, if sustained, will result in hypocalcemia and bone disease. Measurements of vitamin D (25-hydroxyvitamin D, 1,25-dihydroxyvitamin D) levels in patients with the nephrotic syndrome, however, have not consistently shown a reduction.

Nephrotic patients may also have inappropriately low levels of erythropoietin for their level of hematocrit. Erythropoietin appears to be lost in the urine in the nephrotic syndrome. Trace metal–binding proteins such as ceruloplasmin and transferrin can be lost in the urine as well. Nephrotic patients have decreased plasma levels of copper, iron, and zinc.

VIII. TREATMENT

A. Treatment of Proteinuria

The optimal treatment of the nephrotic syndrome is to reverse the primary glomerular abnormality. Unfortunately, such treatment is not available for many of the causes of this syndrome. In the absence of specific therapy, several therapeutic maneuvers can reduce proteinuria. Experimental evidence suggests that proteinuria is not just a manifestation of glomerular injury but is, by itself, a potential cause of continued tubular injury. Thus, reduction of proteinuria not only minimizes the cascade of events that leads to the complications of the nephrotic syndrome but may also minimize renal injury. The goal of therapy is to reduce protein excretion to less than 2 g/24 hours if possible. The two classes of drugs used to reduce proteinuria are angiotensin converting enzyme (ACE) inhibitors and NSAIDs.

ACE inhibitors should always be used first. These agents reduce proteinuria both by altering glomerular hemodynamics (see Chapters 16, 17, and 18) and by directly reducing glomerular permeability to macromolecules. The reduction in proteinuria induced by ACE inhibitors may take weeks to achieve. The beneficial response to ACE inhibitors is augmented by dietary Na^+ restriction, and it is important to educate patients concerning such a diet before starting therapy. A 2 g Na^+ (5 g NaCl) diet is recommended.

The initial dose of the ACE inhibitor should be low (e.g., 5 mg/day of lisinopril or the equivalent dose of another ACE inhibitor) and slowly increased as tolerated. Renal function and serum $[K^+]$ should be monitored to insure that the drug does not cause worsening renal insufficiency or unacceptable hyperkalemia. The response to the ACE inhibitors is dose related. In one study, 5 mg/day of lisinopril decreased proteinuria by 27% and 10 mg/day by up to 63%. Some experts recommend escalating the dose to very high levels to achieve the maximal reduction in protein excretion, but the benefit of such an approach is as yet unproven and this strategy may lead to unacceptable side effects. The pace of dose escalation depends on the level of renal insufficiency, but it would be reasonable to increase the dose every 2–3 weeks. If renal function does worsen significantly on ACE inhibitor therapy, the patient should be evaluated for renal artery stenosis (see Chapter 9). If the patient cannot tolerate an ACE inhibitor because of side effects, such as cough, an angiotensin II receptor blocker can be tried, although the efficacy of this class of drugs remains to be proven.

If a maximal dose of an ACE inhibitor fails to decrease the proteinuria to below 2 g/24 h, then an NSAID can be added to the regimen. Indomethacin has been studied the most extensively in this regard. The beneficial effect of NSAIDs on proteinuria occurs much more rapidly than the effect of ACE inhibitors. The NSAIDs appear to reduce proteinuria primarily by decreasing glomerular capillary hydrostatic pressure. The reduction is achieved by vasoconstriction of the afferent arteriole, leading to a reduction in GFR. As noted earlier, NSAIDs can cause nephrotic syndrome and sodium retention (see Chapter 20). Worsening of proteinuria and renal function needs to be watched for when starting therapy. Great caution should be exercised in using these agents when the creatinine clearance is less than 30 mL/min.

B. Treatment of Edema

The optimal treatment of edema is to reverse the pathological process causing the edema. When this goal cannot be achieved promptly, however, the majority of patients will require specific intervention to minimize their edema. The goal is not to make the patient edema-free but to reduce edema to a level that is tolerable and that minimizes tissue damage and infection. The first approach should always be to restrict dietary Na^+ intake (see earlier for recommendation). If this dietary change is unable to control edema, diuretic therapy should be started.

Patients with the nephrotic syndrome are often very resistant to diuretics, and large doses may be needed to achieve the desired response. This resistance may be due both to the intrinsic renal Na^+ avidity caused by the disease process itself and to the binding of the filtered diuretic agent to albumin in the tubular lumen, preventing it from reaching its site of action. Large doses can help overcome this resistance. When a diuretic agent is needed, most patients require a loop diuretic, particularly when renal insufficiency is present. An appropriate starting dose for the loop diuretic, furosemide, is 40 mg multiplied by the serum creatinine concentration (up to 120 mg as a single dose once or twice daily). In addition to loop diuretics, metolazone can be used to sequentially block Na^+ reabsorption to promote diuresis (see Chapter 2). The use of albumin with diuretics to enhance the diuretic response is not effective.

Some patients, particularly those with albumin levels of less than 2 g/dL, can quickly become intravascularly depleted and develop acute renal failure, particularly on a combination of a diuretic, an ACE inhibitor, and a low Na^+ diet. These drugs can be used safely in combination but should not be started together.

The doses should be escalated slowly, and renal function should be monitored closely. This complication can be avoided if diuretic therapy is not pushed too aggressively. Some patients, such as those with massive edema, will need more urgent diuresis than others. In these individuals, diuretic therapy should be started before using an ACE inhibitor. In patients with only modest amounts of edema, an ACE inhibitor should be tried first without diuretic therapy. All patients receiving diuretic therapy should be taught to weigh themselves daily and to monitor their own edema. When properly educated, patients can regulate their diuretic dose on a day-to-day basis and avoid both under- and overdiuresis.

C. Dietary Protein Intake

Paradoxically, dietary protein restriction is beneficial in patients with the nephrotic syndrome. These patients should not be put on a high-protein diet, despite the loss of protein in the urine. High-protein diets increase albumin synthesis, but this change simply leads to an increase in proteinuria, an effect that can further damage the kidney (see above). When patients are placed on a low-protein diet, proteinuria diminishes and serum albumin levels increase. A protein intake of 0.8–1 g/kg body weight is recommended. Patients placed on such a diet should have nutritional counseling to insure that their diets comply with the restrictions and to insure that they do not become malnourished (see Chapter 16).

D. Treatment of Hyperlipidemia

The risk of atherosclerotic disease as a result of the hyperlipidemia is related to the duration of the nephrotic syndrome. In patients with a short period of illness, hyperlipidemia resolves rapidly, and there is probably little benefit in treating this problem. If the nephrotic syndrome lasts for longer than a few months, the risk of atherosclerotic disease is probably increased. In some patients the nephrotic syndrome can last for years, and these patients should certainly receive lipid-lowering therapy. Treatment should begin with a low-cholesterol diet and exercise. If these measures fail to improve the hyperlipidemia, drug therapy should be initiated. Of the multiple cholesterol-lowering agents available, the HMG Co-A reductase inhibitors (statin drugs) are most effective and best tolerated.

E. Treatment of Hypercoaguable State

No clear recommendations exist for the treatment of the clotting tendency in patients with the nephrotic syndrome. Not all nephrotics are at equal risk of thromboembolic disease. As noted earlier, patients with membranous nephropathy or with albumin levels of <2 g/L appear to be at the greatest risk. At the very least, emphasis needs to be placed on deep vein thrombosis prophylaxis for these patients when their risk is increased (e.g., immobilization, postoperative). Certainly, all nephrotic patients with known deep vein or renal vein thrombosis or pulmonary embolus should be anticoagulated, and the anticoagulation should be continued for the duration of the nephrotic syndrome. As mentioned above, renal vein thrombosis is a problem in patients with membranous nephropathy. There is no consensus for screening renal venograms for patients with membranous nephropathy, but one should maintain a high level of suspicion for renal vein thrombosis in these patients (see below).

IX. ACUTE RENAL FAILURE AND NEPHROTIC SYNDROME

Patients whose renal function has been stable or improving can have a sudden increase in proteinuria or a decrease in renal function. When this happens, it is extremely important to look for an underlying and potentially reversible cause. A common reason for clinical deterioration is overly aggressive diuresis. To the extent that vascular ''underfilling'' is induced (see earlier), renal perfusion will fall, as will the GFR. If the patient is also receiving an ACE inhibitor and/or an NSAID, GFR will fall even more abruptly and oliguric acute renal failure can result. When this complication develops, all drugs should be discontinued immediately and the salt restriction liberalized. As noted earlier, both NSAIDs and ACE inhibitors themselves can cause renal failure even in the absence of overdiuresis.

Acute renal failure can also occur as a result of renal vein thrombosis. Very few patients present with the ''classic'' presentation of flank pain, hematuria, and renal failure. When suspected, the diagnosis is made by renal venography or by magnetic resonance angiography. In nephrotic patients with renal vein thrombosis, thrombolytic therapy may be helpful, but this approach is unproven. All such patients should be anticoagulated. Rarely, nephrotic patients with severe anasarca can develop interstitial edema in the kidney, which can lead to obstruction of the nephrons and acute renal failure. This diagnosis is difficult to make and may require a renal biopsy. Aggressive diuresis or fluid removal by dialysis may be helpful for treating this complication. In patients with renal vein thrombosis and with acute renal failure due to interstitial edema, the loss of renal function is often irreversible.

X. CONCLUSION

Nephrotic syndrome results from a variety of glomerular insults, either from primary renal lesions or from renal effects of systemic illnesses. The goal of therapy is to identify and treat underlying renal dysfunction and reduce proteinuria. Reduction of proteinuria leads to improvement in serum albumin levels. In addition to disease-reversing specific therapy, general approaches that can reduce proteinuria include ACE inhibitors, moderately restricted protein diets, and cautious use of NSAIDs. Diuretic therapy is important for controlling edema.

The most serious complication of the nephrotic syndrome is renal failure. Every attempt should be made to preserve renal function in the nephrotic patient. To assist in achieving this goal, patients with the nephrotic syndrome should be referred to a nephrologist for help with establishing the specific diagnosis and treating this disorder.

SUGGESTED READINGS

Abrass CK. Clinical spectrum and complications of the nephrotic syndrome. J Invest Med 1997; 45:143–153.

Gansevoort RT, De Zeeuw D, De Jong PE. Is the antiproteinuric effect of ACE inhibition mediated by interference in the renin-angiotensin system? Kidney Int 1994; 45: 861–867.

Ginsberg JM, Chang BS, Matarese RA, Garella S. Use of single voided urine samples to estimate quantitative proteinuria. N Engl J Med 1983; 309:1543–1546.

Harris RC, Ismail N. Extrarenal complications of the nephrotic syndrome. Am J Kidney Dis 1994; 23:477–497.

Humphreys MH. Mechanisms and management of nephrotic edema. Kidney Int 1994; 45: 266–281.

Kaysen GA, Gambertoglio J, Jimenez I, Jones H, Hutchinson FN. Effect of dietary protein intake on albumin homeostasis in nephrotic patients. Kidney Int 1986; 29:572–577.

Orth SR, Ritz E. The nephrotic syndrome. N Engl J Med 1998; 338:1202–1211.

Remuzzi G, Bertani T. Pathophysiology of progressive nephropathies. N Engl J Med 1998; 339:1448–1456.

Rodrigo R, Bravo I, Pino M. Proteinuria and albumin homeostasis in the nephrotic syndrome: effect of dietary protein intake. Nutr Rev 1996; 54:337–347.

Smith JD, Hayslett JP. Reversible renal failure in nephrotic syndrome. Am J Kidney Dis 1992; 14:201–213.

Venkatachalam MA, Rennke HG. The structural and molecular basis of glomerular filtration. Cir Res 1978; 43:337–347.

Vriesendorp R, Donker ABJM, De Zeeuw D, De Jong PE, Van Der Hem GK, Brentjens JRH. Effects of nonsteroidal anti-inflammatory drugs on proteinuria. Am J Med 1986; 81:84–94.

Wheeler DC, Bernard DB. Lipid abnormalities in the nephrotic syndrome: causes, consequences, and treatment. Am J Kidney Dis 1994; 23:331–346.

8
The Nephritic Syndrome

Ann Guillot
University of Vermont, Burlington, Vermont

I. INTRODUCTION

The nephritic syndrome is a constellation of physical and laboratory findings, the definition of which varies. Its most complete description includes hematuria, proteinuria, edema, hypertension, and some degree of renal dysfunction. However, many experts in the field narrow the definition to hematuria (with red cell casts), proteinuria (less than the nephrotic range), and some degree of renal dysfunction. Variations in the definition of this syndrome relate to the variability in patient presentation (see below). It is important when approaching a patient with this syndrome to remember that there are three separate approaches used to describe and categorize nephritis. The first is the clinical presentation and progress, the second the histological appearance, and the third the pathophysiology as understood at the cellular and/or molecular levels.

The clinical presentation of nephritis was recognized as early as the writings of Hippocrates, described by the presence of gross hematuria and decreased urine volume. The syndrome was described more completely in the late eighteenth century as a clinical presentation that developed in association with scarlet fever. With the ability to measure protein in the urine in the nineteenth century, this finding was added to the clinical syndrome. The histological appearances of varying forms of nephritis were described in this century, first by light microscopy and later by immunoflourescent and electron microscopy. The pathophysiology of the various forms of nephritis remains only partly understood, even for those types that have been very well characterized clinically.

Although there are several types of nephritis in which the clinical presentation will usually predict the histology and the pathophysiology, there is never perfect congruity between these three types of descriptors. Our current understanding of the various types of nephritis incorporates clinical, histological, and pathophysiological manifestations and uses information from all three of these sources to try to make rational decisions about treatment and to predict outcome (see Chapter 19). If information is available in only one or two of these areas, predictive ability is less reliable.

II. PATHOPHYSIOLOGY OF THE NEPHRITIC SYNDROME

The clinical features of the nephritic syndrome are the result of acute glomerular and/or tubulointersitial inflammation. Glomerular damage leads to loss of protein into the urine and likely is the cause of the hematuria in most instances (see below). In addition, inflammation reduces glomerular capillary surface area and glomerular filtration rate (GFR) typically falls. Hypertension in this syndrome is caused by the renal ischemia engendered by inflammation, which promotes both renal sodium retention and the release of vasoconstrictor hormones. Intense inflammation of the glomeruli leads not only to a reduction in GFR but also to a decrease in afferent arteriolar blood flow and to increased renin and α-adrenergic hormone release. These hormones, coupled with decreased blood flow, act in concert to promote avid renal sodium retention. Blood pressure elevations appear to be directly related to the degree of sodium retention, but the aforementioned vasoconstrictor hormones may be contributing factors, particularly when the hypertension is severe. The edema seen in the nephritic syndrome is also the result of sodium retention but is not usually associated with hypoalbuminemia, in contrast to the nephrotic syndrome (see Chapters 2 and 7). As a result, its distribution in the body may differ from the edema seen in the nephrotic syndrome (see below).

III. CLINICAL PRESENTATION

Of patients who are documented to have acute glomerulonephritis, virtually all have hematuria, most have proteinuria, well over half have hypertension and edema, and approximately half have clinically significant renal insufficiency. The differences in presenting signs and symptoms are due to the wide variety of causes of the syndrome (see Table 1) and probably to the varying degree of inflammation that occurs with each of the causes as well. This variability is also the source of the difficulty in providing a precise and inclusive definition of the nephritic syndrome. Some experts avoid the term altogether and separate the clinical features of acute glomerulonephritis from the more insidious presentation

Table 1 Causes, Complement Levels, and Systemic Symptoms in Patients with Nephritic Syndrome

Cause	Complement levels	Systemic symptoms
Acute postinfectious GN	Low C3	Nonspecific
IgA nephropathy	Normal	Nonspecific
Henoch-Schönlein purpura	Normal	Lower extremity vasculitic rash Abdominal pain, GI bleeding Arthritis
Goodpasture's syndrome	Normal	Pulmonary hemorrhage
Crescentic GN ("rapidly progressive GN")	Normal	Nonspecific
Lupus nephritis	Low C3 and low C4	Arthritis, leukopenia, anemia, facial rash, serositis, fever
SBE (bacterial endocarditis)	Low C3	Changing heart murmur Fever Janeway lesions, Roth spots
Shunt nephritis	Low C3	Presence of central access
Hemolytic uremic syndrome	Normal	Hemolytic anemia Thrombocytopenia Vascular compromise in other organs
Thrombotic thrombocytopenic purpura	Normal	Large and small vessel thromboses
Wegener's granulomatosis	Normal	Sinusitis, pulmonary infiltrates
Cryoglobulinemia	Normal	Rash, arthritis
HIV nephropathy	Normal	AIDS, AIDS-related complex

of the patient with rapidly progressive glomerulonephritis (see Chapter 19) and the patient with asymptomatic hematuria and proteinuria (see Chapter 6). Despite the varying presentation, however, recognition of the nephritic syndrome is often vital for preserving renal function. The features of this syndrome are discussed below.

A. Hematuria

Hematuria can have its origin anywhere along the entire genitourinary tract, from the glomerulus to the urethral meatus. When red cells in the urine have their origin in the glomerulus, they are usually misshapen and irregular in appearance (dysmorphic). They are also characteristically captured in the cylindrical matrix of casts formed in the tubules (red cell casts).

The site at which red cells cross from the capillary space to the urinary space in glomerulonephritis is not entirely clear, although there have been electron microscopic demonstrations of red cells crossing the glomerular capillary wall. The histology of severe glomerulonephritis often includes breaks in the glomerular basement membrane. Red cells could also cross into the urinary space at the level of the tubule when there is acute tubulointerstitial inflammation. The presence of dysmorphic red cells (see Chapter 6) provides suggestive evidence that glomerular disease is present. The irregular appearance of red cells of glomerular origin should be distinguished from red cells that have been exposed to very concentrated urine and have lost their round, biconcave shape.

1. Red Cell Casts

Red cell casts are the hallmark of the nephritic syndrome. However, not all red cells that are found in casts are glomerular in origin. Some may be the result of severe acute interstitial inflammation, and some may be associated with obstructive or cystic diseases. Most red cell casts, however, are indicative of the presence of acute glomerulonephritis. These casts are most diagnostic when the cells fill the entire cylindrical shape of the cast and are at least partially intact. These red cell casts are typically slightly pigmented (reddish brown). Discovery of the presence of red cell casts requires examination of freshly passed urine. The casts are very fragile and disintegrate in urine samples left standing for a long period of time.

2. Other Cellular Elements

White cells as well as red cells are often present in the urine in acute nephritis, reflective of acute glomerular inflammation. When white cells are included in casts, their presence indicates very active inflammation, either glomerular or tubulointerstitial. If eosinophils are present, they may be a signal of drug-induced interstitial nephritis.

3. Minimal Urinary Findings

There have been several reports of patients who have minimal or absent abnormalities in the urine sediment, but who present with significant hypertension and other renal function disturbances and are discovered by biopsy to have acute glomerulonephritis. This presentation is rare but must be considered, because the nephritic syndrome is so variable.

B. Proteinuria

Patients who present with the nephritic syndrome almost always have abnormal urinary protein excretion (>150 mg/24 hours, or a urinary protein/creatinine ratio >0.15; see Chapter 6). The proteinuria is almost always less than nephrotic range, i.e., 3.5 g/24 hours (urinary protein/creatinine ratio <3.5). The presence of nephrotic range proteinuria in patients with the nephritic syndrome is usually indicative of severe glomerular damage and the ultimate outcome is likely to be poor. Minimal or mild proteinuria (<0.5 g/day, or a protein/creatinine ratio <0.5), by contrast, usually indicates that only mild glomerular damage is present and the outlook is better in most instances.

The amount of proteinuria may also be helpful in predicting the specific cause. For example, children with postinfectious glomerulonephritis usually have only mild proteinuria, whereas patients with membranous nephropathy usually have heavier proteinuria. Unfortunately, this information is neither specific nor sensitive, and other diagnostic tests are needed to make specific diagnoses in almost all patients with the nephritic syndrome.

In addition to the degree of proteinuria at presentation, the duration of the proteinuria provides prognostic information. Rapid resolution of proteinuria (within 1–3 months) is an excellent predictor of a good long-term outcome, whereas its persistence for greater than 3–6 months or its reappearance after months or years suggests a poorer prognosis.

C. Renal Functional Abnormalities

Renal dysfunction in patients with the nephritic syndrome may range from mild to severe and can be manifest as a decrease in GFR or as abnormalities in tubular function. Glomerular filtration rate is virtually always decreased in acute glomerulonephritis (GN) and in tubulo-interstitial nephritis (TIN), but the degree of impairment varies from undetectable to the complete absence of filtration. Patients who have severe acute postinfectious GN, Goodpasture's syndrome, or acute drug-induced TIN may lose their GFR rapidly over a period of a few days. Patients who have idiopathic crescentic GN or Wegener's granulomatosis may lose their GFR over a period of weeks to months. The clinical syndrome "rapidly progressive GN" is used to describe the latter patients, even though their progression is slower than that experienced in some of the more acutely catastrophic forms of nephritis.

Clues to the reversibility of GFR loss can be gained by attention to the histology. Patients who have tremendous inflammation, but no sclerosis, crescent formation, or glomerular collapse, may recover completely. Patients who have the latter three findings, however, are likely to have permanent loss of renal function. Recovery of renal function and risk of subsequent progression (gradual loss of renal function over time) depends not only on whether the inflammation can be expeditiously halted but also on the percentage of glomeruli lost in the initial wave of inflammation caused by the GN or TIN.

Many patients with GN and with TIN have abnormalities in handling of salt and water. Generally, patients with acute glomerulonephritis have difficulty excreting salt and water and therefore become fluid volume overloaded, edematous, and hypertensive. The presentation in patients with acute TIN is more variable, and they may present without either hypertension or edema despite an acute reduction in GFR. In either acute GN or TIN, inflammation can lead to sodium retention even when the fall in GFR is subclinical, that is, when the serum creatinine is still within the normal range. When measured, sodium concentration in randomly acquired urine sample is often but not invariably low (10 mEq/L).

D. Hypertension

As indicated earlier, the presence of hypertension is related to the severity of the glomerular and/or tubulointerstitial inflammation. Because this varies with the cause, the presence of hypertension is dependent to some extent on the cause. Most patients with acute postinfectious GN are hypertensive on presentation, whereas patients with IgA nephropathy or Goodpasture's syndrome are less likely to be hypertensive. Nonetheless, hypertension is not a specific or sensitive finding for the nephritic syndrome or for a particular cause.

Hypertension may be mild in some cases and severe to malignant in others. In most instances the severity of the hypertension is related primarily to the degree of renal sodium retention and to the patient's salt intake. When hypertension is present, both systolic and diastolic pressures are typically elevated. In all instances, the hypertension should be treated promptly and aggressively, as it can rapidly augment renal injury. Although the hypertension may be due in part to increased levels of angiotensin II, the use of angiotensin-converting enzyme inhibitors or receptor blockers should be avoided because they may cause a reduction in GFR that can confuse management. The long-acting calcium channel blockers are very effective and safe to use if the patient is able to take oral medications. If the patient is unable to take oral medications, intravenous labetalol and, in the patient with severe of malignant hypertension, nitroprusside are the drugs of choice.

E. Edema

When present, edema in the nephritic syndrome has a characteristic distribution that is different from the nephrotic syndrome. It typically involves the hands and periorbital areas of the face as much as the lower extremities. The reasons for this distribution are not entirely clear. As noted earlier, the edema is related to sodium retention but does not appear to be due to hypoalbuminemia. However, patients with chronic renal insufficiency without hypoalbuminemia often retain sodium and only rarely have this pattern of edema. Thus one wonders whether a diffuse capillaritis is a component of the edema. Although the periorbital pattern is characteristic, particularly of patients with acute GN, dependent edema can also occur. Moreover, a mild degree of hypoalbuminemia is not uncommon, and if proteinuria is severe enough, more severe hypoalbuminemia can develop.

The edema in patients with the nephritic syndrome requires no specific treatment other than dietary sodium restriction in most instances. Diuretic therapy should be reserved for only those with severe edema or with pulmonary edema, as such treatment can cause a further reduction in GFR and confuse management.

F. Other Systemic Symptoms

Many forms of nephritis are accompanied by systemic symptoms specific to the particular pathophysiologic entity, as noted in Table 1. Several general systemic symptoms, however, are common to the syndrome itself, regardless of the cause. Patients with any form of acute nephritis often have nonspecific abdominal pain, flank pain, anorexia, weight loss, and fatigue. These symptoms may linger for weeks after the acute nephritic episode has substantially resolved. Many of the causes of the nephritic syndrome are associated with anemia, a factor that may contribute to the fatigue caused by the syndrome.

IV. LABORATORY EVALUATION

Initial laboratory evaluation of patients who present with the nephritic syndrome depends to some extent on the presentation but in most instances should include the panel of blood and urine tests outlined in Table 2. In a child or young adult who presents with the typical features of acute postinfectious GN (see Chapter 19), one can focus one's testing to the search for antistreptococcal antibodies and

Table 2 Initial Laboratory Evaluation in Patients with the Nephritic Syndrome

Urinalysis
Urine protein/creatinine ratio
Serum creatinine
Serum electrolytes
Hemagram
Streptozyme titer
C_3 and C_4 complement
Antinuclear antibody (ANA)
Antineutrophil cytoplasmic antibody (ANCA)
Antiglomerular basement membrane (anti-GBM) antibody

serum complement levels. However, when the diagnosis is unclear, the full panel of screening tests should be obtained, to consider entities such as lupus erythematosis, vasculitis, and Goodpasture's disease. As shown in Table 1, the serum complement is quite helpful in narrowing the diagnostic possibilities. In almost all instances (with the exception of acute postinfectious GN in a child or young adult), a renal biopsy is necessary to make a specific diagnosis and to guide therapy. The diagnosis and management of specific causes of the nephritic syndrome is discussed in detail in Chapter 19.

SUGGESTED READINGS

Jennette JC. Diagnosis and management of glomerular diseases. Med Clin North Am 1997; 81:653–677.

Montseny JJ. The current spectrum of infectious glomerulonephritis. Medicine 1995; 74: 63–73.

Rodriguez-Iturbe B, Baggio B, Colina-Chourio J, et al. Studies on the renin-aldosterone system in the acute nephritic syndrome. Kidney Int 1981; 19:445–453.

9
Secondary Hypertension

Jeffrey M. Rimmer
University of Vermont, Burlington, Vermont

I. INTRODUCTION

Secondary hypertension is defined as an elevation of arterial blood pressure due to a known cause. Until recently, consideration of secondary causes for hypertension was relegated to academic discussions for a variety of reasons. Foremost among these was the observation that secondary hypertension appeared to be extremely uncommon among the general population with high blood pressure. As a result, even moderately accurate diagnostic tests had low predictive power when used to screen for secondary hypertension in unselected patients. In addition, surgical repair of renal artery stenosis, the most common correctable cause of hypertension, was hazardous and had equivocal long-term results. At the same time, increasingly potent medications that permitted excellent pharmacological control of hypertension were being introduced. Given the ability to control hypertension with drugs, the assumption of any diagnostic or therapeutic risk and expense was questionable, even in individuals with an increased likelihood of secondary hypertension.

Over the past decade, changes in the prevalence of secondary hypertension have occurred, and newer diagnostic techniques have made it easier (if not less expensive) to uncover known causes of hypertension. Two causes of hypertension, renal artery stenosis and chronic renal disease, have become much more common as the population ages. The recognition that the former problem can progress to renal failure has led to the development of safer and more accurate means of diagnosis and to new, more effective interventions, using either surgery or angioplasty. As discussed further below, the accelerating pace of discovery of new mechanisms of hypertension is also increasing the percentage of high blood pressure that is considered to have a known cause. Based on the results of drug therapy in large population studies, the guidelines for adequate blood pressure control have moved lower and lower, and achieving these goals in patients with secondary hypertension is difficult. Finally, while empirical drug therapy is effective for blood pressure control in most patients, specifically directed drugs can control some forms of secondary hypertension better and also prevent target organ damage.

Because of these considerations, it is important to entertain the possibility that hypertension has a discoverable cause. The diagnosis of secondary hypertension can occasionally lead to the cure of high blood pressure, freeing the patient of the lifelong requirement for medication. More important, it can uncover an underlying abnormality for which targeted treatment may reduce future complications. As discussed below, exploration for the presence of secondary hypertension can be accomplished with economical but powerful tools that include an appropriately directed history and physical examination, supplemented by a modest amount of laboratory testing.

II. KNOWN CAUSES OF HYPERTENSION

A large number of processes have been identified as causal in hypertension. The major ones are listed in Table 1. Despite the impressive number of entities, only a small proportion of the population presenting with uncomplicated, isolated hypertension has one of these defined causes. In adults, six diagnoses encompass almost all patients with definable etiologies for high blood pressure (Table 2). These include intrinsic or obstructive renal disease, renovascular disease, primary aldosteronism, pheochromocytoma, Cushing's syndrome, and drug-induced hypertension. Of these six diagnoses, the first two comprise the vast majority. The incidence of renovascular disease ranges from less than 1% to 5% of unselected patients with hypertension but is much higher in selected populations (see later). Similarly, the incidence of parenchymal renal disease may be as high as 5–10% in certain populations.

III. SPECIFIC DISORDERS

All patients with hypertension should have an initial evaluation, following the guidelines of the Joint National Committee Report (see Suggested Readings at end of chapter), including a directed history and physical examination. The recommended initial laboratory evaluation for patients with hypertension is outlined in Table 3. This initial evaluation will in part direct the physician to further diagnostic testing if there are clues suggesting the presence of secondary hyperten-

Table 1 Known Causes of Hypertension

- Acute and chronic renal diseases
  - Glomerulonephritis
  - Interstitial nephritis
  - Acute renal failure
  - Diabetic nephropathy
  - Polycystic kidney disease
  - Nephrocalcinosis
  - Obstructive uropathy
  - Environmental renal damage
    - Radiation, lead, cadmium
- Syndromes associated with high renin activity
  - Renal artery stenosis
    - Atherosclerosis
    - Fibromuscular dysplasia
    - Aortic aneurysm
    - Extrinsic compression
  - Coarctation
  - Renal trauma—subcapsular hematoma, perinephritis
  - Aortitis, large vessel vasculitis
  - Renin-producing tumors
- Syndromes associated with low renin activity and frequent hypokalemia
  - Primary hyperaldosteronism
    - Aldosterone-producing adenoma
      - Angiotensin unresponsive (APA)
      - Angiotensin responsive (AP-RA)
    - Bilateral adrenal hyperplasia
      - Angiotensin-responsive–idiopathic hyperaldosteronism (IHA)
      - Angiotensin-unresponsive–primary adrenal hyperplasia (PAH)
    - Glucocorticoid-remediable aldosteronism (GRA)
    - Adrenal carcinoma
  - Congenital adrenal hyperplasias
  - Syndrome of apparent mineralocorticoid excess
  - Glycyrrhetenic acid (licorice and derivatives)
  - Massive cortisol excess
  - DOC-secreting tumors
  - Liddle's syndrome
  - Exogenous mineralocorticoids
- Pheochromocytoma and other catecholamine-producing tumors
- Other endocrine disorders
  - Hypothyroidism
  - Hyperthyroidism
  - Acromegaly
  - Hyperparathyroidism (and other hypercalcemias)
  - Carcinoid
  - Cushing's syndrome

Table 1 Continued

Drugs—prescription, nonprescription, recreational (see Table 5)
Other
Gordon's syndrome
Neurogenic
Increased intracranial pressure
Dysautonomia, denervation syndromes
? Sleep disordered breathing
Stress, pain
Acute volume expansion
High cardiac output states

Table 2 Estimated Prevalence of Known Causes of Hypertension[a]

Renal parenchymal disease	20–50
Renovascular disease	2–50
Primary aldosteronism	1–10
Cushing's syndrome	1–2
Pheochromocytoma	0.5–2
Drugs	10?

[a] Per 1000 patients with hypertension.

Table 3 Routine Tests for Evaluation of the Hypertensive Patient[a]

Urinalysis
Complete blood cell count
Serum potassium, sodium, and creatinine
Fasting blood glucose
Total cholesterol
High-density lipoprotein cholesterol
12-Lead electrocardiogram

[a] Guidelines suggested by the Sixth Report of the Joint National Committee on Prevention, Detection, Evaluation and Treatment of High Blood Pressure.

sion. The six most common causes of secondary hypertension are discussed in greater detail below, and the clues that increase the probability of their presence are presented. Table 4 summarizes the approach to these six causes of secondary hypertension.

A. Renal Disease

Underlying acute or chronic renal disease is one of the more common causes of hypertension. A discussion of the mechanisms linking renal disease and hypertension can be found in Chapter 17. Virtually any form of renal disease, including glomerular or interstitial nephritis, toxic or obstructive nephropathy, or hereditary renal disease, may present as hypertension. Acute diseases often present with other signs and symptoms of illness, making the diagnosis of secondary hypertension somewhat easier. In chronic, slowly progressive renal disease, there may be little in the history to suggest an underlying problem. For this reason it is to the examiner's advantage to know the results of the urinalysis, serum creatinine, and electrolytes before undertaking a comprehensive history and physical examination.

The importance of discovering renal disease as the source of high blood pressure is twofold. First, detection of renal disease may lead to treatment strategies that stabilize, improve, or reverse the renal disease itself. Second, even when no specific treatment is available for the underlying renal disease, the rate of progression can be slowed by aggressively controlling blood pressure. In particular, patients with heavy proteinuria (>3 g/24 hr) will have a slower progression to renal failure when their blood pressure is reduced below 135/85 mmHg (see Chapter 16).

1. History

Important elements of the history are diverse when dealing with the broad spectrum of renal diseases that result in hypertension. As with all hypertensive patients, knowledge of when the blood pressure was last found to be normal helps define the chronicity of the process. Other key points are as follows:

1. A detailed history of all prescription and nonprescription drugs to determine whether there are any agents that may cause renal disease (see Chapter 20).
2. Any history of infection, stones, or urinary abnormalities. Pain suggestive of stone, cysts, or tumors should be noted especially if the patient has hematuria (see Chapters 21 and 23).
3. If hematuria is present, history of recent infection or symptoms suggestive of systemic vasculitis or nephritic syndrome (see Chapters 6, 8 and 19).

Table 4 Investigation of Common Causes of Secondary Hypertension

Disorder	Initial screen	Secondary screen	Definitive investigation
Renal disease	History Physical examination Urinalysis Serum creatinine	Directed by initial screen	Directed by secondary screen
Renovascular disease	History Physical examination	CEI renogram Duplex doppler ultrasound Pre/Post-captopril PRA	Aortogram
Primary aldosteronism	History Serum electrolytes (K^+)	Simultaneous plasma aldosterone and plasma renin activity	High sodium intake with 24-hour urine for aldosterone or IV saline With pre/post-plasma aldosterone CT scan of adrenal glands Selective adrenal vein sampling for aldosterone lateralization, genetic testing for GRA
Pheochromocytoma	History Physical examination	Spot urine metanephrine/creatinine ratio, serum normetanephrines	0.3 mg clonidine with pre/post plasma catecholamines, CT scan, MRI scan, ^{131}I-MIBG scan
Cushing's syndrome	History Physical examination	Overnight dexamethasone suppression	Low-dose dexamethasone suppression, high-dose dexamethasone suppression, CT and/or MRI examination of pituitary and adrenal glands
Drugs	History	None	None

4. If proteinuria is present, history of diabetes or diabetic symptoms and those related to myeloma and amyloidosis (see Chapters 6, 7, 18, and 19).
5. If pyuria is present, history or symptoms of urinary tract infection and a review of drugs for those that may cause interstitial nephritis (see Chapters 14 and 20).
6. History of difficulty voiding, frequency, and nocturia that may occur with any renal disease but particularly raises the possibility of obstruction (see Chapter 23).
7. A detailed family history of renal disease to assess the presence of either juvenile or adult polycystic kidney disease, hereditary nephritis (Alport's syndrome), and reflux nephropathy, as well as familial forms of hypertension (see Chapter 24).
8. In all patients, history or symptoms of edema, to assess regulation of extracellular volume and severity of proteinuria (see Chapter 6).
9. History of atherosclerotic vascular disease (including coronary artery disease, stroke, and peripheral vascular disease) to assess likelihood of renovascular disease (see later).

2. Physical Examination

With a few exceptions, the physical examination is not very helpful in pointing to the presence of renal disease. Peripheral edema suggests the presence of nephrotic syndrome but is only rarely present in uncomplicated renal insufficiency. The presence of a rash or arthritis suggests vasculitis or allergic interstitial nephritis. Palpable abdominal masses are felt in patients with polycystic kidneys and rarely in patients with renal tumors or chronic obstruction. When bladder outflow obstruction is present, a suprapubic mass (hugely dilated bladder) can occasionally be felt. Retinopathy is usually seen in patients with underlying diabetic nephropathy. Abdominal bruits suggest the presence of renovascular disease (see later).

3. Laboratory Evaluation

Abnormal blood and urinary laboratory findings define the presence of renal disease and are the key to defining the specific renal disease. Any abnormality in the serum creatinine or urinalysis warrants further investigation in the patient with hypertension. These abnormalities should lead to a renal ultrasound to define the anatomy of the kidneys and upper collecting system. Occasionally obstructive nephropathy can occur with no detectable abnormalities in the urinalysis or creatinine. Therefore, there should be a low threshold for obtaining a renal ultrasound in the hypertensive patient with flank or back symptoms or any abnormality on examination of the abdomen. Beyond this, investigation must be directed toward the specific test findings. Chapters elsewhere in this book direct the reader to the appropriate investigation of hematuria, proteinuria, acute renal failure, or changes suggestive of infection.

B. Renovascular Disease

Renovascular disease is generally taken to mean renal artery stenosis that is causative in the development of hypertension. Following the report of Goldblatt and colleagues in 1934, renovascular disease became the prototypical example of secondary hypertension. The mechanism when one of two kidneys is affected depends on stenosis limiting flow to renal parenchyma, activating the renin-angiotensin-aldosterone system, stimulating a pressor response, and, in some settings, sodium retention.

1. Prevalence

In the young, renal artery stenosis is usually secondary to fibromuscular dysplasia, while in middle-age and older patients it is most frequently due to atherosclerosis. The prevalence of this disorder continues to be debated, most likely due to the variability of populations studied. It is probably present in less than 1% of those presenting with hypertension between the ages of 20 and 40 years who are found to have no other abnormalities. Over the age of 40, the probability of finding renal artery stenosis increases steadily. It reaches rates as high as 75% in those over 60 with hypertension undergoing aortography for reasons other than high blood pressure. This observation correlates with multiple other reports that document the frequent presence of renal artery lesions in patients with other evidence of atherosclerosis, particularly peripheral vascular disease or coronary artery disease with secondary heart failure. Despite the high prevalence of renal arterial lesions, it is not clear what proportion of stenoses is responsible for high blood pressure. It is reasonable to assume that 20–70% of these narrowings play a role in hypertension given the response rate to angioplasty in patients with hypertension treated simply on the basis of finding a greater than 50% narrowing of a renal artery. Prior reports of low prevalence in African American populations are probably incorrect. A rise in the serum creatinine following treatment with an angiotensin-converting enzyme inhibitor and inability to control blood pressure with more than two antihypertensive drugs in effective doses are also frequently associated with renovascular hypertension.

2. Rationale for Evaluation

The major value of detection of renovascular hypertension is that its correction frequently allows for control of hypertension with fewer antihypertensive agents. Renal artery stenosis is often associated with progressive renal insufficiency, and it is frequently found in those with end-stage renal disease. Early discovery and correction of these lesions may preserve renal function in some patients. Studies have noted improved patient survival following renal revascularization independent of blood pressure control. This raises the possibility that decreasing activity of the renin-angiotensin-aldosterone system has physiological benefit in addition to that offered by lowering blood pressure.

3. History

The onset of hypertension before the age of 25 or after age 45 is suggestive of renovascular disease. Hypertension that is difficult to control, either of new onset or superimposed on a history of previous good control, is a common finding. Renal dysfunction following converting enzyme inhibitors or angiotensin II receptor blockers is very suggestive. Evidence of other large vessel disease due to atherosclerosis, dysplasia, or arteritis increases the probability of renovascular disease. Therefore, symptoms of a cerebral transient ischemic attack (TIA), angina, or claudication increase the probability of underlying renal artery stenosis. Recurrent pulmonary edema is a finding reported to suggest renovascular disease.

4. Physical Examination

There are no pathognomonic findings on physical examination, but the presence of Grade III or IV hypertensive retinopathy or an abdominal bruit are suggestive of renovascular disease. Any other evidence of large vessel disease (e.g., aortic aneurysm, carotid or femoral artery bruits) also increases the probability of renal artery stenosis.

5. Routine Laboratory Evaluation

The usual laboratory screening tests are not helpful in uncovering the presence of renovascular disease. Mild hypokalemia can be seen as a manifestation of secondary hyperaldosteronism. In contrast to primary hyperaldosteronism, the low potassium may be associated with a sodium concentration at the lower end of the normal range and a creatinine that is frankly elevated or at the upper end of the normal range. The urinalysis can be completely normal, although proteinuria is not uncommon and nephrotic range proteinuria may rarely be present.

6. Further Evaluation

The decision to undertake further testing to determine whether renovascular disease is present in a patient with hypertension is complex. It should include a consideration of whether the benefit of intervention outweighs the risk in your patient if renovascular disease is found to be present. The decision should also include an assessment of the probability that renovascular disease is present prior to testing, as none of the screening tests currently available is diagnostic. Although the indicators that lead one to proceed with further diagnostic testing (assuming the patient will benefit from intervention) remain controversial, the following are generally accepted:

1. Documented abrupt onset of hypertension
2. Difficult-to-manage hypertension (the need for three or more drugs without achieving blood pressure goals)
3. An abrupt increase in serum creatinine concentration after initiating therapy with an ACE inhibitor
4. Hypertension in the setting of coronary artery and peripheral vascular disease, particularly when recurrent pulmonary edema occurs in the absence of cardiac ischemia
5. Hypertension is a patient with a rising creatinine unexplained by a primary renal disease

In all these settings, the probability that renovascular disease is present is moderate, that is, there is a 20–30% chance of finding it. Although some experts advocate the measurement of plasma renin activity to screen for renovascular disease, this approach has not found wide acceptance. At the present time, either the converting enzyme inhibitor (CEI) renogram or the duplex doppler ultrasound examination are recommended to screen further for renovascular disease.

(a) CEI Renogram. The utility of the CEI renogram is based upon the observation that cortical retention of isotope labeled pharmaceutical, usually ^{99}Tc-MAG_3 (mercaptoacetyltriglycine), is enhanced in renovascular disease, particularly following administration of a converting enzyme inhibitor. A well-described protocol relies on aggressive hydration, IV enalaprilat followed by IV furosemide to enhance distal tubular flow. Such protocols require careful timing for optimal diagnostic results and carry some risk of hypotension. Performed with a standardized protocol, these tests yield reasonable predictive results. When they are done casually or infrequently, the results are less likely to be reliable. An additional problem with the scintigram is that the accuracy of results has not been carefully examined in patients with renal insufficiency.

(b) Doppler Ultrasound. Duplex doppler ultrasonography is based on the principle of physics that flow velocity increases in a tube when the diameter is decreased. Doppler ultrasound is used to determine the flow velocity within the renal artery relative to the flow velocity in the aorta. Most centers that use this test report a ratio of renal artery velocity to aortic velocity. A value of greater than 3.0 for this ratio correlates with a >60% stenosis of the renal artery. The test is highly operator dependent and is only reliable at institutions that have a high level of commitment to quality control. It has the advantage of being unaffected by renal insufficiency.

Neither ultrasound nor scintigram is useful in detecting stenoses of distal renal artery branches or small accessory renal arteries. In this setting measurement of the plasma renin activity before and after a dose of captopril may be useful. It is likely that magnetic resonance angiography (MRA) will ultimately provide a superior screening test. None of these tests easily provides consistent results. It is probably best that they be done at a center that uses them frequently and has a commitment to correlate results with the results of arteriography in order to provide an ongoing estimate of specificity.

(c) Aortography. Aortography is the definitive examination for renovascular disease. Given the availability of immediate angioplasty if a stenosis is discovered, there is seldom utility in renal vein renin measurements unless nephrectomy is contemplated. It is appropriate to obtain an aortogram after a positive screening test or, given false negative rates of 5–10%, after a negative test in patients with a highly suggestive history and poorly controlled hypertension. In many cases the history and physical examination raise the probability of renovascular disease to a level that makes immediate arteriography appropriate. Such unequivocal clinical presentations include the patient with known atherosclerotic vascular disease whose renal function declines with a converting enzyme inhibitor or the patient with grade III retinopathy and an abdominal bruit.

At times, in patients where there is a high probability of renovascular disease, the choice is made to use a screening test because of the perceived risk of contrast nephropathy or atheroembolic disease. In this setting, a negative screening test is likely to give a false sense of security. For example, if clinical findings have raised the probability of underlying renovascular disease to 90%, an excellent screening test with a sensitivity of 95% and a specificity of 95% has a negative predictive value of only 38.5%. Therefore, negative results with the screening test offer no meaningful assurance that renovascular hypertension has been excluded.

C. Primary Hyperaldosteronism

This form of hypertension is secondary to overproduction of aldosterone by the adrenal glands. The initial mechanism of hypertension is sodium retention and volume expansion, but increases in cardiac output and vascular resistance also play a role. Autonomous aldosterone secretion stimulates distal tubular sodium reabsorption and both potassium and acid excretion, resulting in the common findings of hypokalemia and metabolic alkalosis.

Primary hyperaldosteronism represents a heterogeneous group of disorders that are of great interest but are often difficult to differentiate. The most common site of production is an angiotensin-unresponsive aldosterone-producing adenoma (APA), with the next most common disorder being angiotensin-responsive bilateral adrenal hyperplasia (idiopathic hyperaldosteronism, IHA). More than 90% of primary hyperaldosteronism is attributed to these two disorders. The remaining cases are due to renin-sensitive adenomas, angiotensin-unresponsive primary adrenal hyperplasia, adrenal carcinoma, and glucocorticoid-remediable aldosteronism (GRA).

Detection of the specific abnormality is important because it offers the opportunity for surgical cure of hypertension that is often severe and resistant to therapy in some instances and for targeted drug therapy in others. Persistently elevated aldosterone levels have been shown to play a role in cardiac fibrosis independent of blood pressure. It is important to recognize and block the effects of elevated aldosterone production for maximal therapeutic efficacy.

1. History

The history is significant for resistant hypertension that is often severe. Symptoms include parasthesias, weakness, easy fatigability, and polyuria. There is a strong family history of premature severe hypertension in families with GRA, often associated with stroke.

2. Physical Examination

Clinical examination may be unremarkable other than severe hypertension. Occasionally orthostatic hypotension without reflex tachycardia is seen. Retinopathy is reported to often be mild for the degree of blood pressure elevation. A positive Trousseau's or Chvostek's sign may be found.

3. Laboratory Evaluation

Spontaneous hypokalemia is the hallmark of primary hyperaldosteronism occurring in 75–90% of cases on routine laboratory examination. Metabolic alkalosis is also common, as is a sodium concentration at the upper limits of the normal range. As a reflection of volume expansion, the serum creatinine may be at the lower limits of the normal range.

4. Further Workup

A random simultaneous measurement of the plasma renin activity and plasma aldosterone level is probably the most practical screening test in a patient suspected of having the disorder. In a patient with autonomous aldosterone secretion, that is, secretion that is independent of the usual signals, one expects to see volume expansion and suppression of plasma renin activity (PRA). A ratio of aldosterone to PRA (aldosterone/PRA, both in ng/mL) of >20 is strongly suggestive of primary aldosteronism. Aldosterone secretion fluctuates, so the sensitivity of this approach is not clear, and a ratio of less than 20 should not be considered to have excluded the disorder. If the ratio is less than 20, particularly if the PRA is low, a suppression test should be done. One of two tests is generally used. The first is measurement of plasma aldosterone levels before and after the 4-hour infusion of 2 L of saline. Most cases of primary hyperaldosteronism will fail to suppress to below 10 ng/dL. This test guarantees volume expansion and limits the time that the patient is at risk of developing severe hypokalemia. It requires clinic space for the period of the test. An alternative is to use oral sodium loading with a high-sodium, high-potassium diet for 3 days in the absence of diuretic use. A 24-hour urine for sodium and aldosterone is collected. This should document adequate sodium loading, and the aldosterone should be suppressed to below 14 μg/24 hours. This test requires no clinic space, but the sustained sodium loading creates the risk of several days of high blood pressure and hypokalemia, which may be dangerous and confounds the interpretation of the aldosterone excretion. If there is a strong family history of hypertension and stroke, the diagnosis of GRA should be considered. Genetic testing is available for this disorder, but other tests include suppression of aldosterone by dexamethasone and measurement of tetrohydro-18-oxocortisol in a 24-hour urine sample.

Once the diagnosis of primary hyperaldosteronism has been made, the usual next step is to determine the subtype. CT or MR scanning is used to determine whether there is obvious evidence of a unilateral adenoma or bilateral adrenal hyperplasia. If an adenoma is found, it most likely is the cause of hyperaldosteronism, but unfortunately both false-positive and false-negative tests occur. For this reason many centers require demonstration of lateralization of aldosterone production by adrenal vein sampling or evidence of autonomy with elevated serum 18-OH-B levels and increased urinary excretion of 18-oxo-F before committing a patient to adrenalectomy. Even with all these efforts it is difficult to clearly classify some cases of primary hyperaldosteronism. Referral to a center that has extensive experience with hyperaldosteronism is recommended.

D. Pheochromocytoma

Pheochromocytoma is a tumor that results in hypertension through the inappropriate secretion of catecholamines. The majority of these uncommon tumors are solitary, occurring within an adrenal gland. As many as 10% are extra-adrenal in location, being found at any potential site along the sympathetic chain. Terminology can be confusing, and it is probably best to consider any functional tumor of sympathetic origin a pheochromocytoma. Approximately 10% of pheochromocytomas have a familial occurrence. Many of these are found in families that have the multiple endocrine neoplasia syndrome (MEN type 2) or Von Hippel-Lindau disease. These familial diseases have been shown to be associated with mutations of the RET proto-oncogene in the case of MEN type 2 and the VHL tumor suppressor gene in the case of von Hippel-Lindau disease. Pheochromocytomas are truly rare causes of hypertension. As opposed to primary hyperaldosteronism, where the prevalence may be found to be increasing as diagnostic screening methods become more widely available, it continues to be difficult to argue that pheochromocytomas will be found in any more than 5 of 100,000 persons with hypertension.

The principal reason to consider the diagnosis of pheochromocytoma is the frequent catastrophic outcome when the disorder is overlooked. Untreated pheochromocytomas may result in death and disability due to malignant hypertension, heart failure, stroke, and dysrhythmia. Surgical removal of benign tumors results in survival returning to normal.

1. History

The medical history is the major screening tool for the existence of pheochromocytoma in patients presenting with hypertension. Paroxysmal symptoms that include headache, sweating, palpitations, nausea, and anxiety are common in patients with pheochromocytoma. Fewer patients complain of tremor, chest pain, dyspnea, flushing, or fever. Although hypertension may be episodic, more than 50% of patients present with sustained hypertension that is often resistant to treatment. The family history is extremely important. Pheochromocytoma should be strongly considered in hypertensive patients who report a family history of pheochromocytoma, medullary thyroid carcinoma, MEN type 2, or Von Hippel-Lindau disease. The incidental finding of an adrenal mass in the patient with hypertension necessitates testing for pheochromocytoma.

2. Physical Examination

On physical examination hypertension is usually present though orthostatic hypotension may also be noted. Significant hypertensive retinopathy is frequently seen.

3. Laboratory Evaluation

None of the laboratory testing in the initial screening tests for secondary hypertension will provide useful information, although hyperglycaemia may be noted if a glucose has been obtained as part of risk factor analysis.

4. Further Workup

When the findings suggest that a screening test is appropriate, the medical history should be reviewed for medications that may yield inaccurate results. Labetolol will frequently interfere with the measurement of catecholamines and their metabolites. The finding of a total metanephrine-to-creatinine ratio of >1 μg metanephrines/mg creatinine in a random urine specimen is highly sensitive for pheochromocytoma. More recently total plasma metanephrine levels have been reported to be more sensitive than measurement of urinary metanephrines, but this is not a widely available test.

Confirmatory tests usually involve validation of the urine screen with a 24-hour urine collection for total catecholamines and metanephrines and anatomical localization of the tumor. Pheochromocytomas are usually large enough to visualized by CT scan or MRI. Functioning masses can be documented with the isotopically labeled derivative of guanethidine, ^{131}I-MIBG. Provocative tests are dangerous, are rarely done, and should not be performed outside of centers with experience in their use. The clonidine suppression test is the most widely used diagnostic tool. In this test plasma catecholamines are measured before and at 2 and 3 hours following a 0.3 mg dose of clonidine. The sum of the plasma norepinephrine and epinephrine concentrations is expected to fall to below 500 pg/mL and less than 40% of the predose level in one of the two postdose samples. Both false positives and false negatives as well as profound hypotension have been reported with this test. If laboratory testing is equivocal in the face of persistent symptoms or an adrenal mass, it should probably be repeated in several months with every attempt to have the patient off all medications.

E. Cushing's Syndrome

Excess glucocorticoid hormones cause Cushing's syndrome. It can occur as a result of overproduction of endogenous steroids or by exogenous administration. Stimulation of adrenal cortisol secretion by pituitary overproduction of ACTH (Cushing's disease) is responsible for the majority of cases. Ectopic ACTH production and the combination of benign and malignant adrenal tumors produce the syndrome in about 25% of patients. The remaining small percentage of cases is due to primary adrenal hyperplasia. The mechanism of hypertension is not completely characterized. It may be partially due to cortisol binding to mineralocorticoid receptors because supernormal concentrations overwhelm the pathways that convert it to cortisone. The production of other steroid hormones with mineralocorticoid actions has been described in all forms of Cushing's syndrome. An increase in the production of renin substrate has been reported. Increased responsiveness to various pressors and the inhibition of the vasodilating effects of ANP has also been noted.

Discovery of Cushing's syndrome is not only important as a curable cause of hypertension. Its detection allows for potential reversal of multiple other secondary abnormalities. It may also signal the presence of an underlying malignancy at a point at which it is still curable.

1. History

The history is usually positive for vague complaints, sometimes suggestive of neuropsychiatric illness. Proximal muscle weakness may have been noted. Patients also frequently complain of easy bruising. The history may also be positive for symptoms secondary to an ACTH producing malignancy.

2. Physical Examination

Cushing's syndrome is one of the classical exercises in physical diagnosis. The typical list of findings includes moon facies, buffalo hump, central obesity, purple striae, proximal muscle weakness, hirsutism in women, multiple bruises, and edema. Unfortunately, syndromes of inappropriate cortisol production are frequently present without these findings.

3. Laboratory Evaluation

The routine laboratory screening for hypertension is not likely to be helpful.

4. Further Workup

Secondary screening is easily started with the overnight dexamethasone suppression test. A bedtime dose of 1 mg of dexamethasone is given and a next morning 8 a.m. cortisol level is measured. Suppression to a level below 5 μg/dL is generally taken as normal and is quite sensitive in detecting Cushing's syndrome. There is a high false-positive rate and further testing is required. A low-dose dexamethasone suppression test is the next step.

In this test 0.5 mg of dexamethasone is given every 6 hours for 2 days. On the third day, either an 8 a.m. cortisol is measured or a 24-hour urine for cortisol is measured. If these are not suppressed, Cushing's syndrome is very likely to be present. Further investigation is required to determine the cause, and this workup is best supervised by a physician specializing in the area. Testing generally involves imaging the pituitary and adrenal glands looking for adenoma, hyperplasia, and tumor. Baseline ACTH is normally suppressed by cortisol-producing tumors. High-dose dexamethasone usually will not suppress ACTH from an ectopic source, while it will frequently suppress secretion from a pituitary adenoma. If results are equivocal, inferior petrosal sinus blood sampling for ACTH levels may demonstrate that the pituitary is the source.

IV. DRUGS ASSOCIATED WITH HYPERTENSION

Hypertension related to prescription and nonprescription pharmaceuticals and to recreational drug use may represent one of the largest areas of potential remediation available to the clinician. This certainly is the case if, as has been suggested, 10% of hypertension in adult males is related to alcohol intake and 5% of women taking oral contraceptives will become hypertensive during 5 years of use. A careful history is required in order to determine whether the agents listed in

Table 5 are contributing to high blood pressure. This is particularly true for the drugs listed as nonprescription or recreational. Many over-the-counter medications simply may not be thought of as drugs during a medical history, and specific inquiry must be made as to their use. A clear history of drugs with abuse potential such as alcohol, cocaine, amphetamines and phenylpropanoline is sometimes difficult to obtain. If their use is suspected, the topic may need to be revisited on several occasions after trust has been established. Alcohol, oral contraceptives, and nonsteriodal anti-inflammatory drugs deserve special consideration because so many people use them.

A. Alcohol

Excessive alcohol intake is clearly linked with elevated blood pressure. Population studies show a correlation between alcohol consumed and blood pressure. A pressor effect of alcohol has been demonstrated in both normotensive and hypertensive subjects. The response to alcohol appears to be independent of obesity and salt intake. Reductions in alcohol intake have been shown to reduce

Table 5 Drugs Associated with Hypertension

Nonprescription and recreational drugs
Alcohol
NSAIDs
Anabolic steroids
Cocaine
Amphetamines
Phenylephrine
Pseudoephedrine
Phenylpropanolamine
Phencyclidine
Prescription drugs
NSAIDs
Oral contraceptives
Cyclosporine
Tacrolimus
Erythropoeitin
Ergotamines
Bromocriptine
Metoclopramide
Lithium
Tricyclic antidepressants
Monoamine oxidase inhibitors

both systolic and diastolic blood pressure. Numerous mechanisms for the pressor response to alcohol have been postulated, but they continue to be unclear.

B. Oral Contraceptives

Oral contraceptives have been strongly associated with hypertension. Studies from the 1980s have shown the average blood pressure to rise in populations of women placed on oral contraceptives as compared with controls. Early studies showed that 5% of women started on these drugs had an increase in blood pressure to greater than 140/90 during 4 years of follow-up. Estrogen doses have declined since these studies and the incidence of hypertension may be lower as a result, but this remains unproven. One study of a biphasic oral contraceptive showed no clear rise in blood pressure during one and a half years of monitoring. In more than half of women who develop hypertension with oral contraceptives, the blood pressure returns to normal if they are discontinued. Although estrogens are most closely associated with an increase in blood pressure, progesterones may augment the hypertensive effects of estrogens. It is interesting that hypertension has not been reported as a consistent or frequent complication of postmenopausal estrogen-replacement therapy. High blood pressure following oral contraceptives has been attributed to sodium retention, increased angiotensiongen production, and insulin resistance.

C. Nonsteroidal Anti-Inflammatory Drugs

Nonsteroidal anti-inflammatory drugs (NSAIDs) have been widely reported to be associated with hypertension. The proposed mechanism is by causing Na^+ retention as a result of inhibition of cyclooxygenase-dependent prostaglandins that promote natriuresis. It is also possible that they inhibit products of arachidonic acid metabolism that function as vasodilators. Population studies have shown that NSAID usage is correlated with greater use of antihypertensive medications. These drugs increase blood pressure in normotensive individuals and worsen high blood pressure in a group with untreated mild hypertension. NSAIDs have been suggested to inhibit the effects of all categories of diuretics, β blockers, and angiotensin-converting enzyme inhibitors. These drugs should be avoided, except for very short-term therapy in individuals with hypertension, and when used for longer than a few days, blood pressure should be closely monitored.

SUGGESTED READINGS

Clyburn EB, DiPette DJ. Hypertension induced by drugs and other substances. Semin Nephrol 1995; 15:72–86.

Erbslöh-Möller B, Dumas A, Roth D, Sfakianakis GN, Bourgoignie JJ. Furosemide-^{131}I-hippuran renography after angiotensin-converting enzyme inhibition for the diagnosis of renovascular hypertension. Am J Med 1991; 90:23–29.

Gomez-Sanchez CE, Gomez-Sanchez EP, Yamakita N. Endocrine causes of hypertension. Semin Nephrol 1995; 15:106–115.

Hoffmann U, Edwards JM, Carter S, Goldman ML, Harley JD, Zaccardi MJ, Strandness DE. Role of duplex scanning for the detection of atherosclerotic renal artery disease. Kidney Int 1991; 39:1232–1239.

Joint National Committee. The sixth report of the Joint National Committee on prevention, detection, evaluation and treatment of high blood pressure. Arch Intern Med 1997; 157:2413–2446.

Karet FE, Lifton RP. Mutations contributing to human blood pressure variation. Recent Prog Hormone Res 1997; 52:263–276.

Lenders JWM, Keiser HF, Goldstein DS, Willemsen JJ, Friberg P, Jacobs MC, Kloppenborg PWC, Thien T, Eisenhofer G. Plasma metanephrines in the diagnosis of pheochromocytoma. Ann Intern Med 1995; 123:101–109.

McKenna RJ, Sequeira SJ, Heffernan A, Chambers J, Cunningham S. Diagnosis under random conditions of all disorders of the renin-angiotensin-aldosterone axis, including primary hyperaldosteronism. J Clin Endocrinol Metab 1991; 73:952–957.

Mannelli M, De Feo ML, Maggi M, Pupilli C, Opocher G, Valenza T, Baldi E, Serio M. Usefulness of basal catecholamine plasma levels and clonidine suppression test in the diagnosis of pheochromocytoma. J Endocrinol Invest 1987; 10:377–382.

Muller FB, Sealey JE, Case DB, Atlas SA, Pickering TG, Pecker MS, Preibisz JJ, Laragh JH. The Captopril test for identifying renovascular disease in hypertensive patients. Am J Med 1986; 80:633–644.

Neumann HP, Bender B, Zäuner I, Berger DP, Eng C, Brauch H, Zbar B. Monogenetic hypertension and pheochromocytoma. Am J Kidney Dis 1996; 28:329–333.

Preston RA, Singer I, Epstein M. Renal parenchymal hypertension: current concepts of pathogenesis and management. Arch Intern Med 1996; 156:602–611.

Rimmer JM, Plante DA, Madias NE. Therapeutic decision making in renal vascular hypertension. In: Novick A, Scoble J, Hamilton G eds. Renal Vascular Disease. Philadelphia: W.B. Saunders Co., 1996, pp. 245–267.

Svetkey LP, Helms MJ, Dunnick NR, Klotman PE. Clinical characteristics useful in screening for renovascular disease. South Med J 1990; 83:743–747.

Young WR, Hogan MJ, Klee GG, Grant CS, van Heerden JA. Primary aldosteronism: diagnosis and treatment. Mayo Clin Proc 1990; 65:96–110.

10

Urinary Tract Infection: Physical and Laboratory Findings

Mary B. Ramundo, W. Kemper Alston, and Christopher J. Grace
University of Vermont, Burlington, Vermont

I. INTRODUCTION

Urinary tract infection (UTI) represents one of the most common infectious syndromes encountered in medical practice today. Physicians in a variety of fields are called upon to diagnose and treat infections in the urinary system. The morbidity associated with these infections ranges from inconvenience secondary to symptoms to serious disease such as gram-negative sepsis or premature labor in pregnancy. Although most of these patients are treated on an outpatient basis, UTI is one of the most common nosocomial infections contributing to increased length of stay, cost of hospitalization, and mortality. Significant health care dollars are spent on diagnosis and treatment of urinary tract infections each year. This chapter discusses the pathophysiology, clinical presentation, and diagnosis of UTI. Treatment of these disorders is presented in Chapter 22.

II. EPIDEMIOLOGY

Urinary tract infections account for more than 7 million outpatient visits and approximately one million hospitalizations per year in the United States. The problem of urinary tract infection spans all age groups. The frequency of UTI in infants is 1–2%, and it is more common in male infants <3 months of age. In the preschool age group UTI is more common in girls. Urinary tract infections are one of the most common infections of adults for which antimicrobials are used. Most UTIs occur in otherwise healthy individuals. Approximately 5% of women of childbearing age, and 10–20% of women overall will experience at least one UTI in their lifetime. The timing of the first UTI often correlates with the onset of sexual activity in young women. In young adults the risk of bacteriuria is approximately 30-fold greater in women than in men. After the age of 65 the difference in risk for bacteriuria is less pronounced, with estimates of risk of 10% in men and 20% in women.

III. DEFINITIONS

Urinary tract infection is an ill-defined term that is used to cover a wide spectrum of infections and host responses. Infection has been defined as multiplication of organisms in the body. The presence of bacteria in the urine is termed bacteriuria, but organisms other than bacteria can cause infection of the urinary tract. The presence of microorganisms in the urinary tract may or may not stimulate an inflammatory response. The presence of microorganisms and inflammatory cells in the urine (pyuria) is usually accompanied by symptoms. In some cases urinary tract infections are asymptomatic and without significant pyuria. These situations will be discussed under the heading of asymptomatic bacteriuria. For the purposes of our discussion, UTI refers to bacteriuria accompanied by pyuria and symptoms.

Urinary tract infections are stratified by location (upper versus lower tract) and by the presence or absence of structural or functional abnormalities. Cystitis refers to infection of the bladder that involves the superficial mucosa. The term lower urinary tract infection is synonymous with cystitis. Acute pyelonephritis is inflammation of the renal parenchyma, usually due to bacteria, and is also referred to as upper urinary tract infection. Chronic pyelonephritis is a histopathological diagnosis that is not specific for infection.

Urinary tract infections that occur in otherwise healthy individuals without structural or functional abnormalities of the urinary tract or underlying disease are referred to as uncomplicated UTIs. Infections in all other individuals are considered complicated. Examples of structural or functional abnormalities include congenital anomalies of the collecting system, prostatic hypertrophy, calculi, urethral strictures, vesicoureteral reflux, neurogenic bladder, urological manipulation, and pregnancy. Diabetes mellitus and immunosuppressive therapy can be complicating factors. Complications can increase the risk of acquiring new infections, increase the potential of an infection to cause symptomatic or serious disease, and increase the probability of treatment failures.

IV. PATHOGENESIS

The normal urinary tract is sterile except for the distal urethra, which may be colonized with a variety of organisms. Bacteria gain access to the bladder most commonly by ascending the urethra. Bacteria gain access to the kidney via vesicoureteral reflux. Hematogenous seeding of the urinary tract is much less common.

A. Normal Host Defenses

Several characteristics of the normal urinary system provide a defense against infection. Efficient emptying of the bladder is one of the best defense mechanisms. Any factor that interferes with normal urinary flow can increase the risk of infection of the urinary tract. Pregnancy and endotoxin release in gram-negative sepsis have an antiperistaltic effect, which facilitates ascent of bacteria from the bladder to the kidney. The flushing effect of the urinary flow helps to prevent attachment of bacteria and colonization of the urinary epithelium. Incomplete bladder emptying allows bacteria to multiply in the urine. Even transient ureteral obstruction results in enhanced susceptibility to infection.

Urea, organic acids, salts, osmolality, and low urinary pH all are factors in decreasing the risk of infection of the urinary tract. Secreted IgA and soluble receptor analogs in the urine interfere with attachment of bacteria to the urinary epithelium. Alterations in the mucopolysaccharide lining of the normal bladder secondary to chemicals, foreign bodies, or disease can increase the risk for UTI. Most patients with UTI do not have structural or functional abnormalities. Size of bacterial inoculum may also play a role. Instrumentation with urinary catheters helps facilitate ascent of organisms into the bladder resulting in increased risk for UTI. Sexual intercourse helps facilitate ascent of periurethral bacteria into the bladder.

The normal flora of the bowel and vagina play a role in the protection against UTIs. Estrogen replacement in elderly women is associated with an increase in lactobacilli in the vaginal flora and a decreased risk of UTI. Young women who use spermicides have fewer lactobacilli in the vagina and an increased risk of UTI. In males, lack of circumcision may increase colonization at the urethral meatus and increase the risk for UTI. Other host factors have been evaluated such as specific blood group antigens, but studies have failed to document a consistent association with increased risk for UTI and a specific blood group. Persons at increased risk for UTI have increased bacterial colonization of the perineum. Increased affinity of vaginal and urinary epithelium for attachment of uropathogenic bacteria also contributes to an individual's susceptibility for UTI. The nature of the biological predisposition has not been well defined.

B. Bacterial Characteristics

Certain bacterial characteristics have been associated with increased virulence in development of UTI. Encapsulated *Escherichia coli* resist phagocytosis. Uropathogenic *E. coli* have specific type P fimbriae that facilitate attachment to uroepithelial cells. Receptors for P fimbriae are present on intestinal mucosa, and *E. coli* with P fimbriae are more likely to colonize the colon. Hemolysins are cytotoxic proteins that can be toxic to epithelial and inflammatory cells and may aid in the mucosal damage required for invasive disease. *E. coli* strains that cause pyelonephritis are more likely to produce hemolysin. Type 1 pili, which can be expressed on the surface of *E. coli*, facilitate phagocytosis of the organism by polymorphonuclear cells. Organisms can undergo phasic variation, which involves shedding of Type 1 pili resulting in increased ability to invade the renal parenchyma. The pathogenesis of cystitis is less well understood, and no specific characteristics have been shown to identify ''cystogenic'' *E. coli*.

C. Inflammatory Response

Inflammation plays a role in clearance of bacteria from the urinary tract. In addition to bacterial and host factors, the immune response is important in the development of UTI. There is an interaction between the bacteria, the urinary epithelium, and the inflammatory cells that is important in determining the inflammatory response. Attachment of bacteria to urinary epithelium results in release of cytokines that stimulate migration of inflammatory cells to the urinary tract. Inflammatory cells can respond directly to bacterial factors such as lipopolysaccharide. In pyelonephritis inflammatory cells produce free radicals and lysosomal enzymes that help promote tissue destruction. Infection results in altered pattern of intrarenal blood flow, which impairs delivery of phagocytic cells and aids in progression of infection within the kidney. Patients with defects in acute inflammatory response, such as renal transplant patients and patients with neutropenia, have increased risk for UTI. Humoral immunity also plays a role. Even lower tract infections are associated with a bladder mucosa antibody response. Tamm-Horsfall protein produced by tubular cells of the ascending loop and distal convoluted tubule inhibits attachment of fimbriated *E. coli*.

D. Microbiology

The organisms that cause UTI are part of the fecal flora. *E. coli* is the pathogen in greater than 80% of cases. *Staphylococcus saprophyticus* accounts for approximately 15% of cases of acute uncomplicated cystitis. *Enterococcus* and members of the family Enterobacteriaceae such as *Klebsiella*, *Enterobacter*, *Serratia*, and *Proteus* are seen less frequently. The pathogens involved in complicated UTIs vary enormously and tend to be more resistant to antimicrobials. *Candida* can colonize the bladder and can also act as a pathogen in the urinary tract, especially in persons with diabetes mellitus or on immunosuppressive therapy. Viruses are unusual pathogens in the urinary tract.

V. CLINICAL MANIFESTATIONS AND DIFFERENTIAL DIAGNOSIS

A. Cystitis

Inflammation of the bladder (cystitis) usually presents acutely with dysuria, urgency, frequency and suprapubic discomfort. Forty percent of patients also have hematuria. It is generally a disease of sexually active younger women, although increasing reports of cystitis in sexually active men are appearing. Cystitis is common in elderly individuals of both sexes. Fever and flank pain are absent. Risk factors for acute cystitis such as recent sexual intercourse, diaphragm/spermicide use, and past episodes of cystitis should be reviewed. Markers for complicated cystitis should be sought (see above and Fig. 1). Older men and women may present with similar symptoms. In men UTI are usually related to prostatic enlargement. Symptoms of outlet obstruction may predominate with bladder fullness, poor urinary stream, and inadequate emptying. The physical exam is generally not revealing but may demonstrate suprapubic discomfort on palpation.

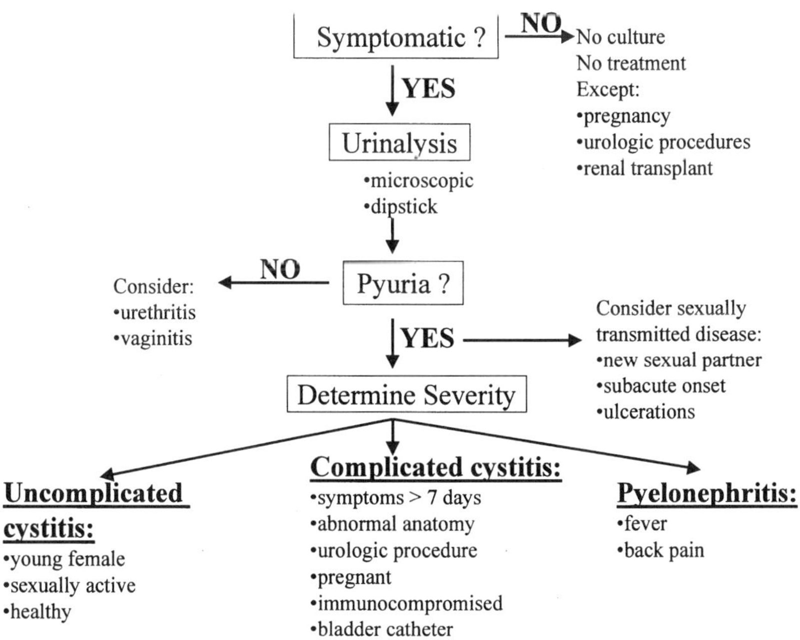

Figure 1 Approach to the adult patient with a suspected UTI.

B. Urethritis

Acute urethritis may mimic cystitis but usually has a more gradual onset with milder symptoms. Common pathogens include *Chlamydia trachomatis*, *Neisseria gonorrhoeae*, and herpes simplex virus. Clues to this diagnosis include new sexual partners and vaginal bleeding secondary to ulcerations and cervicitis. Vaginitis, most commonly caused by *Trichomonas vaginalis* and *Candida* species is associated with the gradual onset of vaginal discharge, pruritis, and dyspareunia but not frequency or suprapubic discomfort. Symptoms of urethritis or vaginitis should prompt a pelvic exam with appropriate cultures.

C. Pyelonephritis

Acute pyelonephritis is characterized by the sudden onset of fever, flank and back pain, and constitutional symptoms including nausea, vomiting, diarrhea or constipation, and weakness. Patients may or may not have dysuria and frequency. Physical examination may reveal high fevers (up to 40.5°C), costovertebral angle (CVA) tenderness, and suprapubic tenderness, although none of these findings is pathognomonic and none may even be present. The illness can span a spectrum from mild symptoms to the toxic patient with frank septic shock. Differential diagnosis includes nephrolithiasis, renal abscess, pelvic inflammatory disease, cholecystitis, appendicitis, and enteritis/colitis.

D. Prostatitis

Prostatic inflammation may be due to bacterial infection (acute and chronic) or to nonbacterial causes. Nonbacterial causes are poorly defined but may include infections from chlamydia, mycoplasma, or ureaplasma, autoimmune disorders, and neuromuscular dysfunction. Men may have pelviperineal pain (sometimes referred to as prostadynia) not related to the prostate. The great majority of men (>90%) with "prostatic" symptoms have nonbacterial prostatitis or pelviperineal pain. Bacterial prostatitis is due to retrograde migration of bacteria from the bladder to the prostate. Acute bacterial prostatitis presents with fever, dysuria, frequency, and perineal and back discomfort. Symptoms of urethral obstruction may predominate. The prostate is firm and tender on rectal exam. Chronic bacterial prostatitis is far more common than acute infection. The prostate gland can be a nidus for persistence of bacteria in the genitourinary tract. Men present with symptoms of recurrent lower tract UTI. Between episodes they are asymptomatic. The prostate gland is nontender on exam.

E. Renal Abscess

Renal abscesses may form within the kidney or in the perinephric space. Intrarenal abscesses may be hematogenous in origin, predominantly in the cortex, or ascending in nature, at the corticomedullary junction. The latter typically arise in the setting of infection with gram-negative bacilli in patients with underlying urinary tract abnormalities such as reflux or obstruction. Cortical abscesses (renal carbuncles), commonly caused by *Staphylococcus aureus*, are generally unilateral, single, and right sided. Perinephric abscesses form in the perinephric fascia as a complication of an intrarenal abscess. The bacteriology is either *S. aureus* or gram-negative rods depending on the site of the intrarenal abscess. Patients with renal abscesses present with subacute onset of fever and back and flank pain. Lower urinary tract symptoms may be absent. Constitutional symptoms including nausea, vomiting, and weakness are common. Past histories of UTIs, renal calculi, or GU instrumentation are often predisposing factors for abscess formation. The patient with persistent fever and toxicity despite appropriate antibiotic therapy should be evaluated with sonography or computerized tomography to rule out an abscess.

F. Asymptomatic Bacteriuria

Asymptomatic bacteriuria is common in the elderly population, both in women and men. The incidence increases with age, progressive debility, fecal incontinence, poor bladder emptying, and Foley catheterization. Thirty to fifty percent of hospitalized patients over the age of 65 years of age have asymptomatic bacteruria. Many of these patients have associated pyuria. Most of these patients do not benefit from antibiotic therapy (see Chapter 22). This needs to be kept in mind when interpreting urine culture results or assessing the febrile patient in order to avoid over treatment of this group of patients. Additionally, many symptoms in elderly patients attributed to a UTI may not be caused by this infection. Signs and symptoms that are not well correlated with UTIs in the elderly population include incontinence, high blood pressure, renal insufficiency, poor sense of well-being, decreased appetite, weakness, and sleep difficulty.

G. Foley Catheter–Related Bacteriuria

Patients with Foley urinary catheters will become colonized with bacteria if the catheter is left in place for more than a few days. Ten to thirty percent of patients undergoing short-term (2–4 days) catheterization will become colonized and 100% of patients with long-term catheters will be colonized within the first month. Most of these patients remain asymptomatic, need not be cultured, and do not require antibiotic treatment. However, up to 30% develop symptoms attributable to UTI, including fever or suprapubic pain, and these patients will require antibiotic treatment. In debilitated patients who are chronically catheterized, one should also think about subclinical bacteremia and cortical renal abscesses of hematogenous origin as potential sources of the bacteriuria.

VI. DIAGNOSIS

The diagnosis of a UTI should be made primarily on clinical grounds. For example, this disorder should be entertained when a patient presents with a characteristic history of dysuria or with the finding of flank tenderness and fever (Fig. 1). In these instances, urinalysis and urine culture serve only a confirmatory role. Pyuria demonstrates the presence of inflammation and a positive urine culture with antibiotic sensitivity testing provides support for therapy. The emphasis on diagnosing UTI clinically is important because the same pitfalls that exist for the diagnosis of community-acquired pneumonia with sputum examination are present with this common infection. Pyuria is not specific for UTIs, and all voided urine specimens are contaminated to some degree. The assumption that a positive urine culture equals a diagnosis of UTI will lead to frequent misdiagnoses and the inappropriate use of antibiotics.

A. Laboratory Evaluation

1. Urinalysis

The first issue to consider in performing a urinalysis is how to obtain the specimen. Although rarely emphasized, all three methods for obtaining urine require adequate attention if useful data are to be gained. The most common, and least invasive, is the midstream, clean-catch urine. Women should wipe the vulva from front to back several times with sterile gauze pads soaked in saline or tap water, with or without a mild soap. Midstream urine should then be carefully collected in a sterile container. In patients unable to provide a clean-catch urine, the bladder may be catheterized to obtain a clean specimen. This technique, however, is more painful and expensive, and improper technique may introduce bacteria into a sterile bladder. Finally, suprapubic aspiration eliminates urethral contamination but is the most invasive and is seldom performed except in pediatric patients.

The finding of pyuria on microscopic examination of urine is the single most important element in the laboratory diagnosis of UTI. Pyuria is defined as greater than 5–10 white blood cells (WBCs) per high-power field (or 10–50 WBCs/mm^3) in the sediment of a urine sample centrifuged at 2000 rpm for 5 minutes. As an alternative, the finding of at least 10 WBCs/mm^3 in an uncentrifuged clean-catch midstream urine indicates the presence of pyuria. Virtually all patients with a clinically significant, symptomatic UTI will have an abnormal number of WBCs in voided urine. As noted earlier, however, pyuria is not specific for UTI. An abnormal number of WBCs may be found in the urine in a wide variety of inflammatory conditions including glomerulonephritis, interstitial nephritis, renal vasculitis, as well as in infections such as vaginitis, prostatitis, and urethritis. The dipstick leukocyte esterase test is a rapid screen for pyuria, and can detect greater than 10 WBCs/mm^3 with a sensitivity of 75–95% and a specificity of 95%. Microscopic or gross hematuria is another finding on urinalysis that may suggest hemorrhagic cystitis in a young woman but lacks specificity.

Establishing the presence of bacteria in a urine sample without using culture techniques is more problematic. Urine may be examined before or after centrifugation with a wet mount or Gram stain. Any bacteria seen under high-power (oil-immersion) magnification in a drop of unspun, clean-catch, midstream urine which has been Gram stained may be significant (one bacterium per high-power field is equivalent to at least 10^5/mm^3). The nitrite dipstick is a specific screening test for bacteria that reduce nitrate, but this rapid chemical test lacks sensitivity. In complicated cases and in hospitalized patients a Gram stain of centrifuged urine can quickly distinguish between enterococci, gram-negative bacilli and fungi and will often help guide empiric therapy. Numerous attempts over the years to localize the site of infection to either the bladder or kidney using voided urine have been unrewarding and are not in routine clinical use. The clinical presentation itself and the response to antibiotic therapy remain the most practical evidence for determining the degree of involvement.

2. Urine Culture

Urine in the kidney and bladder is normally sterile but is frequently contaminated as it exits the urethra. Urine culture allows quantification of bacteriuria as a way of enhancing specificity in the diagnosis of UTI. In addition, culture provides speciation and sensitivity testing, which may be crucial in complicated and nosocomial UTIs. In young women with typical symptoms of uncomplicated cystitis and pyuria on urinalysis, empiric treatment can be undertaken without culture (see Chapter 22). Calibrated loops or pipetting a known volume of urine for culture can provide colony-forming units of bacteria per milliliter of urine. The cost and work involved can be reduced with semiquantitative cultures using an agar-coated slide that is dipped. Unfortunately, numerical cutoffs for defining significant bacteriuria remain controversial and have changed over the years. Data from several decades ago established $\geq 10^5$ bacterial pathogens per mL of voided, midstream, clean-catch urine as diagnostic of UTI. Certainly the higher the colony count, the more likely UTI is to be present. More recent work has concluded that this cutoff lacks sensitivity and that many cases of significant bacteriuria have much lower counts; a cutoff of 10^2 may provide better overall sensitivity and specificity. In addition, traditional colony count cutoffs for young women with *E. coli* cystitis or pyelonephritis may not apply for gram-positive bacteria, yeast, fastidious organisms, male patients, or nosocomial cases with or without an indwelling catheter. The conclusion from this debate is that quantitative colony counts and cutoffs between 10^2 and 10^5 cannot stand alone in the diagnosis of UTI. The history, physical examination, and analysis of a properly obtained specimen of urine for pyuria remain the most important tools available to the clinician.

3. Blood Culture

As with other systemic infections, blood should be obtained for culture prior to administering antibiotics when bacteremia and sepsis are considered possible. In severely ill patients and those being admitted to the hospital, blood cultures provide an invaluable adjunct to urinalysis and culture. Positive blood cultures may have an impact on the management of UTI depending on host factors and the organism involved (see Chapter 22).

4. Prostatic Secretions

Expressed prostatic secretions should be obtained in men with symptoms of chronic prostatitis to enhance the data obtained from voided urine. Prostatic massage performed after midstream urine collection allows comparison of prostatic fluid with voided urine and, when properly performed, can help determine the source of the pyuria and bacteriuria. Prostatic massage is contraindicated in acute prostatitis, which is a straightforward clinical diagnosis.

B. Radiology

Radiology evaluation is not routinely indicated for uncomplicated UTIs. By contrast, radiological techniques are invaluable aids in diagnosing and treating complicated UTIs by uncovering anatomical abnormalities, as well as identifying the presence of obstruction, stone disease, or abscess formation.

1. Plain Radiograph

A flat plate of the abdomen may reveal calculi, gas within the kidney, calcifications, or a soft tissue mass.

2. Intravenous Pyelography

There is little, if any, role for intravenous pyelography in evaluating UTIs. This procedure has been largely replaced by computed tomography (CT) and ultrasound, which can give more anatomical and functional information with less exposure to radiocontrast material and radiation.

3. Renal Ultrasound

The renal ultrasound is an extremely informative noninvasive technique that can be performed rapidly. The technique is particularly useful in evaluating for obstruction and for the presence of stones, abscesses, extrarenal fluid collections, and anatomical abnormalities. The major shortcoming of ultrasonography is that it gives no information about renal function. Transrectal sonography can rapidly exclude prostatic abscess.

4. Computed Tomography

Computed tomography can be performed with or without intravenous (IV) radiocontrast material. Newer helical scanners offer improved imaging over older machines. Blood and calcifications can be demonstrated without contrast, while multiple ''phases'' are obtained with IV contrast. Renal, perirenal, and prostatic abscess are well visualized with contrast. Fluid collections can be delineated and aspirated under CT guidance. At the present time, CT with contrast is considered the study of choice for most cases of complicated UTI.

C. Nuclear Scintigraphy and Magnetic Resonance Imaging

Nuclear scintigraphy adds very little to the diagnosis in complicated UTIs. Radioisotope preparations, such as gallium-67 citrate– or indium-111–labeled white blood cells, may demonstrate renal uptake in upper tract infection but usually do not add any anatomical information to that obtained by CT. Gadolinium-enhanced magnetic resonance imaging is an alternative to CT with contrast but has not been shown to be superior.

SUGGESTED READINGS

Abrutyn E, Mossey J, Berlin JA, Boscia J, et al. Does asymptomatic bacteriuria predict mortality and does antimicrobial treatment reduce mortality in elderly ambulatory women? Ann Intern Med 1994; 120:827.

Andriole VT, ed. Urinary Tract Infections. Philadelphia: W.B. Saunders, 1997.

Baumgarten DA, Baumgartner BR. Imaging and radiologic management of upper urinary tract infections. Urol Clin North Am 1997; 24:545–569.

Fisher JF, Chew WH, Shadomy S, Duma RJ, et al. Urinary tract infections due to *Candida albicans*. Rev Infect Dis 1982; 4:1107–1117.

Hooton TM, Scholes D, Hughes JP, Winter C, et al. A prospective study of risk factors for symptomatic urinary tract infection in young women. N Engl J Med 1996; 335: 468–474.

Kunin CM. Urinary tract infections in females. Clin Infect Dis 1994; 28:1–12.

Kunin CM, White LV, Hua TH. A reassessment of the importance of ''low-count'' bacteriuria in young women with acute urinary symptoms. Ann Intern Med 1993; 119: 454–460.

Lipsky BA. Urinary tract infections in men. Epidemiology, pathophysiology, diagnosis, and treatment. Ann Intern Med 1989; 110:138–150.

Stamm WE. Measurement of pyuria and its relation to bacteriuria. Am J Med 1983; 75(1B):53–58.

Stamm WE, Hooton TM. Management of urinary tract infections in adults. N Engl J Med 1993; 329:1328–1334.

Stamm WE, McKevitt M, Roberts PL, White NJ. Natural history of recurrent urinary tract infections in women. Rev Infect Dis 1991; 13:77–84.

11
Diagnosis of Acid-Base Disorders

F. John Gennari
University of Vermont, Burlington, Vermont

I. INTRODUCTION

This chapter briefly reviews the normal regulation of acid-base balance and focuses on the tools needed to identify and diagnose specific disorders of acid-base equilibrium. The symptoms associated with acid-base disorders are discussed in Chapter 4, and the approach to the treatment of these disorders is discussed in Chapter 28.

II. BASIC CONCEPTS

Blood pH, partial pressure of CO_2 in the blood (PCO_2), and bicarbonate concentration ($[HCO_3^-]$) are normally maintained within a narrow range despite a wide variety of external and internal challenges. Although these three variables, which define acid-base status at any given point in time, are often discussed as though they were independent of each other, they are in fact linked chemically by the Henderson-Hasselbalch equation:

$$pH = 6.1 + \log_{10}([HCO_3^-]/(0.03 \times PCO_2)) \quad (1)$$

For ease of computation and to help understand the nature of the interrelationships between these three variables, this formula is often presented in terms of H^+ rather than pH to remove the logarithms. This form is the Henderson equation:

$$[H^+] = 24 \times (PCO_2/[HCO_3^-]) \quad (2)$$

With either equation, one can see that the pH is determined by the ratio of the PCO_2 to the serum $[HCO_3^-]$. The PCO_2 is regulated by the lungs and serum $[HCO_3^-]$ by the kidneys, resulting in exquisite control of the $[H^+]$ or pH of the body fluids.

In addition to their chemical relationship, pH, PCO_2, and serum $[HCO_3^-]$ are related physiologically. Alterations in serum $[HCO_3^-]$ lead to compensatory adjustments in PCO_2 (through changes in ventilation), minimizing the change in pH that would otherwise occur. This ventilatory response is maintained until the kidney can restore serum $[HCO_3^-]$ to normal. In a similar fashion, any changes in PCO_2 lead to compensatory changes in serum $[HCO_3^-]$ brought about by renal mechanisms, and the renal response is sustained until the PCO_2 is restored to normal. Blood pH is maintained within the normal range on a minute-to-minute basis by adjustments in ventilation, but the kidney is responsible for maintaining acid-base equilibrium on a day-to-day basis by adjusting the rate of bicarbonate reabsorption and acid excretion.

III. MEASUREMENTS AND NORMAL VALUES

A. Serum [Total CO_2] Versus $[HCO_3^-]$

Most commonly, the first indication that an acid-base disturbance is present is an abnormality in the serum [Total CO_2], a component of the serum electrolytes. Serum $[HCO_3^-]$ is not easily measured, and [Total CO_2] is its surrogate. Although [Total CO_2] is commonly referred to as bicarbonate, it is important to emphasize that the two are not precisely equivalent. The [Total CO_2] includes not only $[HCO_3^-]$ but also dissolved CO_2 and other carbonates. As a result, it is normally 1–2 mEq/L higher than serum $[HCO_3^-]$, and the discrepancy increases in direct relation to the PCO_2. Table 1 lists the range of normal for this variable.

Serum $[HCO_3^-]$ is not measured directly but is calculated from measurements of pH and PCO_2 using the Henderson-Hasselbalch equation [Eq. (1)]. Because these measurements are usually made in arterial blood, there is an additional difference between serum $[HCO_3^-]$ and [Total CO_2]. The concentration of bicarbonate increases by 1–3 mEq/L between the arterial and venous blood due to the addition of CO_2 to the blood in the capillaries. Thus, venous [Total CO_2] includes a higher $[HCO_3^-]$ as well as dissolved CO_2 and carbonates. The normal range for arterial $[HCO_3^-]$ is shown in Table 1.

B. pH and PCO_2

As noted earlier, these parameters are usually measured in arterial blood. The reason for this practice is that the pH and PCO_2 of venous blood vary with local venous blood flow rate and thus may not accurately reflect acid-base status, partic-

Table 1 Normal Serum Values

Venous serum	
[Total CO_2][a]	24–30 mEq/L
$[K^+]$	3.5–5.0 mEq/L
Anion Gap	4–16 mEq/L
Arterial blood	
pH[a]	7.38–7.42
PCO_2[a]	35–45 mmHg
$[HCO_3^-]$[a,b]	23–29 mEq/L

[a] Although listed separately, these variables are interrelated. Patients with higher [Total CO_2] or $[HCO_3^-]$ values within the normal range will have higher PCO_2 and pH values.
[b] Calculated from arterial pH and PCO_2.

ularly in the presence of arterial vasoconstriction. Blood pH and PCO_2 are easily measured using electrode techniques that are quite accurate and reproducible. The normal values for these parameters are shown in Table 1.

C. Other Measurements

To assess acid-base status, the above measurements are the only tools necessary. Calculated values such as normalized bicarbonate, blood buffer base, and base excess do nothing but cause confusion when characterizing abnormalities in acid-base status.

IV. NORMAL REGULATION OF ACID-BASE EQUILIBRIUM

In contrast to other ions, H^+ does not normally gain access to our body by ingestion. Instead, this ion is generated primarily by metabolic processes, including the production of strong acids by the breakdown of sulfur-containing amino acids and partial metabolism of fats and sugars to organic acids. Hydrogen ions are also generated by alkali loss in the stool each day. Regardless of its source, any acid produced is buffered immediately by body alkali stores, and eventually an equivalent amount of H^+ is excreted in the urine, regenerating the alkali stores originally consumed in the buffering process. Although the factor or factors regulating the precise balance between acid production and acid excretion are unknown, they allow for wide variations in dietary intake with little or no change in steady-state serum $[HCO_3^-]$. Thus, only minor differences in serum $[HCO_3^-]$

are seen in individuals ingesting a vegetarian diet, which provides a net alkali load to the body, and individuals ingesting a diet high in animal protein, which provides a large acid load to the body.

The regulation of body alkali stores resides within the kidney, which is charged with the dual task of reabsorbing all the filtered HCO_3^- and excreting enough acid (in the form of NH_4^+ and titratable acid, e.g., H_2PO_4) to meet the needs for balance. As discussed later, impairment of either HCO_3^- reabsorption or acid excretion can occur, producing a form of metabolic acidosis termed renal tubular acidosis. Both HCO_3^- reabsorption and acid excretion are accomplished by the secretion of hydrogen ions (H^+) into the tubular lumen through specialized transport proteins located on the lining membrane of tubular epithelial cells. These transporters are the Na^+/H^+ exchanger, which resides in the cells of the proximal tubule and loop of Henle, H^+-ATPase, which is present in cells in both the proximal and distal nephron, and H^+/K^+-ATPase, which is present only in cells in the distal tubule and cortical collecting duct. Secreted H^+ either reacts with filtered HCO_3^-, accomplishing its removal from the urine, or titrates weak acids or ammonia, leading to H^+ excretion in the urine. In addition to these mechanisms for secreting H^+, the distal tubule contains a transport protein that secretes HCO_3^- in exchange for chloride reabsorption to allow for HCO_3^- excretion when the need arises. Some of the hereditary causes of renal tubular acidosis are due to genetic defects in one or more of these transporters.

The CO_2 produced each day by oxidative metabolism is by far the largest source of new H^+ (when hydrated to form carbonic acid), but this source of H^+ has no sustained effect on acid-base balance because it is rapidly excreted by the lungs. Only when ventilation is impaired and CO_2 is retained does this source lead to acidemia.

V. APPROACH TO THE DIAGNOSIS OF ACID-BASE DISORDERS

A. General Considerations

The approach to diagnosing and characterizing disorders of acid-base equilibrium has three components. The first is to identify the primary acid-base abnormality, the second is to determine whether the compensatory response is appropriate, and the third is to determine the cause of the disorder. These three components are discussed separately below.

B. Step 1: Identifying the Primary Disorder

The four primary acid-base disturbances are metabolic acidosis, metabolic alkalosis, respiratory acidosis, and respiratory alkalosis. Table 2 outlines the tools for

Table 2 Characteristics of the four Primary Acid-Base Disorders

	Primary alteration	Effect	Adaptive response	Mechanism
Metabolic acidosis	$\downarrow$ serum $[HCO_3^-]$	$\downarrow$ pH	$\downarrow$ PCO_2	Hyperventilation
Metabolic alkalosis	$\uparrow$ serum $[HCO_3^-]$	$\uparrow$ pH	$\uparrow$ PCO_2	Hypoventilation
Respiratory acidosis	$\uparrow$ PCO_2	$\downarrow$ pH	$\uparrow$ serum $[HCO_3^-]$	Acute: buffer response Sustained: $\uparrow$ acid excretion, $\uparrow$ HCO_3^- reabsorption
Respiratory alkalosis	$\downarrow$ PCO_2	$\uparrow$ pH	$\downarrow$ serum $[HCO_3^-]$	Acute: buffer response Sustained: $\downarrow$ acid excretion, $\downarrow$ HCO_3^- reabsorption

identifying which of these disorders is present. Metabolic acidosis is characterized by a primary reduction in serum [HCO_3^-], causing a reduction in systemic pH. This disorder is usually first identified by the finding of a low [Total CO_2] in a venous blood sample but can only be fully characterized by measurement of pH and PCO_2. Metabolic alkalosis is characterized by an increase in serum [HCO_3^-], causing an increase in systemic pH. Again this disorder can be suspected from abnormalities in the serum electrolytes, but full characterization requires pH and PCO_2 measurements. Respiratory acidosis is characterized by a primary increase in PCO_2, causing a reduction in pH, and respiratory alkalosis is characterized by a decrease in arterial PCO_2, causing an increase in pH. The respiratory disorders are subdivided into acute and chronic disorders, reflecting the delay in the renal compensatory response. The acute disorders are usually suspected on clinical grounds, and the changes in pH are the most dramatic. The chronic disorders are often first recognized by an abnormality in venous [Total CO_2], reflecting the compensatory response (see below). Full characterization, however, requires arterial pH and PCO_2 measurements.

C. Step 2: Determining Whether the Compensatory Response Is Appropriate

Primary perturbations in acid-base equilibrium elicit a predictable compensatory response designed to minimize the change in pH that would otherwise occur (Table 2). When the primary event is a change in serum [HCO_3^-], as in metabolic acidosis or alkalosis, the compensatory response is a change in PCO_2, brought about by a change in ventilation. In metabolic acidosis PCO_2 is reduced by hyperventilation; in metabolic alkalosis PCO_2 is increased by hypoventilation. When the primary event is a change in PCO_2, the acute compensatory response is titration of nonbicarbonate buffers, producing only a minor corrective change in serum [HCO_3^-]. With sustained changes in PCO_2, renal mechanisms are activated, leading to larger changes in serum [HCO_3^-]. This ''chronic'' compensatory response actually begins within 6–12 hours after the onset of hyper- or hypocapnia and is fully expressed within 48–72 hours. Hypercapnia leads to a compensatory response that increases serum [HCO_3^-], and hypocapnia leads to a response that decreases serum [HCO_3^-].

The compensatory responses are predictable, and rules of thumb have been created to allow an assessment of whether the magnitude of the response for a given perturbation is appropriate. This assessment is important because it allows one to make the diagnosis of a so-called ''mixed'' disorder, that is, the concomitant presence of two or more acid-base disturbances at the same time. Such mixed disorders require a different approach to treatment and are discussed later in this chapter and in Chapter 28.

Table 3 Magnitude of Expected Adaptive Responses: Rule of Thumb Formulas[a]

Metabolic acidosis:		Adaptive response: ↓ PCO_2
expected PCO_2	=	$40 - 1.3 \times (24 - [HCO_3^-])$
Metabolic alkalosis:		Adaptive response: ↑ PCO_2
expected PCO_2	=	$40 + 0.7 \times ([HCO_3^-] - 24)$
Respiratory acidosis:		Adaptive response: ↑ $[HCO_3^-]$
Acute:		
expected $[HCO_3^-]$	=	$24 + 0.1 \times (PCO_2 - 40)$
Chronic:		
expected $[HCO_3^-]$	=	$24 + 0.4 \times (PCO_2 - 40)$
Respiratory alkalosis:		Adaptive response: ↓ $[HCO_3^-]$
Acute:		
expected $[HCO_3^-]$	=	$24 - 0.2 \times (40 - PCO_2)$
Chronic:		
expected $[HCO_3^-]$	=	$24 - 0.4 \times (40 - PCO_2)$

[a] $[HCO_3^-]$ (in mEq/L) and PCO_2 (in mmHg) on the right-hand side of these formulas indicate the value in a given patient with either a metabolic or respiratory acid-base disorder.

Table 3 outlines the rules of thumb for the compensatory response to each of the major acid-base disorders. Many variations of these rules are available in various textbooks, but all are based on the same clinical observations. The rules presented here are chosen for their simplicity. With any rule of thumb, one should recognize that it is an approximation and gives no information about variability. As a caution, one should not diagnose the presence of a mixed disorder unless the measured PCO_2 (compensating for a metabolic disturbance) or $[HCO_3]$ (compensating for a respiratory disturbance) varies from the calculated value by more than 5 mmHg or mEq/L. For example, the expected PCO_2 in a patient with a serum $[HCO_3^-]$ of 10 mEq/L calculated by the rule of thumb for metabolic acidosis is 18 mmHg; $18 = 40 - 1.3 \times (24 - 10)$ (see formula 1 in Table 3). Using the caution mentioned above, one should not diagnose a mixed disorder in this instance unless the PCO_2 is less than 13 mmHg (respiratory alkalosis and metabolic acidosis) or greater than 23 mmHg (respiratory and metabolic acidosis).

D. Step 3: Determining the Cause

The remainder of this chapter is devoted to a discussion of the causes of acid-base disturbances and the tools needed for making a specific diagnosis. Two general tools deserve comment here—the anion gap and serum potassium concentration ($[K^+]$). These tools are especially useful in identifying the causes of metabolic acidosis and alkalosis.

1. Anion Gap

The anion gap is calculated as the difference between serum $[Na^+]$ and the sum of serum [Total CO_2] (or $[HCO_3^-]$) and $[Cl^-]$:

$$\text{Anion gap} = [Na^+] - ([\text{Total } CO_2] + [Cl^-]) \tag{3}$$

The anion gap is not really a difference in electrical charge, but reflects the normal presence of unmeasured anions in the serum. The normal value for the anion gap is often given as 12 mEq/L. With the newer autoanalyzer techniques, however, the mean value is 8–10 mEq/L. Because of the variability in the measurements that comprise the anion gap, one should not diagnose an increase in the anion gap unless the calculated value is greater than 16 mEq/L or a decrease unless the value is less than 4 mEq/L. An increase in the anion gap occurs when new unmeasured anions are present in the serum. The most common setting in which this occurs is an organic acidosis (see below). An increase can also occur in severe metabolic alkalosis. Whenever an acid-base disturbance is present, the anion gap should be calculated to help sort out its cause. The only setting in which a decrease in the anion gap occurs is when unmeasured cations are present in serum. This rarely occurs in some monoclonal gammopathies when a new cationic protein accumulates in the blood.

2. Serum $[K^+]$

The serum $[K^+]$ is characteristically increased in certain acid-base disorders and decreased in others. In patients with metabolic alkalosis, serum $[K^+]$ is virtually always low (<3.5 mEq/L), and this finding, coupled with an elevated serum [Total CO_2] often obviates the need for further evaluation (see later). In patients with metabolic acidosis, serum $[K^+]$ may be low, normal, or high, depending on the specific cause. As a result, assessment of the serum $[K^+]$ is extremely useful in sorting out the cause of the acidosis, particularly in the form associated with a normal anion gap. The role of this parameter is discussed further under each of the disorders below.

VI. METABOLIC ACIDOSIS

Metabolic acidosis is defined as a primary reduction in serum $[HCO_3^-]$, and is accompanied by a blood pH of <7.40. The causes of metabolic acidosis are

Table 4 Causes of Metabolic Acidosis

Increased anion gap	Normal anion gap
Diabetic ketoacidosis	Diarrhea
Starvation	Renal tubular acidosis
Alcoholic ketoacidosis	Carbonic anhydrase inhibitors
Lactic acidosis	
Intoxications	
Salicylates	
Methanol	
Ethylene glycol	
Paraldehyde	
Renal failure	

divided into two groups, depending on whether the anion gap is normal or increased (Table 4). The most common causes are discussed below.

A. Increased Anion Gap Metabolic Acidosis

The causes of metabolic acidosis with an increased anion gap are subdivided into (1) the organic acidoses, (2) certain ingestions, such as aspirin, methanol, and ethylene glycol, and (3) renal failure. The first two of these subdivisions are due to a runaway increase in organic acid production, and the last, to a failure to excrete the anions of strong acids that are formed as part of the normal end products of metabolism.

1. Diabetic Ketoacidosis

The metabolic acidosis that develops in patients with uncontrolled diabetes mellitus is caused by the runaway production of β-hydroxybutyric acid. This organic acid is oxidized to acetoacetic acid, so that in the steady state the ratio of β-hydroxybutyrate to acetoacetate in the plasma is 3–5. The H^+ that dissociates from these strong acids at the pH of the body fluids is rapidly buffered by HCO_3^-, and β-hydroxybutyrate and acetoacetate are the organic anions that replace HCO_3 in the serum and cause the increase in the anion gap. The presence of ketoacidosis can be rapidly uncovered by measuring serum ketones, and this measurement should be carried out in all patients with metabolic acidosis who have an increased anion gap. Normal serum has no detectable ketones. The serum ketone test only detects acetoacetate and ketones; it does not detect the presence of β-hydroxybutyrate. In rare instances the ratio of β-hydroxybutyrate to acetoacetate can be increased (e.g., when lactic acidosis is also present), and the serum ketone test can be negative despite the presence of ketoacidosis. In most instances, however, a negative test can safely exclude diabetic ketoacidosis as the cause of the increase in anion gap. The anions produced in diabetic ketoacidosis are excreted rapidly once sodium chloride is administered or ingested. As a result the ketone test can rapidly become negative. In such instances the anion gap also falls to normal.

2. Other Causes of Ketoacidosis

Starvation is associated with an increase in the production of ketoacids and with a mild metabolic acidosis. Typically, however, serum ketones are negative or only slightly positive with starvation, reflecting a much lower rate of production. A more severe metabolic acidosis can occur in so-called alcoholic ketoacidosis. This disorder occurs in heavy drinkers and typically occurs after a spree followed by starvation and vomiting. Excessive ketoacid production and impaired metabolism of ketoacids are responsible, but the serum ketones may not fully reflect the rate of accumulation because the ratio of β-hydroxybutyrate to acetoacetate is increased. Alcoholic ketoacidosis can usually be easily distinguished from diabetic ketoacidosis by history and by the fact that serum glucose levels are normal or low. This disorder is rapidly reversed by the administration of glucose.

3. Lactic Acidosis

Lactic acidosis is caused by the runaway production of lactic acid in amounts exceeding the ability of the body to metabolize this strong acid. This disorder most commonly arises in the setting of tissue hypoxia but can also develop in certain leukemias and when the drug metformin accumulates. In rare instances, no cause can be established. In lactic acidosis, serum ketones are negative and the diagnosis is confirmed by measurement of serum lactate.

4. Salicylate Intoxication

Toxic levels of aspirin cause a metabolic acidosis with an increased anion gap by increasing the production of a wide variety of organic acids. Serum ketones are negative, and lactate levels are typically not increased. Salicylate intoxication produces a unique acid-base disorder because it also stimulates ventilation directly. In fact, most adults who ingest excessive aspirin present primarily with a respiratory alkalosis (see later). When metabolic acidosis is present, it is usually combined with a respiratory alkalosis (see Sec. X). The diagnosis is usually made by measurement of blood salicylate levels.

5. Methanol/Ethylene Glycol Ingestion

Ingestion of either of these toxins leads to life-threatening metabolic acidosis, because their metabolic products are organic acids that accumulate in the body.

Methanol is metabolized to formic acid, and ethylene glycol to glyoxylic and oxalic acid. When these intoxications are suspected, the diagnosis must be made rapidly so that treatment can be initiated promptly (see Chapter 28). Serum ketones are negative, and blood lactate is normal. The diagnosis is made by measuring these substances in the blood. If such tests cannot be done rapidly, one should measure serum osmolality and compare the measured value to the calculated value. The difference, termed the osmolar gap, can identify the presence of an unmeasured solute in the blood.

$$\begin{aligned}\text{Osmolar gap} &= \text{serum osmolality (measured)} \\ &\quad - (2 \times [\mathrm{Na^+}] + \text{glucose}/18 + \text{BUN}/2.8)\end{aligned} \tag{4}$$

In this formula, the units of osmolality are mOsm/kg H_2O, $[Na^+]$ is in mEq/L, and glucose and BUN are in mg/dL. The normal value is 10 or less. The magnitude of the increase in the osmolar gap in intoxications is related to the molecular size of the toxin and its relative toxicity. With methanol, a low molecular weight toxin, the osmolar gap can rise to greater than 50. Ethylene glycol is a larger molecule and, as a result, usually only increases the osmolar gap to 15–25. The osmolar gap should not be confused with the anion gap, discussed earlier. With all intoxications that cause metabolic acidosis, the anion gap is increased and is typically 20–25 mEq/L.

B. Normal Anion Gap Metabolic Acidosis

When metabolic acidosis occurs without an increase in the anion gap, the chloride concentration is typically increased. Two major causes comprise virtually all of this form of metabolic acidosis (see Table 3). The first cause is HCO_3^- loss from the gastrointestinal tract (either pancreatic drainage or diarrhea), and the second is a selective defect in renal acid excretion or HCO_3^- reabsorption, termed renal tubular acidosis. When assessing patients with a normal anion gap acidosis, an additional tool that is sometimes useful in the diagnosis is the urinary cation gap:

$$\text{Urine cation gap} = \text{urine } [\mathrm{Na^+}] + [\mathrm{K^+}] - [\mathrm{Cl^-}] \tag{5}$$

In this formula, [X] is the concentration of each of the ion species of interest in a random urine sample. In a patient with metabolic acidosis, Eq. (5) should yield a value less than zero (the gap is typically greater than -20 mEq/L), reflecting the fact that $[NH_4^+]$ is a major cation that is excreted if renal acidification is normal. A value greater than zero reflects HCO_3^- loss in the urine and is a characteristic finding in certain forms of renal tubular acidosis.

1. Diarrhea

Most of the HCO_3^- secreted by the pancreas into the duodenum is reabsorbed by the end of the ileum, although about 30–40 mEq/day is normally lost in the stool, contributing to endogenous acid production. In most of the diarrhea seen in adults, no acid-base disturbance is present. However, diarrheal diseases that are associated with impaired ileal reabsorption can cause severe metabolic acidosis as a result of selective HCO_3^- loss. Cholera is the paradigm of such a diarrhea, and it is now known that cholera toxin specifically inhibits the cellular signal pathway for ileal HCO_3^- reabsorption. The acidosis due to selective HCO_3^- loss results in volume contraction with an associated increase in serum [Cl^-], so that the anion gap is usually not increased unless a lactic acidosis supervenes. Because large amounts of K^+ are also lost in diarrheal stools, serum [K^+] is characteristically low. The diagnosis is usually easily established by history and by the finding of a metabolic acidosis with a normal anion gap and hypokalemia. Urine pH is maximally acid (<5.5), and, when assessed, the urine cation gap is negative (see above).

2. Renal Tubular Acidosis

Renal tubular acidoses (RTAs) are caused by several defects in renal acid excretion and are categorized according to the specific defect (Table 5). Each of the major types is discussed below.

(a) Type 1 (Distal RTA). Although rare, this form of RTA is perhaps the best studied and understood. The disorder results from a hereditary or ac-

Table 5 Classification and Diagnostic Features of Renal Tubular Acidosis

	Associated features	Diagnostic clues
Type I (distal RTA)	Acidification defect Nephrocalcinosis Hypokalemia	Urine pH > 5.5 Creatinine normal Low [K^+] Nephrocalcinosis
Type II (proximal RTA)	HCO_3^- wasting associated with Fanconi syndrome	Urine pH < 5.5 unless HCO_3^- loaded Creatinine normal [K^+] normal or low Aminoaciduria
Type III	Acidification defect HCO_3^- wasting	
Type IV	Hypoaldosteronism Aldosterone resistance Impaired K^+ excretion Diabetes mellitus	Urine pH < 5.5[a] High [K^+] Creatinine > 1.5 mg/dL

[a] Except in patients with chronic obstructive nephropathy.

quired defect in H^+ secretion (most likely involving H^+-ATPase) in the medullary collecting duct. As a result, the kidney is unable to acidify the urine to the fullest extent. Urine pH is typically >5.5 and often is >6.0, despite systemic acidosis. This defect in H^+ secretion leads to acid retention (due to impaired excretion of ammonium), renal K^+ wasting (due to Na^+ reabsorption not counterbalanced by H^+ secretion), release of calcium from bone, and hypocitraturia. The latter problems promote the development of nephrocalcinosis and stone formation (see Chapter 21). These associated problems are useful in separating type 1 RTA from other causes of metabolic acidosis. The finding of an inappropriately high urine pH, hypokalemia, and nephrocalcinosis in a patient with a normal anion gap metabolic acidosis makes the diagnosis almost certain, and further workup is usually unnecessary. When measured, the urine cation gap (see above) is typically zero or greater, reflecting an inappropriately low rate of ammonium excretion. Type I RTA can occur as an inherited or sporadic isolated disorder. It can also occur in association with a wide variety of inherited or acquired tubulointerstitial diseases and after exposure to certain drugs and toxins, the most common being amphotericin B.

(b) Type 2 (Proximal RTA). Type 2 RTA is primarily a disease of children and only very rarely occurs in adults. In contrast to Type 1 RTA, collecting duct H^+ secretion is normal, but HCO_3^- reabsorption is impaired. Based on indirect observations the defect in reabsorption is presumed to occur in the proximal tubule, but this has not yet been proven for all patients with type 2 RTA. In individuals with type 2 RTA, serum $[HCO_3^-]$ rapidly falls to a level at which tubular reabsorption is complete and then renal acid excretion proceeds normally. Thus, urine pH is normally acid (<5.5) in the steady state, and bicarbonate wasting can only be demonstrated by administering this anion. When the defect is isolated no other laboratory abnormalities are present. More commonly, the defect in renal HCO_3^- handling is a part of the Fanconi syndrome and is accompanied by other defects in proximal tubular reabsorption including phosphate wasting, renal glycosuria, and aminoaciduria. In this clinical setting it is not necessary to bicarbonate load the patient to make the diagnosis. Patients with type 2 RTA should have a normal urinary cation gap. Hypokalemia is not usually a feature of type 2 RTA but develops rapidly when HCO_3^- is administered due to an increase in distal Na^+ delivery with unreabsorbed HCO_3^-. Type 2 RTA can occur either as an isolated defect or in association with other defects in tubular reabsorption. The disease can be inherited or occur sporadically and may develop in a wide variety of renal diseases, including nephrotic syndrome, multiple myeloma, amyloidosis, and Wilson's disease, or after exposure to certain drugs or toxins, including streptozotocin and toluene.

(c) Type 3 RTA. Type 3 RTA is a combined proximal and distal lesion and is often found in children with distal RTA.

(d) Type 4 RTA. Type 4 RTA is perhaps the most common form of RTA seen in adults and is characterized by the associated finding of hyperkalemia. Urine acidification is normal (pH < 5.5). Typically serum $[HCO_3^-]$ is only mildly reduced (to 17–20 mEq/L), and serum $[K^+]$ is 5.0–5.5 mEq/L. Type 4 RTA is caused by hypoaldosteronism or aldosterone resistance. In its most common form, it occurs in patients with mild to moderate chronic renal insufficiency (serum creatinine concentration 2–5 mg/dL). In these patients, renin and aldosterone levels are both low, and thus this syndrome is often termed hyporenin hypoaldosteronism. However, renin and aldosterone levels rarely need to be measured. The diagnosis is made by the finding of renal insufficiency, mild metabolic acidosis (with a normal anion gap), hyperkalemia, and a urine pH of <5.5. Much more rarely the disorder is caused by interference with the action of aldosterone due to a heredity defect in the mineralocorticoid receptor or the epithelial Na^+ channel.

VII. METABOLIC ALKALOSIS

Metabolic alkalosis is defined as a primary increase in serum $[HCO_3^-]$ and is accompanied by an alkaline arterial blood pH (>7.40). It is caused by the addition and abnormal retention of excess alkali in the body fluids. Because the kidney normally responds to an increase in serum $[HCO_3^-]$ by rapidly excreting this anion, sustained metabolic alkalosis by definition occurs only when some additional factor disrupts the normal renal response. The causes of metabolic alkalosis are divided into two groups: those that are correctable by chloride (and ECF volume) repletion and those that are resistant to this form of therapy. Hypokalemia is a feature of all forms of metabolic alkalosis, and its presence can be useful in separating this disorder from chronic respiratory acidosis (see later). The anion gap is usually normal in metabolic alkalosis but can be increased by the disorder is severe.

A. Chloride-Responsive Metabolic Alkalosis

The most common forms of metabolic alkalosis are induced by selective chloride loss from the body, either from the gastrointestinal tract or by the kidney. Chloride depletion alkalosis is almost always associated with some degree of volume depletion, and the combination of chloride and volume depletion induces changes in renal transport processes that lead to abnormal K^+ losses and hypokalemia. The alkalosis is sustained by the combination of chloride and K^+ losses and can rapidly be corrected by chloride and K^+ repletion. Table 6 presents a complete list of the causes. The two most common forms are described below.

Table 6 Causes of Metabolic Alkalosis

Chloride-sensitive	Chloride-resistant
Acid loss from stomach	Mineralocorticoid excess
Vomiting	Primary hyperaldosteronism
Nasogastric suction	Cushing's syndrome
	ACTH-secreting tumor
Diuretic administration	
Thiazides	Glucocorticoid-remediable hypertension
Metolazone	Adrenogenital syndromes
Chloride-depleting diarrhea	Apparent mineralocorticoid excess
Congenital	Licorice
Villous adenoma	Liddle's syndrome
	11β-Hydroxysteroid dehydrogenase deficiency
Recovery from chronic hypercapnia	
	Bartter's syndrome
	Gitelman's syndrome

1. Vomiting/Nasogastric Suction

Loss of HCl from the upper gastrointestinal tract as a result of either vomiting or nasogastric suction increases serum [HCO_3^-] and simultaneously depletes body chloride stores. The chloride losses sustain the metabolic alkalosis by altering renal transport processes, stimulating both H^+ and K^+ secretion into the tubular urine. In the steady state, the serum [HCO_3^-] is elevated, there is associated hypokalemia, and the urine pH is acid. With continued emesis or suction of the upper gastrointestinal tract, serum [HCO_3^-] can rise to very high levels and serum [Cl^-] can fall to very low levels. Bicarbonate levels as high as 80–90 mEq/L have been reported. This is the only form of metabolic alkalosis in which a serum [HCO_3^-] greater than 45 mEq/L can develop. Hypokalemia is a characteristic accompanying feature and the degree of hypokalemia is directly related to the severity of the alkalosis. Sodium and potassium chloride repletion rapidly corrects this disorder.

2. Diuretic Administration

Diuretic agents that specifically inhibit chloride-linked Na^+ reabsorption in the loop and early distal tubule are perhaps the most common causes of metabolic alkalosis. These agents are the loop diuretics (e.g., furosemide, bumetanide), which inhibit the $Na^+/K^+/2\ Cl^-$ transporter, and the thiazides, which inhibit the NaCl cotransporter. These diuretics all cause selective chloride depletion and stimulate H^+ and K^+ secretion. Because volume depletion limits the response of the kidney to these drugs, the degree of alkalosis engendered is also limited. Serum [HCO_3^-] is usually <36 mEq/L and rarely exceeds 40 mEq/L. Hypokalemia is always a prominent feature. Discontinuation of these agents and repletion of chloride and potassium losses corrects the alkalosis. In most cases the diuretic is needed for therapy, and partial correction is induced by KCl administration (see Chapter 28).

B. Chloride-Resistant Metabolic Alkalosis

Chloride-resistant metabolic alkalosis is caused by factors that alter distal tubular H^+ and K^+ transport, independent of chloride depletion. The causes can be subdivided further into those caused by mineralocorticoid excess and those that are the result of primary tubular abnormalities in transport. The most common cause is primary hyperaldosteronism.

1. Primary Hyperaldosteronism

Autonomous aldosterone secretion, due either to an adenoma or to adrenal hyperplasia, produces a characteristic clinical syndrome. The syndrome includes hypertension due to sodium retention, hypokalemia, and metabolic alkalosis (see Chapter 9). In primary hyperaldosteronism the metabolic alkalosis is usually very mild (serum [HCO_3^-] 30–33 mEq/L), and the most striking abnormality is hypokalemia. The serum [K^+] is often <3.0 mEq/L. The volume expansion that is sustained by renal Na^+ retention ensures the continued delivery of excess Na^+ to the distal nephron promoting continued K^+ losses. The metabolic alkalosis is blunted by the volume expansion, which promotes some renal bicarbonate loss. In the steady state urine chloride excretion reflects dietary chloride intake and urine chloride concentration is typically greater than 30–40 mEq/L on a standard North American diet. Persistence of the alkalosis is independent of chloride intake.

2. Other Forms of Mineralocorticoid Excess

A group of much rarer disorders can produce a syndrome identical to that described above for primary aldosteronism. Cushing's syndrome and certain malignant tumors that produce ACTH ectopically can cause the same syndrome. An extremely rare form of hypertension, glucocorticoid remediable aldosteronism, is the result of a genetic mutation that causes aldosterone to be secreted in response to ACTH rather than angiotensin II.

3. Apparent Mineralocorticoid Excess Syndromes

Several newly characterized hereditary abnormalities in distal tubular transport produce a syndrome indistinguishable from primary hyperaldosteronism (i.e., hypertension, hypokalemia, and chloride-resistant metabolic alkalosis) in which serum aldosterone levels are low rather than high. One such genetic defect results in a loss of the ability to downregulate the Na^+ channel in the cortical collecting duct (Liddle's syndrome). A second is a defect that inactivates a critical enzyme associated with the aldosterone receptor, resulting in the receptor being activated by cortisol as well as aldosterone. The metabolic alkalosis seen with heavy licorice use is similar in pathogenesis to the latter genetic defect. These abnormalities can be distinguished from mineralocorticoid excess by the finding of extremely low aldosterone levels.

4. Bartter's and Gitelman's Syndromes

Bartter's and Gitelman's syndromes are rare hereditary disorders manifested by chloride-resistant metabolic alkalosis and hypokalemia, but without hypertension. Bartter's syndrome is usually manifest during childhood and appears to be due to a variety of mutations, all of which have the effect of impeding the chloride-linked Na^+ transporter in the loop of Henle (the $Na^+/K^+/2\,Cl^-$ transporter). Thus, Bartter's syndrome mimics the effect of furosemide. It induces chloride depletion but is paradoxically chloride resistant because the intake of excess chloride is unable to repair the problem caused by the defective loop transport system. Gitelman's syndrome is a milder defect, often not manifest until adulthood, due to a mutation that inactivates the NaCl cotransporter in the early distal tubule. Thus, this disorder mimics the effect of the thiazide diuretics. Both are associated with mild metabolic alkalosis and moderate to severe hypokalemia. They are differentiated by their effects on calcium and magnesium metabolism. Gitelman's syndrome is associated with hypocalciuria and hypomagnesemia, whereas Bartter's syndrome is not.

C. Alkali Administration

The administration of alkali does not normally produce a sustained metabolic alkalosis because the excess alkali is usually excreted rapidly. Nonetheless, it can be a contributing factor in certain circumstances. In patients who are either potassium or chloride depleted, administration of alkali (or alkali precursors such as lactate or acetate) can induce or worsen metabolic alkalosis. In patients with renal insufficiency (either acute or chronic), administration of excess alkali can cause a sustained alkalosis if the alkali cannot be excreted due to a low GFR. Milk-alkali syndrome is an example of the latter problem. This disorder is caused by the concomitant intake of sodium bicarbonate and excess calcium. The alkalinization promotes calcium precipitation, causing renal damage, and the disease is then perpetuated by continued alkalinization and further precipitation of calcium salts.

VIII. RESPIRATORY ACIDOSIS

Respiratory acidosis is caused by CO_2 retention and is manifest by the combination of an increase in PCO_2 and a reduction in pH. The adaptive response to hypercapnia and acidemia is an increase in serum $[HCO_3^-]$. This response occurs as a result of buffer reactions acutely and of renal acid excretion when the hypercapnia is sustained for more than 12–24 hours. Table 3 summarizes the expected adaptive increase in serum $[HCO_3^-]$ for a given increase in PCO_2 in acute and chronic respiratory acidosis. Chronic respiratory acidosis induces an elevation of serum $[HCO_3^-]$ that mimics the pattern seen in metabolic alkalosis. A distinguishing feature, however, is the absence of hypokalemia. To differentiate the two disorders conclusively, measurement of blood pH is necessary. Respiratory acidosis is caused by disorders that impair alveolar ventilation, including upper and lower airway obstructive diseases, restrictive lung disease, central hypoventilation, and neuromuscular disease.

IX. RESPIRATORY ALKALOSIS

Respiratory alkalosis is caused by alveolar hyperventilation and is manifest by a reduction in arterial PCO_2 and an increase in arterial pH. The adaptive response to this hypocapnia and alkalemia is a reduction in serum $[HCO_3^-]$, acutely as a result of body buffer reactions and chronically (when the hypocapnia is sustained for more than 24 hours) by a reduction in renal bicarbonate reabsorption and acid excretion. Table 3 summarizes the expected adaptive reduction in serum $[HCO_3^-]$ for a given reduction in PCO_2 in acute and chronic respiratory alkalosis. The reduction in $[HCO_3^-]$ that occurs with sustained hypocapnia is sufficient to mimic the electrolyte pattern seen in metabolic acidosis. The two disorders can only be differentiated conclusively by measuring arterial pH. In uncomplicated chronic respiratory alkalosis the pH is always greater than 7.40.

A wide variety of diseases and physiological states can cause hyperventilation (Table 7). Respiratory alkalosis is a byproduct of the adaptive hyperventilation induced by hypoxemia. A reduction in PCO_2 occurs when arterial PO_2 falls below approximately 60 mmHg. Hyperventilation and chronic respiratory alkalosis is a normal finding in pregnancy, with PCO_2 falling to 28–30 mmHg in the third trimester. The hyperventilation is stimulated by progesterone, but the reasons for this adaptation are unclear. More commonly, respiratory alkalosis is encountered in severely ill patients with pulmonary injury (e.g., pulmonary embolism) or with central nervous system disease. The disorder is also a feature of sepsis (particularly with gram-negative organisms) and of hepatic failure. Certain drugs can also induce hyperventilation, the best known of these being salicylates.

Table 7 Causes of Respiratory Alkalosis

Hypoxemia
CNS disorders
Cerebrovascular accidents
Infection
Trauma
Tumors
Pulmonary disease
Pulmonary embolism
Pneumonia
Pulmonary edema
Asthma
Interstitial lung disease
Septicemia
Hepatic failure
Pregnancy
Drugs
Salicylates
Nicotine
Xanthines
Progesterone
Anxiety-hyperventilation syndrome

Acute respiratory alkalosis is usually evident to both the patient and the examining physician. Arterial PCO_2, PO_2, and pH should always be measured, however, in the patient who comes to medical attention because of a sudden increase in ventilatory effort. Hypoxemia or metabolic acidosis should always be excluded as the cause of hyperventilation before assuming that anxiety is responsible. Sustained respiratory alkalosis, by contrast, is an often overlooked disorder because appreciation of prolonged hyperventilation on physical examination is difficult. Arterial PCO_2 can be reduced to 30 mmHg if minute ventilation in increased by only 50%, a change that can be achieved without much effort and not be noticed by either the patient or the examining physician. The diagnosis should be suspected in the appropriate clinical setting (see Table 7) when the serum $[HCO_3^-]$ is reduced.

X. MIXED DISORDERS

More than one acid-base disorder can be present at one time. Salicylate intoxication, for example, can cause a combined respiratory alkalosis (by directly stimulating ventilation) and metabolic acidosis (by increasing organic acid production). In most instances, the rules of thumb in Table 3 (see Sec. V.D) can be used to diagnose the presence of a mixed disorder. These rules allow one to determine whether the secondary adaptive response to a given acid-base disorder is in the expected range. If not, then one can conclude that an independent stimulus is operating to alter PCO_2, in the case of a metabolic acid-base disorder, or serum $[HCO_3^-]$, in the case of a primary respiratory disorder. For example, a patient with a serum $[HCO_3^-]$ of 12 mEq/L would be expected to have an arterial PCO_2 of approximately 25 mmHg. If the measured PCO_2 is 35 mmHg, such a finding would indicate an impairment in alveolar ventilation as well and would be defined as a combined metabolic and respiratory acidosis. Perhaps the most common mixed acid-base disturbance is the combination of chronic respiratory acidosis and metabolic alkalosis, the latter induced when diuretics are used to treat cor pulmonale.

The rules of thumb allow the identification of mixed metabolic and respiratory disorders, but some patients can present with a mixed metabolic alkalosis and acidosis. This mixed disorder may develop, for example, in someone with severe nausea and vomiting for several days, who eventually becomes sufficiently volume depleted to develop a superimposed lactic acidosis. Such disorders can be identified by the delta anion gap calculation. This calculation begins with the assumption that the normal anion gap is 12 mEq/L and uses the following formula:

$$\begin{aligned}\text{Preacidosis serum } [HCO_3^-] &= \text{measured } [HCO_3^-] \\ &\quad + (\text{measured anion gap} - 12)\end{aligned} \qquad (6)$$

This calculation is based on the second assumption that the increase in anion gap in a given patient is precisely equivalent to the decrement in serum $[HCO_3^-]$ caused by the addition and retention of acid in the body fluids. Both assumptions are clearly not completely correct, and wide latitude must be given before one makes the assumption that this type of mixed acid-base disorder is present. Thus, the calculated preacidosis serum $[HCO_3^-]$ should always be greater than 31–32 mEq/L before making this diagnosis. However, the disorder should be clearly evident, for example, in the patient who presents with a serum $[HCO_3^-]$ of 18 mEq/L and an anion gap of 30 mEq/L.

Rarely, three acid-base disorders can be present at the same time, termed a "triple disorder." The most common example of such a triple disorder is combined metabolic acidosis and alkalosis coupled to an inappropriate degree of hyperventilation, and thus respiratory alkalosis. In all patients presenting with acid-base disorders, one should use information from the history and physical examination as well as the rules outlined in this chapter to make the appropriate diagnosis. The symptoms associated with these disorders are discussed in Chapter 4, and management of these disorders is discussed in Chapter 28.

SUGGESTED READINGS

Bushinsky D, Coe FL, Katzenberg C, Szidon JP, Parks JH. Arterial PCO_2 in chronic metabolic acidosis. Kidney Int 22:311–314, 1982.

Gabow PA. Disorders associated with an altered anion gap. Kidney Int 27:472–483, 1985.

Gennari FJ. Respiratory acidosis and alkalosis. In: Narins R, ed. Clinical Disorders of Fluid and Electrolyte Metabolism, 5th ed. New York: McGraw Hill, 1994, pp 957–990.

Gluck SL. Acid-base. Lancet 352:474–479, 1998.

Ishihara K, Szerlip HM. Anion gap acidosis. Semin Nephrol 18:83–97, 1998.

Kassirer JP, Schwartz WB. The response of normal man to selective depletion of hydrochloric acid. Am J Med 40:109–118, 1966.

Rimmer JM, Gennari FJ. Metabolic alkalosis. J Intensive Care Med 2:137–150, 1987.

Valtin H, Gennari FJ. Acid-Base Disorders. Boston: Little Brown, 1987.

Weinberger SE, Schwartzstein RM, Weiss JW. Hypercapnia. N Engl J Med 321:1223–1231, 1989.

12
Diagnosis of Tonicity Disorders

Alan S. Segal
University of Vermont, Burlington, Vermont

I. INTRODUCTION

Disorders of salt and water balance are among the most common problems encountered in clinical medicine. It is of utmost importance that these two broad categories be distinguished both physiologically and clinically to prevent confusion between total body sodium (or salt) content and sodium concentration. In the context of this chapter, the term "salt" refers to isotonic saline stores, while "water" refers to solute-free water. Some of the clinical and laboratory distinctions between "salt" and "water" are outlined in Table 1. The normal setpoint for total body salt content is that necessary for normal clinical volume status (euvolemia), while that for water is to have exactly zero net solute-free water with respect to normal tonicity. Solute-free water is defined as the amount of excess water present (positive free water) or water deficiency present (negative free water) to move body tonicity away from the normal value.

Body tonicity is tightly regulated around a setpoint of about 285 mOsm/kg (range: 280–290 mOsm/kg). The homeostatic mechanisms regulating tonicity are:

1. Water gain motivated by the brain and mediated via the GI tract (e.g., thirst → drinking)
2. Water retention signals initiated by the brain and accomplished by the kidney (e.g., exert antidiuretic hormone effect)
3. Water loss (e.g., suppress antidiuretic hormone effect)

Processes that interfere with any of these mechanisms can lead to disturbances of body tonicity. The net gain of water will produce hypotonicity, while net loss of water will lead to hypertonicity.

Table 1 Salt and Water: Clinical and Laboratory Distinctions

	SALT	WATER
	Volume Regulation	*Free Water Regulation*
What is being sensed?	Effective circulating volume	Plasma tonicity
Normal setpoint	Euvolemia	Isotonicity
Sensors	Baroreceptors (e.g., atrial)	Osmoreceptor (hypothalamus)
Effectors	Sympathetic nervous system Renin-Ang II-aldosterone Natriuretic peptides Antidiuretic hormone	Thirst Antidiuretic hormone
What is affected?	Sodium reabsorption Sodium excretion	Free water intake via thirst ADH-dependent free water retention or excretion by the kidney

The clinical relevance of water balance disorders is largely referable to (1) changes in intracellular volume, (2) the cell's volume regulatory response and adaptation to the altered tonicity, and (3) the cellular response to therapeutic interventions. Brain cells constrained within the fixed cranium are at highest risk. Resultant symptoms span the entire neurological spectrum from asymptomatic to comatose (see Chapter 4). Therapeutic complications, which can be catastrophic, include cerebral edema with herniation (during treatment for hypertonicity) and the osmotic demyelination syndrome (during treatment for hypotonicity).

Abnormalities in isotonic saline stores result in either hypovolemia or hypervolemia. It is important to emphasize that ''salt'' problems may occur independently of a ''water'' (tonicity) problem, and vice versa. That is, a patient with a volume disorder may have only that amount of water necessary to make the solute stores isotonic and therefore does not have a water disorder. ''Salt'' is the major determinant of extracellular volume status and is assessed by physical examination. For example, the diagnoses of hypovolemic shock (decreased isotonic saline stores) or hypervolemic edema (increased isotonic saline stores) do not require laboratory studies, just an in assessment of clinical volume status. In this regard it is important to understand that a hypovolemic patient on physical exam is not ''dehydrated'' unless laboratory studies also indicate coexistent hypertonicity. In contrast, ''water'' is the major determinant of intracellular volume status, such that an increase in solute-free water causes cellular swelling without producing a detectable change in clinical volume status. A measurable change in the concentration of any solute (not just extracellular sodium) will also occur.

Abnormalities in water balance are usually first detected clinically by abnormalities in serum sodium concentration. As a result, such abnormalities have traditionally been referred to as ''hyponatremia'' or ''hypernatremia.'' This tradition has created confusion between disorders of sodium content and sodium concentration. I have proposed using the term ''hyperaquaemia'' as an unambiguous alternative for ''hyponatremia'' and the term ''hypoaquaemia'' as an unambiguous alternative for ''hypernatremia.'' Hyperaquaemia and hypoaquaemia focus attention on both the pathophysiological abnormalities in water balance and also indicate that water restriction or administration is the appropriate therapy. In this chapter, the pathogenesis and clinical presentation of the ''dysaquaemias'' are reviewed. Chapter 29 reviews the treatment of these disorders.

II. WATER BALANCE AND REGULATION OF PLASMA TONICITY

Plasma tonicity is controlled by the ability to sense thirst and gain access to water, coupled with the kidney's ability to conserve or excrete water appropriately (see Table 2). Obligate water losses are replaced by water intake, and any water excess is promptly excreted by the kidney to maintain plasma tonicity at a normal level (zero net solute-free water) in the steady state. Disorders of tonicity generally result from a defect in water excretion, although abnormalities of thirst, water intake, and solute excretion can also be pathogenic.

Table 2 Water Balance[a]

	Obligate Daily Water Losses	Totals for 70 kg
Insensible losses via skin and lungs	~10 mL/kg	~700 mL/day
Sensible losses		
Gastrointestinal	~0.6 mL/kg	~ 42 mL/day
Renal	~10 mL/kg	~700 mL/day
Total obligate water loss	~20.6 mL/kg	~1440 mL/day
	Typical Daily Water Intake	**Totals for 70 kg**
Water content of food	~17 mL/kg	~1190 mL/day
Fluid intake	~25 mL/kg	~1750 mL/day
Total typical water intake	~42 mL/kg	~2940 mL/day

Typical Urine Output = Total typical water intake − Total obligate water loss = 2940 − 1440 = 1500 mL/day for a 70-kg person

[a] Based on an obligate solute load of 10 mOsm/kg per day = 700 mOsm/day for 70-kg person. Assumes a maximal urine osmolality of 900 mOsm/kg.

Water losses can be separated into insensible (via skin and lungs) and sensible (via the gut and kidney) components. Usual insensible loss is about 10–15 mL/kg/day, and sensible loss is about 0.6–1 mL/kg/day (gut) plus ~10 mL/kg/day excreted by the kidney. For a 70-kg person, the total water loss is therefore about 1.5 L/day (about 1 mL/min). Over the day, the resultant slight elevation in plasma osmolality stimulates both thirst and the release of antidiuretic hormone (ADH). Thirst provides the drive for water intake that replaces the loss, while ADH allows the kidney to conserve this water by concentrating the urine.

A. Renal Water Handling

There are four requirements for normal regulation of water balance by the kidney (see Fig. 1 and Table 3):

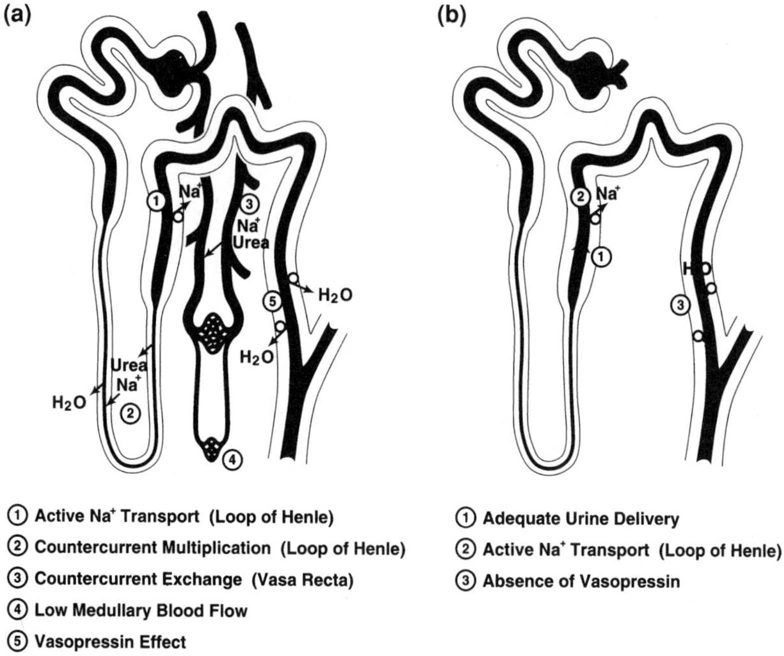

Figure 1 Requirements for maximal water reabsorption (a) and water excretion (b) along the nephron. Both processes depend on (i) adequate delivery of filtrate out beyond the proximal tubule, (ii) intact solute transport without water in the loop of Henle to simultaneously dilute the urine and concentrate the interstitium, and (iii) ability of ADH to either exert a maximal effect to remove water from the urine (a) or to be fully suppressed to maximize water excretion (b).

Table 3 Requirements for Optimal Renal Water Handling

For maximal free water excretion
1. Deliver adequate filtrate to the concentrating/diluting segments beyond the proximal tubule
A problem in renal hypoperfusion or insufficiency
2. Intact function of the concentrating/diluting segments
Ability to separate solute from water to "create" free water
A problem if transport is inhibited by drugs or renal injury
3. Ability to maximally suppress ADH effect
A problem with certain drugs and paraneoplastic syndromes
For maximal free water reabsorption
1. and 2. as above
3. Ability to maximally stimulate ADH secretion
A problem if the posterior pituitary fails to produce enough (central DI)
4. Normal responsiveness of the ADH-sensitive segments of the distal nephron
A problem if anything is wrong with the V_2 receptor, intracellular signal transduction system, or trafficking pathways for the AQP2 water channel, or the AQP2 water channel itself (congenital or acquired nephrogenic DI)

1. Adequate delivery of filtrate to the concentrating/diluting segments of the nephron; a problem in states of renal hypoperfusion or insufficiency
2. Normal function of these nephron segments with the ability to separate solute from water so that free water can be "created" and excreted or conserved as needed; a problem if transport is inhibited by diuretics or renal insufficiency
3. Ability to maximally suppress the release and effect of ADH in order to excrete water; a problem in states of nonosmotic release of ADH (e.g., syndrome of inappropriate ADH), and the ability to maximally stimulate ADH; a problem if the posterior pituitary is damaged as in central diabetes insipidus
4. Normal responsiveness of the ADH-sensitive segments of the collecting duct; a problem in acquired and congenital nephrogenic diabetes insipidus (see later)

B. Antidiuretic Hormone (Vasopressin)

Once released into the blood, the antidiuretic action of vasopressin is mediated through binding to its receptor (the V_2 receptor) in the basolateral membrane of the ADH-responsive cells along the collecting duct. Binding of ADH to the V_2 receptor initiates an intracellular signaling pathway that increases the permeability of the collecting duct to water by inserting water channels into the apical membrane (Fig. 2). The ADH-sensitive water channel protein is aquaporin 2 (AQP2). In addition to the acute regulation of AQP2 by ADH, long-term regulation of water permeability is influenced by the total amount of AQP2 in the cells. Loss-of-function mutations or downregulation of AQP2 may be a feature common to hereditary and acquired forms of urinary concentrating defects (e.g., nephrogenic diabetes insipidus), respectively. Conversely, upregulation of AQP2 may play a key role in the pathogenesis of urinary diluting defects and water retention states (e.g., SIADH, decompensated heart or liver failure).

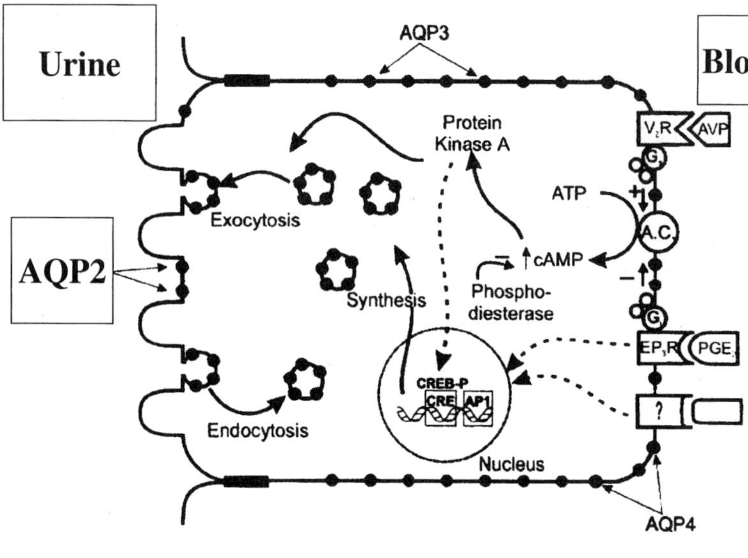

Figure 2 Regulation of water permeability in collecting duct principal cells by aquaporins (AQP). AQP2 is the vasopressin-sensitive water channel that is inserted into the apical (urine) membrane of the cell depending on the level of vasopressin (AVP). In the absence of AVP, most AQP2 water channels are localized to intracellular vesicles, which promotes excretion of a dilute urine. In contrast, AVP in the blood binds to the G-protein (G_s) coupled V_2 receptor (V_2R) and activates adenylate cyclase (A.C.), which catalyzes the production of cAMP and activates the cAMP-dependent protein kinase A (PKA). PKA phosphorylation of AQP2 water channels causes the vesicles to fuse with the apical membrane (exocytosis), greatly increasing apical water permeability, resulting in water reabsorption. The water permeability of the basolateral membrane is always high due to the constitutive presence of AQP3 and AQP4 water channels. When AVP levels fall (and presumably after AQP2 becomes dephosphorylated), AQP2 water channels are retrieved from the apical membrane via endocytosis. Long-term regulation of aquaporins, most notably through a cAMP response element (CRE) and binding protein (CREB), appears to be clinically relevant in a number of conditions including CHF, cirrhosis, DI, and SIADH. (Adapted from Marples et al., 1999.)

C. Regulation of Cell Volume

Maintenance of cell volume is crucial for normal cell functions and is therefore highly regulated. Cells swollen due to hypotonicity will try to restore their volume back towards normal by getting rid of low-molecular-weight solutes (termed osmolytes), a process that allows water to leave the cell down its concentration gradient. Conversely, cells shrunken due to hypertonicity will try to restore their volume back towards normal by taking up osmolytes, a process that allows water to enter the cell down its concentration gradient. Inorganic osmolytes such as Na^+, K^+, and Cl^- can be transported into or out of the cell within seconds or minutes following a change in cell volume. Organic osmolytes are ''nonperturbing'' solutes, including myoinositol, sorbitol, amino acids, and methylamines. In contrast to inorganic osmolytes, volume regulatory accumulation or removal of organic osmolytes is a relatively slow process, usually requiring hours or days to complete. In hypotonic states, swelling activates the passive efflux of organic osmolytes within seconds, but downregulation of their synthesis and uptake is a slow process. In hypertonic states, shrinkage-activated accumulation of organic osmolytes is slow because synthesis of new organic molecules is required, and this activity requires gene transcription and translation. These time-dependent changes in cell volume regulation have clinical implications both for the symptoms associated with disorders of tonicity (see Chapters 4 and 29) and for the treatment of tonicity disorders (see Chapter 29).

III. ASSESSMENT OF TONICITY

The gold standard in diagnosing a tonicity disorder is to assess the effective osmoles, i.e., those osmoles that cause water movement across cell membranes. Whether an osmole is ''effective'' depends not only on what it is, but also where it is. For example, urea is an ineffective osmole in plasma but is a key effective osmole in concentrating the urine. Unfortunately, a convenient method for measuring tonicity is not available, but we can easily measure osmolality, which is an appropriate surrogate if one understands its limitations. Osmolality is a measure of the total number of solutes in a solution regardless of whether they effect water movement across cell membranes. If exogenous osmoles have not been added to the body:

$$\begin{aligned}&\text{Plasma osmolality (mOsm/kg } H_2O)\\&\quad\cong 2 * [Na^+] \text{ (mEq/L)} + [\text{glucose}]/18 \text{ (mg/dL)}\\&\qquad + [\text{BUN}]/2.8 \text{ (mg/dL)}\end{aligned} \tag{1}$$

Although osmolality is a measure of both effective osmoles (usually extracellular ions and sugars) and ineffective osmoles, the latter (e.g., urea) can often be independently measured and subtracted:

$$\text{Plasma tonicity (mOsm/kg } H_2O) = \text{measured plasma osmolality} - [\text{BUN}]/2.8 \text{ (mg/dL)} \quad (2)$$

Because urea is an ineffective osmole in plasma, patients with isolated elevations in BUN (e.g., acute or chronic renal failure) will have a high plasma osmolality but will have no symptoms of dysaquaemia because they remain isotonic.

Alternatively, under most circumstances, plasma tonicity can be calculated:

$$\text{Plasma tonicity (mOsm/kg } H_2O) \cong 2 * [Na^+] \text{ (mEq/L)} + [\text{glucose}]/18 \text{ (mg/dL)} \quad (3)$$

The second term in this equation has two effects on water balance. First, accumulation of glucose (or any other sugar that is an effective osmole such as mannitol) draws water out of cells, simultaneously dehydrating the intracellular compartment and increasing the volume of the extracellular compartment. Second, hyperglycemia leads to glycosuria and a consequent osmotic diuresis, resulting in loss of solute-free water. The approach to assessing the water deficit present in hyperglycemic states is discussed in Chapter 29. Changes in the first term of the above equation are due to changes in water balance, which is the focus of this chapter.

IV. DISORDERS OF THIRST

Osmoreceptors for thirst are localized to the organum vasculosum of the lamina terminalis (OVLT) in the posterior fossa of the brain. This is an area where the blood-brain barrier is discontinuous, which allows fluctuations in body tonicity to be sensed rapidly. The osmoreceptors controlling ADH release are also in the OVLT but are distinct from thirst osmoreceptors.

A. Hypodipsia

Defective thirst (hypodipsia) is a relatively rare disorder that is due to loss of osmoreceptor function. Lesions involving both sets of osmoreceptors (thirst and ADH release) may cause both primary hypodipsia and central diabetes insipidus (see Table 4). Damage to the OVLT may be seen in association with CNS inflammation, tumors, granulomata, trauma, and congenital or degenerative abnormalities. Occlusion of the anterior communicating artery is an important vascular etiology. In severe cases patients will present with symptoms and signs of hypertonicity (e.g., neurological irritability) in addition to those associated with the underlying process. Milder cases may just present with laboratory evidence of hypertonicity (e.g., an elevated serum $[Na^+]$). These patients may have a shift in the threshold of their thirst response and come into a new steady state at a higher

Table 4 Disorders of Water Intake and Causes of Hypertonicity

I. Inadequate water intake (without increased water losses)
   A. Defective thirst or osmoreceptor
      1. Primary hypodipsia: congenital abnormality, idiopathic
      2. Secondary hypodipsia: brain tumors, granuloma, trauma, inflammation, degeneration, occluded anterior communicating artery
   B. Impaired access to water
      1. No source or supply of water: lost in the desert or at sea
      2. Inability to communicate thirst: infants, cognitive impairments (acute or chronic), stroke with expressive aphasia, coma, endotracheal intubation

II. Increased water losses (without adequate water intake)
   A. Extrarenal losses
      1. Insensible (skin and respiratory): increased with fever and hyperventilation states
      2. Skin: sweating
      3. Gastrointestinal: vomiting, diarrhea, laxatives
   B. Renal losses
      1. Normal ADH function: osmotic diuresis (e.g., hyperglycemia, mannitol)
      2. Diabetes insipidus (DI): central DI, congenital or acquired nephrogenic DI, gestational DI

III. Gain of hypertonic solutions
   A. Iatrogenic: hypertonic $NaHCO_3$, NaCl, or mannitol
   B. Accidental ingestion: inadvertent switching of salt for sugar in infant formula
   C. Deliberate (or forced) ingestion: hypertonic emetics or cathartics, ingesting salt without adequate water

plasma tonicity. The absence of thirst differentiates these patients from those with diabetes insipidus.

B. Hyperdipsia (Polydipsia)

Two major types of excess water intake are primary polydipsia and psychogenic polydipsia. Primary polydipsia (also known as dipsogenic polydipsia) is due to defective osmoregulation of thirst, which can be idiopathic or develop in association with CNS diseases (e.g., trauma, multiple sclerosis, tuberculous meningitis, neurosarcoid) or drugs (e.g., lithium therapy). Psychogenic polydipsia (i.e., compulsive water drinking) is much more common and is seen in association with severe emotional or cognitive dysfunction. The thirst center is normal in patients with psychogenic polydipsia, but there is no easy way to test this function and some experts do not distinguish primary from psychogenic polydipsia. The polyuria in primary polydipsia is usually modest and constant over time. In contrast, patients with psychogenic polydipsia often have huge and variable urine flow rates. In extreme cases, their water intake exceeds the maximal rate of solute-free water excretion of the kidney, and hypotonicity supervenes (see later).

V. HYPERTONICITY

Hypertonicity virtually never occurs in an alert adult with (1) a normal thirst mechanism and (2) access to water. Primary hypodipsia, the rare exception to this rule, was discussed above.

A. Increased Water Losses

Conditions associated with excessive free water loss place patients at increased risk of hypertonicity, especially if thirst and/or access to water become impaired (see Table 4). Excess insensible loss (i.e., severe sweating) is usually self-limited and rarely causes severe hypertonicity. Gastrointestinal losses of more free water than solute (e.g., severe diarrhea due to infection or osmotic agents such as lactulose) will increase tonicity and should stimulate both thirst (water intake) and ADH (water retention), but can lead to hypertonicity if intake is impaired or fails to keep pace with losses.

1. Osmotic Diuresis

A major function of the kidney is reabsorption of isotonic solute and water. When nonreabsorbable solutes (e.g., mannitol) are filtered, they provide an osmotic gradient promoting lumenal water entry and inhibiting its reabsorption, resulting in unregulated free water losses into the urine. This ''osmotic'' diuresis will result in hypertonicity if water intake fails to keep up with losses.

Patients with diabetic ketoacidosis (DKA) often present with hypertonicity (and hypovolemia) from increased extrarenal losses (e.g., vomiting) and an osmotic diuresis due both to glycosuria and ketonuria. It is worth mentioning that the convention adopted in this chapter avoids potentially confusing terminology with regard to DKA. For example, the elevated extracellular glucose (an effective osmole) causes water to move out of cells, diluting solutes (including sodium) in the extracellular space. Sodium concentration decreases by approximately 1.6 mmol/L per 100 mg/dL increase in glucose, even though body tonicity is normal or high. A concise description of tonicity, e.g., hypertonic or hypoaquaemic, effectively avoids this problem.

2. Diabetes Insipidus

There are four types of diabetes insipidus (DI): (1) central (neurogenic), (2) renal (nephrogenic), (3) gestational, and (4) dipsogenic (discussed above). Gestational

DI results from the rapid breakdown of ADH due to placental vasopressinase. In most gravid females, an increased rate of secretion keeps pace with metabolism, but occasionally diabetes insipidus occurs, manifest by symptomatic polyuria that improves with ADH analog but not with water deprivation. The remainder of this section will briefly address central and nephrogenic DI.

(a) Central Diabetes Insipidus. Central diabetes insipidus (CDI) results from defective release of ADH from the neurohypophysis. Familial CDI is due to mutations in the gene encoding ADH, usually with an autosomal dominant inheritance. Acquired CDI is due to traumatic injury to the neurohypophysis or pituitary or to certain tumors. Without ADH, solute-free water generated in the loop of Henle is excreted, resulting in a large volume of dilute urine. For example, the obligate daily solute load of ~600 mOsm can be excreted in 0.5 L when the urine is maximally concentrated (1200 mosm/kg), but excretion of the same solute load in the absence of ADH may require ≥12 L if the urine is maximally dilute (≤50 mosm/kg).

Unlike patients with dipsogenic DI who are polyuric because they drink, patients with CDI are polydipsic because they are polyuric. Despite this difference in pathophysiology, there is no difference in serum tonicity if thirst is normal and the patient has access to water. Obviously, water deprivation is not indicated in patients with CDI except for initially making the diagnosis in a monitored setting.

(b) Nephrogenic DI. Conditions associated with an insufficient or absent effect of ADH on V_2 receptors in the distal nephron compromise the ability to concentrate the urine. The inability to optimally transport free water due to abnormalities in renal tubule signal transduction (i.e., functional ADH resistance) results in loss of free water and is known as nephrogenic diabetes insipidus (NDI). NDI can be congenital or acquired.

FAMILIAL NDI. Two types of familial NDI have been described. The most common form is due to a defect in the gene encoding the V_2 receptor. Less often, familial NDI is due to a defect in the gene that encodes the ADH-sensitive water channel, aquaporin 2 (AQP2). The former type is X-linked recessive (affected males and usually asymptomatic carrier females), and the latter is autosomal dominant. Many different mutations have been described in the genes encoding these proteins. Other forms of familial NDI are now being discovered that involve defects in the postreceptor signaling and trafficking systems required for proper insertion and retrieval of otherwise normal AQP2 water channels.

ACQUIRED NDI. Acquired NDI can occur as result of chemical, metabolic (e.g., hypokalemia, hypercalcemia), vascular, infectious, granulomatous (e.g., sarcoid), infiltrative (e.g., amyloid), or malignant renal insults that compromise the AQP2 signaling pathway. Chronic tubulointerstitial renal disease (e.g., sickle cell disease, polycystic kidney disease) or partial obstruction (and post obstructive diuresis) are also associated with defective free water conservation.

Lithium is the most common drug-induced cause of NDI. Up to 20% of individuals receiving this drug have symptomatic polyuria, and defects in urinary concentrating ability can be detected in approximately half. Lithium causes NDI by entering and accumulating in principal cells of the distal nephron and interferes with ADH-induced cAMP production, thereby reducing AQP2 expression in the cell membrane. Lithium can cause hyperparathyroidism, and PTH can also act to decrease ADH-induced cAMP production. In patients who have taken lithium for long periods of time, NDI is often irreversible.

HYPERCALCEMIA. Hypercalcemia is the most common metabolic abnormality associated with acquired NDI. Steady-state calcium concentrations exceeding 11 mg/dL produce a urinary concentrating defect that appears to affect the capacity of the thick ascending loop of Henle to concentrate the interstitium and also interfere with the action of ADH on the collecting tubule. Although the underlying mechanisms have not been completely elucidated, recent studies suggest that the calcium-sensing receptor plays a key role.

B. Impaired Access to Water

Hypertonicity in adults is usually associated with impairment in requesting or gaining access to water, especially in the setting of increased water losses. Common examples include chronically debilitated patients with co-morbid states (e.g., dysphasia following a stroke) and patients on mechanical ventilators during the diuretic recovery phase of acute renal failure. This problem is aggravated in patients with water losses or impaired ADH release or effect, for example, polyuria resulting from the inability to concentrate the urine in diabetes insipidus. Likewise, some elderly persons develop a decrease in the osmotic stimulation of thirst (i.e., the plasma tonicity at which thirst is stimulated is higher than in younger individuals). This change, combined with an age-related decrease in urinary concentrating capacity, places the elderly at increased risk of developing hypertonicity. In particular, patients in nursing homes with neurological impairment are at increased risk for problems with water access. Such patients are also more likely to require additional free water because they are often receiving diuretics, have increased incidence of fever and infection, and may be victims of inadequate care or neglect.

The development of hypertonicity in hospitalized patients is quite common (incidence up to 3–4% of inpatients) and is associated with a mortality rate of 40–60%. In a large retrospective study, hypertonicity (with [Na] $>$ 150 mEq/L) was identified in 3.5% of patients. Only 60% of these patients had hypertonicity on presentation; the remaining 40% developed the problem in hospital. The overall mortality was 50%. Another study demonstrated that almost 90% of patients that develop hypertonicity in the hospital had water access problems. Of those with water access problems, three quarters had less than 1 L of oral water intake per day and almost all had received less than 1 L of free water intravenously.

C. Gain of Hypertonic Solutions

Administration of hypertonic solutions has the potential to increase tonicity and produce negative free water balance. From the perspective of tonicity, the addition of hypertonic solutions to the body can be viewed as equivalent to giving a "dose of negative free water." Indeed, this is the basis for their role in the emergency treatment of symptomatic hypotonicity (see Chapter 29). Oral intake of hypertonic solutes is an everyday occurrence that almost never has significant consequences, again because of the primary defense mechanism of thirst coupled with the ability of the kidney to retain water while excreting the excess solutes. Thus, hypertonicity from the administration or intake of hypertonic solutions is extremely rare. An exception is the patient who has defective thirst mechanisms or who cannot signal their thirst to others. For example, infants have little control over their intake and depend on caretakers to provide proper fluid intake. Despite an ostensibly normal thirst mechanism, infants inadvertently fed high-solute formula have developed fatal hypertonicity.

Large doses of sodium bicarbonate given during resuscitation often produce at least transient hypertonicity. For example, six ampules of sodium bicarbonate (50 mEq/50 mL ampule) adds about 600 effective mOsm to the body, which in a 70 kg man (42 L of total body water) will acutely increase tonicity from 285 to nearly 297 mOsm/kg H_2O. Although this will potently stimulate the release of ADH, hypertonicity will persist if the patient has impaired mental status and is unable to ask for water.

VI. HYPOTONICITY

Hypotonicity is usually due to a defect in water excretion. Three key processes are required to excrete any excess water in the body (see Fig. 1): (1) adequate delivery of solute and water to the concentrating/diluting segments of the nephron (i.e., beyond the proximal tubule), 2) normal function of these segments, and 3) the ability to maximally suppress ADH secretion. Problems excreting a water load occur when any of these key processes are disrupted. Such disruptions may occur in the following settings:

1. States of renal hypoperfusion
2. Decreased GFR

3. Diuretics (especially thiazides) acting in the loop and distal nephron
4. The syndrome of inappropriate ADH secretion/effect due to drugs or paraneoplastic syndromes

Before considering these disorders in detail, the entities of pseudohyponatremia and hyponatremia associated with hypertonicity induced by fluid shifts between body compartments are addressed.

A. Pseudohyponatremia

This term is used to describe a measurement artifact, a reduction in measured serum [Na^+] that does not reflect an actual change in body tonicity in vivo. In this type of ''hyponatremia,'' serum tonicity is normal. Plasma is normally comprised of 93% water and 7% lipids and proteins, so that a [Na^+] of 143 mEq/L in whole plasma actually represents a [Na^+] of 154 mEq/L (i.e., 143/0.93) in plasma water (the same as the [Na^+] of 0.9% isotonic saline). Pseudohyponatremia may occur with severe hyperlipidemia or hyperproteinemia when serum [Na^+] is measured by flame photometry. In these conditions the proportion of plasma comprised of water is reduced. Therefore, when [Na^+] is assessed using flame photometry the value is low because this method measures the concentration in the total volume. Serum [Na^+] falls by ~1 mEq/L for each 460 mg/dL rise in plasma lipids. A direct measurement of osmolality rather than [Na^+] remains accurate because large lipid or protein molecules have negligible effects on the total osmolality of plasma.

This artifact is not a concern when serum [Na^+] is measured with an ion-selective electrode, the method now used in virtually all clinical laboratories in the United States. However, in some laboratories (particularly for stat measurements) the ion-specific electrode technique is used on prediluted specimens instead of on whole blood. Only the [Na^+] measured using an ion-specific electrode on whole blood is accurate in the setting of hyperlipidemia or hyperproteinemia.

B. Hyponatremia Caused by Transcellular Water Movement (Hyperglycemia)

Regardless of the technique used, hyperglycemia lowers serum [Na^+] in the face of a normal or increased serum tonicity because glucose is a low molecular weight solute that increases tonicity in the extracellular compartment and thereby causes a shift of water out of cells. Due to this shift, the measured [Na^+] decreases by about 1.6 mEq/L for each 100 mg/dL rise in plasma [glucose] despite the increase in tonicity. A similar picture may develop during bladder irrigation with glycine-containing solutions or with mannitol therapy if the effective osmole accumulates in the serum. Note that a direct measurement of osmolality or calculation of tonicity will reveal a hypertonic state and eliminate the potential confusion in interpreting the low [Na^+] in these settings.

VII. WATER-EXCRETING DEFECTS

A defect in water excretion can occur whenever blood flow to the kidney is compromised. Clinically, this develops most often in the setting of (1) extracellular volume depletion (i.e., hypovolemia) and (2) states in which there is a decrease in effective circulating volume (e.g., decompensated congestive heart failure, liver failure, and some forms of nephrotic syndrome). See Table 5 for a list of disorders associated with renal hypoperfusion.

Table 5 Causes of Hypotonicity: Hypovolemic and Hypervolemic States

I. True Extracellular Volume Depletion with Renal Hypoperfusion and Physiological ↑ ADH Release
   A. Extrarenal losses of salt and water replaced by water alone
      1. Gastrointestinal: nasogastric suction, vomiting, diarrhea, bleeding
      2. Skin: burns, severe or prolonged sweating (e.g., ultramarathon runners), cystic fibrosis
      3. "Third space": perioperative losses, severe pancreatitis, peritonitis, burns
   B. Renal losses of salt and water replaced by water alone
      1. Diuretics: especially thiazides
      2. Hypoaldosteronism: primary adrenal insufficiency
      3. Renal Na^+ wasting: cerebral salt wasting syndrome, proximal renal tubular acidosis with bicarbonaturia, ↑ atrial natriuretic peptide release, Bartter's syndrome, Gitelman's syndrome
II. Decreased Effective Arterial Flow with ↓ Renal Perfusion and Physiological ↑ ADH Release
   A. Hypervolemic states with peripheral and/or pulmonary edema and/or ascites: $U_{Na} < 20$ mEq/L
      1. Congestive heart failure (decompensated)
      2. Liver failure (e.g., end-stage cirrhosis with portal hypertension)
      3. Nephrotic syndrome with hypoalbuminemia and salt overload
      4. Renal failure with edema
   B. Hypervolemia with hypertension
      1. Acute or chronic renal failure: $U_{Na} > 20$ mEq/L
      2. Bilateral renal artery stenosis: "hyponatremic-hypertensive syndrome": $U_{Na} < 20$ mEq/L

A. Extracellular Fluid Volume Depletion

In any setting in which ECF volume is decreased by more than 10–15%, renal water excretion becomes compromised and hypotonicity will develop if sufficient solute-free water is ingested or administered. The defect is due both to intrarenal factors (i.e., decreased delivery of solute to the diluting segment and collecting duct) and to volume depletion–induced stimulation of ADH secretion. Most commonly this form of hypotonicity develops with gastrointestinal losses (diarrhea or vomiting) followed by increased thirst and water ingestion.

B. Edematous States

Hypotonicity in edematous states indicates excess total body solute-free water in addition to total body salt overload (see Table 5). The development of this form of hyperaquaemia is usually due to a worsening in the underlying pathophysiology.

1. Congestive Heart Failure

The early and compensated phases of congestive heart failure (CHF) are associated with hypervolemia and edema formation, but not with a defect in tonicity regulation. One functional indicator of decompensation in patients with CHF is hypotonicity, due to positive water balance superimposed on positive salt balance. Water retention occurs both through impairment of urinary diluting ability (due to decreased delivery of sodium beyond the proximal tubule) and secretion of ADH. Coupled with this defect in water excretion is an increase in thirst, due at least in part to increased levels of angiotensin II, leading to increased water intake. The sustained presence of hypotonicity is an ominous finding in CHF.

2. Hepatic Failure

As in the case of CHF, patients with compensated cirrhosis may retain salt, but tonicity regulation is normal. When ascites begins to form, however, water excretion becomes impaired both due to low delivery of sodium to the diluting segments and secretion of ADH. The low-flow hemodynamic state of decompensated liver failure is similar to that of decompensated CHF, although the predominant effector in the latter is a primary loss of pressure (due to pump failure), while in the former the underlying cause is loss of resistance (due to vasodilation). As in CHF, elevated angiotensin II levels can stimulate thirst and therefore water intake.

3. Nephrotic Syndrome

Hypotonicity occurs much less often in patients with the nephrotic syndrome than with CHF or cirrhosis, but the mechanisms are the same. When it occurs, the water retention is due to decreased effective circulating volume (secondary to hypoalbuminemia in this instance) and elevated ADH levels. In patients with renal insufficiency, the mechanism discussed below also contributes.

4. Chronic Renal Insufficiency

Patients with chronic renal insufficiency have a decreased capacity for water excretion due simply to a decrease in delivery of urine to the diluting segment. The requirement of the remaining nephrons to excrete sodium may further limit urinary dilution. Typically, hypotonicity is not a problem until the GFR is markedly reduced. For example, if GFR is 10 mL/min (14 L/day) and about 30% of the filtered load is delivered out beyond the proximal tubule, the maximum urine output will be ~4 L/day. Moreover, the urine in this setting is typically isotonic to plasma due to obligate salt losses. In such a patient, hypotonicity will probably develop if more than 2–3 L/day of solute-free water is ingested. In the patient with no renal function, hypotonicity will develop if solute-free water intake exceeds insensible and gastrointestinal water losses.

C. Diuretic-Induced Hypotonicity

The most common cause of hypotonicity is impaired water excretion due to therapy with a loop or thiazide diuretic. In most instances the hypotonicity is mild and reflects the combination of renal hypoperfusion (e.g., the cause of the edema-forming state that led to the use of diuretics), increased thirst, dietary salt restriction, and diuretic-induced impairment of urinary dilution.

Severe hypotonicity can occur in association with the thiazide diuretics, with the highest frequency and severity in elderly women. Thiazide-induced hypotonicity can develop rapidly (within 24–48 hr) and result in death, so a heightened awareness of this complication is appropriate. The pathophysiology of this disorder is not completely clear but probably involves an increase in water intake coupled with thiazide-induced impairment of urinary dilution. The disorder is confined to the thiazide group of diuretics, and this difference is thought to be due to the fact that, in contrast to the loop diuretics, these agents block urinary dilution but not urinary concentrating ability.

There is no effective way to screen for those at risk for this rare complication. However, patients (and especially elderly women) treated with thiazides should not receive any other drugs that might further impair water excretion or stimulate thirst and/or ADH (e.g., nonsteroidal anti-inflammatory drugs). In any case, patients placed on diuretics (especially thiazides) should have their electrolytes monitored closely during the first 3 weeks of therapy.

D. Syndrome of Inappropriate Antidiuretic Hormone Secretion

The syndrome of inappropriate antidiuretic hormone (SIADH) occurs when (1) ADH release from the posterior pituitary cannot be completely suppressed, (2) ADH or ADH-like substances are produced outside the posterior pituitary (i.e., ectopic production by tumors), or (3) the effect of ADH at the level of the kidney is exaggerated. Any of these circumstances will result in retention of solute-free water, promoting positive water balance and hypotonicity. The causes of the SIADH are listed in Table 6.

SIADH due to excess release and/or insufficient suppression of AVP from the posterior pituitary may occur with central nervous system (CNS) disorders, pulmonary processes, endocrine disorders, and with certain drugs.

1. CNS Disorders

SIADH has been reported to occur in a wide variety of CNS disorders, including stroke, seizures, aneurysms, trauma (e.g., hemorrhage, hematoma), infections (e.g., meningitis, encephalitis, brain abscess), brain tumors, vasculitis, acute psychosis, and diseases of uncertain etiology like multiple sclerosis and Guillain-Barré syndrome. The differential diagnosis of hypotonicity in patients with CNS disorders includes the cerebral salt-wasting syndrome, which must be distinguished from SIADH (see later).

2. Pulmonary Processes

Pulmonary processes associated with SIADH include pneumonia, tuberculosis, lung abscess, mechanical trauma (e.g., pneumothorax and positive-pressure ventilation), acute ventilatory failure, cystic fibrosis, and AIDS. Patients suffering from AIDS may also have opportunistic CNS or pulmonary infections. In AIDS patients admitted with an opportunistic infection, almost a third are hypotonic, and most are found to have SIADH.

3. Endocrine Disorders

(a) Hypothyroidism. Patients with hypothyroidism have a diminished capacity for free water excretion. The dominant mechanism, especially in severe cases, is a reduction in GFR. In addition, ADH levels are increased in hypothyroid patients. The cause of the increase in ADH (or failure to suppress the secretion of this hormone in the face of hypotonicity) is unclear.

Table 6 Causes of Hypotonicity: Clinical Euvolemia with ↑ Water Intake and/or ↑ ADH Release/Effect

A. Primary increase in water intake
 1. Primary polydipsia
 2. Psychogenic polydipsia: may also involve changes in thirst, osmostat, and ↑ ADH release/effect
B. Renal failure with net positive water balance
C. Syndrome of inappropriate antidiuretic hormone (SIADH)
 1. Ectopic production by tumors (paraneoplasia): e.g., small cell bronchogenic carcinoma, many others
 2. Pulmonary disease: pneumonia, tuberculosis, asthma, pneumothorax, acute respiratory failure, cystic fibrosis
 3. CNS processes: infections, tumors, trauma, subarachnoid hemorrhage, stroke, Guillain-Barré syndrome, multiple sclerosis, acute psychosis
 4. Drugs potentiating the release and/or effect of ADH
  Sulfonylureas: chlorpropamide, tolbutamide
  Anticonvulsants: carbamazepine, oxcarbamazepine
  Psychotropic agents: phenothiazines (thioridazine, fluphenazine), haloperidol, tricyclic antidepressants (amitryptyline, nortriptyline, desipramine), SSRIs (fluoxetine, sertraline)
  Antineoplastics: cyclophosphamide, ifosfamide, vincristine
  Analgesics: narcotics, nonsteroidal anti-inflammatory drugs, acetaminophen
  Others: clofibrate, ''ecstacy''
  Drugs with ADH-like properties: 8-arginine vasopressin (AVP), 1-deamino-8-D-arginine vasopressin (dDAVP), oxytocin
 5. Stress: emotional or physical (e.g., pain, major surgery)
 6. Glucocorticoid deficiency: cortisol exerts negative feedback on the release of both corticotrophin-releasing factor and ADH; deficiencies of corticotrophin or cortisol rapidly ↑ ADH release
  Primary adrenal insufficiency: cortisol deficiency
  Secondary adrenal insufficiency: corticotrophin deficiency
 7. Hypothyroidism: decreased water excretion may be due to ↓ cardiac output that leads to both ↓ distal delivery and ↑ ADH release; thyroid replacement corrects the water excretion defect
 8. HIV infection
 9. Psychosis
 10. Perioperative hyponatremia
 11. ''Idiopathic''
  Occult tumor (e.g., small cell bronchogenic cancer)
  Temporal arteritis (especially in the elderly)
  Reset osmostat

(b) Adrenal insufficiency. Hypotonicity is the most common electrolyte abnormality seen in patients with adrenal insufficiency. As with any volume-depleted state, GFR and distal delivery decrease and nonosmotic release of ADH is stimulated, both of which impair water excretion, resulting in hypotonicity if water intake continues. It is important to emphasize that cortisol secretion normally inhibits both the synthesis and secretion of ADH. Therefore, even relatively euvolemic patients with cortisol deficiency may develop hypotonicity due to inadequate suppression of ADH.

4. Drugs

(a) ADH-Like Drugs. Obviously, drugs that have intrinsic antidiuretic properties can cause SIADH (see Table 6). The major ADH-like drugs are 8-arginine vasopressin, 1-deamino-8-D-arginine vasopressin (dDAVP, desmopressin), and oxytocin. Patients with central diabetes insipidus taking dDAVP, which is more potent and longer acting than vasopressin, must carefully regulate their water intake to avoid hypotonicity.

(b) Sulfonylureas. Chlorpropamide and tolbutamide cause hypotonicity in up to 7% of patients (severe in 2%) by amplifying the effect of ADH on collecting duct water permeability. Interestingly, this complication does not occur with the newer sulfonylureas such as glyburide and glipizide. These agents actually increase water excretion and are preferable, especially in diabetics with congestive heart failure.

(c) Anticonvulsants. Carbamazepine and oxcarbamazepine may also potentiate the effect of ADH on the kidney. These agents rarely cause clinically significant hypotonicity.

(d) Psychotropic Agents. Phenothiazines, fluphenazine, tricyclic antidepressants, haloperidol, and selective serotonin reuptake inhibitors (e.g., fluoxetine, sertraline) have all been rarely associated with hypotonicity. It is important to remember that psychosis itself can stimulate release of AVP.

(e) Antineoplastic Agents. Cyclophosphamide, especially at high intravenous doses, may potentiate the effect of ADH on the kidney. Hypotonicity is a special problem with this drug because it is usually given with large amounts of free water. Ifosfamide is a related drug that can also cause the syndrome. Vincristine can cause SIADH by a direct effect on the neurohypophysis, and vinblastine may do the same.

(f) Analgesics. Opiates (morphine, meperidine) cause release of AVP in rats, but direct evidence for this in humans is rather scant. Indeed, effects of narcotics on ADH release in humans vary from stimulation to inhibition.

(g) Clofibrate. This triglyceride-lowering agent has been reported to cause SIADH in much the same way as chlorpropamide.

(h) "Ecstasy." Hypotonicity is associated with the hallucinogen 3,4-methylenedioxy-methamphetamine (3,4-MDMA or "ecstasy"). At least 3 deaths from cerebral edema occurred in the first 15 reported cases. The postulated mechanism is SIADH due to drug-induced vasopressin secretion, although there is some controversy.

5. Ectopic ADH Production

SIADH due to ADH or ADH-like substances produced outside the posterior pituitary may occur in association with a wide variety of tumors. The first description of SIADH was due to ectopic ADH production in two patients with bronchogenic carcinoma. Since that time, ectopic ADH production has been observed in association with a wide variety of carcinomas, lymphomas, sarcomas, and mesotheliomas, although lung cancer remains the most common etiology.

E. Diagnostic Criteria for SIADH

To make the diagnosis of SIADH, the hypotonic patient must be clinically euvolemic. Therefore, blood pressure should be normal or increased without any postural changes and the patient should have no edema. Recall that these patients actually have a slight increase in ECF volume due to the retained water, which is manifested by an increase in GFR. Serum creatinine, BUN, and uric acid should all be normal or low. Surreptitious polydipsia can be excluded by the finding that the urine is not maximally dilute (i.e., specific gravity greater than 1.005 or urine osmolality greater than 100 mOsm/kg H_2O). Although not required for the diagnosis, a urine $[Na^+]$ of >20 mEq/L supports the finding that the patient is euvolemic. However, it should be noted that in the steady state urine $[Na^+]$ will just reflect sodium intake. Other disorders associated with water excretion defects—cardiac, liver, thyroid, adrenal, and renal diseases—must all be excluded. Moreover, the patient should not be taking any medications known to interact with water metabolism independent of ADH (e.g., thiazides). Measurement of serum ADH levels is not helpful because ADH may be increased in other disorders associated with a water-excreting defect (e.g., ECF volume depletion).

F. Other Causes of Dysregulation of ADH Secretion

1. Perioperative Hyperaquaemia

Hypotonicity following surgery is a complication that can have a disastrous outcome. Typically, the syndrome develops in the first 48–72 hours after surgery, and serum [Na^+] may fall rapidly to levels of <110 mEq/L. Cerebral edema with generalized convulsions and ventilatory arrest are commonly the first indications that hypotonicity is present. Although gender may not determine who gets POH, the outcome appears to be much worse in women of childbearing age. Prepubertal children of both genders are also at increased risk.

Key factors in the pathogenesis of POH are (1) perioperative administration of hypotonic solutions, (2) nonosmotic stimuli for ADH release (e.g., nausea, pain, stress, drugs), (3) volume depletion, (4) specific procedures (e.g., transurethral resection of the prostate, gynecological procedures, orthopedic surgery, and transsphenoidal surgery), and (5) predisposing risk factors (e.g., menstruant women, preoperative use of thiazides or nonsteroidal anti-inflammatory drugs, intraoperative use of oxytocin to treat bleeding). The syndrome can be avoided if hypotonic solutions are not administered in the postoperative period.

2. Reset Osmostat

In some patients with hypotonicity, water balance, when tested, appears to be normal. Such patients maintain salt and water balance, but they do so around a serum tonicity that is clearly lower than normal. This phenomenon is a normal feature of pregnancy. The osmotic thresholds for both thirst and ADH release each decrease by ~10 mOsm/kg within the first few weeks after conception, possibly due to an effect of chorionic gonadotropin and relaxin. This ''parallel'' shift in osmostats leads to increased water intake that results in ''permissive'' hyperaquaemia until the tonicity once again falls below the thirst threshold. As a result, serum [Na^+] decreases by ~5 mEq/L during pregnancy. The osmostat resets to normal in the postpartum period. With the exception of normal pregnancy, most patients with a ''reset osmostat'' have a debilitating illness such as tuberculosis, quadriplegia, malnutrition, or cancer. Because they can excrete excess water when they are below their ''setpoint,'' these patients typically have a stable mild hypotonicity and are not at risk for developing symptoms of water intoxication.

3. Hypotonicity Associated with Inadequate Solute Intake

The daily urine solute load sets the upper limit on urine volume in the face of excess water intake. Normal individuals ingesting a typical Western diet usually produce 10–15 mOsm/kg body weight per day resulting in an obligate solute load of 600–900 mOsm per day. Excretion of this solute load in a maximally dilute urine (50–60 mOsm/kg H_2O) allows for a urine volume of 10–15 L/day, well in excess of the volume of water normally ingested. However, individuals consuming primarily beer (''beer potomania'') or ingesting a high water, low protein diet may have very low solute loads. Although these individuals can excrete a maximally dilute urine, the total amount of water they can excrete is limited by the lack of solute. For example, a solute load of <240 mOsm per day will lower the maximal urine flow rate to less than 4 L per day. Hypotonicity is unavoidable if more than this volume of water is ingested. Beer drinkers and so-called "tea and toasters" are at highest risk to develop hypotonicity on this basis.

4. Hypotonicity Associated with Sports and Exercise

Hypotonic sweat losses during exercise typically lead to mild hypertonicity that stimulates thirst and ADH release. However, the sodium content of sweat increases at higher rates of sweating, and if these volume losses are replaced only with water, hypotonicity may develop. Severe hypotonicity has been reported to occur particularly during intensive events such as ultramarathons. Although the pathogenesis is not known with certainty, replacement of extrarenal salt and water losses with water alone probably plays a key role. Stress and volume related release of ADH is likely to be a contributing factor, impairing the ability of the kidney to excrete the excess water rapidly. Although less common than hypertonicity, hypotonicity is a greater threat to the life of these athletes.

5. Hypotonicity in the Neurosurgical Patient: The Cerebral Salt Wasting Syndrome

The course of patients suffering head injuries, brain tumors, stroke, intracranial infections, and subarachnoid hemorrhage (SAH) is not infrequently complicated by hypotonicity. Up to one third of patients with SAH may develop hypotonicity. Although hypotonicity in the setting of head trauma is often associated with increased ADH release, under certain circumstances it may be a result of the cerebral salt wasting syndrome (CSWS). Although not proven, this disorder is thought to arise as a result of the secretion of a natriuretic peptide from the damaged brain (brain natriuretic peptide, BNP). A working definition of the CSWS is ECF volume depletion and hypotonicity as a direct result of the renal loss of NaCl. This disorder is most often seen in patients with acute neurological or neurosurgical crises. CSWS is sometimes difficult to separate from SIADH; indeed, some experts in the field dispute whether CSWS actually exists. However, most agree that it is a separate entity and that one should attempt to distinguish it from SIADH because the approach to therapy is quite different (see Chapter 29). The critical distinction is that ECF volume is reduced in CSWS and normal or slightly increased in SIADH. Therefore, treatment with isotonic saline will correct the hypotonicity in CSWS but may exacerbate it in SIADH.

G. Clinical Approach to Hypotonicity

In most clinical settings, the laboratory finding of a low serum [Na^+] first suggests the diagnosis of hypotonicity. The first step in assessment is to calculate plasma tonicity [see Eq. (3)] or measure serum osmolality and correct for urea [see Eq. (2)]. If serum [Na^+] is measured by the electrode technique on whole blood, one need not be concerned about pseudohyponatremia and serum osmolality does not need to be measured. If the calculated tonicity is low, then the patient has a water excretion defect. The following diagnostic steps will in most instances lead to the cause of the hypotonicity:

1. Assess clinical volume status. If the patient is volume depleted, isotonic saline should correct the hypotonicity.
2. If the patient is edematous, further diagnostic attention should be directing at seeking the cause of the edema and correcting the underlying problem if possible.
3. If the patient is neither volume-depleted nor edematous (i.e., is euvolemic), assess serum creatinine concentration to determine whether renal failure is present.
4. If renal function is normal and the patient is euvolemic, carefully review medications to determine whether a drug-induced cause of hypotonicity is present.
5. If no drug can be implicated, then a primary dysregulation of ADH is likely the cause. Consider the diseases associated with SIADH, reset osmostat, and the relationship to surgery.

Therapy for the specific causes of hypotonicity is discussed in detail in Chapter 29.

SUGGESTED READINGS

Ashraf N, Locksley R, Arieff AI. Thiazide-induced hyponatremia associated with death or neurologic damage in outpatients. Am J Med 70:1163–1168, 1981.

Bartter FC, Schwartz WB. The syndrome of inappropriate secretion of antidiuretic hormone. Am J Med 42:790–806, 1967.

Deen PM, Verdijk MA, Knoers NV, Wieringa B, Monnens LA, van Os CH, van Os BA. Requirement of human renal water channel aquaporin-2 for vasopressin-dependent concentration of urine. Science 264:92–95, 1994.

Gennari FJ. Current concepts. Serum osmolality. Uses and limitations. N Engl J Med 310: 102–105, 1984.

Goldman MB, Luchins DJ, Robertson GL. Mechanisms of altered water metabolism in psychotic patients with polydipsia and hyponatremia. N Engl J Med 318:397–403, 1988.

Harrigan MR. Cerebral salt wasting syndrome: a review. Neurosurgery 38:152–160, 1996.

Lang F, Busch GL, Ritter M, Völkl H, Waldegger S, Gulbins E, Häussinger D. Functional significance of cell volume regulatory mechanisms. Physiol Rev 78:247–306, 1998.

Marples D, Frokiaer J, Nielsen S. Long-term regulation of aquaporins in the kidney. Am J Physiol 276:F331–339, 1999.
McManus ML, Churchwell KB, Strange K. Regulation of cell volume in health and disease. N Engl J Med 333: 1260–1266, 1995.
Nielsen S, Kwon TH, Christensen BM, Promeneur D, Frokiaer J, Marples D. Physiology and pathophysiology of renal aquaporins. J Am Soc Nephrol 10:647–663, 1999.
Oelkers W. Hyponatremia and inappropriate secretion of vasopressin (antidiuretic hormone) in patients with hypopituitarism. N Engl J Med 321:492–496, 1989.
Palevsky PM, Bhagrath R, Greenberg A. Hypernatremia in hospitalized patients. Ann Intern Med 124:197–203, 1996.
Papadakis MA, Fraser CL, Arieff AI. Hyponatraemia in patients with cirrhosis. Q J Med 76:675–688, 1990.
Peters JP, Welt LG, Sims EAH, Orloff J, Needham J. A salt wasting syndrome associated with cerebral disease. Trans Assoc Am Physicians 63:57–64, 1950.
Robertson GL. Syndrome of inappropriate antidiuresis. N Engl J Med 321:538–539, 1989.
Rose BD. New approach to disturbances in the plasma sodium concentration. Am J Med 81:1033–1040, 1986.
Schrier RW. Pathogenesis of sodium and water retention in high-output and low-output cardiac failure, nephrotic syndrome, cirrhosis, and pregnancy (2). N Engl J Med 319:1065–1072, 1127–1134, 1988.
Schrier RW, Howard RL. Unifying hypothesis of sodium and water regulation in health and disease. Hypertension 18:III164–168, 1991.
Schwartz WB, Bennett W, Curelop S, Bartter FC. A syndrome of renal sodium loss and hyponatremia probably resulting from inappropriate secretion of antidiuretic hormone. Am J Med 23:529–542, 1957.
Segal AS. Salty language is confusing. Hosp Pract (Off Ed) 31:81–84, 1996.

13
Diagnosis of Disorders of Potassium Balance

James A. Strom and Geetha Narayan
St. Elizabeth's Medical Center and Tufts University School of Medicine, Boston, Massachusetts

John T. Harrington
Tufts University School of Medicine, Boston, Massachusetts

I. INTRODUCTION

Total body potassium content is approximately 2500–5000 mEq (35–55 mEq/kg). About 90% of the total is within cells and less than 0.5% is within the plasma. Daily potassium metabolism can be summarized as consisting of oral or intravenous intake, absorption into an extracellular space of about 14 L, partial uptake into a larger intracellular space, and ultimate near-total excretion into the urine. About 10% of the total intake is excreted in stool and sweat. Hypo- and hyperkalemia can result from derangements in intake, abnormal shifts into and out of cells, or derangements in excretion. Clinically, excesses or deficits in excretion are of greatest importance.

II. NORMAL INTAKE AND BALANCE

Typical western diets provide 50–100 mEq of K^+ daily. Great variation exists, however, with some poor diets providing 25 mEq/day or less and diets rich in certain fruits and vegetables containing several hundred mEq/day. After absorption, variable degrees of cellular potassium uptake (''redistribution'') take place. Factors influencing cellular uptake include insulin, catecholamines (β-adrenergic stimulation promoting K^+ entry and α-adrenergic stimulation inhibiting K^+ entry), serum potassium concentration, abnormalities of acid-base status, and plasma osmolality. Normally, ingested potassium is balanced by excretion in the urine, with small contributions from sweat and fecal excretion. Large potassium loads produce slight rises in serum K^+ concentration ($[K^+]$) and significant transfer to the intracellular space. This potassium is slowly released and excreted over several hours.

A. Intracellular Stores

The intracellular space is not only twice as large as the extracellular space, but its K^+ concentration is much higher: 130–150 versus 3–5 mEq/L. It thus has the capacity to buffer potassium deficits or excess without life-threatening changes in serum $[K^+]$. By contrast, relatively small changes in serum $[K^+]$ often betray large changes in total body potassium. A reduction in serum $[K^+]$ from 4 to 3 mEq/L typically reflects a deficit of 200–400 mEq, and a reduction to 2 mEq/L, a deficit of 600–800 mEq. The capacity to buffer excess potassium is more limited; an increase in serum $[K^+]$ to 5 mEq/L typically reflects an increase in total body potassium of 100–200 mEq. However, many factors affect transcellular K^+ distribution and may alter these relationships (see later).

B. Renal Excretion

Potassium is freely filtered by the glomerulus, reabsorbed in the proximal tubule and Henle's loop, and its ultimate excretion fine-tuned by secretion or further reabsorption in the distal tubule and collecting duct. Secretion of K^+ is accomplished by specialized cells, termed principal cells, in the collecting duct and can increase, sometimes up to >400 mEq/day, in response to increased intake. When potassium stores are depleted, urinary K^+ loss can be limited to about 20 mEq/day by reabsorption of K^+ by different specialized cells, termed intercalated cells, in the collecting duct. Urinary K^+ concentration usually is quite low in this situation, but it may exceed 20 mEq/L if daily urine volume is low.

The major factors that influence the secretion of K^+ by the collecting duct cells are serum $[K^+]$, aldosterone, tubular fluid sodium delivery to the collecting duct, and tubular fluid flow rate. Although an increase or decrease in any of these will tend to increase or decrease urinary K^+ losses, a reciprocal interaction among the factors often serves to prevent K^+ deficits or surfeits. For instance, sodium loading increases both sodium delivery and flow rate to the distal nephron but suppresses the renin/angiotensin/aldosterone system. Conversely, sodium deficits reduce sodium delivery and flow rate but stimulate renin/angiotensin/aldosterone. Thus, potassium balance tends to be normal in both circumstances. In contrast, hypo- or hyperkalemia frequently results when tandem increases or decreases in these stimuli occur. For example, patients with hypoaldosteronism due to diabetic nephropathy are often normokalemic when volume replete. However, when sodium intake is restricted, the decreased tubular fluid sodium delivery and flow rate, coupled with aldosterone deficiency, may provoke hyperkalemia. By the same token, patients with primary hyperaldosteronism will have more severe hypokalemia when volume is expanded.

Aldosterone plays a pivotal role in both the physiology and pathophysiology of potassium metabolism. It increases K^+ secretion by the principal cells by several mechanisms. It increases sodium reabsorption, generating an electrochemical gradient for K^+ secretion. It stimulates the Na^+/K^+ ATPase, moving Na^+ out of and K^+ into tubular cells for secretion, and it opens channels for K^+ secretion. Tubular fluid sodium delivery plays its role in K^+ secretion by offering increased substrate for Na^+ reabsorption, and flow rate is important in ''washing away'' secreted K^+ to maintain a gradient from cell to tubular lumen for K^+ movement.

III. HYPOKALEMIA

Hypokalemia, defined as a serum $[K^+]$ of <3.6 mEq/L, can be caused by reduced intake, by increased cellular uptake, or by increased losses of K^+. Of these three possibilities, the vast majority of patients with hypokalemia have abnormal losses, and of these almost all are due to abnormal renal losses. In most instances, the cause of the hypokalemia is obvious, e.g., diuretic use. At other times, this disorder is a diagnostic puzzle. Measurement of blood pressure, acid-base status, urinary K^+ excretion, and, sometimes, urinary chloride excretion will provide clues to the diagnosis. Table 1 presents an extensive differential diagnosis of hypokalemia. The more important entities are discussed below.

A. Inadequate Intake

Reduced K^+ intake rarely causes hypokalemia because the kidney can reduce urinary K^+ losses to less than 20–25 mEq per day when K^+ intake is low. Thus, a markedly restricted diet over a prolonged period is necessary to cause K^+ depletion. Nonetheless, the kidney does not conserve potassium completely and an obligate loss of 20–25 mEq per day may contribute to K^+ depletion, particularly when other losses have occurred. For example, multiple factors are present in alcoholism and eating disorders, where vomiting, diarrhea, increased aldosterone secretion, laxative abuse, and sometimes diuretics are intertwined with poor intake of K^+. In some of these scenarios, urine K^+ values may be confusing, but

Table 1 Causes of Hypokalemia

1. *Poor intake*	
"Tea and toast" diets	
Alcoholism	
Eating disorder	
Clay ingestion	
2. *Redistribution*	
Insulin	
Catecholamines and beta agonists	
Theophylline intoxication	
Alkalemia	
Periodic paralysis	
Aldosterone	
Increased blood cell production	
Chloroquine or barium intoxication	
Hypothermia	
3. *Nonrenal K^+ Loss*	
Diarrhea	
Laxative abuse	
Sweat	
Alcoholism, eating disorders	
4. *Renal K^+ losses*	
Associated with metabolic alkalosis	Associated with metabolic acidosis
Diuretics	Distal RTA
Vomiting and NG suction	Amphotericin
Primary aldosteronism	Proximal RTA
Cushing's syndrome	Glue-sniffing (toluene)
Ectopic ACTH production	Diabetic ketoacidosis
Nonreabsorbable anions including penicillins	
Bartter's and Gitelman's syndromes	
Congenital adrenal hyperplasia	
Apparent mineralocorticoid excess	
Licorice	
Liddle's syndrome	
11 β-Hydroxysteroid dehydrogenase deficiency	
No predictable acid-base disorder	
Magnesium depletion	
Aminoglycosides	
Cisplatin	
Renal artery stenosis	
Malignant hypertension	
Marked polyuria	

in general, urine K^+ is <20 mEq/day with poor intake. Acid-base status is usually normal, although profound hypokalemia (serum $[K^+]$ < 2.0 mEq/L) can cause metabolic alkalosis (see Chapter 11).

B. Transcellular K^+ Shifts

1. Insulin

Exogenous or endogenous increases in plasma insulin lead to cellular K^+ uptake (by increasing the synthesis and insertion of Na^+/K^+ ATPase in cell membranes). Insulin administration predictably decreases serum K^+ by approximately 0.5 mEq/L within 15–30 minutes, and endogenous insulin release is a key part of the normal response that transiently moves K^+ into cells after absorption of this ion from the gut. The effect is acute but not chronic, as hypokalemia is not a feature of patients with insulinomas. Hypokalemia due to insulin administration is a well-recognized event during the treatment of diabetic ketoacidosis.

2. Catecholamines and β Agonists

Endogenous increases in epinephrine and exogenous administration of epinephrine, dopamine, dobutamine, albuterol, and terbutaline all produce transient hypokalemia by stimulating the entry of K^+ into cells. Potassium uptake is stimulated specifically by the β_2 catecholamine receptor. Of note, mildly hypokalemic patients may experience arrhythmias during acute myocardial infarction, when catecholamine release further lowers serum K^+. Similarly, asthmatics treated with β agonists can acutely develop significant hypokalemia. In fact, this phenomenon underlies the treatment of hyperkalemia with β agonists (see Chapter 30). Hypokalemia is a feature of theophylline toxicity due to catecholamine-mediated K^+ redistribution as well as direct effects on cellular second messenger activity.

3. Alkalemia

Metabolic alkalosis causes cellular K^+ uptake as H^+ exits cells, but the magnitude and time course of this response is variable. This effect is rather small and does not explain the substantial hypokalemia that is characteristic of sustained metabolic alkalosis. Rather, urinary K^+ losses are responsible (see below), and the degree of hypokalemia is actually mitigated somewhat by the movement of K^+ from the intracellular to the extracellular compartment. The alkalemia associated with respiratory alkalosis causes no shift of K^+ into cells.

4. Periodic Paralysis

The hypokalemic form of periodic paralysis is caused by paroxysmal episodes of cellular K^+ uptake and presents with episodes of muscle weakness, sometimes progressing to flaccid paralysis. Attacks generally last from hours up to 1 day and especially affect the limbs and trunk. Serum K^+ may be reduced to 2 mEq/L or less. Attacks are often recurrent and often follow carbohydrate loads (insulin release) or factors that increase catecholamines such as exercise, severe stress, or epinephrine administration. The genetic form of this disease is due to a mutation in the gene encoding the dihydropyridine receptor, a voltage gated calcium channel, and is transmitted in an autosomal dominant or, rarely, an X-linked inheritance. A similar clinical presentation is seen in patients with thyrotoxicosis, particularly in Asian males. In both the familial and sporadic forms, urine K^+ excretion falls during attacks and acid-base status remains normal. This combination often helps to distinguish the sporadic case of periodic paralysis from the severe hypokalemia sometimes seen with diuretics, eating disorders, or laxative abuse. Clinical history, including the acuity of the muscle weakness and the spontaneous resolution, is also helpful in making a diagnosis.

C. Nonrenal Potassium Losses

1. Diarrhea

Short-lived, mild episodes of diarrhea generally do not lead to major K^+ losses in the stool. However, severe watery diarrhea, chronic diarrhea, or chronic laxative abuse often produces significant hypokalemia. Examples are cholera, VIP-secreting tumors, and villous adenomas of the rectum. The hypokalemia seen in diarrhea is often, but not always, associated with metabolic acidosis due to concomitant HCO_3^- loss. Some patients with hypokalemia due to losses in the stool present with a normal serum [HCO_3^-] (typically with laxative abuse), and some even manifest metabolic alkalosis (when associated with selective chloride losses such as caused by a villous adenoma). Patients with laxative abuse frequently deny the usage, and sigmoidoscopy or chemical tests on the stool may be required for diagnosis.

2. Sweat

Intense exercise in hot, dry climates may cause enough sweat loss to produce K^+ depletion. Curiously, hypokalemia is rarely seen.

3. Eating Disorders/Alcoholism

In patients with these disorders, multiple causes of hypokalemia may be present. These include various combinations of poor intake, vomiting, diarrhea, diuretic abuse, laxative abuse, catecholamine release, and secondary hyperaldosteronism.

As a result, urinary K^+ excretion and acid-base status are variable. The diagnosis usually is made on the basis of the clinical history.

D. Renal Potassium Losses

Abnormal renal loss of K^+ is the most common cause of hypokalemia. In this setting, urinary K^+ excretion generally is greater than 20–25 mEq/day despite the presence of hypokalemia. For diagnostic purposes, it is useful to categorize hypokalemia from renal K^+ losses according to the accompanying acid-base disturbance: metabolic alkalosis, metabolic acidosis, or no acid-base disturbance (Fig. 1). Of these three groups, metabolic alkalosis encompasses the most frequent causes of hypokalemia. Metabolic alkalosis itself causes K^+ depletion and hypokalemia by accelerating renal K^+ excretion. Thus, the coexistence of metabolic alkalosis in a patient with hypokalemia substantially narrows the differential diagnosis and practically eliminates the need to measure urinary K^+, as it is almost invariably elevated. Finding the root cause of the metabolic alkalosis identifies the cause of the hypokalemia. Because the measurement of urinary chloride concentration is useful in the differential diagnosis of metabolic alkalosis (see Chapter 11), we have categorized the renal K^+ losses associated with metabolic

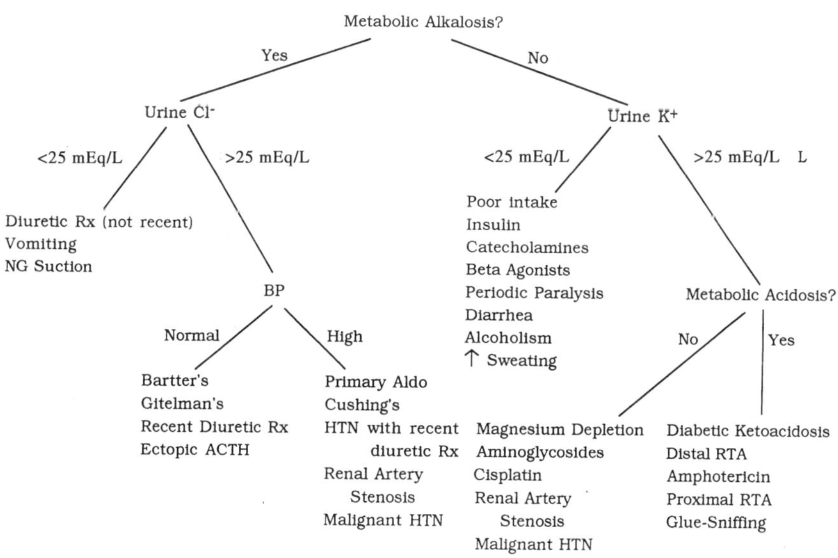

Figure 1 Diagnosis of relevant causes of hypokalemia.

alkalosis into those in which chloride depletion is the cause of the alkalosis (low urinary chloride excretion) and those in which chloride depletion is not the cause of the alkalosis (normal chloride excretion).

1. Renal K^+ Loss with Metabolic Alkalosis Due to Chloride Depletion

(a) Thiazide and Loop Diuretics. These drugs are undoubtedly the most frequent causes of hypokalemia and metabolic alkalosis. By inhibiting Na^+ reabsorption more proximally, they increase Na^+ delivery and flow rate to the cortical collecting duct, promoting K^+ secretion and excretion into the urine. In addition, these drugs stimulate aldosterone secretion by reducing extracelluar volume, further promoting K^+ secretion. Hypokalemia can be quite severe in some patients, especially those taking frequent, high doses of loop diuretics for congestive heart failure or a combination of a loop diuretic and metolazone. The urinary chloride concentration is low ($<$20 mEq/L) in these patients, reflecting their chloride depletion, except during the period of pharmacological action of the diuretic. If surreptitious diuretic abuse is a potential cause of unexplained hypokalemia, multiple urine chloride determinations may be needed to detect the occasionally depressed urinary chloride level. An urinary assay for diuretics also may be helpful.

(b) Vomiting and Nasogastric Suction. The hypokalemia that results from the loss of gastric contents is not due to the gastric fluid loss itself, because the concentration of K^+ in gastric juice usually is less than 10 mEq/L. Instead, the loss of HCl from the stomach causes a metabolic alkalosis that increases K^+ secretion by the collecting duct. (The pathophysiology of metabolic alkalosis is reviewed in Chapter 11.) Urinary chloride concentration is invariably low, and this finding can be helpful in the diagnosis of hypokalemia and metabolic alkalosis due to surreptitious vomiting.

2. Renal K^+ Loss with Metabolic Alkalosis Independent of Chloride Depletion

(a) Primary Aldosteronism. Patients with this disorder have single or multiple, generally benign, adrenal adenomas or bilateral adrenal hyperplasia. They present with hypertension, spontaneous hypokalemia, metabolic alkalosis, and urinary chloride levels of $>$20–30 mEq/L. The concomitant Na^+ retention cannot be detected clinically. Mild hypernatremia ($\sim$144 mEq/L) may be present. Serum or urine aldosterone levels are generally elevated and nonsuppressible with saline administration. Plasma renin activity is invariably suppressed, usually to $<$1 ng/mL/hr, and a ratio of plasma aldosterone to plasma renin of $>$30–50 is present in the majority of such patients (see Chapter 9).

(b) Glucocorticoid-Responsive Aldosteronism. This rare hereditary disorder is caused by a fusion genetic mutation that links stimulation of aldosterone secretion to ACTH rather than angiotension. Clinically these patients present in a fashion identical to that seen with primary hyperaldosteronism due to a tumor or hyperplasia. In contrast, however, there is a strong family history of early onset hypertension and its complications. The diagnosis is made by gene analysis of affected families.

(c) Cushing's Syndrome and Ectopic ACTH Production. In patients with these disorders, plasma aldosterone and renin levels are generally normal. The mineralocorticoid effect stems from enormous overproduction of either cortisol or other nonaldosterone mineralocorticoids like corticosterone. Hypokalemia is more common with ectopic ACTH since cortisol levels are much higher than in patients with Cushing's syndrome. Patients with Cushing's generally have the obvious clinical features of the syndrome, while muscle weakness and wasting predominate in patients with cancer-induced ectopic ACTH production.

(d) Bartter's and Gitelman's Syndromes. These rare disorders are caused by defects in sodium chloride reabsorption in the loop of Henle or distal tubule, causing mild to moderate volume depletion and increased secretion of renin/angiotensin/aldosterone. The increased presentation of sodium to the collecting duct along with the increased levels of aldosterone cause increased urinary excretion of K^+ and H^+ with resulting hypokalemia and metabolic alkalosis. Patients with Bartter's syndrome typically present in childhood with polyuria, volume depletion, growth retardation, and occasionally mental defects. Patients with Gitelman's syndrome usually present later in life, often in adulthood. The similarity of the latter disorder to that induced by diuretics can cause confusion. Severe, sometimes symptomatic, hypomagnesemia can be a clue to Gitelman's syndrome. In addition, patients with Gitelman's syndrome have a low urinary calcium excretion in contrast to the high urinary calcium excretion seen in patients with Bartter's syndrome. Because of the tendency toward volume depletion, the blood pressure is normal or even low in Bartter's and Gitelman's syndromes in contrast to the hypertension seen in patients with primary aldosteronism or Cushing's syndrome. In both these syndromes, the urinary chloride levels reflect intake and, unless the patient is ingesting a diet with little chloride, will be $>$20–30 mEq/L. This distinction helps distinguish these disorders from the metabolic alkalosis of vomiting.

(e) Syndromes of Apparent Mineralocorticoid Excess. Two rare genetic diseases cause hypertension, hypokalemia, and metabolic alkalosis with low rather than elevated aldosterone levels. Both are due to mutations that promote Na^+ reabsorption and K^+ secretion in the collecting duct independent of aldosterone. Liddle's syndrome is caused by a mutation that prevents inactivation of

the apical membrane sodium channel (EnaC), causing it to be continually open and stimulating Na^+ reabsorption. The second disorder, often termed syndrome of apparent mineralocorticoid excess, is due to a mutation that inactivates 11β-hydroxysteroid dehydrogenase. This enzyme normally prevents cortisol from binding to the mineralocorticoid receptor. Without this enzyme, cortisol binds to the receptor and stimulates Na^+ reabsorption and K^+ secretion. In both disorders, renin and aldosterone levels are extremely low, and thus they can easily be dissociated from primary hyperaldosteronism.

3. Renal K^+ Loss with Metabolic Acidosis

Although less common, some causes of metabolic acidosis cause K^+ loss and are important to recognize.

(a) Distal Renal Tubular Acidosis (Type 1). In this disorder, failure of normal distal tubular H^+ secretion or back leakage of H^+ results in metabolic acidosis with a normal anion gap (see Chapter 11). Hypokalemia regularly develops as a result of increased K^+ secretion in the collecting duct and loss into the urine. Alkali therapy tends to reduce K^+ wasting. Distal renal tubular acidosis can be induced by the antifungal agent amphotericin B, and both hypokalemia and metabolic acidosis can occur as a complication of treatment with this drug.

(b) Proximal Renal Tubular Acidosis (Type 2). Failure to reabsorb HCO_3^- normally in the proximal tubule leads to a ''flood'' of anion delivered distally, favoring increased K^+ secretion. In the steady state of acidosis, K^+ excretion returns to control levels and hypokalemia may not be present. When alkali therapy is given, however, K^+ secretion is stimulated and hypokalemia can develop or worsen. Glue-sniffing (toluene intoxication) produces a syndrome that resembles proximal renal tubular acidosis. The metabolism of toluene to hippuric acid causes metabolic acidosis. The delivery of hippurate, a nonreabsorbable anion, to the collecting duct stimulates K^+ secretion; hypokalemia often results.

(c) Diabetic Ketoacidosis. K^+ wasting due to both polyuria and increased excretion of nonreabsorbable ketoacid anions is the rule in diabetic ketoacidosis. The magnitude of the potassium depletion may exceed 200–300 mEq. Hypokalemia may be masked by the shift of K^+ out of cells caused by hyperglycemia and insulin lack and by a concomitant fall in GFR due to volume depletion, but it generally becomes apparent when insulin therapy is initiated.

4. Renal K^+ Loss with No Predictable Acid-Base Disturbance

(a) Magnesium Depletion. Magnesium depletion, manifested by hypomagnesemia, is a common concomitant abnormality in hypokalemic patients. Hyperaldosteronism, diuretics, diarrhea, cisplatin, and Gitelman's syndrome cause

wasting of both potassium and magnesium. In addition, hypomagnesemia itself causes renal K^+ wasting. As a result, magnesium depletion often needs repair before hypokalemia will correct with K^+ supplementation. Postulated mechanisms for the pathogenesis of hypokalemia include the opening of K^+ channels for secretion and the induction of increased aldosterone secretion by hypomagnesemia. Aminoglycosides appear to cause hypokalemia by producing hypomagnesemia. Hypomagnesemic patients may develop hypocalcemia as well, providing a clue to the presence of the underlying hypomagnesemia.

(b) Renal Artery Stenosis. The increases in renin/angiotensin/aldosterone seen with renal artery stenosis (or other high renin states like malignant hypertension) often produce mild hypokalemia. Though metabolic alkalosis can be seen, it is generally quite mild. Normal acid-base status is the rule.

E. Approach to the Diagnosis of Hypokalemia

A diagnostic algorithm for diagnosing the causes of hypokalemia is shown in Figure 1. As stated earlier, we prefer to initially categorize patients as to the presence or absence of metabolic alkalosis. The data to facilitate this evaluation are readily available, and metabolic alkalosis is most often present in patients with hypokalemia. When alkalosis is present, the patients can be further subdivided based on urine chloride levels and the presence or absence of hypertension. In the absence of metabolic alkalosis, patients are subdivided by urine K^+ excretion into nonrenal or renal sources of hypokalemia and the renal sources in turn divided into those with metabolic acidosis and those with normal acid-base status. Analysis of 24-hour urine chloride and potassium excretion is the more rigorous method to determine their levels, but measurement on a "spot" urine sample may provide sufficient information.

IV. HYPERKALEMIA

Patients with hyperkalemia, defined as a serum [K^+] of >5.0 mEq/L, may have abnormalities in K^+ intake, abnormal transcellular shifts of K^+, or defects in renal K^+ excretion. Of these possibilities, renal excretory defects are the most common. Large increases in potassium intake or shifts rarely produce significant hyperkalemia in the absence of excretory defects. Before reviewing the causes of hyperkalemia, we first discuss spurious or factitious hyperkalemia.

A. Spurious Hyperkalemia

Patients with spurious hyperkalemia have increased serum K^+ levels that do not accurately reflect in vivo circulating plasma [K^+]. The most obvious cause is hemolysis of red cells and the release of their intracellular K^+ into the serum. Hemolysis tints the serum pink and is almost always reported by the laboratory. Less obvious is the release of intracellular K^+ from the normal clotting of blood in a "red-top" tube. Serum $[K^+]$ is thus always slightly higher than plasma $[K^+]$ (usually by less than 0.5 mEq/L) because platelets and white cells release K^+. However, major increases in platelet or white cell count can cause worrisome but spurious increases in measured serum $[K^+]$. The increase in serum $[K^+]$ is directly related to the number of platelets or white blood cells (WBC). Platelet counts of $>$500,000/μL or WBC counts of $>$100,000/μL are necessary to spuriously raise serum $[K^+]$ to abnormal levels. The diagnosis of spurious hyperkalemia should be suspected when the platelet or WBC count is high, the electrocardiogram shows no signs of hyperkalemia, and there are no clinical manifestations of hyperkalemia. If thrombocytosis is the cause, the diagnosis can be confirmed by measuring plasma (i.e., heparinized blood) rather than serum $[K^+]$. A less appreciated cause of spurious hyperkalemia stems from repetitive fist clenching by the patient with "difficult" veins before phlebotomy. Forearm muscles may release enough potassium to raise the measured serum $[K^+]$ by about 1 mEq/L. This artifact can be produced by fist clenching alone.

B. Increased K^+ Loads

The principal cells of the cortical collecting duct normally have an enormous adaptive capacity to increase K^+ secretion. For example, the typical Irish peasant diet just prior to the potato famine in the mid-nineteenth century consisted of approximately 15 pounds of potatoes per day, resulting in a daily K^+ intake of nearly 500 mEq. To cause hyperkalemia, an exogenous or endogenous K^+ load thus must be massive or acute or, more commonly, be coupled with a defect in potassium secretion. For instance, patients with stable, mild hyperkalemia due to diabetic nephropathy may develop significant clinical problems if they ingest a salt substitute (which contains K^+) or suffer tissue gangrene. Likewise, previously normal patients frequently develop hyperkalemia when acute renal failure is coupled with muscle damage due to rhabdomyolysis. KCL supplementation of patients taking thiazide or loop diuretics represents one of the most frequent causes of drug-induced hyperkalemia. Clinically important sources of external or internal K^+ loads are presented in Table 2.

C. Transcellular K^+ Shifts

A number of clinical circumstances, summarized in Table 3 and discussed below, cause hyperkalemia because of significant shifts of K^+ from cells to the extracellular compartment.

Table 2 Potassium Loads

External	Internal
Diet	Tissue necrosis
Salt substitutes	Hematoma resorption
Potassium supplements	Tumor lysis
Low-sodium canned foods	Rhabdomyolysis
Potassium penicillin	Hemolysis
Stored blood for transfusion	
Collins' solution for organ preservation	

Table 3 Transcellular K^+ Shifts

Insulin deficiency
Hyperosmolality
β Blockers
Exhaustive exercise
Hyperkalemic periodic paralysis
Mineral acids
Rare drug-induced
Digitalis intoxication
Succinylcholine
Arginine HCL

1. Insulin Deficiency, Hyperosmolality

The pathogenesis of the hyperkalemia frequently associated with diabetic ketoacidosis is quite complex. The insulin deficiency and hyperosmolality that accompany the disorder combine to move K^+ from cells and raise serum K^+ even in the presence of K^+ depletion. Because insulin plays a key role in facilitating K^+ entry into cells, a deficiency of this hormone is associated with reduced K^+ entry and an increase in serum [K^+]. Hyperosmolality causes K^+ movement by increasing the [K^+] gradient between the interior and exterior of the cells as water moves out and by "solvent drag" of K^+ by water movement. Some patients with diabetic ketoacidosis also have renal insufficiency and hypoaldosteronism, all contributing to the hyperkalemia (see later).

2. β-Blockers

Because β_2 adrenergic receptors facilitate K^+ entry into cells, an increase in serum [K^+] due to nonselective β blockers is not surprising. The effect is trivial in individuals with no other defect in K^+ homeostasis, as other mechanisms (such as increased tubular secretion) compensate. When other abnormalities in K^+ metabolism are present, however, such as renal transplant tubular dysfunction (e.g., from cyclosporine or tacrolimus), chronic renal insufficiency, or hypoaldosteronism, a significant increase in serum $[K^+]$ can occur. Even in otherwise normal individuals, intense exercise can result in significant hyperkalemia in the presence of nonselective β blockade. Selective (β_1) adrenergic blockers do not have the same effect.

3. Exercise

Vigorous exercise causes an increase in serum $[K^+]$ due to muscle cell K^+ release. The hyperkalemia is generally minor and is quite transient, although increases of 1–2 mEq/L have been reported with exhaustive exercise. Patients with other abnormalities such as renal failure or β blockade are particularly susceptible.

4. Hyperkalemic Periodic Paralysis

This form of periodic paralysis results from a rare autosomal dominant defect of the skeletal muscle Na^+ channel. Affected patients have attacks of weakness or even paralysis varying in frequency and duration. Hyperkalemia is often but not invariably observed, and T-wave ECG changes may be present. Respiratory paralysis is not seen. Cold exposure, potassium intake, or recovery from exercise often triggers an attack.

5. Mineral Acids

Administration of HCl or NH_4Cl causes a fall in pH coupled with the movement of K^+ out of cells, acutely increasing serum $[K^+]$ by approximately 0.5 mEq/L for each 0.1 fall in pH. With the exception of experimental models, however, this form of acidosis is extremely rare. Clinical acute metabolic acidosis is almost always due to overproduction of organic acids, and in this setting no transcellular K^+ shift occurs as a result of the acidosis per se. With sustained metabolic acidosis, other factors (e.g., changes in renal K^+ transport) are of overriding importance in determining serum $[K^+]$.

D. Defective Renal Excretion and Renal Failure

Because K^+ excretion is dependent on the secretion of this ion in the distal nephron rather than filtration, a major reduction in renal function is necessary to produce a clinically significant impairment in K^+ excretion. In the absence of excessive K^+ intake, decreased distal Na^+ delivery, or other complicating features, a fall in GFR to less than 5–10 mL/min is required to cause hyperkalemia. In experimental models of renal insufficiency, the principal cells of the cortical collecting duct undergo anatomical and functional changes that allow major increases in K^+ secretion per nephron, helping to forestall K^+ retention and hyperkalemia. Severe chronic renal failure, oliguric acute renal failure (especially with tissue catabolism), and moderate chronic renal failure associated with hypoaldosteronism (see below) are common renal causes of hyperkalemia. Colonic K^+ secretion increases in chronic renal failure to up to 20 mEq/day. Thus, constipation may cause hyperkalemia in this population. Occasionally patients with only modest increases in serum creatinine concentration manifest hyperkalemia that is ultimately demonstrated to be due to renal failure alone. These patients are generally quite elderly, have little muscle mass, and often have been at prolonged bed rest or have received steroids. Their serum creatinine level poorly reflects the severity of their renal failure, which can be clarified by measurement or appropriate calculation of GFR (see Chapter 5).

E. Aldosterone Deficiency

Apart from severe renal failure, the most common and clinically important causes of hyperkalemia result from disorders characterized by aldosterone deficiency. These disorders include congenital and acquired primary adrenal disease and intrinsic as well as drug-induced abnormalities of the renin/angiotensin/aldosterone system. The differential diagnosis of aldosterone deficiency is presented in the top half of Table 4 and the key causes are discussed below.

1. Hyporeninemic Hypoaldosteronism

Hyporeninemic hypoaldosteronism (HRHA) accounts for most of the instances of hyperkalemia that cannot be explained by severe renal failure. It is often, but not always, accompanied by a mild to moderate metabolic acidosis with a normal anion gap, termed Type 4 renal tubular acidosis (see Chapter 11). Renal insufficiency (serum creatinine, 2–5 mg/dL) is almost always seen in association with the hypoaldosteronism and is likely a contributing factor in the hyperkalemia. Diabetic nephropathy is the most common underlying cause, with various forms of interstitial renal disease accounting for most of the other cases. Damage to the juxtaglomerular apparatus with resulting deficits in renin, angiotensin, and aldosterone production has been offered as the explanation for the syndrome. Some observations suggest that other mechanisms may be involved, including intra-adrenal abnormalities, chronic volume expansion (which suppresses renin), increases in ANP (which suppress aldosterone), and abnormalities in prostaglandin metabolism. Unlike addisonian patients, HRHA patients present with mild volume overload, not salt depletion. Hyponatremia is unusual. The classic case of hyporenin-hypoaldosteronism comprises hyperkalemia, metabolic acidosis, renal

Table 4 Abnormal Potassium Secretion

Aldosterone deficiency
Primary adrenal disease
Addison's disease
Congenital enzymatic defects
Hyporeninemic hypoaldosteronism
Diabetic nephropathy
Other renal diseases, especially tubulointerstitial
Drugs
NSAIDs
ACE inhibitors
Angiotensin receptor antagonists
Heparin
Cyclosporine and tacrolimus
Primary defect in tubular K^+ secretion
Tubulointerstitial disease, especially urinary tract obstruction
Gordon's syndrome
Drugs
Spironolactone
Triamterene
Amiloride
Trimethoprim

insufficiency, a normal cortisol level, low plasma renin and aldosterone levels, and a urine pH of <5.5. If the diagnosis is in doubt, measurements of cortisol, renin, and aldosterone can be very helpful. Because hyperkalemia is a strong stimulus to the release of aldosterone, a low or low-normal aldosterone level in the face of hyperkalemia is highly suggestive of this syndrome. Volume depletion, drugs that further inhibit aldosterone secretion (e.g., ACE inhibitors), or other causes of decreased distal tubular sodium delivery often exacerbate hyperkalemia in patients with this disorder.

2. Addison's Disease

Patients with primary adrenal disease have deficiencies in both cortisol and aldosterone production and often manifest hyperkalemia. Hyponatremia, salt wasting, and metabolic acidosis are frequent associated abnormalities. Because the clinical presentation of primary adrenal failure is quite variable and the disorder is so readily treatable with appropriate steroid replacement therapy, however, one should have a low threshold for pursuing the possibility in patients with hyperkalemia. The diagnosis is made by a Cortrosyn test that indicates abnormal glucocorticoid secretion. Causes include autoimmune and granulomatous diseases and adrenal hemorrhage. In addition, AIDS patients frequently demonstrate hyperkalemia, and these individuals may develop adrenal insufficiency due to tuberculosis or CMV. Alternatively, cortisol secretion may be normal and the hyperkalemia may be due to hypoaldosteronism or to a drug-induced tubular defect, e.g., trimethoprim (see below).

3. Drug-Induced Hypoaldosteronism

Several drugs impair the normal responsiveness of the renin/angiotensin system or the adrenal production of aldosterone. Hyperkalemia frequently is the result, especially if there is at least mild-moderate renal insufficiency present as well. Nonsteroidal anti-inflammatory drugs (NSAIDs) impair renin release via prostaglandin inhibition. They also may reduce distal tubular sodium delivery and reduce GFR. In patients with underlying renal insufficiency, hyperkalemia and hypoaldosteronism may result. Angiotensin-converting enzyme (ACE) inhibitors and receptor blockers cause similar reductions in plasma aldosterone and predispose patients with renal insufficiency to hyperkalemia. Salt depletion, underlying hyporenin-hypoaldosteronism due to diabetic nephropathy, and concurrent NSAID use are additional risk factors. Heparin impairs adrenal aldosterone biosynthesis by enzyme inhibition. Low molecular weight heparin has a similar effect. Even doses of heparin in the range of 10,000 U/day can gradually reduce aldosterone secretion. However, hyperkalemia affects only a small fraction of heparin-treated patients, and additional predispositions to hyperkalemia are usually present. Cyclosporine and tacrolimus (FK506) are associated with hyperkalemia in organ transplant recipients. Hyporeninemic-hypoaldosteronism appears to be the major cause, though a direct suppressive effect on tubular K^+ secretion also has been recognized.

F. Tubular Defects in Potassium Secretion

Abnormalities in K^+ secretion manifest abnormalities similar to those described above for aldosterone deficiency but, by definition, are associated with normal or elevated aldosterone levels. Unfortunately, distinguishing aldosterone deficiency from a renal tubular K^+ secretory defect is not always straightforward. Some disorders (e.g., chronic obstructive nephropathy) are associated with both hypoaldosteronism and tubular secretory defects. Maneuvers such as evaluating the ratio of plasma aldosterone to serum [K^+], reducing serum [K^+] to normal and remeasuring plasma aldosterone, stimulating aldosterone secretion with diuretics and upright posture, or assessing the therapeutic response to mineralocorticoid replacement have been advocated. None of the maneuvers is well standardized or widely accepted however. Similarly, measurement of the transtubular [K^+] gradient (TTKG): (urine/serum [K^+]) divided by (urine/serum osmolality), envisioned as a means of quantifying distal tubular K^+ secretion, does not differentiate between the two disorders.

When plasma aldosterone levels are frankly elevated or reduced, the distinction of aldosterone deficiency from a tubular defect is not difficult. In the classic case of a tubular secretory defect, plasma renin and aldosterone levels are elevated, cortisol is normal, and urine pH is >5.5 despite metabolic acidosis. Chronic renal insufficiency is usually present due to urinary obstruction, systemic lupus erythematosus (SLE), sickle cell nephropathy, amyloidosis, or other causes of tubulointerstitial disease. A defect in sodium transport in the collecting duct, reducing luminal electronegativity, probably explains the abnormality in potassium secretion in most patients. A rare genetic disease, Gordon's syndrome, presents with hypertension and hyperkalemia, usually with an associated metabolic acidosis, despite normal adrenal and renal function.

Potassium-sparing diuretics impair distal K^+ secretion without suppressing aldosterone levels or plasma renin and are among the most common causes of drug-induced hyperkalemia. Spironolactone competitively inhibits the action of aldosterone in the distal tubule. Triamterene and amiloride block the Na^+ channel at the luminal membrane of the tubular cell, thereby removing the electrochemical driving force for K^+ secretion. The antibiotic agent trimethoprim acts in an identical fashion and can cause hyperkalemia when given in high doses. Hyperkalemia is unusual with any of these drugs unless renal insufficiency or another predisposition to potassium intolerance is present.

V. APPROACH TO THE DIAGNOSIS OF HYPERKALEMIA

In most patients, the underlying cause of hyperkalemia is obvious. Examples include oliguric acute renal failure, end-stage chronic renal failure, and diabetic ketoacidosis. Many other causes are due to moderate chronic renal disease coupled with an acute change that reduces distal tubular sodium delivery or impairs the renin/angiotensin/aldosterone system. Examples include volume depletion and a number of drugs including NSAIDs, ACE inhibitors, angiotensin receptor antagonists, heparin, and K^+-sparing diuretics. Beta blockers or high K^+ intake occasionally cause hyperkalemia in patients with renal insufficiency.

Patients with unexplained, asymptomatic, reproducible hyperkalemia in the setting of normal renal function may have spurious hyperkalemia. Workup should include an EKG (which should be normal), phlebotomy repeated without fist-clenching, measurement of WBC and platelet counts, and sometimes simultaneous serum and plasma $[K^+]$.

Chronic, reproducible hyperkalemia in patients with mild-moderate CRF, no volume status abnormality, and no drug toxicity or unusual intake suggests aldosterone deficiency or a primary defect in tubular K^+ secretion. Workup includes plasma cortisol, renin and aldosterone levels, urine pH, and a renal ultrasound.

SUGGESTED READINGS

Alappan R, Perozella M, Buller GK. Hyperkalemia in hospitalized patients treated with trimethoprim-sulfamethoxale. Ann Intern Med 1996; 124:316–320.

Allon M. Hyperkalemia in end-stage renal disease: mechanisms and management. J Am Soc Nephrol 1995; 6:1134–1142.

Batlle DC, Arruda JA, Kurtzman NA. Hyperkalemic distal renal tubular acidosis associated with obstructive uropathy. N Engl J Med 1981; 304:373–380.

Bettinelli A, Bianchetti MG, Girardin E, et al. Use of calcium excretion values to distinguish two forms of primary renal tubular hypokalemic alkalosis: Bartter and Gitelman syndromes. J Pediatr 1992; 120:38–43.

Blumenfeld JD, Sealey JE, Schlussel Y, et al. Diagnosis and treatment of primary hyperaldosteronism. Ann Intern Med 1994; 121:877–885.

Carlisle EJ, Donnelly SM, Vasuvattakul S, et al. Glue-sniffing and distal renal tubular acidosis. Sticking to the facts. J Am Soc Nephrol 1991; 1:1019–1027.

Castellino P, Bia M, DeFronzo RA. Adrenergic modulation of potassium metabolism in uremia. Kidney Int 1990; 37:793–798.

DeFronzo RA. Clinical disorders of hyperkalemia. In: Seldin DW, Giebisch G, eds. The Kidney. New York: Raven Press, 1992:2279–2337.

DeFronzo RA, Nephrology Forum. Hyperkalemia and hyporeninemic hypoaldosteronism. Kidney Int 1980; 17:118–134.

DuBose TD, Nephrology Forum. Hyperkalemic hyperchloremic metabolic acidosis: pathophysiologic insights. Kidney Int 1997; 51:591–602.

Ethier JH, Kamel KS, Magner PO, et al. The transtubular potassium gradient in patients with hyperkalemia and hypokalemia. Am J Kidney Dis 1990; 15:309–315.

Fontaine B, Lapie P, Plassart E, et al. Periodic paralysis and voltage-gated ion channels. Kidney Int 1996; 49:9–18.

Gennari FJ. Hypokalemia. New Engl J Med 1998; 339:451–458.

Glassock RJ, Cohen AH, Danovitch G, et al. Human immunodeficiency virus (HIV) infection and the kidney. Ann Intern Med 1990; 112:35–49.

Kurtz I, Nephrology Forum. Molecular pathogenesis of Bartter's and Gitelman's syndrome. Kidney Int 1998; 54:1396–1410.

Mitchell JE, Seim HC, Colon E, et al. Medical complications and medical management of bulimia. Ann Intern Med 1987; 107:71–77.

Morris AI, Turnberg LA. Surreptitious laxative abuse. Gastroenterology 1979; 77:780–786.

Oster JR, Singer I, Fishman LM. Heparin-induced aldosterone suppression and hyperkalemia. Am J Med 1995; 98:575–586.

Rose BD. Clinical Physiology of Acid-Base and Electrolyte Disorders. 4th ed. New York: McGraw-Hill, 1994.

Rose BD. Causes of hyperkalemia. In: Rose BD, ed. UpToDate. 1999.

Tannen RL. Potassium disorders. In: Kokko JP, Tannen RL, eds. Fluids and Electrolytes. 3rd ed. Philadelphia: W.B. Saunders, 1996:111–199.

Weiner ID, Wingo CS. Hypokalemia—consequences, causes, and corrections. J Am Soc Nephrol 1997; 8:1179–1188.

Whang R, Whang DD, Ryan MP. Refractory potassium depletion. A consequence of magnesium deficiency. Arch Intern Med 1992; 152:40–45.

Wingo CS, Armitage FE. Potassium transport in the kidney: regulation and physiological relevance of H^+-K^+–ATPase. Semin Nephrol 1993; 13:212–224.

14

Diagnosis of Disorders of Calcium, Phosphorus, and Magnesium Metabolism

F. John Gennari
University of Vermont, Burlington, Vermont

I. INTRODUCTION

Calcium, phosphorus, and magnesium are key elements for normal cellular function, intracellular signaling, and, in particular, for normal bone metabolism. Calcium and phosphorus (as phosphate) metabolism are regulated by the same hormonal factors, and their regulation is inextricably intertwined. Less is known about the regulation of magnesium balance, but this ion plays a key role in the regulation of extracellular calcium as well. Depletion or excess of each of these ions in the body fluids has significant clinical effects. Thus an understanding of their normal regulation and how this can be disrupted in disease states is essential for the management of these disorders. Although their regulation is linked in the body, each of these ions is discussed separately for ease of entry into the subject. When appropriate, their linkages are discussed.

II. CALCIUM

It is well recognized that calcium salts are a major component of bone. Of the approximately 1.3 kg of calcium contained in the body, 99% resides in bone. What is less well recognized is that calcium is a key ion for intracellular signaling. Unlike all other ions in the body, the concentration of calcium in cell cytoplasm is much less than 1 mEq/L. Micromolar changes in cytoplasmic calcium concentration cause profound effects on cell function, including muscle contraction, nerve conduction, and transcellular ionic transport. Calcium is also unique in that it is the only ion for which a cell membrane receptor exists. Thus, extracellular calcium, by binding to its receptor, can signal regulatory events within the cell. Given its key role in cell function, it is not surprising that the concentration of ionized calcium in the ECF is rigorously controlled. The normal value is maintained within the narrow range of 1.1–1.3 mmol/L. Unfortunately, total calcium, not just the ionized fraction, is what is routinely measured. Thus, in order to understand disorders of calcium metabolism, one first needs to understand the relation between the normal range reported by the laboratory, 9–10.5 mg/dL, and ionized calcium.

A. Interpretation of Serum Calcium Concentration

Extracellular calcium exists in three states. Approximately 40% is bound to albumin, 10% is complexed with organic anions such as citrate, and 50% exists as the free cation. From a homeostatic perspective, only free ionized calcium is regulated. Routine laboratory measurement of calcium, however, measures total calcium, including the bound and complexed species. Both protein binding and complexing of calcium are affected by serum pH, but by far the largest factor influencing serum calcium concentration is the prevailing albumin concentration. Protein binding of calcium is directly related to the concentration of albumin. As a result, an abnormal value for serum calcium concentration most commonly reflects changes in serum albumin concentration rather than any abnormality in the regulation of ionized calcium.

In recognition of this fact, many laboratories report a ''corrected'' or ''calculated'' serum calcium concentration, using one of a series of formulas derived to correct for serum albumin concentration. The simplest of these is:

$$\text{Corrected [calcium]} = \text{measured [calcium]} + (4.4 - \text{serum albumin (g/dL)}) \tag{1}$$

Another widely used correction is to increase serum [calcium] by 0.8 mg/dL for each 1 g/dL reduction in serum albumin concentration (using 4.2 g/dL as the starting point). Unfortunately, none of these formulas (more than 10 variations of the above have been developed) fully account for variations in serum [calcium]. In fact some studies report that the corrected [calcium] adds little of significance to the measured value reported by the laboratory. Nonetheless, evaluation of serum [calcium] should always include a simultaneous evaluation of serum albumin. Moreover, when one has a clinical concern about calcium homeostasis and, particularly when the value is only slightly elevated or decreased, one should consider measuring ionized [Ca^{2+}] to assess whether an abnormality is present. As a general rule, one need not measure ionized calcium if the serum calcium concentration, corrected for albumin, is greater than 13 mg/dL or less than 8 mg/dL. The ionized calcium, however, is the gold standard for assessing abnormalities in extracellular [Ca^{2+}].

A final problem with interpreting serum [calcium] is the variety of units used for this parameter. Ionized calcium is reported in mmol/L or mEq/L, whereas total calcium is reported in mg/dL. For calcium, 1 mmol = 2 mEq = 4 mg/dL. Thus, normal ionized [Ca^{2+}] is 4.5–5.3 mg/dL, 2.25–2.65 mEq/L, or 1.1–1.3 mmol/L.

B. Regulation of Calcium Homeostasis

Calcium is the only ion for which major regulation of body stores begins at the epithelium of the gut. Under normal conditions, only about 20% of ingested cal-

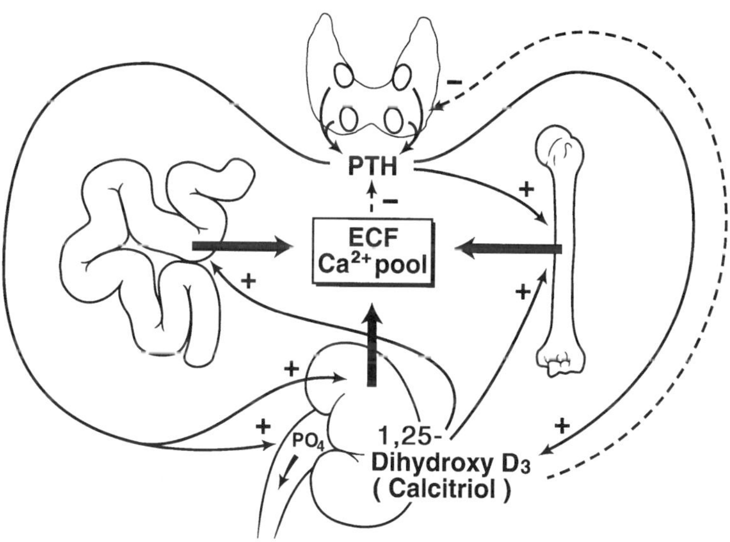

Figure 1 Interactions between ionized calcium concentration ([Ca^{2+}]), parathyroid hormone (PTH), and calcitriol in the normal regulation of serum [Ca^{2+}]. The lines indicate the feedback connections and sites of action, with the dashed lines denoting inhibition (−) and the solid lines denoting stimulation (+). PTH stimulates Ca^{2+} release from bone and calcitriol production by the kidney, and it inhibits phosphorus reabsorption by the kidney. Calcitriol stimulates Ca^{2+} absorption from the gut, facilitates PTH-induced stimulation of Ca^{2+} release from bone, and directly inhibits PTH secretion. An increase in serum [Ca^{2+}] also directly inhibits PTH secretion.

cium is absorbed, and this fraction is closely controlled by the active form of vitamin D (1,25-dihydroxycholecalciferol, or calcitriol). A portion of absorbed calcium is exchanged for bone calcium in its continual remodeling. In the steady state, however, absorbed calcium is balanced by the renal excretion of calcium. These events are regulated by the interplay between parathyroid hormone (PTH), calcitriol, and serum phosphorus concentration (Fig. 1). Through its receptor, extracellular Ca^{2+} directly regulates the secretion of PTH. An elevated [Ca^{2+}] inhibits the secretion of this hormone by saturating the calcium receptors on parathyroid gland cells. PTH stimulates the release of Ca^{2+} from bone and reabsorption of Ca^{2+} by the kidney. PTH also stimulates the production of calcitriol by the kidney. Calcitriol in turn stimulates Ca^{2+} absorption from the gut, facilitates PTH-mediated Ca^{2+} release from bone, and inhibits the release of PTH, creating both a direct and indirect negative feedback loop. Phosphate concentration also participates in this regulatory cascade. Hyperphosphatemia blocks the inhibitory effect of calcium on PTH secretion and inhibits the production of calcitriol by the kidney, removing another feedback inhibitor of PTH secretion. To complete this feedback loop, PTH promotes phosphate excretion by the kidney, reducing its concentration in the body (see later). Both PTH and calcitriol act to maintain extracellular [Ca^{2+}], but there is no counterbalancing system to reduce the concentration of this ion. Calcitonin has this effect but appears to play little role in normal calcium homeostasis. In individuals eating a normal North American diet, approximately 200 mg of calcium is absorbed each day, and renal calcium excretion is approximately 200 mg/day.

III. DISORDERS OF CALCIUM HOMEOSTASIS

A. Hypercalcemia

An abnormal increase in serum ionized [Ca^{2+}] produces a wide variety of nonspecific symptoms (see Chapter 4). When ionized [Ca^{2+}] increases to >1.6 mmol/L (reflected as a serum [calcium] corrected for albumin concentration of greater than 13–14 mg/dL), however, confusion and acute renal failure can develop rapidly. As a result, the concentration of this ion should always be measured in any patient with altered mental status of unclear cause and in particular in the patient with accompanying acute renal failure. Multiple drugs and clinical conditions can cause mild hypercalcemia ([calcium] 11–13 mg/dL), but more severe hypercalcemia is virtually always due to unregulated secretion of PTH or to the production by certain malignancies of a peptide with similar effects (PTH-related peptide). Table 1 summarizes the causes of hypercalcemia, and the key causes are discussed below.

Table 1 Causes of Hypercalcemia

Primary hyperparathyroidism
Malignancies
PTH-related peptide (solid tumors)
Osteoclast activating factors (leukemias, multiple myeloma)
Bone destruction (prostate cancer)
Calcitriol-mediated (lymphomas)
Granulomatous disease
Sarcoidosis
Tuberculosis
Fungal infections
Vitamin D intoxication
Familial hypocalciuric hypercalcemia
Renal failure (autonomous hyperparathyroidism)
Hyperthyroidism
Drugs
Lithium
Thiazide diuretics
Vitamin A intoxication
Immobilization
Pheochromocytoma

1. Primary Hyperparathyroidism

Primary hyperparathyroidism occurs when the secretion of PTH no longer responds to its controlling factors (Fig. 1). This disorder is most commonly caused by a parathyroid adenoma, but it also can be caused by idiopathic diffuse hyperplasia. Primary hyperparathyroidism is uncovered by the presence of persistent hypercalcemia. If renal function is normal, serum phosphorus concentration is commonly low, but this finding is not always present. When renal function is impaired, hypophosphatemia is not usually present. Typically, serum [calcium] is only mildly elevated, and the patient is either asymptomatic or has nonspecific symptoms. However, acute episodes of severe hypercalcemia ([calcium] $>$ 15 mg/dL) can occur. These episodes are presumably related to volume contraction, although in some instances the cause is unclear. When severe hypercalcemia occurs, immediate treatment is necessary to prevent permanent renal damage (see Chapter 31).

The diagnosis of primary hyperparathyroidism is made simply and directly by measuring the serum PTH level. The finding of a level that is inappropriately high for the prevailing serum [Ca^{2+}] makes the diagnosis. The one exception to this rule is the patient with renal insufficiency (see below). Although there are a wide variety of indirect tests available, none is sufficiently specific or sensitive and serum PTH levels are now measured quite reliably.

2. Hypercalcemia of Malignancy

Malignant tumors can cause hypercalcemia by a number of mechanisms. Certain solid tumors (e.g., breast, lung) can produce a peptide that binds to certain PTH receptors in the body (PTH-related peptide). Production of this peptide produces the same clinical features as primary hyperparathyroidism. Tumoral hypercalcemia is probably the most common cause of severe hypercalcemia. The diagnosis is made by direct measurement of PTH-related peptide. PTH levels by contrast will be vanishingly low in this disorder. In contrast to primary hyperparathyroidism, serum phosphorus levels are not usually reduced and vitamin D levels are not increased.

Other tumors, most notably bone marrow tumors such as multiple myeloma, cause hypercalcemia by the release of cytokines that promote osteolytic activity directly. These cytokines include TGF-α, interleukin-1α, and tumor necrosis factor. These osteoclast-activating cytokines are sometimes termed as a group osteoclast-activating factors (OAF). Typically the hypercalcemia caused by these tumors is only mild to moderate, but severe hypercalcemia can occur as well. In these disorders both PTH and PTH-related peptide levels will be low.

Some tumors that characteristically metastasize to bone (e.g., prostate cancer) cause hypercalcemia by destruction of bone and release of calcium. In rare instances lymphomas are associated with hypercalcemia as a result of autonomous calcitriol production by the tumor, analogous to that seen with granulomas (see below).

3. Granulomatous Disease

Certain granulomatous diseases, most notably sarcoidosis, are associated with hypercalcemia. In these disorders, the granulomas produce calcitriol in an unregulated fashion. The hypercalcemia is usually mild and is a diagnostic clue to the presence of the disease but also usually requires therapeutic attention. In addition to sarcoidosis, hypercalcemia has been reported with tuberculosis and with granulomatous fungal infections.

4. Vitamin D Intoxication

Deliberate or inadvertent overdosage of any of the vitamin D preparations available can cause hypercalcemia. The hypercalcemia can be severe and, when caused by excess ingestion of long-acting forms of vitamin D (e.g., cholecalciferol), can persist for as long as several weeks after the drug is discontinued. Calcitriol is safer in this regard because the hypercalcemia produced is rapidly reversed on discontinuation of the drug.

5. Familial Hypocalciuric Hypercalcemia

This rare familial disorder causes hypercalcemia that is sometimes difficult to distinguish from primary hyperparathyroidism. PTH levels can be slightly increased. The characteristic feature is a low renal calcium excretion (usually <150 mg/day coupled with hypercalcemia) and of course the positive family history.

6. Renal Failure

In renal failure the ''setpoint'' at which serum [Ca^{2+}] inhibits PTH secretion is altered so that PTH is secreted at higher serum levels. Although historically this was thought to be due to parathyroid hyperplasia secondary to an initial period of hypocalcemia, it can be demonstrated even in the absence of hypocalcemia. Because patients with renal failure are now usually treated with dietary calcium supplements and calcitriol, hypercalcemia has become a more common finding than hypocalcemia.

7. Drugs

A variety of drugs can cause mild hypercalcemia. Lithium causes hypercalcemia by inducing parathyroid hyperplasia. The thiazide diuretics decrease renal calcium excretion but do not cause hypercalcemia in the absence of some other defect in calcium homeostasis.

B. Hypocalcemia

Hypocalcemia (defined as a serum [Ca^{2+}] < 1.1 mmol/L, or a serum [calcium], corrected for albumin, of < 9 mg/dL) occurs only in a few settings (Table 2). These are discussed below.

1. Hypoparathyroidism

Hypoparathyroidism is a rare condition that can be congenital or can develop later in life, occurring either in a familial or a sporadic pattern. Patients with hypoparathyroidism typically present with symptomatic hypocalcemia and have associated hyperphosphatemia. These manifestations of altered calcium homeostasis are often associated with other findings in the idiopathic form of the disease including dry and scaly skin, scant axillary, pubic, and eyebrow hair. In addition, idiopathic hypoparathyroidism can be associated with other endocrine abnormalities, including adrenal, thyroid, or gonadal failure. Hypoparathyroidism can also be acquired as a result of surgical parathyroidectomy. In patients with renal fail-

Table 2 Causes of Hypocalcemia

Hypoparathyroidism
Idiopathic
Postparathyroidectomy
Calcitriol deficiency
Renal failure
Nutritional deficiency
Lack of exposure to sunlight
Pseudohypoparathyroidism
Magnesium deficiency
Renal failure
Acute pancreatitis
Citrate administration
Anticonvulsant therapy

ure, this is not an uncommon procedure that leads to symptomatic hypocalcemia. In this instance, the hypocalcemia is aggravated by the enhanced uptake of calcium by bone that has been calcium depleted by prior hyperparathyroidism (so-called hungry bone syndrome). In all instances the diagnosis of parathyroid hormone deficiency can be made by finding a PTH level that is lower than expected for the prevailing ionized serum [Ca^{2+}].

2. Impaired Tissue Responsiveness to PTH

In this group of disorders, the PTH level is high despite the presence of hypocalcemia. Thus, the calcemic response to PTH is impaired. This impairment could be due to a receptor defect or to events occurring after PTH binds to its receptor. Except in rare instances, PTH resistance is a postreceptor problem. The most common cause of hypocalcemia is acute or chronic renal insufficiency. The skeletal resistance to PTH in renal disease is multifactorial, including a component of calcitriol deficiency (see below) and direct tissue unresponsiveness. Hypocalcemia is present in only a minority of patients with renal insufficiency. Hypomagnesemia is associated with hypocalcemia due to both impaired PTH release and impaired tissue responsiveness to PTH (see later).

Pseudohypoparathyrodism is a rare hereditary disorder associated with tissue unresponsiveness to PTH. The cause of the unresponsiveness is not known, but is likely due to a defective PTH receptor.

3. Calcitriol Deficiency

Calcitriol deficiency leads to hypocalcemia both by impairing intestinal calcium absorption and by reducing skeletal responsiveness to PTH. Deficiency in the active form of vitamin D can be the result of many factors, including poor nutrition, lack of exposure to sunlight, and liver and kidney disease. The basic precursor for calcitriol, cholecalciferol, can be ingested and absorbed from certain foods or dietary supplements or can be synthesized in the skin, a process stimulated by exposure to sunlight. The liver hydroxylates cholecalciferol, producing 25-hydroxyl cholecalciferol in an unregulated fashion. This compound circulates in the blood and is the substrate for the renal production of calcitriol, 1,25-dihydroxycholecalciferol. The 1α-hydroxyl enzymatic step in the kidney is regulated both by PTH and serum phosphate concentration. Thus low PTH levels (as in hypoparathyroidism) or hyperphosphatemia can lead to a functional calcitriol deficiency.

The most common cause of calcitriol deficiency is renal disease, which results in the loss of the synthetic enzyme necessary for the production of this hormone. Liver disease only rarely causes impaired 25 hydroxylation. Nutritional deficiency has been overcome in most developed countries by the addition of vitamin D to milk. In contrast to hypoparathyroidism, the hypocalcemia seen with calcitriol deficiency is not associated with hyperphosphatemia (with the exception of the functional form that is caused by hyperphosphatemia or when coexistent renal disease impedes phosphate excretion by the kidney). Isolated calcitriol deficiency impairs renal phosphate reabsorption and increases its excretion. As a result, hyophosphatemia can occur.

4. Calcium Precipitation/Complexing

Hypocalcemia can result from acute precipitation of calcium salts in necrotic tissue, such as occurs with acute pancreatitis or with acute hyperphosphatemia. In either instance, for the hypocalcemia to persist there must be some skeletal resistance to PTH or accompanying PTH deficiency. A transient reduction in ionized [Ca^{2+}] can be caused by administration of citrate (with blood transfusions or plasmapheresis), which complexes calcium in the blood.

IV. PHOSPHORUS

Phosphorus exists in the body as inorganic and organic phosphate. Approximately 90% of the phosphate in the body is in the bones. Of the remaining 10%, most resides intracellularly. Phosphate in serum and body tissues is measured as elemental phosphorus and expressed as mg/dL. In the serum, it exists only as inorganic phosphate, and the normal concentration is 2.5–4.5 mg/dL (0.8–1.5 mmol/L). Phosphorus is contained in most of the foods we eat, and approximately 60% of ingested phosphorus is absorbed, primarily in the small intestine. Although absorption is largely unregulated, calcitriol stimulates phosphorus absorption from the gut. In addition, phosphorus absorption is increased in states of phosphorus depletion by a calcitriol-independent mechanism. Once absorbed, phosphates participate in cell and bone turnover, but in the steady state phosphate absorption is balanced by renal phosphate excretion. Phosphate is freely filtered by the glomerulus, and approximately 80% is reabsorbed. Phosphate reabsorption is confined almost entirely to the proximal tubule, and its reabsorption there is linked to sodium by an apical membrane cotransporter. Phosphate reabsorption is regulated by PTH; PTH specifically inhibits the contransporter and reduces phosphate reabsorption. In addition, renal phosphate handling is regulated by phosphate intake. A high phosphate intake inhibits reabsorption, and phosphate depletion promotes reabsorption. A variety of other factors influence renal phosphate handling, including acid-base status, calcitriol, growth hormone, and thyroid hormone.

V. DISORDERS OF PHOSPHATE HOMEOSTASIS

A. Hyperphosphatemia

Hyperphosphatemia is virtually always the result of impaired renal phosphate excretion. The most common cause is renal failure. As renal function declines, the ability to excrete phosphate, even in the presence of adequate PTH, becomes progressively impaired. With continued dietary phosphate intake, hyperphosphatemia develops, contributing to disordered calcium homeostasis (see earlier). The diagnosis is made by measurement of serum phosphorus; there are few symptoms save for pruritis when serum calcium concentration is not low (see Chapter 4). The causes of hyperphosphatemia are listed in Table 3. As mentioned earlier, PTH deficiency and tissue unresponsiveness to PTH (pseudohypoparathyroidism) are associated with hyperphosphatemia in the absence of renal insufficiency. Increased tissue breakdown or treatment of malignancies can lead to the release of large amounts of intracellular phosphate into the extracellular fluid. However, significant hyperphosphatemia occurs in this setting only when there is an associated reduction in renal function. Administration of large amounts of exogenous phosphate (e.g., laxatives) to patients with renal insufficiency can also cause hyperphosphatemia.

B. Hypophosphatemia

Hypophosphatemia, defined as a serum phosphorus concentration of <2.5 mg/dL, is a relatively unusual finding because of the ubiquity of phosphates in the food we eat. In most instances, hypophosphatemia is a reflection of phosphate depletion (Table 3). The exceptions are acute respiratory alkalosis and treatment

Table 3 Disorders of Phosphate Homeostasis

Hyperphosphatemia
Renal failure
Hypoparathyroidism
Pseudohypoparathyroidism
Cell destruction
Rhabdomyolysis
Cancer chemotherapy
Phosphate administration
Laxatives/enemas
Hypophosphatemia
Hyperparathyroidism
Fanconi syndrome
Antacid abuse
Vitamin D deficiency
Chronic alcoholism
Uncontrolled diabetes mellitus
Acute respiratory alkalosis
Hyperalimentation

of diabetic ketoacidosis. In both these settings hypophosphatemia occurs because of a sudden shift of phosphate into cells. The diagnosis of hypophosphatemia is made by measurement of serum phosphorus concentration. Only with severe hypophosphatemia (phosphorus < 1.0 mg/dL) are clinically significant adverse effects seen (see Chapter 4).

Hyperparathyroidism causes hypophosphatemia by increasing urinary phosphate excretion, but this finding is not always present in this disorder. PTH-independent urinary phosphate wasting occurs in some forms of proximal (type 2) renal tubular acidosis (Fanconi syndrome) and following renal transplantation. Calcitriol deficiency impairs phosphate absorption from the gut. The overuse of antacids can also lead to hypophosphatemia by impairing phosphate absorption.

Severe hypophosphatemia can occur in chronic alcoholism and is usually multifactorial in origin. It may be due to poor dietary intake, gastrointestinal disorders that impair phosphate absorption, and hyperventilation occurring with cirrhosis or alcohol withdrawal. During hyperalimentation or during a nutritional recovery syndrome, phosphate depletion is coupled with a sudden shift of phosphate into recovering cells and can lead to severe hypophosphatemia. In most instances, however, patients receiving parenteral nutrition are catabolic and hypophosphatemia does not occur.

VI. MAGNESIUM

Magnesium is a key intracellular ion, activating enzymes and playing a role in protein and DNA synthesis. Unlike calcium and phosphorus, however, magnesium is contained in only a subset of foods including cereals, nuts, dairy products, and green leafy vegetables. As a result, many Americans ingest suboptimal amounts of this key substance. Much less is known about the regulation of magnesium balance than other ions. It appears that about 30–70% of ingested magnesium is absorbed, primarily in the small intestine. Absorption may be affected by calcitriol, but the major determinant appears to be magnesium intake. Once absorbed, magnesium is maintained primarily as an intracellular ion. The normal serum concentration is 0.7–1.3 mmol/L (1.5–2.5 mEq/L). By contrast, the concentration of magnesium in metabolically active cells is as high as 15–20 mEq/L. Approximately 30% of serum magnesium is protein-bound (primarily with albumin), and the remainder exists as the free ion.

The major determinant of magnesium balance is the kidney. Magnesium is filtered and has a unique pattern of reabsorption along the nephron. In contrast to most other ions, only approximately 25% of filtered magnesium is absorbed in the proximal tubule. The primary site for magnesium reabsorption is the ascending limb of Henle's loop, where approximately 65% is reabsorbed. Its reabsorption at this site appears to be regulated by serum calcium concentration, magnesium concentration, and PTH. Both hypercalcemia and hypermagnesemia depress magnesium reabsorption. PTH increases magnesium reabsorption.

A. Hypomagnesemia

Hypomagnesemia, defined as a serum magnesium concentration of <1.5 mEq/L, is a very common abnormality, occurring in up to 10% of hospitalized patients. The causes are listed in Table 4 and include poor dietary intake, impaired gastrointestinal absorption, and abnormal renal losses. Severe hypomagnesemia can occur in chronic alcoholism and is usually multifactorial in origin. It may be due to poor dietary intake, gastrointestinal disorders that impair magnesium absorption, and renal magnesium losses. Diarrheal states, malabsorption, and laxative abuse are all associated with impaired absorption of dietary magnesium and can result in hypomagnesemia. Hypercalcemia from any cause promotes renal magnesium losses and can cause hypomagnesemia. Hypomagnesemia is a typical finding in patients treated with loop or thiazide diuretics, as these agents impair renal magnesium reabsorption. Other drugs, including the antirejection agents cyclosporine and tacrolimus, cause renal magnesium wasting. Commonly, patients with hypomagnesemia have magnesium depletion secondary to more than one of the above factors. Primary hyperaldosteronism is associated with abnormal

Table 4 Disorders of Magnesium Homeostasis

Hypomagnesemia
Malnutrition
Chronic alcoholism
Malabsorption syndrome (e.g., sprue)
Diarrhea
Laxative abuse
Hypercalcemia
Primary hyperaldosteronism
Hyperthyroidism
Gitelman's syndrome
Idiopathic hypomagnesemia (familial)
Drugs
Diuretics
Gentamicin
Cyclosporine
Tacrolimus
Cisplatinum
Hypermagnesemia
Renal failure
Magnesium administration
Antacids
Laxatives
Treatment of eclampsia

renal magnesium losses, as is Gitelman's syndrome, a rare genetic disorder of distal tubular transport. Isolated hypomagnesemia is a rare hereditory disorder.

Magnesium depletion may be more common than the subset defined by a low serum magnesium concentration. Research studies have shown that magnesium depletion may exist in the absence of a low serum magnesium concentration. Nonetheless, the clinical diagnosis is made by measuring serum magnesium concentration and finding a level lower than 1.5 mEq/L. As discussed earlier, the diagnosis may be suspected in patients with the combined findings of hypokalemia and hypocalcemia. Hypomagnesemia inhibits PTH release and can produce hypocalcemia by this mechanism. The mechanism by which it produces hypokalemia that is resistant to potassium replacement therapy is unknown.

B. Hypermagnesemia

Hypermagnesemia ($[Mg^{2+}] > 2.5$ mEq/L) is a potentially life-threatening electrolyte abnormality when severe, causing hypotension, paralysis, and severe bradycardia (see Chapter 4). Because the kidney ordinarily excretes excess magnesium rapidly, sustained hypermagnesemia is a disorder confined to patients with renal insufficiency. Even in these individuals, hypermagnesemia is usually not a significant problem unless magnesium intake is unusually high. The most common sources of excess magnesium are the magnesium-containing antacids and laxatives. Both products should be avoided or used with caution in patients with renal insufficiency. Hypermagnesemia is a goal in the treatment of eclampsia, but overzealous treatment can lead to symptomatic hypermagnesemia. In elderly patients, the excessive use of magnesium-containing laxatives can also lead to hypermagnesemia.

SUGGESTED READINGS

Bilezikian JP. Management of acute hypercalcemia. N Engl J Med 1992; 326:1196–1203.

Brown EM, Pollak M, Hebert SC. The extracellular calcium-sensing receptor. Its role in health and disease. Ann Rev Med 1998; 49:15–29.

Bourke E, Delaney V. Assessment of hypocalcemia and hypercalcemia. Clin Lab Med 1993; 13:157–181.

Mundy GR. The hypercalcemia of malignancy. Kidney Int 1987; 31:142–155.

Quamme GA. Renal magnesium handling: new insights in understanding old problems. Kidney Int 1997; 52:1180–1195.

Weisinger JR, Bellorin-Font E. Magnesium and phosphorus. Lancet 1997; 352:391–396.

15
Acute Renal Failure

Matthew G. Chaffin
Androscoggin Clinical Associates, Lewiston, Maine

Jonathan Himmelfarb
Maine Medical Center, Portland, Maine

I. INTRODUCTION

Acute renal failure (ARF) is a clinical syndrome characterized by an abrupt and severe deterioration of renal function over a period of hours to days. As a result, patients with ARF are unable to maintain fluid and electrolyte homeostasis and have a diminished capacity to excrete nitrogenous wastes. Serum creatinine concentration may rise as rapidly as 2.0 mg/dL/day, and oliguria (urine output of <400 mL/day) (see Chapter 1) is present in 40–75% of patients. As many as 60% of patients with ARF may require hemodialysis. Acute renal failure is an important syndrome for the clinician to recognize both because of its high mortality and because many causes of acute renal dysfunction are either spontaneously reversible or reversible with appropriate intervention.

II. EPIDEMIOLOGY

A. Acute Renal Failure in the Community

There are remarkably few studies examining the incidence of ARF in the community. A prospective study encompassing two health districts in Devon, England, identified 172 cases of severe acute renal failure (serum creatinine concentration > 500 μM, i.e., >5.5 mg/dL) per million adults per year. Age-related incidence rose from 17 per million yearly in adults under the age of 50 to 949 per million yearly in the 80- to 89-year age group. A community study from Spain identified 209 cases of acute renal failure per million population per year. Although there are no similar data from the United States, it is likely that 300–700 cases per million adults occur annually in this country.

B. Acute Renal Failure in Hospitalized Patients

More information is available about the incidence of ARF in hospitalized patients in the United States. The incidence varies widely, depending on the definition of ARF. Commonly used definitions include an increase in serum creatinine concentration of >0.5 mg/dL or an increase of more than 50% over the baseline value. Some studies require the need for dialysis in their definition of ARF. Despite this variability, ARF appears to occur in approximately 1% of patients on admission to the hospital, in 5–7% during the course of hospitalization for general medical or surgical problems, and in as many as 23% of patients undergoing cardiopulmonary bypass surgery. Major risk factors include advanced age, diabetes, and underlying renal insufficiency.

III. DIAGNOSIS

When ARF develops in a hospitalized patient, it is usually easily recognized by a sudden increase in the serum creatinine concentration or, when oliguria develops, by an abrupt decrease in urine output. More difficult to diagnose is the patient who is first evaluated with an elevation in the serum creatinine concentration. The limitations of serum creatinine concentration in assessing GFR are discussed below, after which the approach to the patient first seen with an elevated creatinine concentration is reviewed.

A. Assessment of Renal Function

The uses and limitations of the serum creatinine concentration as an estimate of GFR are discussed in detail in Chapter 5. The primary requirement for the serum creatinine to be used to estimate GFR, however, is that the patient be in a steady state of creatinine production and excretion. In ARF, because of ongoing alterations in creatinine production, volume of distribution, and excretion, this requirement is almost never met, and therefore one cannot use serum creatinine concentration as an index of GFR (Fig. 1). The rate of change in this parameter from day to day, however, can be used to estimate whether renal function is improving or deteriorating. More exact measurements of GFR include iothalamate and inulin clearance, but these techniques are too cumbersome for routine clinical use. There are several additional reasons why creatinine may not be a good indicator of renal function in patients with acute renal failure (Table 1). Urea, commonly

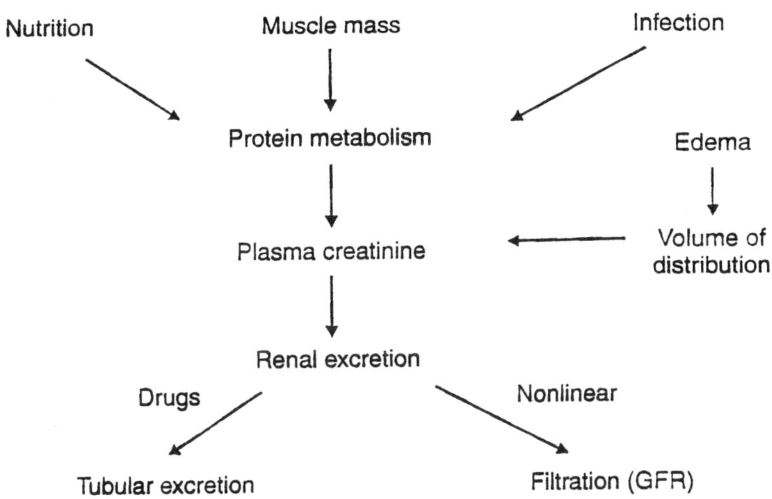

Figure 1 Confounding influences on serum creatinine concentration that may obscure its relationship to GFR in acute renal failure (ARF). (From Star RA. Treatment of acute renal failure. Kidney Int 54:1817–1831, 1998.)

measured as a low molecular weight uremic toxin, is freely filtered but is reabsorbed to a variable extent. Therefore, blood urea nitrogen (BUN) concentration is not a good estimate of renal function even under steady-state conditions. In ARF, both its production and excretion rates are altered. This is especially true in critically ill patients where BUN can be elevated for a number of reasons (Table 1).

Table 1 Causes of Elevated BUN and Creatinine Not Associated with Loss of GFR

BUN	Creatinine
Increased protein intake	Increased muscle release
Upper GI bleeding	Decreased tubular secretion
Corticosteroids	Cimetidine
Increased catabolism	Trimethoprim
Prerenal azotemia	Interference with measurement (Jaffe reaction)
	Ketones
	Cephalosporins

B. Acute vs Chronic Renal Failure

In any patient who is first seen with an elevation in serum creatinine concentration, chronic renal failure must be considered in addition to ARF, particularly when previous measurements of renal function are not available. The duration of symptoms of uremia, such as a decrease in appetite, polyuria, nocturia, and pruritis, may be helpful but are often not present in any direct relationship to the onset of renal failure. A renal ultrasound showing bilaterally atrophied or hyperechoic kidneys is strong evidence of a chronic problem. Detection of renal osteodystrophy by radiographic means in the hands or clavicle can be helpful. With the exception of a historical record of serum creatinine values demonstrating an abrupt increase over a short period of time, there are no laboratory tests that are reliable in distinguishing acute from chronic renal failure. Hypocalcemia, hyperphosphatemia, and anemia all may occur in either acute or chronic renal failure.

C. Approach to Determining the Cause of ARF

Once the diagnosis of ARF has been established, the approach to determining its cause is to consider three major categories: prerenal, intrinsic, and postrenal (or obstructive). By definition, prerenal causes are reversible with treatment that restores renal perfusion. In postrenal disease, renal function will return to normal after the obstruction has been removed if the obstruction has been acute. If the obstruction is a chronic problem then there may be some permanent loss of kidney function. Intrinsic renal failure has many causes, the most common hospital-acquired cause being acute tubular necrosis (ATN).

D. Initial Evaluation

Patients with acute renal failure should be approached in the same manner whether they are inpatients or outpatients. The medical history, including thorough examination of the medical record, is crucial. Nephrotoxin exposure needs to be searched for by history and hospital record (see Chapter 20 for an extensive discussion of nephrotoxic renal injury). Prerenal and obstructive causes (see below and in Chapter 23) should be sought for first, because these are in most instances rapidly reversible problems. Physical examination should focus on assessment of extracellular fluid (ECF) volume and effective circulating blood volume (EBV). Changes in body weight, daily intake and output, and other hemodynamic measures such as pulmonary capillary wedge pressure and cardiac output should be assessed when available. Urinalysis should always be a part of the initial assessment because it frequently can provide supportive evidence for various forms of intrinsic renal causes of ARF. Anuria (urine output < 50 mL/day) (see Chapter 1) is suggestive of obstruction because it only rarely occurs in patients with intrinsic renal disease or prerenal azotemia.

IV. CAUSES OF ACUTE RENAL FAILURE

A. Prerenal Azotemia

Prerenal azotemia is defined as any state in which an acute deterioration in renal function is caused by decreased renal blood flow (Table 2). In patients with prerenal azotemia, correction of the cause of the decrease in renal perfusion should reverse the ARF because there is no structural abnormality in the kidney. Prerenal azotemia can be considered as being caused by decreased effective blood volume (EBV), defined as the volume of arterial blood required to perfuse vital organs. This volume cannot be measured precisely but signs of inadequate volume can be assessed clinically (see below). The causes of ineffective or inadequate circulating blood volume can be either absolute or relative. Absolute causes include any cause of direct decrease in blood volume such as dehydration, ECF volume depletion, bleeding of any cause, or fluid accumulation in a so-called "third space" such as occurs in pancreatitis. EBV can also be decreased when blood volume is normal or increased but circulating arterial volume is reduced in settings such as congestive heart failure, liver disease, and septic states. Finally, EBV may be normal but renal hemodynamics can be altered by a variety of drugs, including nonsteroidal anti-inflammatory drugs (NSAIDs), drugs that interfere with the action of angiotensin II (ACE inhibitors or receptor blockers), radiocontrast agents, and calcineurin inhibitors (cyclosporine and tacrolimus), leading to prerenal azotemia.

Findings on physical examination supportive of ECF volume depletion include low or undetectable venous pressures in the jugular veins and orthostatic hypotension or tachycardia. Dry oral mucosa and decreased skin turgor are not good indicators of volume status. If available and reliable, the patient's recent changes in weight, intake, and output are also important in defining ECF volume status. Assessing ECF volume in a postsurgical patient is notoriously difficult, and physical exam alone cannot be relied upon to identify subtle volume deple-

Table 2 Pathophysiology of Prerenal Azotemia

Decreased extracellular volume	Decreased intravascular volume (third spacing)	Decrease effective circulating volume	Renal vasoconstriction
Hemorrhage	Pancreatitis	CHF	Sepsis
GI losses	Postsurgical	Sepsis	Cirrhosis
Renal losses	Burn injury	Cirrhosis	NSAIDs
Skin losses	Nephrotic syndrome	Renal artery stenosis	Cyclosporine
			Radiocontrast agents
			Hypercalcemia

tion. Central venous pressure can be measured with invasive hemodynamic monitoring if there is question. A trial of isotonic saline is frequently used with 250–500 mL administered rapidly followed by reassessment of clinical signs as well as changes in urine output.

1. BUN/Creatinine Ratio

One laboratory finding that is suggestive of prerenal azotemia is a BUN value that is increased out of proportion to the increase in serum creatinine concentration, expressed as a BUN/creatinine ratio (both in mg/dL) > 20. The physiological response of the kidney to a decrease in blood flow is to increase the reabsorption of both water and urea from the collecting ducts, and this change in transport reduces urea clearance to a greater extent than the reduction in creatinine clearance. However, it should be emphasized that this finding is neither very sensitive nor specific. In catabolic states an increase in urea production can cause the same finding even when intrinsic renal disease is the cause of the acute renal failure. A similar finding can also be seen in obstructive uropathy, as a result of urea reabsorption from the renal pelvis and ureters.

2. Urine Sodium Excretion

Urinary sodium excretion may also be used to determine whether ARF is due to a prerenal cause as opposed to intrinsic renal disease. The most useful test is to measure the fraction of filtered sodium that is excreted in the urine (FE_{Na}). FE_{Na} is the ratio of urinary to plasma sodium concentration divided by the ratio of urinary to plasma creatinine concentration multiplied by 100 $[(U_{Na}/S_{Na})/(U_{Cr}/S_{Cr}) \times 100]$. The normal response of the kidney to a reduction in renal blood flow is to avidly recapture all the filtered sodium, and therefore in prerenal states FE_{Na} should be $<1\%$. A FE_{Na} of $>2\%$ suggests the presence of tubular damage, that is, ATN (see below). There are, however, several clinical situations where the FE_{Na} will misrepresent the actual physiology. These are listed in Table 3.

B. Postrenal (Obstructive) ARF

The kidneys are able to compensate to a degree such that near normal renal function can be obtained if one kidney is completely obstructed. Therefore, postrenal causes of ARF are due to either bilateral obstruction of the ureters or obstruction at the bladder outlet. There are many processes that can cause either problem (see Chapter 23). A good history is the most useful tool to uncover the etiology prior to any further testing. A history of nephrolithiasis, prostatic hypertrophy, or systemic symptoms of tumor are suggestive of an obstructive cause of ARF. ARF with anuria also suggests obstruction, but partial obstruction may present with polyuria. If, on physical examination, the patient has suprapu-

Table 3 Syndromes with a Misleading FeNa

Low FeNa and ARF	High FeNa and prerenal azotemia
Intrarenal vasoconstriction	Prior diuretic use
Radiocontrast	Chronic renal insufficiency
Severe burns	
Sepsis	
Pigment nephropathy	
NSAIDs	
Amphotericin B	
Cyclosporine	
Liver disease	
Vasoconstrictor drugs	
Inflammatory states	
Acute glomerulonephritis	
Acute vasculitis	
Renal transplant rejection	

bic distention or tenderness, the diagnosis is straightforward and an attempt at bladder catheterization should be made immediately. Examination of the prostate in men to assess size and check for masses is essential. In women, a pelvic examination may delineate etiologies of obstruction from either the cervix or the uterus.

1. Radiological Evaluation

In all patients with ARF, a renal ultrasound should be performed to determine whether hydronephrosis is present (prior to placement of a Foley catheter if possible). In volume-depleted patients, the severity of hydronephrosis may not be appreciated until the patient is fluid repleted. If an ultrasound does not show hydronephrosis and obstruction is still a strong consideration, additional radiological studies should be undertaken. A CT scan can demonstrate pelvicalyceal dilatation with the added benefit of examining the retroperitoneum and bladder for masses. A retrograde ureterogram is the definitive study for identifying obstruction, but it requires general anesthesia. Intravenous pyelography should not be attempted in ARF because it requires a nephrotoxin (radiocontrast) and will not visualize the kidney well if the serum creatinine concentration is >2.5 mg/dL. A radionucleotide study such as $^{99}Tc^{m}$-DTPA may not be useful if renal dysfunction is marked, as sufficient isotope will not accumulate in the kidneys for adequate visualization.

2. Management of Obstructive ARF

All patients with ARF due to obstruction should have the obstruction released as soon as possible to minimize damage of the renal parenchyma. In the case of bladder neck obstruction, a suprapubic catheter may be placed until definitive work-up and/or surgery can be performed. With bilateral ureteral obstruction either percutaneous nephrostomies or retrograde ureteral stenting should be performed in a timely fashion by a radiologist or urologist. Once the obstruction is relieved, the patient needs to be monitored closely for a postobstructive diuresis (see Chapter 23). This can occur in the setting of both acute and chronic obstruction. Diuresis may initially be as brisk as 2–3 L/hr, leading to rapid volume depletion and exacerbation of renal dysfunction. Electrolytes, volume status, and renal function need to be followed closely.

C. Intrinsic ARF

Intrinsic causes of acute renal failure can be conveniently divided anatomically into glomerular, interstitial, vascular, and tubular etiologies (Table 4). Intrinsic renal disease accounts for 20–30% of all ARF in hospitalized patients, with ATN being the most common diagnosis.

1. Glomerular Disease

Acute renal failure secondary to glomerular disease can occur with acute postinfectious or rapidly progressive glomerulonephritis (RPGN). RPGN can occur as an isolated renal disease or can be associated with a systemic vasculitis (see Chapter 19). Other primary glomerular diseases rarely cause ARF. Membranous nephropathy can cause nephrotic range proteinuria and hypertension, but the associated renal insufficiency usually does not progress to acute renal failure. Minimal change disease with severe nephrotic syndrome (>10 g proteinuria/day with serum albumin <2.0 mg/dL) can cause interstitial parenchymal edema leading to ARF. A small subset of patients with IgA nephropathy and Henoch-Schönlein purpura can progress rapidly and present with ARF.

Glomerular disease should be suspected as a cause of ARF when hematuria, red cell casts, and heavy proteinuria are found on urinalysis. In most cases in which glomerular disease is suspected, renal biopsy is needed to make a precise diagnosis. Screening laboratory tests are sometimes helpful. A low serum complement level is expected in postinfectious glomerulonephritis, in lupus nephritis, and in cryoglobulinemic vasculitis. A positive antineutrophil cytoplasmic antibody titer (ANCA) is seen in polyarteritis, in Wegener's granulomatosis, and in some forms of idiopathic RPGN. An antiglomerular basement membrane antibody (anti-GBM) is seen in Goodpasture's syndrome and in one form of idiopathic RPGN. Nonetheless, because of the types of interventions considered, a

Table 4 Etiology of Acute Intrinsic Renal Failure

Rapidly progressive glomerulonephritis	Tubulointerstitial	Vascular	ATN
Type I—linear deposits	Drug-induced	Large vessel vasculitis	Ischemic
Antiglomerular basement disease	Beta-lactams (methacillin, ampicillin, penicillin)	Cholesterol emboli	Hypotension
Goodpasture with pulmonary hemorrhage	Rifampin	Renovascular disease	Sepsis
Type II—glomerular deposits	Ciprofloxacin	NSAIDS	Toxin
Postinfection	Cephalosporins	Coagulopathic	Pigment nephropathy (myoglobin/hemoglobin)
Systemic lupus erythematosis	Infection	HUS/TTP	Drug-induced (aminoglycosides, heavy metals, cisplatin)
Type III—no deposits or pauci-immune	Staphylococcus	DIC	Crystal-induced
Wegener's	Infiltration		Uric acid
PAN	Lymphoma		Oxalate
	Leukemia		Drug-induced (acyclovir, indivir)
	Sarcoid		

renal biopsy reviewed by a skilled nephropathologist is the standard of diagnostic care for glomerular disease associated with ARF. The diagnosis and management of these disorders is discussed in detail in Chapter 19.

2. Tubulointerstitial Disease

Allergic interstitial nephritis (AIN) is an unusual cause of ARF, accounting for only 1–3% of ARF. AIN can be caused by a wide variety of insults. These can be divided into infectious, drug-related, infiltrative, and rheumatological causes. A complete history of recent exposures and medications is very important. The classic description of AIN includes fever, rash, and eosinophilia, but all of these findings are present in only approximately 25% of patients. Identification of eosinophils in the urine sediment has been advocated by some as useful in the diagnosis of AIN, but this test requires special preparation of the urine by the laboratory and is neither sensitive nor specific. Urinalysis typically shows pyuria and white cell casts but may also demonstrate hematuria.

Although a wide variety of drugs have been reported to produce AIN (see Chapter 20), the best characterized cases are caused by the use of semi-synthetic penicillins such as methacillin. Although the disease can be suspected on clinical grounds, a renal biopsy is necessary to make a definitive diagnosis. The characteristic pathological lesion is an inflammatory interstitial infiltrate containing abundant eosinophils.

A different form of AIN is caused by the use of NSAIDs. Fever, rash, and eosinophilia are rare in the AIN caused by NSAIDs, and the disease usually develops after months of use (with the mean onset at 5–6 months), as opposed to several days with antibiotic-induced AIN. Dialysis may be required in up to 40% of these patients, and complete return to baseline renal function can take up to a year. Nephrotic range proteinuria is seen in up to 80% of cases. Urinalysis typically shows pyuria and white cell casts. The histological glomerular lesion is minimal change disease in conjunction with interstitial inflammation. Chronic NSAID use, especially with phenactin, can cause also papillary necrosis (see Chapter 20), which if severe can also result in ARF.

3. Acute Tubular Necrosis

The most common cause of intrinsic ARF is due to renal tubular injury from ischemia and/or nephrotoxin exposure and is termed acute tubular necrosis (ATN).

Ischemia from any cause leads to a common pathway of injury in the kidney. Initially, hypoxic injury causes ATP depletion in renal tubular epithelial cells followed by loss of cell polarity and ability to maintain electrochemical gradients. An early manifestation of this hypoxic injury is a loss of the ability to concentrate and dilute urine. Eventually the tubular epithelial cells swell as they are unable to maintain their internal osmolality. Up to this point, cell damage is rapidly reversible if perfusion is restored. If hypoxia persists, however, tubular cell necrosis and detachment from the basement membrane occurs. Recovery then requires the regeneration of new epithelial cells under the influence of cytokines and growth factors. In contrast to ischemia, nephrotoxins cause damage directly to the tubular cell. Many nephrotoxins are concentrated in the renal tubular epithelium. When nephrotoxins reach critical intracellular levels, cell injury and death from either necrosis or apoptosis may occur. Clinically important nephrotoxins include heavy metals, organic compounds such as toluene, and antibiotics such as aminoglycosides (see Chapter 20).

The susceptibility of the tubules of the kidney to hypoxic injury is due to the unique blood supply in the kidney. All blood flow to the tubules and renal interstitium is postglomerular, and in the deep cortex and medulla the arterioles and veins are arranged in adjacent columns to facilitate countercurrent exchange of solutes. Although this exchange process is essential for urinary concentrating ability and for acid excretion, it also creates an oxygen gradient between the cortex and medulla, with oxygen tension falling to low levels in the renal medulla. The limited delivery of oxygen to the renal medulla contributes to the special susceptibility to hypoxic injury, especially in the thick ascending limb where transport demands for oxygen are relatively high.

4. Evaluation of the Patient with ATN

Acute tubular necrosis is the most common cause of ARF in hospitalized patients, and many of these cases are iatrogenic. History may provide evidence of either an ischemic or a toxic event leading to ATN. Especially important is evaluation for previous nephrotoxins, including aminoglycosides, NSAIDs, intravenous contrast, cyclosporine, and cisplatinum. Additionally, the use of ACE inhibitors and competitive angiotensin II blockers may reduce blood flow and enhance the likelihood of hypoxic injury.

On physical examination, there are no characteristic findings to assist in the diagnosis of ATN. Urine output can be low or normal. Urinalysis may reveal muddy brown casts, presumably representing free hemoglobin precipitated into casts, but this finding is present only in 50–70% of cases, and it is not entirely specific for ATN. In ATN, the FE_{Na} is characteristically >1%, reflecting tubular damage. Again, however, this finding is not pathognomonic. Both previous diuretic use and acute on chronic renal failure can lead to a ''falsely'' elevated FE_{Na}.

In the absence of pathognomonic findings, the diagnosis is often based on a priori probability and on a combination of findings. The diagnosis is confirmed in many instances only retrospectively when the patient has an abrupt and rapid recovery. Renal biopsy is only rarely indicated, but when performed, characteristic abnormalites, confined to the renal tubules, are usually seen.

V. SPECIAL ETIOLOGIES OF ARF

A. Atheroembolic Acute Renal Failure

The incidence of atheroembolic renal failure has increased dramatically with more aggressive and invasive treatments of coronary, renal, and peripheral vascular disease. Atheroembolic disease rarely occurs spontaneously, and most cases are associated with angiographic or surgical procedures involving the aorta or the use of fibrinolytic therapy. Characteristically, renal function declines several days to 1–2 weeks after the procedure that induced the atheroembolic shower. The renal failure is thought to be induced by the inflammatory response to the shower rather than by the shower itself.

The disease can be asymptomatic but in many instances is associated with abdominal or lower extremity pain. Atheroembolic showers can cause pathology in almost any organ system, including acute renal failure, pancreatitis, GI bleeding, and gangrene in the extremities. Skin manifestations include livedo reticularis, palpable purpura, and necrosis. Funduscopic exam may reveal so-called Hollenhorst plaques, which are cholesterol emboli lodged in the retinal arterioles. There are no pathognomonic laboratory findings, although over half of the patients with atheroembolic renal failure have an elevated eosinophil count and reduced serum complement, and most patients have an elevated erythrocyte sedimentation rate. Urinalysis can show microscopic hematuria, granular and hyaline casts, and proteinuria. Infrequently, nephrotic-range proteinuria may develop. There is no specific treatment for atheroembolic renal failure, and the renal failure is often irreversible. Aggressive lowering of serum cholesterol may improve the outcome. Prognosis is extremely poor when multiple organs are affected, but when the damage is primarily confined to the kidneys, long-term survival may occur and, on occasion, renal function may show partial recovery after several months.

B. Pigment Nephropathy

Pigment nephropathy is a toxic tubular injury caused by myoglobin or hemoglobin. The most common cause is rhabdomyolysis, which causes myoglobin-induced ARF. Rhabdomyolysis is a syndrome of muscle injury and necrosis with release of intracellular components. Muscle necrosis occurs with crush injuries, with prolonged loss of consciousness or stupor, particularly when the patient is found lying on a hard surface. It can also be drug-induced and has been increasingly reported with the use of cholesterol-lowering drugs. Typically, renal function declines abruptly, with oliguria a common presentation. On laboratory testing, rhabdomyolysis is manifested by an elevated creatine kinase, and the value is usually >3000 u/L in patients with pigment-induced ARF. Hyperkalemia, acidemia, hyperphosphatemia, and hypocalcemia frequently develop due to the massive release of intracellular contents. The urine is strongly positive for blood by dipstick, but red cells are either not seen or are few in number on microscopic examination of the urine sediment. If the disease is recognized early, alkalinization of the urine, using intravenous bicarbonate, may be helpful. The risk of the treatment is fluid overload and systemic alkalinization if renal failure is already established. In most instances, supportive care is all that is necessary, and recovery of renal function is the rule. Hemoglobin is a much rarer cause of pigment nephropathy, causing ARF only in the setting of massive hemolysis.

C. Hepatorenal Syndrome

Hepatorenal syndrome (HRS) is a vasoconstrictive cause of acute renal failure that occurs in the setting of advanced liver disease. The syndrome is characterized by renal vasoconstriction in the setting of systemic vasodilation. The cause of the isolated renal vasoconstriction remains unclear, but it is thought to be a physiological response to the generalized vasodilation that results in arterial underfilling. When examined, minimal structural damage to the kidneys is found despite marked deterioration in function. This has been shown both anatomically at autopsy and functionally by demonstrating that the kidneys function well when transplanted to patients without hepatic disease. Furthermore, patients with HRS who receive a liver transplant can recover their renal function completely. The cause of the generalized vasodilation that leads to an irreversible decrease in effective arterial volume is also unknown.

HRS most commonly occurs in the setting of cirrhosis but can also occur with fulminant hepatitis. Ascites and jaundice are almost always present. Renal function usually deteriorates rapidly over a number of days, and the decline in renal function is virtually always accompanied by progressive oliguria and avid sodium retention. Cirrhotic patients are especially susceptible to developing hepatorenal syndrome after aggressive paracentesis or diuresis. Although volume depletion may be a contributing factor, hepatorenal syndrome is separable from prerenal azotemia by the fact that renal function does not improve with expansion of ECF volume or other maneuvers to increase effective vascular volume. The renal failure is irreversible and the outcome is usually fatal. Most patients with hepatorenal syndrome die of complications of cirrhosis before dying of uremia.

Treatment includes excluding all other causes of prerenal azotemia. Volume status should be assessed as previously described, and hypovolemia should be gently corrected. Colloids are an excellent choice for volume expanders. Renal replacement therapy (including peritoneal dialysis, hemodialysis, or continuous hemofiltration) has not been shown to improve outcome, but it can be used as a temporizing measure if liver transplant is imminent. There have been two prospective randomized studies of the use of peritoneovenous shunts, neither of which demonstrated improved outcome. Only orthotopic liver transplantation has been shown to reverse hepatorenal syndrome.

D. Thrombotic Microangiopathy

Thrombotic microangiopathy, including both hemolytic uremic syndrome (HUS) and thrombotic thrombocytopenic purpura (TTP), is a pathological process of hyaline and fibrin thrombi within arterioles and capillaries (see Chapter 19). In HUS, this process is largely confined to the kidney, whereas in TTP it is more generalized. HUS is an illness that commonly occurs in children and is characterized by renal failure, hemolytic anemia, and thrombocytopenia. ARF is preceded from 3 days to 3 weeks by abdominal pain, vomiting, and diarrhea. As many as 40% of patients may only develop mild renal dysfunction. In adults, postpartum women and women on contraceptives are most commonly affected. Interestingly, HUS can be familial and recurrent. Urinalysis reveals hematuria, proteinuria, and red cell casts. ARF is frequently irreversible in adults, and dialysis support is necessary. TTP more frequently affects adults and includes neurological symptoms (60%), fever, bleeding (44%), microangiopathic hemolytic anemia, and less frequently ARF (12%). Exam reveals purpura, pallor, and neurological abnormalities. Treatment of thrombotic angiopathy includes aggressive plasma exchange, sometimes accompanied by high-dose corticosteroids (see Chapter 19).

E. Pregnancy-Associated ARF

Pregnancy is associated with a special risk for ARF, particularly in the setting of uncontrolled hypertension or with infection associated with abortion. With the advent of better understanding of this complication and a decline in septic abortions, the incidence of pregnancy-associated ARF has declined dramatically in the past 20 years. Causes of ARF include acute pyelonephritis, preeclampsia, HELLP (hemolysis, elevated liver functions, and low platelets) syndrome, idiopathic postpartum renal failure, and cortical necrosis of pregnancy. The renal complications of pregnancy are reviewed in detail in Chapter 25.

VI. TREATMENT OF ARF: GENERAL CONSIDERATIONS

Treatment of ARF depends upon establishing the cause (Table 5). As indicated earlier, prerenal causes of ARF should be addressed by repleting ECF volume

Table 5 Approach to the Patient with Acute Renal Failure

Review medical record
Exposure to nephrotoxins
Arterial angiography
Hypotension
Sepsis
Abnormal fluid losses
Assess hemodynamic status
Arterial blood pressure
ECF volume
Clinical assessment
Central venous pressure
Swan line
Assess urine volume and sediment
"Muddy brown" casts
Other formed elements
Assess for obstruction
Renal ultrasound
CT scan if indicated
Assess urine sodium excretion (FeNa) if diagnosis unclear (see text)

or correcting the underlying abnormality if possible. Relief of obstruction can rapidly reverse obstructive uropathy. The management of intrinsic glomerular and vascular diseases is addressed in Chapter 19. At present there is no specific treatment available for the most common cause of ARF, that is, ATN. Because ATN is, by definition, a reversible condition, the general approach to the management of this disorder is directed at preventing complications from developing while awaiting recovery of renal function.

A. Conservative Support

Conservative support for the patient with ATN includes general care of the inciting event and treatment of the metabolic alternations, nutritional deficiencies, and volume changes engendered by renal failure. Specific attention should be paid to following blood pressure and daily weights as well as daily intake and both urinary and nonurinary losses. Serum electrolytes should be evaluated daily, with particular attention to serum potassium and bicarbonate concentrations. Calcium and phosphate should be monitored daily during the initial phase and then every 2–3 days afterward. BUN and creatinine concentrations should be measured daily. In patients with ATN, serum creatinine concentration often increases by 1–2 mg/dL daily. Stabilization of serum creatinine in the absence of renal replacement therapy is usually an indicator of imminent renal recovery. Remember, however, that serum creatinine concentration is determined both by muscle mass and renal function (see Fig. 1 and Table 1). Thus, an elderly malnourished patient may have a serum creatinine concentration as low as 2 mg/dL with little change from day to day and still have ARF.

1. Metabolic Considerations

Hyperkalemia can be life-threatening and should be treated aggressively (see Chapter 30). In general a serum [K^+] of >6.5 mEq/L or lesser degrees of hyperkalemia associated with evidence of A-V or intraventricular conduction abnormalities are indications for emergency treatment. Treatment should be initiated to stabilize cardiac membrane potential (intravenous calcium) and to transfer potassium from the extracellular to the intracellular compartment (insulin and glucose, nebulized albuterol and bicarbonate administration if acidosis is present). If these measures do not rapidly control hyperkalemia, then renal replacement therapy should be initiated.

Metabolic acidosis is a common feature of ARF and is usually caused by multiple factors. Acidemia with pH < 7.20 refractory to treatment with bicarbonate is an indication for renal replacement therapy. Hypocalcemia and hyperphosphatemia are common abnormalities, particularly in the catabolic patient with ATN. In most instances specific treatment of these abnormalities is unnecessary. However, some patients may develop seizures from severe hypocalcemia, and in these instances intravenous calcium and initiation of renal replacement therapy are indicated.

2. Nutrition

In the patient with ATN who is not catabolic and who is eating a 2 g potassium, 2 g sodium, 1 g phosphorus diet should be initiated, and fluid intake should be limited to urine output plus insensible losses. In most instances, fluid intake should be limited to 1–1.5 L/day. Protein intake should not be restricted. In many patients with ATN, an extremely hypercatabolic state is a concomitant feature. Malnutrition can develop rapidly due to inadequate protein and calorie intake as well as diminished utilization of available nutrients. Malnutrition is common, occurring in 30–60% of patients, and is associated with a significant increase in mortality. Protein catabolic rates range from 1.4 to 2.0 g/kg body weight per day (normal 0.8–1.0). Considering that a 70-kg man has 6 kg of noncollagenous protein, this can amount to a loss of 15% of total body noncollagenous protein per week. During hemodialysis, as much as 5–8 g of free amino acids are lost with standard dialysis membranes. With newer high-flux dialysis membranes, 30% more amino acids can be lost. Even larger losses can occur with continuous venovenous hemofiltration techniques (see below). Thus, nutritional status should be carefully monitored and nutritional support (i.e., adequate intake of protein or amino acids) started early in the course of acute renal failure.

B. Maneuvers to Increase Urine Output

Although there are no convincing data to conclude that increasing urine output in the oliguric patient with ATN improves outcome, initial management is often directed at attempting to restore an adequate urine output. Intravenous mannitol, furosemide, and "renal dose" (0.5–2 μg/kg/min) dopamine have all been used for this purpose. Loop diuretics, especially furosemide and bumetanide, have been used to increase urine flow in the hope of flushing out plugged tubules and in an attempt to decrease oxygen demand in the medullary thick ascending limb of the nephron by reducing the "work" of the Na/K ATPase. Mannitol has been used to induce a natruresis and diuresis for similar reasons, but it also may reduce cellular swelling and influx of calcium into the cell. In addition it has been shown that mannitol acts as a free-radical scavenger. Dopamine has receptors in the renal vasculature, when activated cause vasodilation and increase renal blood flow, GFR, and sodium excretion. When using any of these agents it is critically important to first assure that filling pressures and effective vascular volume have been restored to normal levels and that prerenal causes of ARF have been excluded. If prerenal causes have been excluded, a brief trial of any of these approaches has become standard of care, but they should not be continued if no response occurs. Atrial natriuretic peptide has also been used to try to increase urine output and speed recovery from ATN, but a recent controlled trial has shown no benefit of this therapy.

C. Renal Replacement Therapy

Renal replacement therapies currently available include conventional hemodialysis, continuous venovenous hemofiltration (with or without added dialysis), and acute peritoneal dialysis. The latter therapy is no longer used in most hospitals, largely due to the availability and familiarity with hemodialysis and continuous renal replacement therapy in the acute setting. Although there are no clear-cut guidelines, renal replacement therapy should be initiated in most instances if metabolic acidosis and hyperkalemia (unresponsive to other interventions), ECF volume overload, or mental status changes attributable to uremia are present. In addition, renal replacement therapy is indicated specifically for the treatment of certain drug intoxications associated with ATN, including methanol and ethylene glycol ingestions. In patients with multiorgan failure, dialysis is generally initiated promptly once the diagnosis of ATN is established to try to avoid the potential additive complications of rapidly developing uremia, acidosis, and fluid volume overload.

The choice of replacement therapy initiated depends upon local considerations (particular expertise) as well as the specific needs of the patient with renal failure. No therapy has been shown to be more efficacious. Complications of renal replacement therapy include hypotension, arrhythmias, ''dysequilibrium'' syndromes, bleeding, infection, and dialyzer reactions. The use of biocompatible dialysis membranes that do not activate the complement system appear to improve outcome. Regardless of the mode of intervention, mortality for the patient who develops ATN in the intensive care unit is very high—50–80%. Even in the patient on the general hospital ward who develops ATN as a result of drug or radiocontrast nephrotoxicity, mortality is increased and may be as high as 30–40%.

VII. PREVENTION

Although there have been great strides in our understanding of the pathogenesis of ATN, there has been little progress in our ability to reverse this disorder once it is established. The most important consideration, therefore, is to prevent an inciting event from developing in patients at risk. Preventive measures include dosing all medications appropriately for GFR, careful avoidance of unnecessary nephrotoxins, and maintaining ECF volume at an appropriate level. In particular, patients at risk with planned exposure to nephrotoxic radiocontrast agents should be appropriately prepared. Diuretic medication should be held, as well as any nonsteroidal anti-inflammatory drugs, prior to the procedure, and administration of half-isotonic or isotonic saline administered around the time of the procedure. Transplant patients receiving either cyclosporine or tacrolimus should have a dose withheld prior to any angiographic procedure as well. With careful attention to these issues, the likelihood of developing ARF can be minimized.

SUGGESTED READINGS

Alkhunaizi AM, Schrier RW. Management of acute renal failure: new perspectives. Am J Kidney Dis 28(3):315–328, 1996.

Himmelfarb J, Safirstein R. Acute renal failure: from bench to bedside. ARRT 4(suppl 1): S1–S101, 1997.

Star RA. Treatment of acute renal failure. Kidney Int, 54:1817–1831, 1998.

Thadhani R, Pascual M, Bonventre JV. Acute renal failure. N Engl J Med 334(22):1448–1460, 1996.

16
Chronic Renal Insufficiency

Robert N. Santella
University of South Dakota School of Medicine, Sioux Falls, South Dakota

I. INTRODUCTION

Chronic renal insufficiency is a functional diagnosis characterized by a sustained and irreversible decrease in glomerular filtration rate. Patients with chronic renal insufficiency typically are asymptomatic until the damage to the kidney is far advanced, but the disease can progress rapidly to end-stage renal failure if no intervention is undertaken. Early diagnosis and treatment are of paramount importance in order to slow, or arrest, the progression of kidney damage. This chapter focuses on the management of patients with glomerular filtration rates that are irreversibly reduced to between 15 and 50 mL/min, defined by serum creatinine concentrations between approximately 2 and 5 mg/dL.

Although few data exist regarding the prevalence of mild chronic renal insufficiency, accurate data are available for end-stage renal disease (ESRD). At the end of 1995 there were over 270,000 patients in the United States with ESRD. For every patient with ESRD, there are at least eight patients with chronic renal insufficiency not yet having reached end stage. The number of patients reaching ESRD increases significantly with age. In 1995 the incidence rate was 384 per million population for 50-year-olds but greater than 1000 per million population for those over age 65 (see Fig. 1). In addition, the number of new patients needing chronic dialysis has been increasing at a rate of 6–10% per year. Although annual growth in the renal failure population is occurring at all ages, most of the increase is in the elderly. The number of ESRD patients is increasing at a rate of 7.5%

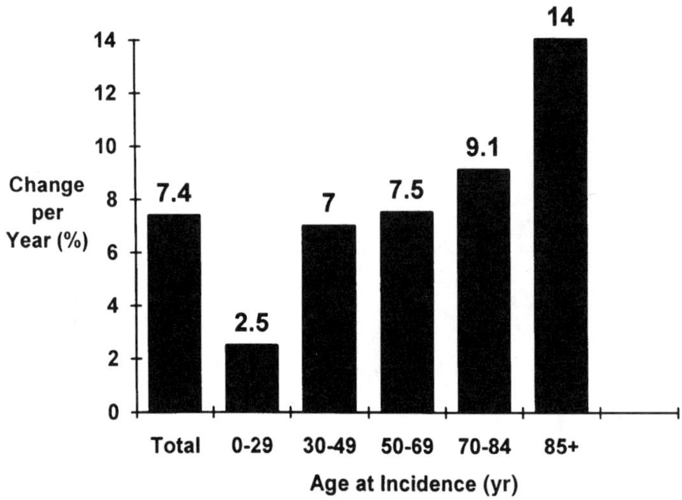

Figure 1 Annualized percent increase in reported ESRD point prevalence rates between 1994 and 1995, by age at onset of ESRD. (Adapted from U.S. Renal Data System, 1997.)

per year in those aged 50–69 years, 9.1% per year in those aged 70–84 years, and 14% per year in those over age 85.

Chronic renal insufficiency and eventual ESRD impart huge financial and human costs. As renal function deteriorates, quality of life diminishes concomitantly. With renal failure comes the fatigue of anemia, an increase in vascular events with hypertension and accelerated atherosclerosis, extracelluar fluid volume overload, left ventricular dysfunction, malnutrition, and bone disease from secondary hyperparathyroidism. Dietary changes are imposed and multiple medications are necessary. Half of all dialysis patients are functionally disabled, and the majority are financially burdened. Most concerning is the dramatic impact of renal failure on mortality rates. As shown in Table 1, a 50-year-old white woman in the United States without renal disease has 31 years of remaining lifetime, but a 50-year-old woman with ESRD has only 5 years of life remaining. High rates of cardiovascular disease are responsible for this excess mortality. ESRD mortality rates are dramatically influenced by age and comorbid disease, especially diabetes. Finally, in terms of financial cost, the 1995 total direct medical payments for ESRD by public (mostly Medicare) and private sources exceeded 13 billion dollars.

Table 1 Expected Remaining Lifetimes for U.S. Population (1990) and Dialysis Patients (1995) by Age, Race, and Sex

Age	U.S. population, 1990				ESRD population, 1995[a]				Dialysis population, 1995			
	Black		White		Black		White		Black		White	
(yr)	M	F	M	F	M	F	M	F	M	F	M	F
30–34	38.2	44.6	44.6	50.4	13.4	13.2	14.8	14	11.6	11.5	9.5	8.8
35–39	34.1	40.6	40	45.6	11.8	11.7	12.4	11.9	10.4	10.4	8	7.6
40–44	30.1	36.8	35.4	40.8	10.2	10.2	10.1	9.2	9.2	9.2	6.7	6.8
45–49	26.2	32.4	30.9	36.1	8.9	8.8	8.4	8.3	8.1	8.1	5.9	6.1
50–54	22.5	28.2	26.5	31.5	7.5	7.3	6.8	6.6	6.9	6.8	5.1	5.1
55–59	19.1	24.3	22.4	27	6.3	6.1	5.4	5.3	5.9	5.8	4.2	4.3
60–64	16	20.9	18.6	22.8	5.3	5.3	4.3	4.3	5.1	5.1	3.6	3.7
65–69	13.3	17.2	15.2	18.9	4.3	4.4	3.4	3.4	4.2	4.3	3.1	2.8
70–74	10.8	14.2	12	15.2	3.5	3.5	2.8	2.9	3.5	3.5	2.7	2.5
75–79	8.8	11.3	9.3	11.8	3	2.9	2.4	2.5	3	2.9	2.4	2.5
80–84	6.9	8.7	7	8.8	2.4	2.4	2	2	2.4	2.4	2	2
85+	5.4	6.5	5.1	6.1	1.9	2.1	1.6	1.8	1.9	2.1	1.6	1.7

[a] Includes patients treated with either dialysis or transplantation.
Source: Adapted from U.S. Renal Data System, 1997.

$$C_{cr}\ (\text{cc/min}) = \frac{(140 - \text{age}) \times \text{lean body weight (kg)}}{P_{cr} \times 72} \quad (\times\ 0.85 \text{ for women})$$

Figure 2 Cockcroft-Gault formula for estimate of creatinine clearance (C_{cr}). P_{cr} = Plasma creatinine. The value is multiplied by 0.85 for women because they have less muscle mass.

II. MEASUREMENT OF RENAL FUNCTION

A thorough discussion of measurement of renal function is presented in Chapter 5, but two important points bear emphasizing. First, although serum creatinine concentration is simple to measure and readily available, it is a poor tool for detecting early renal insufficiency. For example, in an individual with a baseline glomerular filtration rate (GFR) of 100 mL/min and a serum creatinine concentration of 0.9 mg/dL, a 30% decline in GFR to approximately 70 mL/min will increase serum creatinine to only 1.3 mg/dL, a value still within the normal range. A serum creatinine of 1.7 mg/dL in the same patient corresponds to a GFR of 50 mL/min, a loss of half of his or her renal function (see Chapter 5). Second, while renal function declines with age, the serum creatinine does not increase in the absence of kidney disease. This paradox is explained by a decrease in creatinine production with aging, offsetting the fall in creatinine excretion that occurs when GFR decreases. Therefore, an increase in creatinine concentration in an elderly individual indicates a major decrease in renal function, superimposed on the reduction due to renal senescence. Estimating glomerular filtration rate from the patient's age, body weight, and serum creatinine using the Cockcroft-Gault formula (Fig. 2) provides a more accurate estimate of renal function than does the serum creatinine alone. To make the diagnosis of chronic renal insufficiency, one must assure oneself that the fall in GFR is due to structural renal damage, and not to hemodynamic changes or to drug-induced interference with creatinine excretion (see Chapter 5). As discussed in Chapter 5, BUN is a poor measurement of kidney function because urea generation and excretion are influenced by many factors that are independent of GFR.

III. CAUSES OF CHRONIC RENAL INSUFFICIENCY

The most common cause of chronic renal insufficiency in the United States is diabetes mellitus, accounting for almost 40% of all renal failure (see Table 2). Between 20 and 40% of patients with type 1 diabetes develop renal damage. A lower fraction of patients with type 2 diabetes develop renal insufficiency, probably because many patients develop type 2 diabetes later in life. The predisposition

Table 2 Causes of Chronic Renal Failure

Diabetes	37%
Type 1	15%
Type 2	22%
Hypertension (includes renal artery stenosis)	29%
Glomerulonephritis	11%
Tubulointerstital disease (includes obstruction)	4.5%
Cystic/Hereditary/Congenital	3.5%
Secondary glomerulonephritis (includes vasculitis)	2.4%
Neoplasms (includes multiple myeloma)	1.6%
HIV nephropathy	1%
Miscellaneous/Unknown	5–10%

Source: Adapted from U.S. Renal Data System, 1997.

to accelerated cardiovascular disease in type 2 diabetes often leads to premature death before renal failure develops. In populations in which type 2 diabetes occurs at younger ages, the prevalence of nephropathy is similar to that of type 1 diabetes. Despite the lower prevalence of renal failure in type 2 diabetes, there are more renal failure patients with type 2 diabetes than type 1 because most patients with diabetes have type 2 disease.

Hypertension is recorded as the second most common cause of renal failure. However, because renal insufficiency of any etiology commonly leads to hypertension (see later), many of these cases may be misclassified. A substantial number of cases of renal failure labeled as being hypertensive in etiology are in reality caused by renal artery atherosclerotic occlusive disease. Various forms of glomerulonephritis such as idiopathic membranous nephropathy, IgA nephropathy, and lupus nephritis make up the third most common cause of renal failure. Together diabetes, hypertension, and glomerulonephritis are responsible for nearly 80% of renal failure. Numerous other diseases make up the remaining causes of renal failure. The etiology is categorized as unknown in approximately 5% of cases.

IV. DIAGNOSTIC APPROACH

When presented with a patient with renal insufficiency, an effort should be undertaken to make a specific diagnosis. Many causes of renal insufficiency are associated with significant systemic disease and/or have specific treatments. As with any other disease state, obtaining a thorough history from the patient can provide important clues to the cause of renal insufficiency. Systemic diseases such as diabetes, lupus, and amyloidosis reveal themselves as the patient relates his or her story. New bone pain in an elderly individual suggests multiple myeloma. Frequent but weak urinary stream in an elderly man suggests prostatic bladder outlet obstruction and obstructive nephropathy. A history of multiple urinary tract infections as a child suggests the possibility of reflux nephropathy. The presence of coronary and peripheral vascular disease should lead the physician to consider renovascular disease. A family history of renal failure suggests polycystic kidney disease or hereditary nephritis. The patient's history of drug usage can lead the physician to consider analgesic nephropathy, lithium-induced renal disease, or renal damage due to interstitial inflammation from nonsteroidal anti-inflammatory drugs. Similarly, the physical exam is an essential component of the diagnostic work-up. Physical examination can uncover clues of systemic disease, identify the enlarged kidneys of polycystic disease, and assess the presence and severity of hypertension.

Laboratory evaluation is the central technique for diagnosing the causes of renal insufficiency. In addition to determining the degree of renal insufficiency by measuring the serum creatinine concentration (see Chapter 5), laboratory evaluation allows elucidation of the degree of proteinuria and the nature of the inflammatory changes in the urine sediment. Hematuria may or may not be an indicator of the presence of glomerular disease, but red blood cell (RBC) casts are virtually pathognomonic of a glomerular etiology. Heavy proteinuria (>2000 mg per 24 hours) usually indicates glomerular disease, and nephrotic range proteinuria (>3500 mg per 24 hours) always indicates glomerular disease. At this point the etiology may be quite clear. For example, a patient with long-standing diabetes who has a history of progressive proteinuria and who develops an increase in the serum creatinine almost certainly has diabetic nephropathy. However, in many patients, the etiology is not at all clear. Certain laboratory studies help narrow the differential diagnosis of glomerular disease. Low complement levels are seen with infection-related glomerulonephritis, membranoproliferative glomerulonephritis (MPGN), cryoglobulinemia, and lupus nephritis. Antinuclear antibody testing screens for lupus. Hepatitis C is associated with MPGN. A patient with significant proteinuria or RBC casts in which the diagnosis is uncertain should be referred to a nephrologist for consideration for a renal biopsy in hopes of diagnosing a treatable form of glomerular disease.

A search for treatable renal insufficiency is also indicated in patients with nonglomerular disease. All patients should be screened for obstructive nephropathy with a renal ultrasound. Obstructive nephropathy can occur along with another cause of chronic renal insufficiency. For example, neurogenic bladder dysfunction secondary to diabetic neuropathy can worsen renal function in patients with diabetic nephropathy. The renal ultrasound is useful both for diagnosis and for prognosis. Small echogenic kidneys generally indicate long-standing, advanced disease with little hope of reversibility. Many patients with nonglomerular disease have hypertensive nephrosclerosis for which there is no specific therapy.

However, hidden in this group of patients with hypertension, a benign urinalysis, minimal proteinuria, and unexplained renal insufficiency are a substantial number of patients with potentially reversible renovascular disease. Silent multiple myeloma (without hypercalcemia or bone pain) is not uncommon, especially in the elderly population. All patients over age 40 with renal insufficiency should be screened for myeloma with both serum and urine protein electrophoresis or immunofixation.

V. INTERVENTIONS TO SLOW THE PROGRESSION OF CHRONIC RENAL INSUFFICIENCY

Chronic renal insufficiency is by definition a progressive disease. Some causes of chronic renal disease have specific treatments, and these are described in the appropriate disease chapters. However, many diseases have no definitive therapy. In addition, once nephron loss has occurred, hemodynamic and metabolic factors influence a complex pathophysiological process that leads to progressive nephron loss and fibrosis, progressive renal insufficiency, and eventual ESRD. This progression occurs even if the original renal insult is no longer active. Of course, the earlier the original insult is treated, the more nephrons are preserved, the slower the chronic progression, and the less likely it is that the patient will reach ESRD. Fortunately, several interventions have been demonstrated to slow progression of chronic renal insufficiency (see Table 3).

A. Blood Pressure Control

Studies in animals and in human subjects indicate that renal disease advances more rapidly when blood pressure is elevated and that antihypertensive therapy slows progression of disease. The renal protective effect of antihypertensive ther

Table 3 Therapies to Slow Progression of Chronic Renal Insufficiency

Confirmed	Speculative
Aggressive blood pressure control (<130/85)	Control of hyperlipidemia
	Smoking cessation
Aggressive glycemic control in patients with diabetes	
Use of ACE inhibitors	
Dietary protein restriction	

apy in patients with malignant hypertension was shown many years ago. More recently, antihypertensive therapy has been shown to exert beneficial effects on proteinuria and renal function in patients with only mild elevations in blood pressure. These beneficial effects appear to be proportional to blood pressure reduction. The Joint National Committee for the Detection, Evaluation, and Treatment of High Blood Pressure recommends a target blood pressure of 130/85 mmHg or less for patients with renal disease. This recommendation is based on the results of the Modification of Diet in Renal Disease (MDRD) study. Although this study was designed to examine the effects of dietary protein restriction on progression of renal disease, it also assessed the effect of blood pressure control on the rate of decline in GFR. Patients were randomized either to usual blood pressure control (mean blood pressure = 107 mmHg, or 140/90) or more aggressive blood pressure control (mean = 92 mmHg or 125/75). In patients with a baseline GFR between 25 and 55 mL/min, the decline in GFR was initially more rapid in the 4 months after randomization, but significantly slower thereafter (mean follow-up of 2.2 years) in the group whose blood pressure was maintained at the lower levels. The effect of aggressive control of blood pressure was most striking in patients with heavy proteinuria (>1 g/24 hr).

Nephron loss as a result of any disease results in compensatory glomerular hypertension and hyperfiltration in the unaffected nephrons. This compensatory process, unfortunately, can lead to further nephron loss by promoting glomerulosclerosis and more nephron loss, initiating a relentless cycle of continued nephron destruction even if the initial disease process is arrested. Angiotensin-converting enzyme (ACE) inhibitors lower glomerular capillary pressure as well as systemic blood pressure, thus ameliorating this detrimental glomerular hemodynamic process. The renal protective effect of ACE inhibitors was initially demonstrated in various animal models, but it has now been substantiated in human trials. The most dramatic effect of ACE inhibitors is in patients with diabetic nephropathy. In patients with type 1 diabetes and proteinuria, captopril reduces the risk of death, dialysis, or transplantation by almost half (see Fig. 3). In patients with type 2 diabetes and microalbuminuria, enalapril decreases albumin excretion and arrests the decline in renal function over a 5-year period. More recently, the ACE inhibitor benazepril was shown to reduce the risk of doubling the serum creatinine or the need for dialysis in patients with a wide variety of renal diseases by 53%. The risk reduction is greater if ACE inhibitor therapy is instituted when the renal disease is less severe and appears to be the greatest in those with glomerular disease and heavy proteinuria. A recent meta-analysis found ACE inhibitors beneficial for the treatment of renal disease of any etiology, delaying the onset of clinically important outcomes by 33–60%. In most of the ACE inhibitor trials the renal protective effects are independent of the hypertensive effects. In patients with diabetes and proteinuria, ACE inhibitors are protective even in patients with-

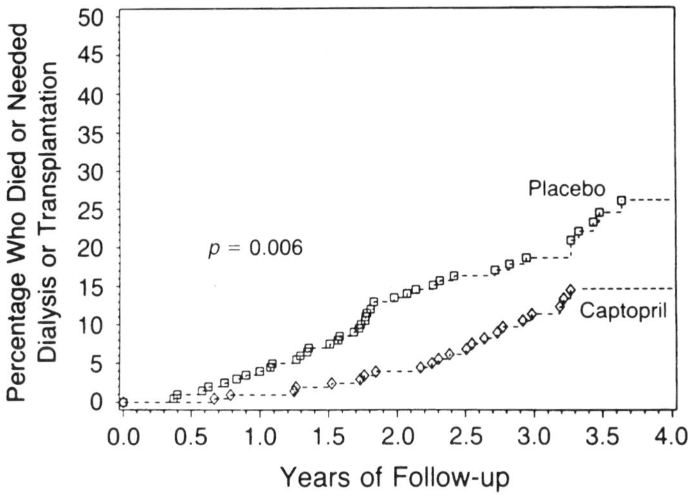

Figure 3 Cumulative percent of patients with type 1 diabetes and nephropathy who died or required dialysis or renal transplantation among 409 patients randomly assigned to receive captopril or placebo. (From Lewis EJ, et al., N Engl J Med 329(20):1459, 1993.

out hypertension. Although not yet rigorously proven in clinical trials, angiotensin II receptor blockers (e.g., losartan) confer the same protection as ACE inhibitors in animal trials and are likely to be effective in slowing the progression of renal disease in humans.

B. Intensive Treatment of Diabetes Mellitus

Evidence from a variety of studies has shown that aggressive efforts to lower blood glucose concentrations in patients with type 1 diabetes reduce the incidence of microalbuminuria as well as overt diabetic nephropathy. The Diabetes Control and Complications Trial (DCCT) is perhaps the largest and best designed of these studies. In this study, a reduction in hemoglobin A_1 by 2% reduced the incidence of diabetic nephropathy by 54% over an average of 6.5 years of follow-up. In another small cohort study from Sweden, the incidence of diabetic nephropathy fell from 30% to zero over 20 years in young type 1 diabetic patients who had sustained hemoglobin A1C levels of 7.0% during the entire course of their illness. Based on evidence such as this, early and aggressive control of blood glucose in patients with type 1 diabetes is perhaps the best intervention available to reduce the likelihood of developing renal disease and to slow its progression when already present. Similar evidence is now available for the much larger group of patients who have type 2 diabetes. As a result, current recommendations are to reduce HbA_1C levels to below 8.0% and ideally to reach a goal of 7.0% in both type 1 and type 2 diabetes.

C. Protein Restriction

Following the initial observations associating a high-protein diet with progressive nephropathy in rats, many studies in animals have shown an impressive benefit of dietary protein restriction on renal function. The results in human studies are less clear. Several small studies suggested a benefit of dietary protein restriction on progression of renal insufficiency in humans, prompting the MDRD study mentioned earlier. This large randomized study showed only a minimal benefit for dietary protein restriction. However, when the effect of the amount of protein actually ingested, rather than the amount prescribed, was evaluated in a reanalysis of the data, a clear benefit was shown for lower protein intake. In patients with a GFR of <25 mL/min, the rate of decline in renal function was slowed by 1 mL/min per year for each 0.2 g/g reduction in dietary protein intake. Although this reduction appears small, it results in a 51% prolongation of the time before initiation of renal replacement therapy. It has been argued that all studies of the effects of dietary protein restriction on the progression of renal disease, including the MDRD study, have been too small to have statistical significance. For this reason, two meta-analyses of the role of dietary protein restriction in renal disease have been published, both of which concluded that dietary protein restriction is beneficial in slowing both diabetic and nondiabetic chronic renal disease.

The recommended target for prescribed dietary protein is 0.6 g/kg body weight per day, a prescription that usually achieves a dietary protein intake of 0.7 g/kg body weight per day. Although this degree of protein restriction is beneficial, it is extremely difficult to adhere to and requires a compliant and motivated patient. Dietary protein restriction carries with it a risk of malnutrition, especially as the need for dialysis approaches. As renal disease progresses, a subtle anorexia develops, and protein intake may spontaneously fall to as low as 0.5 g/kg/day when the creatinine clearance falls below 10 mL/min. Protein malnutrition is strongly associated with mortality in dialysis patients. Although the MDRD study found the prescribed diet to be safe, without significant malnutrition, study conditions ensured frequent dietary counseling and monitoring of nutritional parameters. Regular follow-up with a skilled dietitian and frequent monitoring of protein intake and nutritional status are essential to achieve compliance with the diet yet avoid malnutrition. Thus, from a practical perspective, protein restriction is not feasible in most patients with chronic renal insufficiency. A general approach is to reduce protein intake to 1g/kg/day, which may have a partial beneficial effect.

D. Hyperlipidemia

Hyperlipidemia is common in patients with renal disease. This finding is most prominent in the nephrotic syndrome (see Chapter 7). Hypercholesterolemia is also very common in nonnephrotic diabetic nephropathy. Other forms of renal insufficiency have less effect on total cholesterol but are associated with elevations in triglyceride levels and reductions in HDL cholesterol levels. The high rate of cardiovascular events in patients with chronic renal insufficiency alone is reason for treatment of hyperlipidemia, but treatment may also slow the progression of chronic renal disease. In animal models, high-lipid diets exacerbate and low-lipid diets or lipid-lowering agents slow the rate of progression of renal disease. In diabetic nephropathy, total and low-density lipoprotein (LDL) cholesterol levels are independent risk factors for progression. In nondiabetic patients with hypercholesterolemia and hypertriglyceridemia, the rate of loss of renal function is twice that of patients without hyperlipidemia. No long-term studies examining the effects of lipid-lowering agents on progression of renal insufficiency in humans have been published. Short-term trials have shown that antilipemic agents are safe and effective. Lipid-lowering agents have been shown to reduce proteinuria in diabetic nephropathy. The greatest and most consistent reductions in total and LDL cholesterol are seen with 3-hydroxy-3-methylglutaryl co-enzyme A (HMG-CoA) reductase inhibitors. Fibric acid analogs cause greater reductions in triglycerides. Given the association of hyperlipidemia with progression of renal disease and the very high cardiovascular event rate in this population, it seems prudent to treat the lipid disorders aggressively.

E. Other Factors

The adverse effects of smoking are widely known, but the effects of smoking on the kidney are underappreciated. Although not extensively studied, some interesting associations have been found. Smoking shortens the time between onset of diabetes and onset of proteinuria and accelerates the rate of progression of diabetic nephropathy to ESRD. In addition, there is evidence that smoking cessation is beneficial for renal function. One study found progression of diabetic nephropathy in 53% of current smokers, 33% of patients who had stopped smoking, and 11% of nonsmokers. Smoking is a predictor of significant renal artery stenosis. In addition, smoking has been linked to progression of disease in polycystic kidney disease and lupus nephritis.

F. Conclusions

Given the high morbidity and mortality that accompanies ESRD, every effort should be made to slow the progression of chronic renal insufficiency. Aggressive blood pressure control, use of an ACE inhibitor, and monitored dietary protein restriction are effective measures used to slow the decline in renal function. In patients with diabetes mellitus, aggressive control of blood sugar can reduce the likelihood of diabetic nephropathy. Treatment of hyperlipidemia and smoking cessation are prudent interventions utilized to reduce vascular events and may be effective in preserving renal function as well.

VI. TREATMENT OF COMPLICATIONS OF CHRONIC RENAL INSUFFICIENCY

The common fluid and electrolyte disorders that complicate chronic renal insufficiency include extracellular fluid volume overload, hyperkalemia, and metabolic acidosis. It is important to anticipate these complications and initiate early treatment to avoid serious consequences (see Table 4).

A. Edema

Salt and water retention occurs with even mild to moderate renal insufficiency and is probably the main factor responsible for the hypertension that almost invariably accompanies renal insufficiency. Clinically evident edema is uncommon, however, unless the nephrotic syndrome is present, until the GFR falls to less than 10–15 mL/min. Patients with lesser degrees of renal insufficiency are usually able to maintain sodium balance despite a large loss of functioning nephrons because the remaining nephrons can substantially increase sodium excretion by reducing renal tubular sodium reabsorption. The signal for this change in sodium transport, however, is ECF volume expansion. As GFR falls, the range of sodium intakes at which sodium balance is maintained is progressively restricted. Intake

Table 4 Common Complications of Chronic Renal Insufficiency

Edema
Hyperkalemia
Metabolic acidosis
Hyponatremia
Anemia
Renal osteodystrophy
Hypertension

of large amounts of salt can easily overwhelm the excretory capacity of the failing kidneys. The superimposition of left ventricular dysfunction predisposes to symptomatic pulmonary congestion earlier in the course of renal insufficiency. More commonly peripheral edema is the first clinical manifestation of salt and water retention. Because cardiac disease is quite common in this population of patients, an episode of pulmonary edema should prompt an evaluation of cardiac function.

Dietary sodium restriction to <100 mEq/day (2–2.5 g) is the centerpiece of the treatment for both hypertension and edema in patients with renal insufficiency. This change in diet is difficult for most individuals and requires counseling by a trained dietitian. If dietary restriction is not effective or not attained, diuretic therapy is necessary. Thiazide diuretics are usually ineffective if the serum creatinine is >3 mg/dL, and therefore the loop diuretics are the agents of choice in patients with chronic renal insufficiency. It is important to remember that these diuretics are short acting and that higher doses are required to achieve an effect when the GFR is reduced. The initial aim of loop diuretic therapy is to find the effective threshold dose. If 20 mg of furosemide does not induce a diuresis, then 20 mg three times per day will be ineffective as well. With normal renal function an effective diuresis starts with only 10 mg of furosemide, but patients with advanced chronic renal insufficiency may require doses up to 400 mg/day. Once an effective dose is found it is important to understand the time course of the diuretic response. Diuresis from a loop diuretic lasts approximately 6 hours. Because of the rapid intravascular volume loss the renal tubules become sodium avid after the effect has abated. If the patient is not adequately restricting sodium intake, this postdiuretic period of sodium retention can equal the sodium losses induced by the diuretic, resulting in no change in sodium balance, weight, or edema. In such cases twice daily dosing along with dietary sodium restriction can be very effective.

In patients who appear to be resistant to even high doses of furosemide, the cause is always excessive dietary intake. Nonetheless, because these patients often cannot reduce their intake even when counseled, a greater diuresis can be achieved by the combination of a thiazide diuretic or metolazone with a loop diuretic. When using this combination, the maximum benefit is achieved when the thiazide or metolazone is taken 30 minutes before the loop diuretic. This combination invariably causes large potassium losses and often produces hyponatremia, and patients should be monitored frequently for hypokalemia and hyponatremia.

Intravenous loop diuretics are often more effective than oral dosing because more drug is delivered rapidly to its site of action. The onset of action is more rapid with intravenous dosing, but the time course of diuretic response is the same with either the oral or intravenous route. Potassium-sparing diuretics should not be used in chronic renal insufficiency because of the risk of significant hyperkalemia.

B. Hyperkalemia

Mild to moderate hyperkalemia (5–5.5 mEq/L) is a common feature in patients with renal insufficiency and requires no intervention, except for restriction of potassium intake to 2–3 g (50–75 mEq) per day. Despite the presence of hyperkalemia, potassium balance is usually well maintained until GFR decreases to less than 20 mL/min. In some forms of kidney disease, most notably diabetic nephropathy and tubulointerstitial diseases, aldosterone levels are low and more severe hyperkalemia can occur earlier in the course of renal disease. The majority of patients with this problem, termed hyporeninemic hypoaldosteronism, are elderly and hypertensive, and half have diabetic nephropathy. This form of hyperkalemia is associated often, but not always, with a mild to moderate degree of metabolic acidosis with no increase in unmeasured anions (type 4 renal tubular acidosis) (see later and Chapter 11). Unfortunately, ACE inhibitors also lower aldosterone levels and can exacerbate existing hyperkalemia. This problem sometimes forces the discontinuation of these beneficial agents in patients with renal insufficiency. Obstructive nephropathy can also cause hyperkalemia relatively early in the course of renal disease. Volume depletion and sodium restriction can reduce potassium excretion by impairing adequate distal delivery of sodium. Diuretics that inhibit renal potassium excretion (spironolactone, triamterene, and amiloride) can cause severe hyperkalemia and should be not be used in renal insufficiency. Trimethoprim has effects similar to amiloride and can cause hyperkalemia in patients with renal insufficiency. Nonsteroidal anti-inflammatory drugs reduce GFR and can also exacerbate hyperkalemia. In patients with diabetes, hyperglycemia causes a shift of potassium out of cells. In the presence of renal insufficiency the resultant hyperkalemia is sustained and can be life-threatening.

If the problem of hyperkalemia is anticipated and serum levels are monitored, emergency situations are easily avoided. The first intervention, as indicated earlier, is dietary potassium restriction. Identification and discontinuation of offending medications is the next step (see Table 5). An often unrecognized source of excess potassium intake is the salt substitute available in the supermarket. Since colonic potassium secretion plays an increased role in potassium homeostasis as renal function declines, preventing constipation may be helpful in managing hyperkalemia in chronic renal insufficiency.

Hyperchloremic acidosis is commonly associated with hyperkalemia, and treatment with alkali therapy will decrease serum potassium concentration. Since many patients with chronic renal insufficiency and hyperkalemia have edema, use of loop diuretics is often an effective therapy. Mineralocorticoid therapy in the form of fludrocortisone (0.2–1 mg/day) is effective in patients with hyperkalemia due to low aldosterone levels. However, most patients with hyporeninemic hypoaldosteronism have hypertension and edema, which is exacerbated by mineralocorticoid therapy. Almost all pre-ESRD patients can maintain acceptable se-

Table 5 Medications That Cause Hyperkalemia

Potassium chloride (including K^+-containing salt substitutes)
Potassium-sparing diuretics (spironolactone, triamterene, amiloride)
Angiotensin-converting enzyme inhibitors
Nonsteroidal anti-inflammatory drugs
Heparin
Beta-adrenergic antagonists
Digoxin/Digitalis intoxication
Trimethoprim
Cyclosporine/Tacrolimus
Pentamidine

rum potassium levels with the above interventions. Chronic use of the potassium exchange resin kayexelate is rarely necessary. Patients with chronic renal insufficiency certainly are susceptible to acute, severe hyperkalemia, the treatment of which is described in Chapter 30.

C. Acidosis

A small but significant reduction in serum bicarbonate concentration occurs in most patients with chronic renal insufficiency who are ingesting a typical North American diet. It remains unclear whether acid balance is maintained in chronic renal insufficiency, but regardless of whether balance is achieved, the mild hypobicarbonatemia appears to have deleterious effects on bone and muscle metabolism. In patients with mild to moderate renal insufficiency, serum bicarbonate ranges from 18 to 24 mEq/L and the anion gap is normal. Once the GFR falls below 25 mL/min, retention of the anions of metabolic acids occurs and the anion gap increases. The degree of acidosis for any degree of renal dysfunction is quite variable, depending primarily on dietary intake of protein and to a lesser extent on the preservation of tubular function and acid excretion. Diseases associated with renal tubular acidosis cause more serious problems. As the patient approaches ESRD, plasma bicarbonate concentrations often fall to between 12 and 20 mEq/L.

Mild to moderate metabolic acidosis is usually asymptomatic, but there are several reasons why normalizing serum bicarbonate and pH may be beneficial. Acidosis probably exacerbates hyperparathryoid-induced bone disease and causes negative calcium balance. Acidosis also promotes muscle breakdown and catabolism. In children, acidosis is a potent inhibitor of growth. There are some preliminary data suggesting that alkali therapy slows the progression of chronic renal insufficiency. Certainly treatment of acidemia provides a margin of protection against a superimposed independent acidosis. Alkali therapy should always be instituted in children to minimize growth retardation.

Although there is some controversy, maintenance of the serum bicarbonate level at greater than 20 mEq/L generally is recommended for adults with renal insufficiency. Serum bicarbonate can be maintained by administering enough sodium bicarbonate to offset the daily acid load, approximately 0.5–1 mEq/kg/day. Higher doses may be necessary initially in order to correct the alkali deficit. Each 650 mg sodium bicarbonate tablet contains 8 mEq of each of sodium and bicarbonate. The extra sodium can exacerbate edema and hypertension, and additional diuretic therapy may be necessary. Sodium bicarbonate therapy is sometimes poorly tolerated due to production of CO_2 gas in the stomach. An alternative oral alkali therapy is sodium citrate. Citrate is rapidly metabolized to bicarbonate (1 mL of sodium citrate = 1 mEq alkali). Although citrate does not produce the gastric bloating associated with bicarbonate therapy, some find its taste intolerable. More concerning, citrate enhances intestinal aluminum absorption and cannot be used in patients taking aluminum-containing antacids due to the risk of developing aluminum intoxication. Calcium carbonate therapy, often used in chronic renal insufficiency as a phosphate binder (see later), can contribute to control of acidemia as well.

D. Water Balance

Patients with chronic renal insufficiency have a limited ability to excrete or conserve water, predisposing them to both hypo- and hypernatremia. A similar impairment of water balance occurs with aging, and therefore the elderly patient with chronic renal insufficiency is particularly susceptible. Thirst is usually adequate in maintaining the plasma sodium concentration within the normal range. However, if a patient with chronic renal insufficiency is debilitated and unable to take in enough water or is not given enough water to offset losses in the hospital setting, hypernatremia can result. More commonly, hyponatremia develops in patients with chronic renal insufficiency who either drink or are given hypotonic fluids in excess of their ability to excrete water. In hospitalized patients with renal insufficiency, intravenous administration of 5% dextrose and water or half-isotonic saline should be avoided. Patients with chronic renal insufficiency frequently have mild, asymptomatic, chronic hyponatremia due to chronic excess water intake.

E. Anemia

Anemia commonly develops with chronic renal insufficiency when the serum creatinine rises above 3 mg/dL (see Fig. 4). The anemia is normochromic and normocytic with a low reticulocyte count and is primarily due to erythropoietin

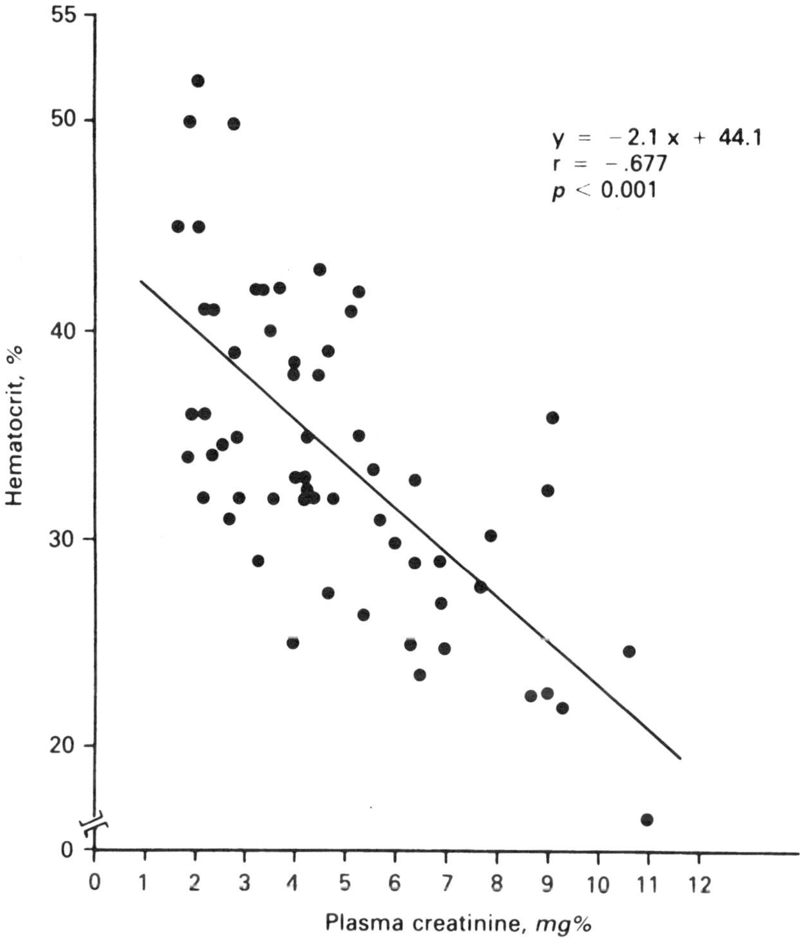

Figure 4 Relationship between hematocrit and plasma creatinine concentration in 60 patients with varying degrees of renal insufficiency. (Reproduced from McGonigle RJS, et al., Kidney Int 25:439, 1984.)

deficiency. Although erythropoietin deficiency (due to decreased synthesis and secretion of this hormone by the kidney) is always present, one should always ensure that other treatable causes of anemia are not present. Most importantly, one should assess iron stores to exclude iron deficiency. Administration of recombinant human erythropoietin (EPO) readily corrects the anemia of chronic renal insufficiency but is extremely expensive. Before embarking on EPO treatment, one should be certain the patient has appropriate insurance coverage (see later). This therapy is an integral part of treatment of patients with ESRD, but it is clear that therapy earlier in the course of renal insufficiency is beneficial, reducing symptoms of fatigue, pruritus, sexual dysfunction in men, and anorexia. Erythropoietin has been shown to reduce left ventricular hypertrophy (LVH), a common complication of chronic renal insufficiency and a strong predictor of mortality. Correction of anemia with EPO significantly improves energy, physical function, home management, social activity, and cognitive function. While EPO clearly reduces morbidity, no randomized, controlled trials have been conducted to assess its effects on mortality. One risk of EPO therapy is more severe hypertension, and close attention should be paid to blood pressure when using this drug. Erythropoietin eliminates the need for blood transfusions, an important goal, as it is desirable to avoid blood transfusions to reduce the risk of sensitization in patients who are future renal transplant candidates.

Although no clear guidelines exist for EPO use in predialysis patients, it is prudent to initiate erythropoietin therapy once the anemia causes significant symptoms, usually when the hematocrit is less than 30%. Erythropoietin therapy is expensive ($10 per 1000 units, $2,000–$5,000 per year) and is unaffordable for most individuals unless covered by health insurance. If the patient is Medicare eligible, Medicare will pay for 80% of the cost if the serum creatinine is >3 mg/dL and if the drug is administered at a health care facility. Medicare does not pay for self-administration unless the patient is receiving chronic home dialysis therapy. If the patient has private insurance for medications, the cost of erythropoietin is frequently covered.

Chronic administration of pharmacological doses of EPO are required for the correction of anemia. The starting dose in pre-ESRD patients is 50 units/kg body weight administered subcutaneously, once or twice weekly. Hematocrit and blood pressure should be monitored every 2 weeks. The hematocrit usually rises several weeks after starting therapy, and the dose is adjusted monthly if necessary. The target hematocrit is somewhat controversial. Medicare will not reimburse for EPO if the average of the last three hematocrits is >36.5%. However, most symptoms are relieved once the hematocrit is >33%. In dialysis patients, survival declines as the hematocrit decreases below a range of 30–33%. Such studies in predialysis patients have not been performed. Therefore, the recommended target hematocrit is 33–36%.

There are several causes of resistance to EPO, including chronic inflammation of any cause, aluminum toxicity, and bone marrow failure, but the most common cause is iron deficiency. For an adequate response to EPO, satisfactory iron stores must be maintained. Iron (Fe), total iron-binding capacity (TIBC), and ferritin should be monitored every 3 months. Patients with chronic renal insufficiency absorb oral iron poorly, and intravenous iron dextran therapy is frequently necessary. Intravenous iron replacement therapy is indicated when the iron saturation (Fe/TIBC × 100) is <20% or the serum ferritin is <100 ng/mL, despite oral iron administration. After a 25 mg test dose and observation for an allergic reaction, 500 mg of iron dextran may be administered intravenously in a single slow infusion and repeated as needed. Testing the stool for occult blood is indicated in any patient not responding to erythropoietin adequately.

F. Bone disease

Renal osteodystrophy is the collective term used to describe three major skeletal disorders that occur in chronic renal insufficiency: osteitis fibrosa due to secondary hyperparathyroidism, adynamic bone disease, and osteomalacia.

Osteomalacia is characterized by reduced bone turnover with an increase in osteoid (unmineralized bone). Most cases of osteomalacia in chronic renal insufficiency were probably due to aluminum deposition in bone. With the dramatic reduction in the use of aluminum containing phosphate binders, osteomalacia is now an uncommon cause of renal osteodystrophy. Osteomalacia is more common in chronic renal insufficiency patients with metabolic acidosis and is one reason for correcting the acidosis.

Adynamic bone disease occurs in about one third of patients with renal insufficiency. Bone turnover is reduced in this disorder, but unlike osteomalacia, there is no increase in osteoid formation. As with osteomalacia, adynamic bone disease can result from aluminum toxicity. Parathyroid hormone (PTH) levels are relatively low in adynamic bone disease, and excess suppression of PTH with calcitriol may be responsible for many cases. Most patients with adynamic bone disease are asymptomatic and require no specific therapy. Avoiding aluminum-containing medications and taking care not to oversuppresss PTH are important considerations.

The most common form of renal osteodystrophy is osteitis fibrosa due to secondary hyperparathyroidism. The histological picture is that of high-turnover bone disease: increased number and activity of osteoclasts, increased bone resorption, and marrow fibrosis. Osteoid is increased in a haphazard arrangement. Phosphate retention and calcitriol [1,25$(OH)_2$ vitamin D] deficiency are the most important factors in the pathogenesis of secondary hyperparathyroidism. As GFR falls in chronic renal insufficiency, phosphate retention occurs. An increase in PTH secretion initially maintains phosphate balance by increasing release from bone and enhancing urinary excretion. However, once the GFR falls to <30 mL/min, serum phosphate levels increase. Hyperphosphatemia promotes PTH release by both decreasing calcitriol and directly increasing PTH synthesis. Calcitriol levels begin to fall when the GFR falls to <40 mL/min, due to both phosphate retention and reduction in functioning renal tissue. Calcitriol exerts a direct inhibitory effect on PTH synthesis. In addition to low circulating calcitriol levels in chronic renal insufficiency, vitamin D receptors in the parathyroid gland are reduced.

In patients with renal insufficiency, hyperparathyroidism is usually asymptomatic until it is quite severe. Eventually, however, it can cause bone pain, premature fractures, myopathy, and metastatic calcifications. Hyperparathyroidism has also been implicated as a cause of uremic pruritus. Early treatment is necessary to avoid these complications. Treatment is directed first at control of hyperphosphatemia with phosphate binders and thereafter at control of PTH secretion with calcitriol supplementation. Reduction in plasma phosphorus to normal levels will prevent most of the abnormalities of hyperparathyroid bone disease. Restricting dietary phosphorus is difficult, but because most foods high in protein content are also high in phosphorus, dietary protein restriction can also achieve a reasonable reduction in dietary phosphorus intake. As discussed earlier, malnutrition becomes a concern as the need for dialysis approaches. When the GFR is >15 mL/min, dietary protein is no longer restricted. In this setting it is reasonable to avoid nonessential foods that are excessively high in phosphorus, such as milk, cheese, and cola, without restricting foods with high biological value protein such as meat. Consultation with a trained dietitian is the optimal approach.

Most patients will eventually need oral phosphate binders to control hyperphosphatemia. Although it is a very effective phosphate binder, aluminum hydroxide is no longer used in most patients because of the potential for aluminum toxicity, manifested as osteomalacia and encephalopathy. Calcium carbonate and calcium acetate are now the phosphate binders of choice. Calcium carbonate is more palatable but is a less potent phosphate binder than calcium acetate. Calcium carbonate is readily available over the counter. The dose needed to adequately control serum phosphorus varies with the patient's diet and degree of renal insufficiency, ranging between 2 and 10 g of binder per day. The initial dose is one or two tablets three times per day with meals, increasing until the plasma phosphorus falls to <5.5 mg/dL.

Hypercalcemia may become a problem with use of calcium salts, especially with concomitant use of calcitriol supplementation. Taking the binder with meals (between 30 minutes before and 30 minutes after each meal) minimizes calcium absorption and maximizes phosphate binding. While calcium citrate will also bind dietary phosphorus, care must be exercised because citrate will increase gastrointestinal aluminum absorption.

Treatment with oral calcitriol [1,25$(OH)_2$ vitamin D] will reduce PTH levels and prevent bone pathology. Patients with chronic renal insufficiency and intact PTH levels >200 pg/mL should be treated with calcitriol. While the upper limit of normal for intact PTH is 65 pg/mL, there is substantial resistance to PTH in renal failure patients and a concern that adynamic bone disease will develop if the intact PTH level is reduced to ''normal'' levels. Prevention of hyperparathyroidism is much more effective than treatment of established bone disease. Therefore, all patients with advancing chronic renal insufficiency should have a measurement of PTH performed. Pulse calcitriol therapy (two to three times per week) has been popularized but is probably no more effective than daily therapy. Pulse therapy may induce less hypercalcemia. Low-dose calcitriol (0.25 μg/day) should be started when the intact PTH is >200 pg/mL. If the patient does not become hypercalcemic, the dose should be slowly increased with a goal PTH level of 130–200 pg/mL. The calcitriol dose should be reduced by half for mild hypercalcemia (10.5–11.5 mg/dL) and should be temporarily discontinued with restarting at a lower dose for more severe hypercalcemia. Changing to twice weekly dosing with the same total weekly dose is equally effective in reducing PTH and may cause less hypercalcemia. If the PTH level falls to <130 pg/mL (twice the upper limit of normal), the dose should be reduced by half. If the PTH level remains <130 pg/mL, calcitriol should be discontinued to avoid precipitation of adynamic bone disease. Supplemental calcitriol therapy should not be started until the plasma phosphorus level has been controlled to <6.5 mg/dL. If the plasma calcium level rises in the setting of significant hyperphosphatemia, metastatic calcification can occur. For the same reason, the calcitriol dose should be reduced if the calcium-phosphorus product (serum calcium in mg/dL multiplied by the serum phosphorus in mg/dl) exceeds 75. New analogs of vitamin D that do not induce hypercalcemia are currently in clinical trials and will soon be available. Such agents will be easier to use and will allow for better PTH control.

Aggressive control of PTH levels over recent years in dialysis patients has dramatically reduced skeletal morbidity due to osteitis fibrosa and has nearly eliminated the need for parathyroid surgery. Earlier aggressive control of hyperphosphatemia and hyperparathyroidism in the pre-ESRD population will aid in eliminating the clinical effects of the disease entirely.

G. Hypertension

Hypertension has been addressed in Chapter 17, but several important points need to be emphasized with regard to hypertension in the setting of chronic renal insufficiency. In addition to being an important modifiable cardiovascular risk factor, aggressive control of blood pressure can slow the progression of renal disease. As discussed earlier, the blood pressure goal in patients with chronic renal insufficiency is less than 130/85. An ACE inhibitor should be considered the first drug used to lower blood pressure (see earlier discussion). Although most patients tolerate these drugs well, serum potassium and creatinine levels should be checked. An increase in serum potassium concentration does not necessarily require discontinuation of an ACE inhibitor. The addition of a loop diuretic can increase potassium excretion and ameliorate the hyperkalemia. ACE inhibitors should also not be discontinued if serum creatinine increases by a small amount. Although patients with severe left ventricular failure or renovascular disease are at risk for developing an abrupt decline in renal function, most patients with chronic renal insufficiency do not experience any decline. These agents should only be discontinued if there is an acute and substantial decline in renal function associated with their use. In addition to heart failure and renal artery stenosis, an ACE inhibitor–induced decline in renal function can occur if there is an acute fall in intravascular volume such as with a large diuresis or from gastrointestinal volume losses or with concomitant use of prostaglandin-inhibiting nonsteroidal antiinflammatory drugs.

When treating hypertension in the setting of chronic renal insufficiency, it is often not appreciated that the presence of edema indicates that sodium retention is contributing significantly to the hypertension. A loop diuretic in this setting will help to reduce blood pressure. Although thiazides are more effective in essential hypertension, they are ineffective antihypertensive agents in patients with chronic renal insufficiency. Most patients with chronic renal insufficiency will require the addition of a loop diuretic to control their blood pressure.

VII. REFERRAL TO A NEPHROLOGIST

Optimal predialysis care includes early intervention aimed at delaying progression of chronic renal insufficiency, prudent management of the complications of chronic renal insufficiency, early placement of dialysis access, and timely initiation of dialysis and/or preparation for renal transplantation. Management of chronic renal insufficiency requires active interventions and is not simply a monitoring exercise. Referral to a nephrologist is indicated if the cause of chronic renal insufficiency is uncertain so that specific therapy is not overlooked. If blood pressure cannot be controlled to optimal levels or if there is difficulty regulating any of the complications of chronic renal insufficiency, one should seek the help of a renal physician.

Several studies have examined the issue of early versus late referral of chronic renal insufficiency patients to a nephrologist. Late referral increases hospital length of stay at initiation of dialysis 2- to 10-fold compared to early referral. If renal replacement therapy commences within 3 months of referral, hospitalization time is increased, even if dialysis is started electively rather than emergently. Delayed referral carries heavy financial costs. Studies show \$20,000–\$40,000 additional cost for each patient referred late. Complications of chronic renal insufficiency are less severe in patients referred early. One study reported the one-year mortality rate for patients referred late to be three times higher than those referred early. However, this 12-month mortality rate may reflect initiation of dialysis at an earlier stage in the natural history of the disease rather than actually altering the course of disease. Further study is needed to determine whether predialysis care impacts on long-term mortality following initiation of dialysis. Only 20–25% of patients with chronic renal failure are referred to a renal physician prior to initiation of dialysis.

Education of patients with chronic renal insufficiency helps them prepare for end-stage renal disease and has been shown to help maintain employment and delay the need for renal replacement therapy. Referral to a nephrologist insures proper timing of placement of dialysis access. The National Kidney Foundation Dialysis Outcomes Quality Initiative guidelines recommend placement of hemodialysis vascular access when the serum creatinine rises above 4 mg/dL, the creatinine clearance falls to <25 mL/min, or dialysis is anticipated within one year. Transplantation is less costly than dialysis, reduces morbidity, and extends life. The waiting time for a cadaveric renal transplant now averages 2–4 years. Unfortunately, most renal failure patients do not start the process of pretransplant work-up until already on maintenance dialysis. Early referral and timely work-up for transplantation may reduce or eliminate the time on dialysis, particularly if living kidney donors are available. Therefore, referral to a nephrologist is recommended when the measured or estimated (by Cockcroft-Gault) creatinine clearance is <25 mL/min or the decline in renal function is rapid.

VIII. SUMMARY

Care of the patient with chronic renal insufficiency starts with a search for the specific cause of renal disease and its treatment. Therapies aimed at slowing progression of renal insufficiency can delay the development of end-stage disease significantly. Diligent treatment of complications, prudent referral to a renal physician, and timely preparation for renal replacement therapy can reduce financial and human costs substantially.

SUGGESTED READINGS

Alpern RJ, Sakhaee K. The clinical spectrum of chronic metabolic acidosis: homeostatics mechanisms produce significant morbidity. Am J Kidney Dis 1997; 29(2):291–302.

Baker LR, Abrams L, Roe CJ, Faugere MC, Fanti P, Subayti Y, Malluche HH. 1,25(OH)2D3 administration in moderate renal failure: a prospective double-blind trial. Kidney Int 1989; 35(2):661–669.

Brater DC, Voelker JR. Use of diuretics in patients with renal disease. In: Bennett WM, McCarron DA, eds. Contemporary Issues in Nephrology. Pharmacotherapy of Renal Disease and Hypertension, Vol 17. New York: Churchill Livingstone, 1987.

Eadington DW. Delayed Referral for dialysis: higher morbidity and higher costs. Semin Dialysis 1995; 8(5):258–260.

Hamdy NA, Kanis JA, Beneton MN, et al. Effect of alfacalcidol on natural course of renal bone disease in mild to moderate renal failure. Br Med J 1995; 310:358.

Hasslacher Ch, Ritz E, Wahl P, Michael C. Similar risks of nephropathy in patients with type I or type II diabetes mellitus. Neph Dialysis Trans 1989; 4:859–864.

Jungers P, Zingraff J, Page B, Albouze G, Hannedouch T, Man NK. Detrimental effects of late referral in patients with chronic renal failure: a case-control study. Kidney Int 1993; 43(suppl 41):S170–S173.

Keane WF. Lipids and the kidney. Kidney Int 1994; 46:910–920.

Kupin WL, Narins RG. The hyperkalemia of renal failure: pathophysiology, diagnosis and therapy. Contrib Nephrol 1993; 102:1–22.

Levey AS, Adler S, Caggiula AW, England BK, Greene T, Hunsicker LG, Kusek JW, Rogers NL, Teschan PE. Effects of dietary protein restriction on the progression of advanced renal disease in the modification of diet in renal disease study. Am J Kidney Dis 1996; 27(5):652–663.

Maki DD, Ma JZ, Louis TA, Kasiske BL. Long-term effects of antihypertensive agents on proteinuria and renal functions. Arch Intern Med 1995; 155:1073–1080.

Maschio G, Alberti D, Janin G, Locatelli F, Mann J, Motolese M, Ponticelli C, Ritz E, Zucchelli P, and The Angiotensin-Converting-Enzyme Inhibition in Progressive Renal Insufficiency Study Group. Effect of the angiotensin-converting-enzyme inhibitor benazepril on the progression of chronic renal insufficiency. N Engl J Med 1996; 334(15):939–945.

Massy ZA, Ma JZ, Louis TA, Kasiske BL. Lipid-lowering therapy in patients with renal disease. Kidney Int 1995; 48:188–198.

Mountokalakis TD. The renal consequences of arterial hypertension. Kidney Int 1997; 51: 1639–1653.

Orth SR, Ritz E, Schrier RW. The renal risks of smoking. Kidney Int 1997; 51:1669–1677.

Pedrini MT, Levey AS, Lau J, Chalmers TC, Wang PH. The effect of dietary protein restriction on the progression of diabetic and nondiabetic renal diseases: a meta-analysis. Ann Intern Med 1996; 124:627–632.

Peterson JC, Adler S, Burkart JM, Greene T, Hebert LA, Hunsicker LG, King AJ, Klahr S, Massry SG, Seifter JL. Blood pressure control, proteinuria, and the progression of renal disease. Ann Intern Med 1995; 123(10):754–762.

Portoles J, Torralbo A, Martin P, Rodrigo J, Herrero JA, Barrientos A. Cardiovascular effects of recombinant human erythropoietin in predialysis patients. Am J Kidney Dis 1997; 29(4):541–548.

Revicki DA, Brown RE, Feeny DH, Henry D, Teehan BP, Rudnick MR, Benz RL. Health-related quality of life associated with recombinant human erythropoietin therapy for predialysis chronic renal disease patients. Am J Kidney Dis 1995; 25(4):548–554.

Rimmer JM, Horn JF, Gennari FJ. Hyperkalemia as a complication of drug therapy. Arch Intern Med 1987; 147(5):867–869.

Suki WN. Use of diuretics in chronic renal failure. Kidney Int 1997; 51(suppl 59):S33–S35.

U.S. Renal Data System: USRDS 1997 Annual Data Report. Bethesda, MD: The National Institutes of Health, National Institute of Diabetes and Digestive and Kidney Diseases, 1997.

17
Hypertension in Patients with Renal Disease

Stephen C. Textor
Mayo Medical School and Mayo Clinic, Rochester, Minnesota

I. INTRODUCTION

Hypertension and renal disease are closely interconnected disorders. Most diseases that impair glomerular filtration rate lead to disturbances in Na^+ and extracellular fluid volume regulation, and these disturbances ultimately raise arterial pressure. Indeed, some investigators argue that any sustained rise in pressure requires "resetting" of the kidney. In recent years, studies of isolated genetic mutations of renal tubular Na^+ reabsorption, such as Liddle's syndrome, have reemphasized the dominant role of the kidney in regulating blood pressure. Conversely, hypertension plays a major role in progressive renal injury and the cardiovascular morbidity that accompanies advanced renal failure. Hence, understanding the principles and effective management of hypertension in the setting of renal disease is essential for clinicians caring for such patients. This chapter summarizes current concepts regarding the pathophysiology and treatment of these disorders.

II. PREVALENCE OF HYPERTENSION IN RENAL DISEASE

A. Unilateral Renal Injury

Some forms of unilateral renal injury, such as trauma or vascular occlusion, can induce hypertension by activating pressor systems such as the renin/angiotensin system. In the absence of renal artery occlusive disease, however, injury-stimulated hypertension is uncommon. Unilateral lesions such as slowly developing ureteral obstruction or renal hypogenesis usually have little effect on blood pressure. By contrast, unilateral renal artery stenosis routinely leads to hypertension (see Chapter 9).

B. Bilateral Renal Parenchymal Disease

Most renal parenchymal diseases affect both kidneys and produce loss of functioning nephrons, eventually associated with interstitial fibrosis. Acute renal failure due to tubular damage commonly leads to volume expansion, which usually resolves after recovery of renal function. Despite recovery from the renal injury, disturbed Na^+ and volume control with residual hypertension persists in some patients. Hypertension is a cardinal feature of many acute glomerular diseases, even those with only moderate loss of glomerular filtration. Children with acute glomerulonephritis, for example, demonstrate evidence of ECF volume expansion and incomplete suppression of the renin-angiotensin-aldosterone system.

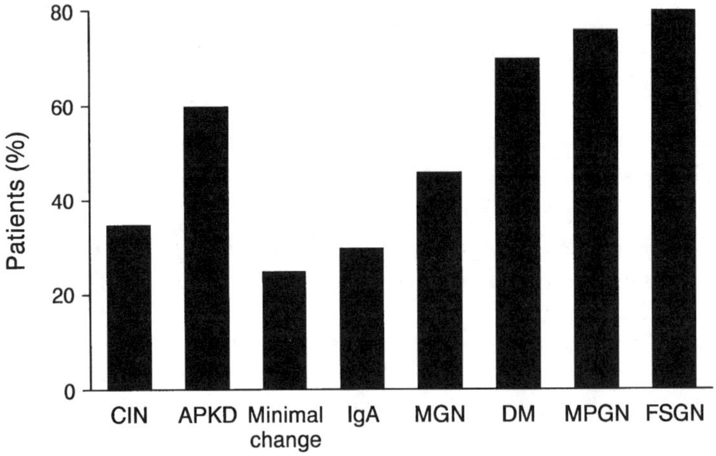

Figure 1 Prevalence of hypertension in various forms of chronic renal failure: these estimates indicate that most glomerular diseases are characterized by hypertension, even at early stages of renal dysfunction. Tubulo-interstitial disease and minimal change nephropathy are notable exceptions early in their course. As the loss of GFR becomes more severe (<35 mL/min), most forms of renal disease lead to hypertension regardless of their etiology. (Data modified from Smith and Dunn, 1995). IgA, IgA nephropathy; APKD, autosomal dominant polycystic kidney disease; MGN, membranous glomerulopathy; DM, diabetic nephropathy; CIN, chronic interstitial nephropathy MPGN, membranoproliferative glomerulopathy; FSCG, focal sclerosing glomerulonephritis.

Hypertension is almost an invariable consequence of chronic bilateral renal damage. Patients with chronic renal insufficiency due to primary glomerular diseases have associated hypertension in 75–90% of cases (Fig. 1). A notable exception is minimal change nephropathy, in which nephrotic syndrome develops with normal arterial pressure. Diseases considered interstitial in origin, such as analgesic nephropathy, are less uniformly associated with elevated blood pressures. The prevalence of hypertension rises as the severity of renal insufficiency progresses. This feature is illustrated by the rise in hypertension from 80 to 91% in the Modification of Diet in Renal Disease (MDRD) trial between Study A (mean GFR 39 mL/min/1.73 m^2) and Study B (mean GFR 19 mL/min/1.73 m^2). Hypertension is nearly universal in patients with advanced renal disease.

C. Obstructive Uropathy

Obstructive uropathy is frequently associated with hypertension, although this relationship is not as clearly defined as for other renal diseases. An example of this process may be seen in patients with ureteral obstruction associated with a pregnant uterus or endometriosis. Relief of obstruction leads to resolution of hypertension in this instance. Some older men with benign prostatic hypertrophy require less intensive antihypertensive therapy after transurethral resection of the prostate.

III. PATHOPHYSIOLOGY OF HYPERTENSION IN RENAL DISEASE

The hemodynamic determinants of blood pressure are cardiac output and total peripheral vascular resistance (Fig. 2). Many of the central elements regulating these components are deranged with renal disease. Cardiac output is determined primarily by cardiac filling volume, which in turn is a reflection of extracellular fluid (ECF) volume.

A. Regulation of Extracellular Volume in Patients with Renal Disease

Disturbed Na^+ excretion is a fundamental characteristic of renal disease. As a result, salt and water retention occurs, although it may be insufficient to cause clinically apparent edema. Nonetheless, ECF volume expansion is present when measured by ''Na^+ space'' or the volume of distribution of an extracellular marker, such as iothalamate or inulin. Many cardiovascular regulatory systems, such as the renin-angiotensin system (RAS) or atrial natriuretic peptide (ANP) are modulated by ECF volume. In the presence of renal disease, the relationship

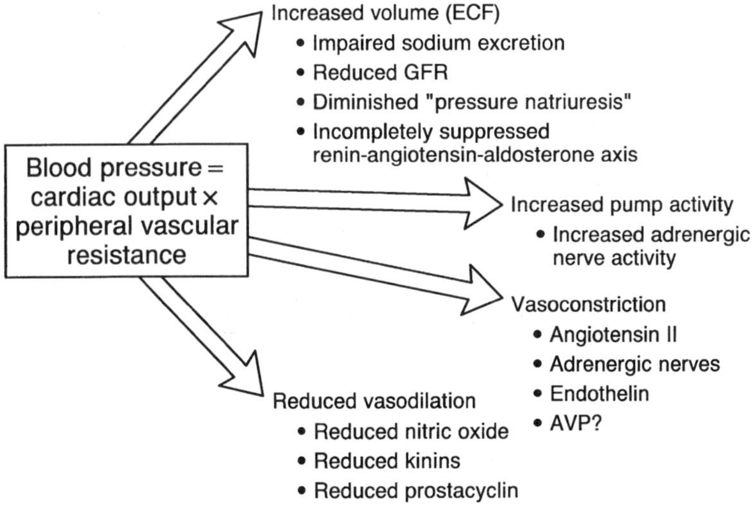

Figure 2 Overview of pathophysiological mechanisms that contribute to hypertension in patients with chronic renal disease. Both expanded extracellular fluid volume and disturbed regulation of vascular tone participate in its pathogenesis.

between ‘‘exchangeable Na^+’’ and the RAS, for example, is disturbed, with plasma renin activity remaining elevated despite persistently expanded ECF volume. When these individuals are further volume expanded, moreover, the RAS fails to be completely suppressed. This abnormal responsiveness is further exaggerated with progression of renal disease. As noted above, the majority of patients with reduced glomerular filtration have clinically significant hypertension. An important corollary to this observation is that blood pressure is often more easily controlled after starting dialysis therapy and removing excess Na^+ and water (Fig. 3).

1. Pressure Natriuresis

The key role of the kidney in long-term blood pressure regulation may be seen in terms of the relationship between arterial pressure and Na^+ excretion, termed ‘‘pressure natriuresis’’ by Guyton (Fig. 4). A rise in arterial pressure normally induces an increase in urinary Na^+ and water excretion until pressure falls to its normal ‘‘setpoint.’’ Conversely, a fall in arterial pressure, such as observed after fluid removal or hemorrhage, results in avid Na^+ retention until renal perfusion pressure is restored. Several important clinical features are consistent with such

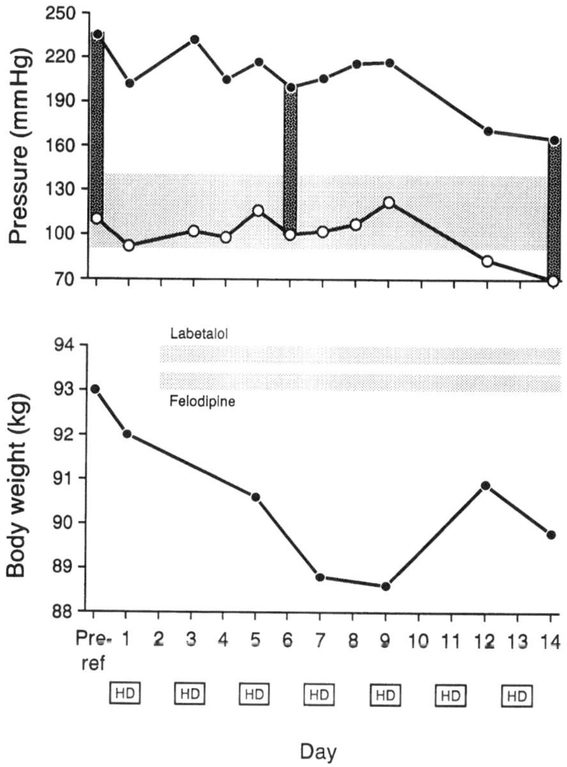

Figure 3 Body weight and blood pressure in a patient with chronic renal failure undergoing hemodialysis. Antihypertensive medications (labetalol and felodipine) were of limited effectiveness while volume expansion persisted. As body weight was reduced by ultrafiltration, blood pressures fell toward normal, reflecting a fall toward more normal extracellular fluid volume. Some component of ECF expansion is present in nearly all patients with chronic renal failure.

a mechanism. First, sustained impairment of Na^+ excretion, induced by mineralocorticoid excess or inhibition of prostaglandin synthesis by nonsteroidal anti-inflammatory agents, leads to a rise in arterial pressure until a natriuresis is achieved. Second, achieving long-term Na^+ balance, i.e., excretion at lower renal arterial pressures, is critical to effective blood pressure control. The role of diuretic therapy in treating hypertension is perhaps best explained as a means of "resetting" the ability of the damaged kidney to excrete Na^+ at a lower perfusion

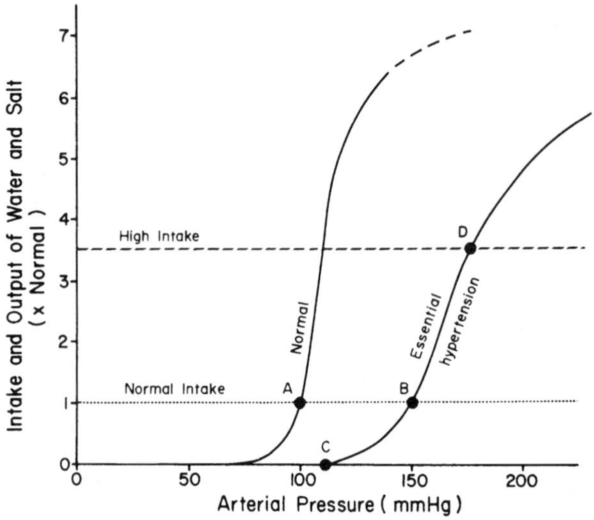

(a)

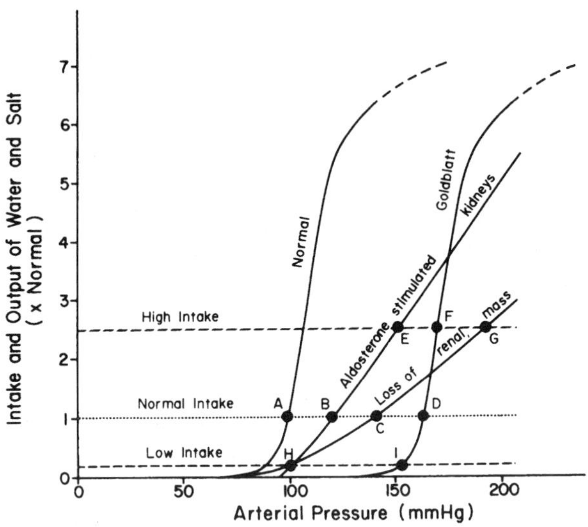

(b)

Figure 4 (a) Pressure natriuresis: normal subjects maintain Na^+ balance, e.g., excrete the daily intake of Na^+, within a narrow range of renal artery perfusion pressures. Alterations in renal artery pressure change the rate of Na^+ excretion sharply. Individuals with essential hypertension require higher pressures to maintain Na^+ balance (as shown for point B). This relationship between Na^+ balance and arterial pressure is believed to reflect a fundamental property of the kidney in regulating blood pressure, as illustrated by transplanting ''resistant'' and ''sensitive'' kidneys (see text). (b) The effect of various kidney disturbances upon the ''pressure-natriuresis'' relationship, indicating that loss of nephron mass, excessive aldosterone production and activation of the renin-angiotensin system (Goldblatt hypertension). All of these disturbances shift the curve to the right, thereby requiring higher arterial pressures to maintain Na^+ excretion. (From Guyton, 1991, with permission.)

pressure. Third, failure to achieve blood pressure reduction despite administration of potent antihypertensive agents such as minoxidil is often the result of inadequate Na^+ excretion.

An interesting corollary to this paradigm is that blood pressure level follows the kidney when transplanted. In ''salt-sensitive'' Dahl hypertensive rats, the presence of hypertension is determined by the genetic origin of the transplanted kidney. Hence, a salt-sensitive rat may be rendered normotensive after implantation of a ''resistant'' kidney. Similar observations have been reported in patients reaching end-stage renal disease (ESRD) on the basis of hypertensive nephrosclerosis who were later transplanted with kidneys from normotensive donors. Such patients achieved normal blood pressures without requiring antihypertensive therapy, indicating that the presence of a ''normotensive kidney'' was the primary determinant of systemic blood pressure.

The mechanisms responsible for altered ''pressure natriuresis'' in renal disease are varied and complex. They include disturbances in renal sympathetic nervous function, local alterations in the renin-angiotensin system, and altered balance between nitric oxide and other endothelial-derived vasoactive systems.

2. Primary Hyperaldosteronism and Liddle's Syndrome

Primary hyperaldosteronism and Liddle's syndrome are examples of isolated hormonal or Na^+ transport disorders producing hypertension. Primary overproduction of aldosterone due to the presence of an adrenal adenoma or adrenal hyperplasia leads to hypertension with enhanced renal Na^+ reabsorption and potassium excretion (see Chapter 9). The curability of this disorder by resection of the causative adrenal adenoma emphasizes how a single mechanism can disturb the com plex balance of cardioregulatory forces in blood pressure control.

Liddle's syndrome, an autosomal dominant form of hypertension associated with hypokalemia, provides further support for the concept that renal Na^+ handling is a primary mechanism of blood pressure regulation. The disorder is characterized by a genetic mutation that alters the collecting duct epithelial Na^+ channel (EnaC) in a manner that prevents its deactivation. As a result, Na^+ reabsorption is abnormally enhanced just as in hyperaldosteronism. Enhanced Na^+ reabsorption leads to suppression of both renin and aldosterone and to the development of elevated arterial pressure, K^+ wasting, and hypokalemia. Liddle's syndrome is one of several genetically transmitted forms of renal hypertension now identified. While single gene mutations producing hypertension are rare, they provide models for the study of nephron functional abnormalities leading to hypertension.

B. Regulation of Vascular Resistance in Renal Failure

In addition to volume expansion, systemic vascular resistance is elevated in hypertensive patients with renal disease. Several mechanisms may participate in developing vasoconstriction. The level of activation of the renin-angiotensin system remains "inappropriate" in such patients, partly due to derangements of the normal relationships between the juxtaglomerular apparatus and stimuli that regulate renin release, including arterial baroreflexes, adrenergic nervous system activity, and tubular Na^+ delivery. Adrenergic nerve traffic in peripheral nerves increases in patients with renal disease, a phenomenon that decreases after removal of native kidneys. Thus it is likely that diseased kidneys cause afferent nerve stimulation, an effect that subsequently increases central nervous system activity and efferent sympathetic nerve stimuli to peripheral vascular beds. Circulating levels of another potent vasoconstrictor, endothelin, are elevated in some forms of renal injury. In some experimental models, blockade of endothelin improves arterial pressure and increases both renal blood flow and glomerular filtration. Its role in human disease is not yet established clearly.

Elevated vascular resistance also may derive from impaired vasodilation. Nitric oxide is an important local regulatory agent to maintain vasodilation, and its production may be disturbed in the presence of renal injury. Inhibition of nitric oxide produces profound vasoconstriction within both the kidney and peripheral vascular circulation, and reduces Na^+ excretion and glomerular filtration. Drugs that impair nitric oxide production, such as cyclosporine, produce similar effects. Several other vasodilating hormones, such as prostacyclin or atrial natriuretic peptides, are increased in many forms of renal disease. Hence, it is unlikely that they are directly responsible for the abnormal vasoconstriction. Apparently, however, they are not sufficient to counteract the net effects of vasoconstricting forces.

C. Summary

Taken together, patients with renal disease have derangements both in the regulation of Na^+ balance by the kidney, leading to expansion of extracellular fluid volume, and in the regulation of vascular resistance, leading to abnormal vasoconstriction. As a result of these abnormalities, elevated arterial pressures are nearly universal.

IV. CLINICAL MANIFESTATIONS OF HYPERTENSION IN PATIENTS WITH RENAL DISEASE

A. Risks of Hypertension

The risks of hypertension in patients with renal disease are at least as great as in other patients with hypertension. These risks are due to hypertension-induced target organ injury, specifically left ventricular hypertrophy and vascular disease affecting the brain, heart, and other beds. High blood pressure itself causes few symptoms, until a stroke or myocardial infarction occurs. Hypertensive target organ damage, including left ventricular hypertrophy and small vessel cerebral infarction, develops more rapidly and more frequently in the absence of the normal nocturnal fall in blood pressure. This normal circadian pattern is commonly disturbed in patients with impaired renal function. An example of such a patient is shown in Figure 5. Instead of a fall in blood pressure, nocturnal readings may be as high or higher than daytime readings. This change can lead to reversal of day-night patterns of Na^+ excretion, manifested as nocturia. Patients with essential hypertension without this nocturnal fall are more likely to develop microalbuminuria, an early marker of renal damage.

In patients with advanced renal failure needing dialysis or transplantation, complications of atherosclerosis are common sources of morbidity and mortality. Cardiac and vascular events together account for more than half of deaths in ESRD populations. The prevalence of left ventricular hypertrophy in patients starting dialysis is estimated to exceed 35%, and left ventricular hypertrophy is the strongest predictor of congestive heart failure. This risk is compounded by the presence of other known cardiovascular risk factors, including diabetes mellitus, smoking, and age. Hence, vigorous intervention to delay progression of hypertensive target organ damage is warranted to reduce long-term cardiovascular morbidity and mortality.

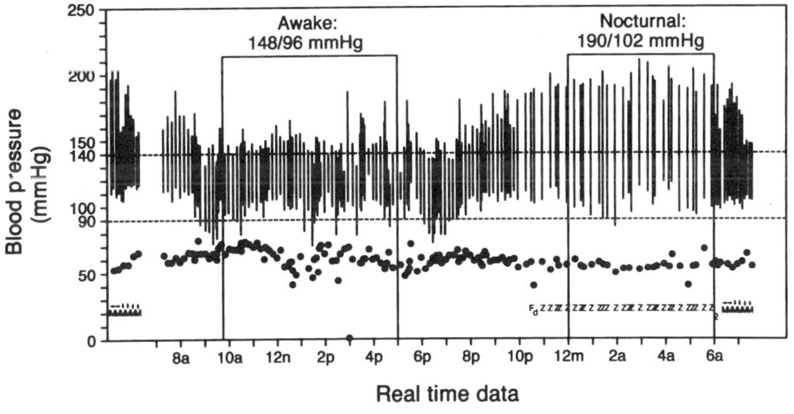

Figure 5 Altered circadian rhythm in patients with chronic renal failure: blood pressure levels during a 24-hour period are shown here in a patient with renal dysfunction (GFR = 42 mL/min) undergoing treatment with corticosteroids. The normal 10–15% fall in blood pressure during the nocturnal hours is absent, a feature that has been associated with accelerated target organ injury, including left-ventricular hypertrophy, small vessel ischemic strokes, and increased proteinuria.

B. Risk of Renal Injury

In addition to the harm it causes to the heart and brain, hypertension accelerates the progression of renal injury in patients with kidney disease. When severe and untreated, malignant hypertension can lead to proteinuria and progressive renal failure. Treatment of severe hypertension materially improves survival and retards progression to end-stage renal disease. Whether milder forms of ''benign essential hypertension'' in patients without kidney disease lead to parenchymal renal injury is controversial. In several large, randomized treatment trials of essential hypertension, no differences were found in the incidence of ESRD between placebo and treated groups. By contrast, blood pressure level in large population studies was found to be a major independent risk factor for ESRD. The risks of renal disease and hypertension are greater in African-American subjects than in Caucasians. It is difficult to exclude the presence of unidentified renal disease, which itself predisposes to long-term hypertension, in such population-based surveys. One explanation of such data is that ''two hits'' may be necessary, one of which is intrinsic renal injury or genetic predisposition to renal injury, and the second of which is the simultaneous presence of hypertension.

C. Risk of Accelerating Renal Injury in Patients with Preexisting Renal Disease

Extensive studies in both patients and experimental animals indicate that a the progression of renal parenchymal disease is accelerated in the presence of elevated arterial pressure. This may be due in part to the hemodynamic effects of elevated intraglomerular pressures, causing direct hydraulic injury to the glomerulus in addition to the primary disease process, which may be mediated by other mechanisms. The mediators of this ''hydraulic'' injury are not known but may include release of local factors, such as endothelin, inflammatory cytokines, and mediators of oxidative stress.

The rate of decline of kidney function in patients reaching end-stage renal disease (ESRD) is related to arterial pressure during the course of their disease. Effective blood pressure reduction reduces the rate of disease progression of many glomerular diseases. This effect is manifest as reduced glomerulosclerosis and interstitial damage, as well as a reduction in the rate of decline in GFR. Such evidence provides strong support for the interaction between arterial pressure and progressive renal injury.

V. TREATMENT OF HYPERTENSION IN PATIENTS WITH RENAL DISEASE

The principles of effective blood pressure reduction are based on our understanding of the pathophysiology of hypertension in patients with renal disease, as discussed earlier in this chapter. They include the need to reverse ECF volume expansion, to facilitate Na^+ excretion at lower arterial pressures, and to lower peripheral vascular resistance. In most respects, these principles are similar to those applied to the treatment of essential hypertension. There are, however, some elements of particular importance to patients with impaired renal function.

A. Diuretic Therapy

Selection of a diuretic agent should include consideration of the level of glomerular filtration. Thiazide diuretics have limited effects on Na^+ reabsorption and may be ineffective in patients with reduced GFR. Some experts recommend limiting their use to patients with serum creatinine levels below 2.0 mg/dL. Some members of this class, specifically metolazone and indapamide, appear to retain efficacy at somewhat higher levels of creatinine. Loop diuretics, such as furosemide and bumetanide, are more appropriate for patients with low GFR and have a longer duration of action in such patients than in patients with normal kidney function. Because these diuretics must be secreted into the tubular urine to be effective, higher doses are often needed to achieve a satisfactory diuretic response.

Maintaining K^+ excretion becomes more difficult as GFR falls, particularly in patients with tubular function disturbances, such as obstructive uropathy (see Chapters 13 and 23). As a result, supplemental K^+ is usually not needed when diuretic therapy is used. In addition, K^+-sparing agents such as triamterene, amiloride, or spironolactone should be avoided or be used with great caution in patients with renal insufficiency to avoid hyperkalemia. An important corollary to this principle is that the presence of hypokalemia in patients with renal insufficiency, particularly when seen in association with ACE inhibition (see below), even in the presence of modest diuretic use, is "inappropriate" and may reflect K^+ wasting, usually due to aldosterone excess.

B. α- and β-Adrenergic Blockade

α-Blockers (e.g., terazocin), β-blockers, combined α-β-blockers, and adrenergic agonists are all effective agents in patients with chronic renal insufficiency. Some consideration must be given to accumulation of metabolites, particularly with long-acting agents, which may potentiate both efficacy and duration of side effects. All these agents may reduce Na^+ excretion further, requiring an increase in dosage requirements for diuretics.

C. Calcium-Channel Blockers

Calcium-channel blocking (CCB) drugs have been an important addition to effective antihypertensive therapy for patients with renal disease. In addition to reducing peripheral arterial resistance, these agents have effects within the kidney, lowering renal vascular resistance and sometimes producing a diuretic effect. Hence, some patients will report increased urine flows and will have increased Na^+ excretion when receiving CCB treatment. These agents, however, are not a substitute for diuretics. CCBs commonly produce arteriolar vasodilation in local vascular beds, predisposing to edema formation. This property of calcium antagonists tends to limit the reliability of edema as a sign of ECF volume expansion and the edema usually does not respond to diuretic therapy. In experimental animals, diltiazem-class CCBs modify mesangial expansion and reduce proteinuria, perhaps independently of systemic pressure reduction. This property may provide an additional advantage for renal protection. This effect, unfortunately, is not seen with the more potent and therefore more useful dihydropyridine class of CCBs. In fact the dyhydropyridine CCBs occasionally increase proteinuria, most likely through the same arteriolar vasodilation that produces local tissue edema elsewhere.

D. Angiotensin-Converting Enzyme Inhibitors/AII Receptor Blockers

Angiotensin-converting enzyme (ACE) inhibitors and angiotensin receptor antagonists are key agents for treating hypertension in patients with renal disease. These drugs act primarily by interrupting the renin-angiotensin system, both within the systemic circulation and within the kidney. The degree of blood pressure reduction by these agents is magnified when ECF volume is reduced by diuretic use or when high-grade renal artery stenosis is present leading to underpefusion of the kidney. ACE inhibitors have been shown in multiple studies to reduce the rate of progression of both diabetic and nondiabetic renal disease. This effect appears to be greater than can be explained by the reduction of systemic arterial pressure. Although angiotensin receptor antagonists have not been studied extensively in this regard, they appear to have a nearly identical protective effect.

A major element of their application in patients with renal disease reflects the importance of angiotensin II as a factor that maintains efferent arteriolar tone within the kidney. Efferent vascular tone is the principal regulator of glomerular hydrostatic pressure, particularly when afferent arteriolar tone is limited. ACE inhibitors lower efferent vascular resistance and thereby decrease glomerular filtration pressure. This effect reduces GFR but also decreases glomerular injury and proteinuria. Whether the reduction in glomerular hydrostatic pressure or some other factor is the cause of the protective effect seen in humans is unknown. Because angiotensin is a growth factor, interference with its actions may also slow the production of collagen and fibrosis that occurs with chronic renal injury.

ACE inhibitors and angiotensin II receptor antagonists must be considered a "double-edged sword," however. Under conditions of compromised afferent arteriolar circulation to the kidney, such as occurs in the presence of renal artery stenosis, severe volume depletion, or heart failure, a reduction in efferent arteriolar tone may produce a sharp fall in filtration and cause acute renal failure. If detected early, this effect is nearly always reversible. In patients with renal artery stenosis, sensitivity to ACE inhibition in this manner reflects "critical" renal artery stenosis that is best managed by renal revascularization (see Chapter 9). Hence, the property of ACE inhibitors to reduce efferent arteriolar tone both leads to a special role in protection against progressive renal failure in renal disease and to a special caution against excessive reduction in GFR in patients with renal arterial disease. A second problem with this class of drugs is hyperkalemia. By both reducing GFR and removing the main signal for aldosterone release, these agents produce a functional hypoaldosteronism, impairing K^+ excretion and causing hyperkalemia.

VI. TARGET BLOOD PRESSURE AND PROGRESSION TO RENAL FAILURE

Effective antihypertensive therapy in patients with renal failure has several important dimensions. As noted above, the ubiquity of hypertension in patients with renal disease adds a major level of cardiovascular risk, particularly when combined with additional risk factors such diabetes mellitus and hyperlipidemia. Reduction of cardiovascular risk, particularly the risk of stroke, myocardial infarction, and congestive heart failure, is a major objective of therapy in this setting, as in any patient with hypertension.

The additional dimension in patients with renal disease is slowing the progression to renal failure. Despite major reductions in the mortality rates of stroke and coronary artery disease observed since widespread application of the antihypertensive therapy, no similar reduction in the incidence rate of ESRD has occurred. While epidemiological observations suggest that risk of ESRD is closely related to arterial pressures, intervention trials until now have provided less uniform evidence that the levels of arterial pressure usually achieved slow progressive renal injury (Fig. 6). Some experts argue that the level of blood pressure needed to achieve this benefit is not commonly attained in patients with renal disease. Hence, more vigorous efforts at "strict" blood pressure control may be required, particularly in some forms of renal disease, such as nephrosclerosis in African Americans. The benefits of lower arterial pressures are evident from results in the MDRD trial, in which one aim was to compare disease progression in patients with lower mean arterial pressures (MAP < 92 mmHg) to those with more conventional levels of achieved pressures

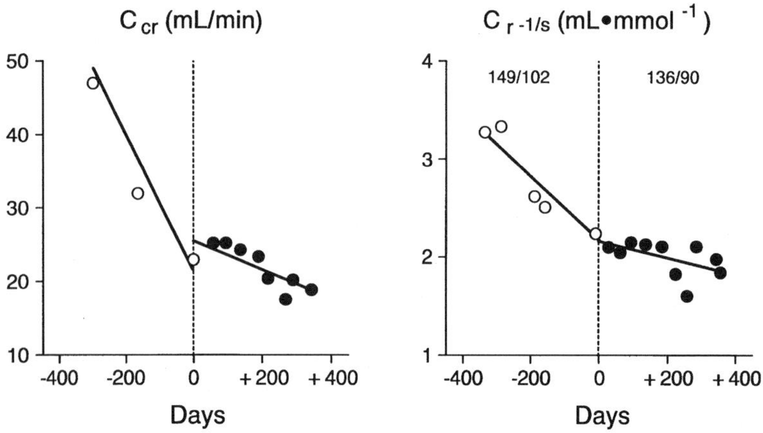

Figure 6 Slowing of progressive renal failure after antihypertensive therapy: these figures illustrate changes in the rate of decline of GFR, expressed either as creatinine clearance or reciprocal creatinine (1/creatinine) after reducing BP from 149/102 mmHg to 136/90 mmHg in patients with chronic glomerulonephritis. Data from many sources underscore the association of elevated arterial pressures with a rapid decline in renal function to end-stage renal failure. Recent trials underscore the fact that progression can be slowed with "strict" blood pressure control levels, i.e., 135/85 mmHg, in some forms of renal disease, particularly diabetic nephropathy and glomerular diseases characterized by heavy proteinuria. These benefits are most apparent with administration of agents that block the renin-angiotensin system, such as ACE inhibitors (see text).

(MAP $<$ 107 mmHg). When stratified according to the degree of proteinuria, patients excreting more than 3.0 g/day had lower rates of disease progression in the strict blood pressure group. Patients with lesser degrees of proteinuria had less benefit, at least during the limited period of follow-up (2 years). These results led the Joint National Committee of the National High Blood Pressure Education Program to recommend vigorous blood pressure control in patients with kidney disease and proteinuria. Several trials are currently in progress to examine whether lower arterial pressures may offer renal protection during longer periods of follow-up.

VII. SUMMARY

Hypertension is a nearly universal abnormality in patients with chronic renal insufficiency and failure. The elevated blood pressure is due to derangements in control of both ECF volume and vascular resistance. Hypertension accelerates both progression of renal injury and morbidity related to atherosclerosis in this population, which is the largest cause of death in patients with ESRD. Effective blood pressure control can reduce cardiovascular morbidity and mortality and, when pursued aggressively, can reduce the rate of disease progression. Blood pressure control is a key element of the management of patients with renal disease.

SUGGESTED READINGS

Beevers DG, Lip GYH. Does non-malignant essential hypertension cause renal damage? A clinician's view. J Human Hyper 1996; 10:695–699.

Brazy PC, Stead WW, Fitzwilliam JF. Progression of renal insufficiency: role of blood pressure. Kidney Int 1989; 35:670–674.

Converse RL, Jacobsen TN, Toto RD, et al. Sympathetic overactivity in patients with chronic renal failure. NEJM 1992; 327:1912–1918.

Cowley AW, Roman RJ. The role of the kidney in hypertension. JAMA 1996; 275:1581–1587.

Curtiss JJ, Luke RG, Dustan HP, et al. Remission of essential hypertension after renal transplantation. N Engl J Med 1983; 309:1009–1015.

Davies DL, Schalekamp MA, Beevers DG, et al. Abnormal relation between exchangeable sodium and the renin-angiotensin system in malignant hypertension and in hypertension with chronic renal failure. Lancet 1973; i:683–687.

Gansevoort RT, Navis GJ, Wapstra FH, de Jong PE, de Zeeuw D. Proteinuria and progression of renal disease: therapeutic implications. Curr Opin Nephrol Hyper 1997; 6: 133–140.

Guyton AC. Dominant role of the kidneys in long-term regulation of arterial pressure and hypertension: the integrated system for pressure control. In: Guyton AC, ed. Textbook of Medical Physiology. Philadelphia: W.B. Saunders Company, 1991, pp. 205–220.

Klag MJ, Whelton PK, Randall BL, Neaton JD, Brancati FL, Stamler J. End-stage renal disease in African-American and white men. JAMA 1997; 277:1293–1298.

Klahr S, Levey AS, Beck GJ, et al. The effects of dietary protein restriction and blood-pressure control on the progression of chronic renal disease. N Engl J Med 1994; 330:877–884.

Levin ER. Mechanisms of disease: endothelins. N Engl J Med 1995; 333:356–363.

Mountokalakis TD. The renal consequences of arterial hypertension. Kidney Int 1997; 51: 1639–1653.

National High Blood Pressure Education Program Working Group: 1995 Update of the Working Group Reports on Chronic Renal Failure and Renovascular Hypertension. Arch Intern Med 1996; 156:1938–1947.

Perry HM, Miller JP, Fornoff JR, et al. Early predictors of 15-year end-stage renal disease in hypertensive patients. Hypertension 1995; 25(part 1):587–594.

Peterson JC, Adler S, Burkart JM, et al. Blood pressure control, proteinuria and the progression of renal disease. Ann Intern Med 1995; 123:754–762.

Rodriguez-Iturbe B, Baggio B, Colina-Chourio J, et al. Studies on the renin-aldosterone system in the acute nephritic syndrome. Kidney Int 1981; 19:445–453.

Satin AJ, Seiken GL, Cunningham FC. Reversible hypertension in pregnancy caused by obstructive uropathy. Obstet Gynecol 1993; 81:823–825.

Smith MC, Dunn MJ. Hypertension in renal parenchymal disease. In: Hypertension: Laragh JH, Brenner BM, eds. Pathophysiology, diagnosis and management. New York: Raven Press, 1995, pp. 2081–2102.

Textor SC. Renal failure related to ACE inhibitors. Semin Nephrol 1997; 17:67–76.

Warnock DG. Liddle syndrome: an autosomal dominant form of hypertension. Kidney Int 1998; 53:18–24.

Wilcox CS. Diuretics. In: Brenner BM, ed. The Kidney. Philadelphia: W.B. Saunders, 1995, pp. 2299–2330.

Wise HM. Hypertension resulting from hydronephrosis. JAMA 1975; 235:491.

18
Diabetic Nephropathy

Gerald C. Groggel
University of Nebraska Medical Center, Omaha, Nebraska

I. INTRODUCTION

Diabetic nephropathy is a histologically characteristic glomerular disease found in patients with diabetes mellitus. Diabetes mellitus is now classified into two types based on pathogenetic mechanisms rather than on the type of therapy. Type 1 diabetes (old type I or insulin-dependent diabetes mellitus, IDDM) encompasses most cases resulting from pancreatic islet beta cell destruction by immune mechanisms. Type 1 is characterized by absolute insulin deficiency and, as a result, type 1 patients are more prone to ketoacidosis. Type 2 (old type II or non–insulin-dependent diabetes mellitus, NIDDM) includes all forms of diabetes resulting from insulin resistance coupled with an insulin secretory defect.

The newly established diagnostic criteria for both types of diabetes mellitus include a fasting serum glucose ≥126 mg/dL, a random serum glucose ≥200 mg/dL with symptoms, or an oral glucose tolerance test with a 2-hour serum glucose ≥200 mg/dL. Type 2 diabetes accounts for 90–95% of all diabetic patients. The long-term complications of diabetes mellitus can be subdivided into microvascular (involving arterioles and capillaries) and macrovascular (involving medium and large arteries). The microvascular complications include diabetic nephropathy, diabetic retinopathy, and diabetic neuropathy. Diabetes mellitus is also an important risk factor for macrovascular complications, which include coronary artery disease, peripheral vascular disease, and cerebrovascular disease.

II. DIABETIC NEPHROPATHY: CLINICAL PRESENTATION

A. Incidence

Diabetic nephropathy is the leading cause of end-stage renal disease (ESRD) in the United States, accounting for almost 40% of all cases. Both type 1 and type 2 diabetics develop this complication. After 10–20 years, 30–40% of all type 1 diabetic patients will develop diabetic nephropathy. Although the incidence of nephropathy in type 2 diabetes and the time course to its development is less clearly defined, it appears to be in a similar range, 5–30%. Presently, the number of diabetic patients with ESRD is evenly divided between type 1 and type 2 patients. The number of type 2 patients with ESRD is growing rapidly, however, and shortly these patients will exceed type 1 patients. The annual cost of treating diabetic ESRD is over $4 billion. In addition to diabetic nephropathy, diabetic men have a threefold increase in relative risk of developing ESRD from other causes, according to a recent analysis of diabetic participants in the Multiple Risk Factor Intervention Trial (MRFIT).

B. Diagnosis

Diabetic nephropathy is diagnosed by the presence of proteinuria (>300 mg/24 hr) in a patient with longstanding diabetes mellitus. In most instances, further diagnostic workup is not necessary (see below). Before the development of overt proteinuria, diabetic patients destined to develop diabetic nephropathy excrete abnormal, albeit small, amounts of albumin in their urine. This abnormality is termed ''microalbuminuria.'' Detection of microalbuminuria requires an assay specific for albumin; it is not detected by dipstick or by the measurement of total urinary protein. Diabetic patients with more than 30 mg/24 hr of albumin in the urine have microalbuminuria. When the urinary albumin excretion exceeds 300 mg/24 hr, the patients have overt proteinuria and the dipstick will be positive. The definitions of normal albuminuria, microalbuminuria, and macroalbuminuria (clinical proteinuria) are shown in Table 1.

1. Screening Tests for Microalbuminuria

All patients with type 1 diabetes of greater than 5 years duration should have their urine screened annually for microalbuminuria, according to the recommendations of the American Diabetes Association. Type 2 diabetic patients should be screened at the time of diagnosis and yearly thereafter. Microalbuminuria can be assessed by collecting a 24-hour urine sample, by a timed collection over a shorter interval of time, or by measuring the albumin and creatinine concentrations in a random urine sample and calculating an albumin/creatinine ratio (see

Table 1 Proteinuria: Definitions

	24-hr urine albumin (mg/24 hr)	Albumin(mg/dL)/ Creatinine(mg/dL) ratio	Timed urine albumin (μg/min)
Normal albumin excretion	<30	<0.03	<20
Microalbuminuria[a] (dipstick negative)	30–300	0.03–0.30	20–200
Macroalbuminuria (clinical proteinuria)	>300	>0.30	>200

[a] Detected by albumin antibody technique.

Table 1). For patient convenience and accuracy, the random urine sample is now the recommended approach. A ratio of albumin (mg/dL) to creatinine (mg/dL) of >0.03 is indicative of microalbuminuria and a ratio of >0.3 indicates the presence of clinical proteinuria. If microalbuminuria is found, persistent microalbuminuria should be demonstrated with two to three other collections over the next 3–6 months. Transient microalbuminuria can occur in association with severe hyperglycemia, heart failure, fever, exercise, urinary tract infection, and uncontrolled hypertension. Most of these are thought to cause a transient increase in albumin loss into the urine by altering glomerular hemodynamics.

2. Further Diagnostic Workup

Proteinuria in patients with diabetes mellitus who have concurrent diabetic retinopathy, neuropathy, and diabetes of at least 10 years duration is so likely to be due to diabetic nephropathy that no further workup is necessary. One should consider other causes for the proteinuria, however, if the urinary sediment shows evidence of inflammation (red cells, white cells, cellular casts) or if screening tests show low complement levels or other abnormal serologies. Over 95% of type 1 patients with diabetic nephropathy, but only 50–75% of the type 2 patients with nephropathy, also have diabetic retinopathy. In type 1 patients without retinopathy, other causes for the proteinuria should be investigated (see Chapter 19). In such instances a nephrology consult should be obtained to assess whether a renal biopsy is indicated. Because diabetic nephropathy is so common, diabetic patients with atypical presentations are still more likely to have diabetic renal disease rather than other rarer causes of proteinuria. In the vast majority of diabetic patients, clinical proteinuria signals the presence of diabetic nephropathy. A quarter of these patients will have the nephrotic syndrome as well.

III. TREATMENT

Treatment of diabetic nephropathy is intended to slow progression of the renal damage. Major treatments for diabetic nephropathy include meticulous control of blood pressure, use of an angiotensin-converting enzyme (ACE) inhibitor, glycemic control, low-protein diet, and control of hypercholesterolemia (Table 2). Treatment should also include smoking cessation, dietary sodium restriction, regular exercise, prompt diagnosis and management of urinary tract infections and obstruction, and avoidance of nephrotoxins. Each of these therapies is discussed below. Many of these same interventions, if begun early in the course of diabetes, may actually delay the development of diabetic nephropathy.

A. Blood Pressure Control

The most important treatment for the patient with diabetic nephropathy is to control blood pressure. Antihypertensive therapy slows the progression of renal disease from all causes. In prospective trials in patients with type 1 diabetes, combination therapy (furosemide, metoprolol, and hydralazine in two studies) or single-agent therapy (propranolol, metoprolol, or captopril) resulted in a decrease in albuminuria and a lower rate of decline in the glomerular filtration rate. One European study showed that triple drug therapy decreased the rate of decline in glomerular filtration rate from 0.89 to 0.22 mL/min/month. Based on these results, aggressive treatment of hypertension could extend the time from the onset of hypertension and nephropathy to ESRD by 14 years.

Table 2 Recommended Treatments to slow the Progression of Diabetic Nephropathy

Proven benefit[a]
Blood pressure control
Blood glucose control
Blockade of renin/angiotensin system
Probable benefit[b]
Cholesterol control
Low-protein diet
Smoking cessation

[a] Benefit demonstrated in large-scale prospective randomized studies.

[b] Benefit demonstrated in animal studies or in small-scale studies in humans.

1. Blood Pressure Goals

The definition of hypertension is undergoing continual revision. The sixth report of the Joint National Commission, published in 1997 (see Chapters 9 and 17), now defines optimal blood pressure as <120/80, normal blood pressure as <130/85, and hypertension as 140/90 or higher. Many epidemiological studies have demonstrated that the risk of cardiovascular and cerebrovascular disease is a continuous function of both systolic and diastolic pressure and that lower blood pressures are beneficial. Based on the evidence currently available, the Joint National Commission recommends reduction in blood pressure in patients with diabetes mellitus to below a systolic blood pressure of 130 mmHg and a diastolic blood pressure of 85 mmHg. For patients with isolated systolic hypertension, the initial goal of therapy should be to reduce the systolic blood pressure to <160 mmHg and/or to lower the systolic blood pressure by 20 mmHg. If these goals can be achieved and well tolerated, further lowering of the systolic blood pressure should be attempted.

2. Nonpharmacological Interventions

In patients with mild to moderate hypertension and normal renal function, the recommended initial treatment is nonpharmacological therapy involving lifestyle modifications. These include weight loss if the patient is obese, dietary Na^+ restriction, regular exercise, moderation of alcohol intake, and smoking cessation. In patients with hypertension, reducing Na^+ intake to <100 mEq per day (2.3 g Na^+ or 5.8 g NaCl) is recommended. Reducing daily sodium intake by as little as 40 mEq per day, however, can significantly lower blood pressure. Excessive alcohol intake has been shown to raise blood pressure and cause resistance to antihypertensive therapy. Daily alcohol intake should be limited to no more than one ounce of ethanol (eight ounces of wine or 24 ounces of beer). Regular physical activity not only increases exercise capacity, an effect that plays an important role in the prevention of cardiovascular disease, but also lowers blood pressure and improves glycemic control. Regular exercise is also an important component in a weight reduction program. Patients should engage in moderate aerobic exercise three to four times a week. Cigarette smoking is a major risk factor in cardiovascular disease and may also accelerate the progression of diabetic nephropathy. All diabetic patients should be strongly advised to stop smoking. If these measures do not control blood pressure within 6 months, drug therapy is indicated. In patients with more severe hypertension, or those in whom renal insufficiency is already present, the same lifestyle modifications should be undertaken in combination with drug therapy.

3. Drug Therapy

The antihypertensive drug of first choice in all diabetic patients is an angiotensin-converting enzyme (ACE) inhibitor (see below for specific rationale). The goal of therapy is a blood pressure of 130/85 mmHg or less. In patients who tolerate this blood pressure well, one may try to reduce the blood pressure even lower to 120/80 mmHg. Care should be taken in achieving this goal in patients with underlying diabetic neuropathy, cardiovascular disease, or cerebrovascular disease who are at particular risk for orthostatic hypotension or cerebral hypoperfusion.

The classes of antihypertensive drugs available, in addition to ACE inhibitors, include diuretics, β blockers, calcium channel blockers, α-adrenergic blockers, and angiotensin II receptor blockers. All are effective agents in patients with diabetes. The choice of drug should be dictated by patient acceptance as well as by coexistent medical problems. For example, a selective β_2 blocker should be used if the patient has coronary artery disease. In most patients with renal insufficiency, diuretic therapy is necessary for blood pressure control. These agents are particularly useful as adjunctive therapy with ACE inhibitors (see Chapter 17 for a discussion of the treatment of hypertension in patients with renal insufficiency). In patients with serum creatinine concentrations greater than 2–3 mg/dL, thiazide diuretics are ineffective and a loop diuretic should be used. Potassium-sparing diuretics should probably be avoided in diabetic patients because of the high risk of developing hyperkalemia.

The dihydropyridine class of calcium channel blockers (e.g., nifedipine) are effective, well-tolerated antihypertensive drugs, but there is some controversy concerning whether these agents have special risks in diabetic patients. In a study of type 2 diabetic patients treated with nisoldipine, there was a significantly higher incidence of myocardial infarction compared to those treated with enalapril. Results such as these have raised the concern that the dihydropyridines may be harmful in diabetic patients with underlying coronary artery disease and should be used with caution.

B. Reducing Glomerular Injury

1. ACE Inhibitors

In patients with diabetic nephropathy, ACE inhibitors reduce the level of albuminuria and slow the rate of loss of glomerular filtration to a greater degree than other antihypertensive agents that lower blood pressure to a similar level (see Chapter 17). Because ACE inhibitors selectively reduce efferent arteriolar resistance and thereby decrease glomerular hydrostatic pressure, their added benefit supports the hypothesis that hyperglycemia produces glomerular injury in part by causing afferent arteriolar vasodilation and thereby increasing glomerular capillary hydrostatic pressure. The resultant glomerular capillary hypertension is manifest initially as hyperfiltration and then, as injury develops, as proteinuria and eventually as a loss of functioning nephron units. Inhibition of angiotensin

II lowers glomerular capillary pressure by reducing efferent arteriolar tone in experimental animals with diabetes and slows the progression of renal injury. The same effect is presumed to occur in humans.

Further evidence for a special beneficial effect of ACE inhibitors in patients with diabetes mellitus comes from studies in normotensive type 1 diabetics with microalbuminuria. In one large,randomized, prospective trial, albumin excretion increased from 52 to 76 mg/min in placebo-treated diabetic patients over 2 years, while those treated with captopril experienced a reduction in albumin excretion from 52 to 41 mg/min. In a second trial, captopril reduced the risk of progressing from microalbuminuria to overt proteinuria by 69%. The rate of fall of the creatinine clearance also tended to be faster in the placebo-treated group.

Similar studies have also been performed in type 2 diabetic patients. In a 5-year controlled clinical trial of normotensive patients with type 2 diabetes and microalbuminuria, enalapril stabilized microalbuminuria and serum creatnine concentration, while in the control group there was progression. In a second trial, treatment with enalapril produced a decrease in microalbuminuria while the placebo group had an increase. Within 5 years, 8% of the enalapril treated group, as compared with 23.5% of the placebo group, progressed to clinical proteinuria. Based on these data, all diabetic patients with microalbuminuria should be treated with an ACE inhibitor if they can tolerate this drug. ACE inhibitor may also delay the progression of diabetic retinopathy.

ACE inhibitors have few adverse effects and may even have beneficial effects on lipid metabolism and insulin sensitivity. Significant adverse effects include hyperkalemia, cough, and a rapid decline in renal function. Hyperkalemia may be a particular problem in patients with advanced renal insufficiency or patients with the hyporeninemic hypoaldosterone syndrome (see Chapter 11). If a rapid decline in renal function occurs, patients should be investigated for bilateral renal artery stenosis (see Chapter 9). These agents are also contraindicated during pregnancy.

One cannot assume that the angiotensin II receptor blockers have similar effectiveness until controlled trials demonstrate this to be the case. However, studies in experimental animals with diabetes suggest that this new class of angiotensin blockers will likely have the same or similar beneficial renal effects. Based on data from animal studies, the angiotensin II receptor blockers (e.g., losartan, valsartan, irbesartan) are reasonable alternatives for the patient who is unable to tolerate an ACE inhibitor.

2. Calcium Channel Blockers

Some studies have shown that the benzothiazepine (diltiazem) and the phenyalkylamine (verapamil) classes of calcium channel blockers reduce the level of albuminuria in patients with diabetic nephropathy, but no studies to date have demonstrated a reduction in the rate of fall of the glomerular filtration rate with their use. The dihydropyridine (e.g., nifedipine) class of calcium channel blockers has not been shown to have any beneficial effects on proteinuria in diabetic patients. Thus, although useful for blood pressure control, the calcium channel blockers are not proven to have any additional benefit for the treatment of diabetic nephropathy.

C. Glucose Control

As discussed earlier, hyperglycemia causes glomerular injury in part by increasing glomerular capillary hydrostatic pressure. In addition, it injures the glomerular basement membrane directly by glycosylating key structural proteins. Finally, hyperglycemia stimulates secretion of growth factors that promote mesangial cell proliferation and collagen production. Studies in both experimental animals and in humans with diabetes mellitus have shown that intensive efforts to control blood glucose concentration slow the progression and delay the development of diabetic nephropathy. The Diabetes Control and Complication Trial (DCCT) showed that intensive diabetic treatment delays the onset and slows the progression of microalbuminuria. In this trial, the intensive treatment goal was to maintain preprandial blood glucose between 70 and 125 mg/dL and 90-minute postprandial glucose between 106 and 180 mg/dL. Intensive treatment decreased the risk of microalbuminuria in patients without retinopathy by 34% and in patients with mild retinopathy by 43%. Clinically significant albuminuria (300 mg/24 hr) developed in twice as many patients in the conventionally treated group. In a second large randomized trial with 7½ years of follow-up, nephropathy developed in 18% of the standard treated group and 2% of the intensified treatment group. A large trial done in the United Kingdom has shown beneficial effects of intensive treatment in patients with type 2 diabetes mellitus.

The question remains whether intensive therapy, as carried out in the DCCT trial, can be applied to large numbers of diabetic patients. In that trial, the risk of severe hypoglycemia increased two- to threefold in the intensive treatment group, and averaged 0.54 events per patient per year. Thus, physicians must be aware of the potential for profound hypoglycemia when attempting to aggressively control blood glucose. Data from a number of studies, however, suggest that benefits are seen when the hemoglobin A_1C is lowered by as little as 1%. Thus, improvement in serum glucose control is recommended in all diabetics to slow or delay the renal injury caused by hyperglycemia

D. Protein Restriction

Restricting dietary protein reduces the rate of glomerulosclerosis in rats by preventing glomerular capillary hypertension. High dietary protein intake accelerates the loss of renal function. Protein restriction in humans is an attractive nonpharmacological approach to treatment of diabetic nephropathy and other forms of chronic renal insufficiency. In the modification of diet in renal disease study (see Chapter 17), dietary protein restriction slowed the progression of renal disease in patients with chronic renal insufficiency, but only to a small degree. Only 3% of the subjects were diabetic in this large clinical trial. Several other small studies in patients with diabetic nephropathy have suggested a beneficial effect of a low-protein diet. In a meta-analysis of five such trials in patients with type 1 diabetes, a low-protein diet reduced the relative risk for progression to 0.56. Current guidelines from the American Diabetes Association recommend a protein intake of 0.8 g/kg body weight in patients with diabetic nephropathy. Nutritional deficiency may occur in some patients, and all patients should be monitored for evidence of malnutrition. Ideally, patients on a protein-restricted diet should be followed by an experienced dietitian.

E. Treatment of Hyperlipidemia

Lipid abnormalities are frequently found in diabetic patients with albuminuria. These include elevations of total cholesterol, low-density lipoprotein (LDL) cholesterol, and triglycerides and a reduction of high-density lipoprotein (HDL) cholesterol levels. In a study of 19 normotensive type 2 diabetic patients with hypercholesterolemia and microalbuminuria, simvastatin treatment decreased microalbuminuria from pretreatment levels by 25%. This small study suggests that control of plasma cholesterol may reduce urinary albumin excretion and slow the progression of diabetic nephropathy.

Dictary fat intakc should thc follow the nutritional guidelines of the American Diabetes Association. The hydroxyl-methyl-glutaryl-coenzyme A (HMG CoA) reductase inhibitors (statins) are effective in controlling the dyslipidemia in diabetic patients. Certainly, diabetic patients with LDL cholesterols >130 should be treated. If there are other significant risk factors for coronary heart disease such as smoking, hypertension, family history of premature coronary heart disease, and HDL cholesterol <35 mg/dL, therapy for dyslipidemia should be instituted at LDL cholesterol levels >100. Because diabetic glomerulosclerosis appears to be very similar to atherosclerosis in other vasculatures, control of these risk factors should benefit the progression of diabetic nephropathy.

F. Modification of Other Risk Factors

Modification of other risk factors is also important in the diabetic patient with nephropathy. Smoking cessation appears to be beneficial in slowing the progression of diabetic nephropathy. In a one-year study of patients with type 1 diabetes, hypertension, and diabetic nephropathy, progression of the nephropathy was less common in nonsmokers (11%) and in patients who had quit smoking (33%), than in smokers (50%). Benefits of a regular exercise program include better control of blood pressure, improved insulin sensitivity and glycemia, and better control of the dyslipidemia.

Other potential sources of renal injury should be avoided as much as possible. Autonomic neuropathy can contribute to obstructive uropathy and pyelonephritis. Diabetic patients should be screened for obstructive uropathy with a renal ultrasound as part of their initial evaluation, and ultrasonography should be repeated anytime there is an unexpected increase in serum creatinine concentration. Urinary tract infections should be diagnosed and treated appropriately. Nonsteroidal anti-inflammatory agents and aminoglycoside antibiotics should be avoided if possible (see Chapter 20). Intravascular volume depletion due to excessive diuresis should also be avoided. Because diabetic patients are at high risk to develop vascular complications, they are often candidates for radiocontrast administration for cardiac catheterization or other diagnostic procedures. Exposure to radiocontrast media should be minimized as much as possible in these patients to preserve residual renal function. If the diabetic patient is to receive a radiocontrast agent, intravascular volume should be optimized before the study is undertaken by discontinuing diuretics and administering saline solutions intravenously (see Chapter 20 for recommendations).

G. Planning for End-Stage Renal Disease

Despite instituting the therapies outlined above, patients with established diabetic nephropathy will eventually progress to end-stage renal disease and need dialysis and/or transplantation for continued survival. It is important to emphasize that patients with diabetic nephropathy often develop uremic symptoms and require renal replacement therapy earlier than patients with other forms of renal disease. As a result, they should be referred to a nephrologist early in their course, preferably when the serum creatinine first rises to >2.0 mg/dL or when the glomerular infiltration rate falls to <70 mL/min. Because vascular access can be a particularly vexing problem in diabetic patients, preservation of the vasculature should be attempted as much as possible. This includes minimizing intravascular catheters and needle sticks for blood drawing.

IV. SUMMARY

Diabetic nephropathy is the leading cause of end-stage renal disease, accounting for over 40% of all new cases. The major clinical manifestation of diabetic nephropathy is proteinuria. Treatments to delay the onset and to control the progression of diabetic nephropathy include glucose control, excellent control of the blood pressure, and blockade of the renin-angiotensin system. A reasonable parameter to follow in the patient with diabetic nephropathy is the degree of proteinuria with therapy aimed at reducing this as much as possible. When the serum creatinine rises to >2 mg/dL, these patients should be referred to a nephrologist for evaluation and for preparation for the eventual need for renal replacement therapy and/or transplantation,

SUGGESTED READINGS

American Diabetes Association. Report of the expert committee on the diagnosis and classification of diabetes mellitus. Diabetes Care 1997; 20:1183–1197.

American Diabetes Association. Management of dyslipidemia in adults with diabetes. Diabetes Care 1998; 21:179–182.

Anderson S, Brenner BM. Intraglomerular hypertension: implications and drug treatment. Ann Rev Med 1993; 39:243–253.

Bennett PH, Haffner S, Kaiske BL, Kean WF, Mogensen CE, Parving H-H, Steffes MW, Striker GE. Screening and management of microalbuminuria in patients with diabetes mellitus. Am J Kidney Dis 1995; 25:107–112.

Chaturvedi M, Sjolie A-K, Stephenson JM, Abrahamian H, Keipes M, Castellarin A, Peponik ZR, Fuller JH. Effect of lisinopril on progression of retinopathy in normotensive people with type I diabetes. Lancet 1998; 351:28–31.

Diabetes Control and Complications Trial Research Group. The effect of intensive treatment of diabetes on the development and progression of long-term complications in insulin-dependent diabetes mellitus. N Engl J Med 1993; 329:977–986.

Diabetes Control and Complications Trial (DCCT) Research Group. Effect of intensive therapy on the development and progression of diabetic nephropathy in the Diabetes Control and Complications Trial. Kidney Int 1995; 47:1703–1720.

Groggel GC. Diabetic nephropathy. Arch Fam Med 1996; 5:513–520.

Kasiske BL, Kabil RSN, Na JZ, Liao M, Keane WF. Effect of antihypertensive therapy on the kidney in patients with diabetes: a meta-regression analysis. Ann Int Med 1993; 118:129–138.

Klahr S, Levey AS, Beck BJ, Caggiula AW, Hunsicker L, Kusek JW, Striker G. The effects of dietary protein restriction and blood-pressure control on the progression of chronic renal disease. N Engl J Med 1994; 330:877–884.

Lewis EJ, Hunsicker LG, Bain RP, Rohde RD. The effect of angiotensin-converting-enzyme inhibition on diabetic nephropathy. N Engl J Med 1993; 329:1456–1462.

Magensen CE, Keane WF, Bennett PH, Jeruns G, Parving H-H, Passa P, Steffes MW, Strobes GE, Viberti GC: Prevention of diabetic renal disease with special reference to microalbuminuria. Lancet 1995; 346:1080–1084.

Microalbuminuria Captopril Study Group. Captopril reduces the risk of nephropathy in IDDM patients with microalbuminuria. Diabetologia 1996; 39:587–593.

Perneger TV, Brancati FL, Whelton PK, Hlag MI. End-stage renal diseases attributable to diabetes mellitus. Ann Intern Med 1994; 121:912–918.

Ravid M, Savin H, Jutrin I, Bental T, Katz B, Lishner M. Long-term stabilizing effect of angiotensin-converting enzyme inhibition on plasma creatinine and on proteinuria in normotensive type II diabetic patients. Ann Intern Med 1993; 118:577–581.

Ritz E, Stefanski A. Diabetic nephropathy in type II diabetes. Am J Kidney Dis 1996; 27:167–194.

Steffes MW, Osterby R, Chavers B, Mauer SN. Mesangial expansion as a central mechanism for loss of kidney function in diabetic patients. Diabetes 1989; 38:1077–1081.

Tonolo G, Ciccarese M, Brizzi P, Puddu L, Secchi G, Calvia P, Atzeni MM, Melis MG, Maioli M. Reduction of albumin excretion rate in normotensive microalbuminuric type 2 diabetic patients during long term simvastatin treatment. Diabetes Care 1997; 20:1891–1985.

UK Prospective Diabetes Study (UKPDS) Group. Intensive blood glucose control with sulphonylureas or insulin compared with conventional treatment and risk of complications in patients with type 2 diabetes (UKPDS 33). Lancet 1998; 352:837–852.

19

Primary and Secondary Glomerular Diseases

Laura M. Dember
Boston University School of Medicine, Boston, Massachusetts

I. INTRODUCTION

This chapter covers diseases of the glomerulus or its blood supply. A review of normal glomerular anatomy and function, clinical syndromes, and treatment-associated toxicities precedes the discussion of specific diseases.

A. Structure and Function of the Glomerulus

The glomerulus consists of a capillary network interposed between an afferent and an efferent arteriole. The capillary surface is formed by a thin, uniquely fenestrated endothelium. The mesangium, comprised of mesangial cells and their extracellular matrix, lies in a central region between the capillary loops. Bowman's capsule surrounds the capillary network, and the cavity between the parietal epithelial cells of Bowman's capsule and the visceral epithelial cells (podocytes) surrounding the capillary walls is called Bowman's space. Also known as the urinary space, Bowman's space is continuous with the proximal tubule.

The principal function of the glomerulus is to produce an ultrafiltrate from circulating blood. The glomerular "filter" consists of three layers: the endothelium, the glomerular basement membrane, and the visceral epithelial cells. Water and small solutes pass freely through this filter, while larger molecules are filtered to a lesser extent or not at all. In addition to size, filtration is also dependent on the ionic charge of a substance.

The rate of ultrafiltrate production, or the glomerular filtration rate (GFR), determines the kidney's capacity for solute and water clearance. As in other capillary beds, fluid transport across the glomerular capillaries is mediated by hydrostatic and oncotic forces, ultrafiltration surface area, and ultrafiltration surface permeability. Alterations in each of these determinants of GFR occur in glomerular disease. Elucidation of the structural and functional abnormalities that underlie the diseases described in this chapter has enabled more accurate diagnosis and more successful treatment approaches.

B. The Renal Vasculature

The main renal arteries branch successively into the segmental, interlobar, arcuate, and intralobular vessels. The absence of anastomoses between the branches effectively renders the vessels end arteries and increases the potential for parenchymal damage with compromise of any component of the arterial supply. Because of involvement of both the macro- and micro-vasculature in many renal diseases, categorization of disease as either ''glomerular'' or ''vascular'' is somewhat arbitrary. Several of the diseases included in this ''glomerular disease'' chapter could be considered to be primary vasculopathies.

C. The Renal Biopsy

A renal biopsy is often required to diagnose or guide management of glomerular disease. In most patients the renal biopsy can be performed percutaneously with minimal or no sedation. Ultrasound localization, real-time ultrasound guidance, and computed tomography are the most frequently utilized radiological imaging methods. Many nephrologists prefer automated spring-loaded biopsy needles to manual needles because less dexterity is needed to obtain renal tissue and the cutting blade is exposed to renal tissue for a shorter time. The risks of percutaneous renal biopsy include parenchymal or subcapsular hemorrhage, arteriovenous fistula formation, and puncture of adjacent organs. The risk of complications is increased in patients with uncontrolled hypertension, uremia, or fibrotic kidneys.

Light microscopy, immunofluorescence, and electron microscopy provide complementary information and, therefore, are all routinely performed on renal biopsy specimens. Light microscopy assesses glomerular size, cellularity, capillary patency, capillary wall thickness, and extent of sclerosis. Immunofluorescence with fluorescein-labeled antibodies is used to detect the presence and deposition pattern of immunoglobulin, complement, or fibrin. Electron microscopy enables examination of ultrastructural features of the podocytes, basement membrane, and immune complexes or fibrillary deposits. Due to the complexity and, in many cases, subtlety of renal biopsy findings, it is critical that biopsy specimens be processed in a properly equipped laboratory and interpreted by a pathologist experienced in nephropathology.

D. Definition of Clinical Syndromes

Patients with glomerular disease can present with a variety of clinical syndromes including asymptomatic proteinuria with or without hematuria, the nephritic syndrome, and the nephrotic syndrome. (These syndromes are discussed in detail in Chapters 6–8.) The terms ''nephrotic-range proteinuria'' and ''subnephrotic-range proteinuria'' refer to urinary protein excretion of ≥3 g/day and 0.2–3 g/day, respectively. Glomerulonephritis may manifest as full-blown acute nephritic syndrome (gross hematuria, red cell casts, hypertension, edema, and elevated serum creatinine) or it may be indolent. ''Rapidly progressive glomerulonephritis'' (RPGN) refers to glomerular disease characterized by extracapillary cell proliferation (i.e., crescent formation) and rapid deterioration of renal function over days to months. This relatively uncommon, but fulminant, complication of several of the diseases discussed in this chapter (see Table 1) must be recognized and treated promptly in order to prevent irreversible renal injury. Systemic vasculitis, a generalized inflammation of blood vessels, often involves the kidney and is discussed later in this chapter.

E. Treatment of Glomerular Disease: General Principles and Drug Toxicities

Treatment of glomerular disease is one of the most challenging and controversial areas of nephrology. The variability of disease course and treatment response,

Table 1 Diseases Associated with Rapidly Progressive Glomerulonephritis

Anti-GBM disease/Goodpasture's syndrome
Microscopic polyangiitis
Wegener's granulomatosis
Idiopathic crescentic glomerulonephritis
Systemic lupus erythematosis
Henoch-Schönlein purpura
Postinfectious glomerulonephritis
IgA nephropathy
Membranous nephropathy
Membranoproliferative glomerulonephritis
Cryoglobulinemia

the limitations of existing clinical studies, and the toxicities associated with immunosuppressive drugs all contribute to the complexity of managing these diseases. Although the initial evaluation of glomerular disease is often conducted by primary care physicians, prompt referral to a nephrologist is strongly recommended for both diagnosis and treatment.

Symptomatic treatment for patients with nephrotic syndrome and nephritic syndrome are discussed in Chapters 7 and 8, respectively. Tight blood pressure control is recommended in all patients with glomerular disease. Because of their antiproteinuric effect, angiotensin-converting enzyme (ACE) inhibitors should be used whenever possible in patients with proteinuria (Table 2). The newer angiotensin II receptor antagonists are alternatives for patients who develop ACE inhibitor–induced cough; however, it is not yet known whether these agents have the renal protective effects of the ACE inhibitors. Close monitoring for hyperkalemia and GFR reduction is recommended after initiation of either ACE inhibitors or angiotensin II receptor antagonists, particularly in patients with underlying renal insufficiency.

Several of the immunosuppressive agents used to treat glomerular disease are reviewed in Table 2 and discussed below. This material is intended to familiarize the reader with these agents but should not be viewed as a comprehensive review of drug toxicities or administration practices. The immunosuppression and bone marrow suppression associated with these drugs requires that patients be closely monitored for infection and cytopenias.

1. Glucocorticoids

Because of their potent anti-inflammatory effects, glucocorticoids are frequently used in the treatment of glomerular disease either as monotherapy or in conjunction with cytotoxic agents. Glucocorticoid toxicities include hyperglycemia, hyperlipidemia, cataract formation, central obesity, osteoporosis, avascular necrosis, myopathy, and psychosis. Since most of the toxicities of glucocorticoids are dependent upon dosage and duration of use, effort should be made to use the lowest effective dose for the shortest duration possible. It is important, however, to avoid premature discontinuation of these agents since relapse may require repeated courses and a greater cumulative dose. It has become increasingly common practice to prescribe bisphosphonates, hormonal therapy, or calcium and vitamin D for prophylaxis against osteoporosis in patients receiving extended courses of glucocorticoids. In many centers *Pneumocystis carinii* pneumonia prophylaxis with trimethoprim-sulfamethoxazole is now advised for patients receiving combination therapy with a cytotoxic agent and glucocorticoids.

2. Cyclophosphamide

Cyclophosphamide is reserved for patients with disease that is refractory to glucocorticoids, rapidly progressive, or life-threatening. Cytopenias occur

Table 2 Medications Used to Treat Glomerular Disease

Drug	Proposed mechanism of action	Toxicities	Comments
ACE inhibitors	Reduces intraglomerular capillary pressure and possibly fibrosis	Hyperkalemia, hemodynamic reduction in glomerular filtration rate, acute renal failure	Monitor serum potassium and creatinine
Glucocorticoids	Inhibits transcription of pro-inflammatory cytokines	Immunosuppression, glucose intolerance, central obesity, cataracts, osteoporosis, avascular necrosis, hyperlipidemia, psychosis	Consider calcium and vitamin D supplementation, bone densitometry, bisphosphonates, and hormone replacement
Cyclophosphamide	Alkylating agent	Immunosuppression, bone marrow suppression, hemorrhagic cystitis, late hematologic malignancy, bladder carcinoma, alopecia, sterility	Hydrate prior to dose; closely monitor blood count; administer *Pneumocystis carinii* pneumonia prophylaxis; consider ova or sperm storage; reduce dose in renal insufficiency
Cyclosporine	Prevents T-cell activation by inhibiting interleukin-2 transcription	Immunosuppression, hyperkalemia, hypertension, nephrotoxicity, hirsutism, neurotoxicity, gingival hyperplasia	Monitor renal function, blood pressure, and blood drug level
Azathioprine	Competitively inhibits *de novo* pathway of purine synthesis	Bone marrow suppression, hepatotoxicity, late malignancies, macrocytosis	Monitor blood count and liver function tests
Mycophenolate Mofetil	Noncompetitively inhibits *de novo* synthesis of guanine nucleotides	Bone marrow suppression, nausea, diarrhea	Monitor blood count
Methotrexate	Inhibits dihydrofolate reductase and methylation of deoxynucleotides	Bone marrow suppression, nausea, oral ulcers, hepatotoxicity, macrocytosis	Supplement folate, monitor blood count and liver function tests, avoid ethanol, reduce dose in renal insufficiency

commonly with use of this agent and should be anticipated. Cyclophosphamide-induced hemorrhagic cystitis may be prevented with vigorous hydration and possibly co-administration of the detoxifying agent mesna. The risk of irreversible gonadal failure increases with patient age (particularly for women) and cumulative dose. Bladder carcinoma and hematological malignancy are not uncommon among patients treated with extended courses of cyclophosphamide.

3. Cyclosporine

Cyclosporine is being used with increasing frequency as treatment for primary glomerulopathies and systemic autoimmune diseases. The potential for chronic cyclosporine nephrotoxicity warrants close monitoring of renal function and probably blood drug levels in patients with underlying renal disease. Hypertension, acute renal failure, hyperkalemia, gingival hyperplasia, and hirsutism are all common adverse effects of this drug.

4. Azathioprine

Azathioprine is used as a glucocorticoid-sparing agent in patients with systemic autoimmune diseases. It has not been found to be particularly effective for primary glomerulopathies. Patients treated with this drug should be monitored for cytopenias and hepatotoxicity.

5. Mycophenolate Mofetil

Mycophenolate mofetil is a relatively new immunosuppressive agent that is now used routinely in organ transplant recipients but is only beginning to be studied in glomerular disease. Nausea and diarrhea are common side effects, but they often resolve with dose reduction or with continued use. Cytopenias may also occur with use of this medication.

6. Methotrexate

Methotrexate is being used with increasing frequency in the treatment of systemic vasculitis. The major toxicities of methotrexate include hepatotoxicity that may lead to cirrhosis, bone marrow suppression, oral ulcers, and idiosyncratic pulmonary infiltrates. Folic acid supplementation may reduce the incidence of some of these adverse effects.

II. PRIMARY GLOMERULAR DISEASES

A summary of the features of primary glomerular diseases is shown in Table 3.

Table 3 Clinical and Laboratory Features of Primary Glomerular Diseases

Characteristic	Minimal change disease	FSGS	Membranous nephropathy	Membrano-proliferative GN	IgA nephropathy
Creatinine	Usually normal	Elevated	Normal or elevated	Normal or elevated	Normal or elevated
Urinalysis	Protein, ± rbcs	Protein, ± rbcs	Protein, rbcs	Protein, rbcs, ± rbc casts	Protein, rbcs, rbc casts
Urine protein[a]	Nephrotic	Nephrotic	Nephrotic	Nephrotic or sub-nephrotic	Nephrotic or sub-nephrotic
Complements	Normal	Normal	Normal	Low	Normal
Serologies	Negative	Negative	Negative	± C3 nephritic factor	± IgA immune complexes
Associated findings	Edema	Edema, hypertension	Edema, hypertension	Edema, hypertension	Edema, hypertension

Abbreviations: FSGS, focal and segmental glomerulosclerosis; GN, glomerulonephritis; rbcs, red blood cells.

[a] Nephrotic refers to urinary protein excretion of ≥ 3 g/day. Subnephrotic refers to urinary protein excretion of 0.2–3 g/day.

A. Minimal Change Disease

Minimal change disease (MCD) is an idiopathic glomerular disease characterized by the rapid onset of severe, symptomatic nephrotic syndrome. The name minimal change disease has largely superseded the older terms lipoid nephrosis and nil disease because it more accurately describes the histological findings. Although marked responsiveness to glucocorticoids distinguishes MCD from other glomerular diseases, the high relapse rate and toxicity associated with repeated courses of glucocorticoids can pose challenges in its management.

1. Epidemiology and Pathogenesis

MCD is the most common cause of idiopathic nephrotic syndrome in children, accounting for approximately 80% of cases. Although often thought of as a childhood disease, MCD occurs in adults as well, particularly, but not exclusively, in the elderly. The etiology of MCD is not known. An immunological basis of the disease is suggested by the clinical response to immunosuppressive agents, by in vitro functional abnormalities in T lymphocytes, and by its association with Hodgkin's disease.

2. Pathology

By light microscopy the glomeruli appear normal, hence the name MCD. In a minority of cases, a slight increase in mesangial cellularity is present, the visceral epithelial cells may be swollen, and glomerular capillaries may be somewhat dilated. Immunofluorescence studies are usually negative, but in some cases mesangial IgM, IgG, or C3 deposits are found, which likely result from nonspecific trapping of circulating immunoglobulins. Electron microscopy reveals the major morphological features of MCD: effacement of the glomerular visceral epithelial cells and obliteration of the slit pore complex. These abnormalities are not unique to MCD and occur in other conditions associated with heavy proteinuria.

3. Clinical and Laboratory Features

The clinical presentation of MCD is nephrotic syndrome (see Chapter 7). Moderate hypertension may accompany the nephrotic syndrome and is more common in adults than in children. Serum creatinine may be slightly elevated at presentation, but this elevation tends to resolve with remission of the nephrotic syndrome. Urinalysis shows oval fat bodies and, in some patients, red cells. Macroscopic hematuria is rare, and red cell casts are not seen. Acute renal failure occasionally occurs in MCD, more often in adults than in children, and appears to be associated with ischemic injury to the tubules. The long-term renal outcome of MCD is excellent, with fewer than 5% of patients developing end-stage renal disease.

4. Treatment

The impetus for treating MCD arises from the deleterious consequences of the nephrotic state. Because persistent nephrotic syndrome is considered especially harmful in children, most pediatric nephrologists promptly treat initial episodes and relapses. The decision to begin treatment in adults is less straightforward because the consequences of nephrotic syndrome are less harmful and the therapy is less well tolerated. Glucocorticoid treatment produces remission of the initial episode of nephrotic syndrome in greater than 90% of children and in 80–90% of adults. The response occurs within 8 weeks in children but may be delayed until 12–16 weeks in adults. Sixty to 80 percent of patients have at least one relapse, and approximately one third have frequent relapses during glucocorticoid tapering or following drug discontinuation. Because of the toxicity associated with repeated courses of glucocorticoids, alternative treatments are often used in frequently relapsing patients. Cylophosphamide or chlorambucil can induce remission in steroid-resistant patients and may reduce the relapse rate. Cyclosporine may be an effective alternative to cytotoxic therapy. Although cyclosporine treatment courses of up to 1–2 years are often necessary to prevent relapse after discontinuation of the drug, the gonadal toxicity associated with cyclophosphamide or chlorambucil is avoided.

5. Secondary MCD

MCD may occur in association with Hodgkin's disease, leukemia, nonsteroidal anti-inflammatory drugs (NSAIDs), lithium, and ampicillin. Unlike idiopathic MCD, NSAID-associated glomerulopathy is usually accompanied by a prominent interstitial inflammatory infiltrate and acute renal insufficiency. Resolution of secondary forms of MCD occur with treatment of the underlying condition or discontinuation of the causative drug.

B. Primary Focal and Segmental Glomerulosclerosis

Focal and segmental glomerulosclerosis (FSGS) is a histological pattern of glomerular injury consisting of segmental sclerosis in some but not all glomeruli. The disease can be idiopathic or secondary (see Table 4).

1. Epidemiology and Pathogenesis

Primary FSGS accounts for 5–20% of cases of idiopathic nephrotic syndrome in children and adults. Because many children with nephrotic syndrome are not biopsied prior to treatment, the true incidence in children is not known. FSGS occurs more often in young adults than in the elderly and is more prevalent in African Americans than in whites. Its etiology is not well under-

Table 4 Causes of Secondary Focal and Segmental Glomerulosclerosis

Unilateral renal agenesis
Unilateral nephrectomy
HIV-associated nephropathy
Heroin nephropathy
Obesity
Sickle cell disease
Reflux nephropathy
Reduction in number of functioning nephrons

stood, but the initial glomerular epithelial cell injury may be mediated by cytokines or other circulating factors. Segmental scar formation ultimately leads to global sclerosis and a progressive reduction in the glomerular filtration rate (GFR).

2. Pathology

The name FSGS describes the light microscopic findings that define this disorder. ''Focal'' lesions involve some but not all glomeruli, and ''segmental'' lesions involve only a portion of the glomerular tuft. Sclerosis is an irreversible pathological process characterized by an increase in extracelluar matrix material that results in collapse of capillary lumens. Immunofluorescence microscopy is either negative or may show IgM and C3 deposition in regions of sclerosis, a finding thought to reflect nonspecific trapping of these molecules. Widespread or segmental epithelial foot process effacement is evident by electron microscopy. Because of the focal nature of the sclerotic changes, the renal biopsy in FSGS occasionally may be misinterpreted as minimal change disease.

3. Clinical and Laboratory Features

Patients with FSGS present with either asymptomatic proteinuria or nephrotic syndrome. Hypertension and microscopic hematuria are usually present, and approximately one third of patients have renal insufficiency when first seen. The degree of proteinuria is an important predictor of outcome. Fifty percent of nephrotic patients require dialysis or renal transplantation within 6–8 years, and the percentage is much greater if protein excretion is greater than 10 g/day. In contrast, renal survival is greater than 80% at 10 years in nonnephrotic patients. An elevated serum creatinine concentration, significant tubulointerstitial fibrosis on renal biopsy, and failure of the nephrotic syndrome to remit with treatment are all predictors of poor renal outcome.

4. Treatment

Although the response rate of FSGS to glucocorticoids was previously thought to be extremely low, it is now apparent that 45–60% of adults may have complete or partial remission if treatment is continued for as long as 9 months. Most patients who respond to steroid treatment have some reduction in proteinuria within 3–4 months. Cyclophosphamide can be used as a glucocorticoid-sparing agent in patients who are steroid-responsive but relapse frequently. Among those who are steroid-resistant, the response to cyclophosphamide is poor. Cyclosporine may decrease proteinuria in steroid-dependent and steroid-resistant patients, but both the relapse rate after discontinuation of the medication and the risk of cyclosporine nephrotoxicity seem to be greater in FSGS than in MCD.

5. Collapsing Glomerulopathy

Collapsing glomerulopathy is a variant of FSGS characterized histologically by extensive segmental and global glomerular capillary collapse with epithelial cell swelling and hyperplasia. The lesion can be seen in HIV-associated nephropathy (see later) or can be ''idiopathic.'' The collapsing variant of FSGS, more common in African Americans than in white individuals, is often associated with massive proteinuria and a more rapid progression to end-stage renal failure.

C. Membranous Nephropathy

Membranous nephropathy is an immune complex-mediated disease, which can be idiopathic or associated with underlying disease or medication (see Table 5). The variable course of this disease and the difficulty in identifying patients at risk for poor renal outcome have contributed to an ongoing controversy regarding its treatment.

Table 5 Causes of Secondary Membranous Nephropathy

Malignancies:	solid tumors, non-Hodgkin's lymphoma, leukemia
Drugs:	penicillamine, gold, captopril, probenecid
Infections:	hepatitis B, malaria, syphilis, schistosomiasis, filariasis
Autoimmune diseases:	systemic lupus erythematosis, Hashimoto's thyroiditis, bullous pemphigoid, rheumatoid arthritis, Sjögren's syndrome, dermatitis herpetiformis, myasthenia gravis
Miscellaneous:	renal allografts

1. Epidemiology and Pathogenesis

Membranous nephropathy is the cause of approximately 10–25% of cases of adult nephrotic syndrome and a somewhat greater proportion in adults over the age of 50. In children the disease occurs most often in the setting of chronic hepatitis B antigenemia. Subepithelial immune deposits are the pathological hallmark of this disease. The nature of these deposits and the mechanisms underlying their development remain elusive.

2. Pathology

Histologically, the disease is defined by the presence of diffuse subepithelial immune deposits containing IgG. These deposits result in a uniform thickening of the glomerular basement membrane that is sometimes evident by light microscopy. Immunofluorescence is positive for IgG and C3 in the capillary walls, and the deposits may be directly visualized by electron microscopy.

3. Clinical and Laboratory Features

The majority of patients with membranous nephropathy come to medical attention because of nephrotic syndrome, although some present with asymptomatic proteinuria. Hypertension is often a concomitant feature. Urinalysis reveals microscopic hematuria in up to 50% of patients. Red cell casts are unusual and serum complement levels are normal except in patients with membranous nephropathy associated with systemic lupus erythematosis. The natural history is variable and difficult to predict. Spontaneous remission of the nephrotic syndrome and stable renal function characterizes the course in many patients; however, progressive renal impairment leading to end-stage renal disease occurs in approximately one third of patients. The patients most likely to have progressive loss of renal function are those with persistent, heavy proteinuria (>8–10 g/day), hypertension, renal insufficiency, male gender, and age greater than 50 years. Glomerular sclerosis and interstitial fibrosis are renal biopsy features associated with poor outcome.

4. Treatment

Virtually all patients with membranous nephropathy should receive aggressive treatment of hypertension, ACE inhibition, lipid-lowering therapy, and diuretics if necessary (see Chapter 7). Because of the high rate of spontaneous remission, some feel that specific treatment of membranous nephropathy should be reserved for those with the highest risk of progressive disease. The efficacy of glucocorticoid treatment is debated but is considered by many to be a reasonable option in patients at low risk of progression who continue to have nephrotic-range proteinuria on ACE inhibitors. For patients with unfavorable risk profiles, treatment with a cytotoxic agent, cyclophosphamide or chlorambucil, together with glucocorticoids should be considered. The most widely publicized protocol consists of alternate monthly courses of prednisolone and chlorambucil for up to 6 months. In patients with marked impairment in GFR, the risk of cytotoxic therapy may outweigh the potential benefit. The efficacies of alternative treatments such as cyclosporine and mycophenolate mofetil have not been established but are under investigation.

5. Secondary Membranous Nephropathy

Secondary causes should be considered in all patients with membranous nephropathy (Table 5). If a secondary cause is identified treatment should be directed at the underlying disease. Malignancy, present in 5–10% of cases, is usually evident at the time of diagnosis of membranous nephropathy but may be occult. Similarly, membranous nephropathy may be the first manifestation of systemic lupus erythematosis.

D. Membranoproliferative Glomerulonephritis

Membranoproliferative glomerulonephritis (MPGN) is a morphological entity associated with a chronic and usually progressive glomerulonephritis. Idiopathic MPGN is subdivided into three types on the basis of morphological features. The secondary forms, more common than the idiopathic variety, are listed in Table 6. Several of these are addressed in detail elsewhere in this chapter.

1. Epidemiology and Pathogenesis

Idiopathic MPGN occurs most often in older children or young adults. Approximately 80% of patients have the Type I variant, 10–20% have Type II, and less than 5% have Type III. MPGN accounts for approximately 7% and 12% of cases

Table 6 Causes of Secondary Membranoproliferative Glomerulonephritis

Systemic lupus erythematosis
Cryoglobulinemia
Hepatitis B
Hepatitis C
Leukemia
Lymphoma
Paraproteinemias

of idiopathic nephrotic syndrome in children and adults, respectively. Both the idiopathic and secondary forms appear to be mediated by immune complex formation and complement activation, although the pathogenesis remains unclear.

2. Pathology

Mesangial proliferation, basement membrane thickening, and a "double contour" appearance of the capillary walls due to immune deposits and mesangial cell interposition are the characteristic morphological features of MPGN. Subendothelial and mesangial electron-dense deposits containing immunoglobulin and the C3 complement component are present in Type I MPGN, while intramembranous deposits are found in Type II MPGN, also termed "dense deposit disease." Type III MPGN disease is a less universally accepted variant with subepithelial, subendothelial, and mesangial deposits.

3. Clinical and Laboratory Features

Type I MPGN is a slowly progressive disease, which usually presents as nephrotic syndrome. Although remission from nephrotic syndrome is rare, the majority of patients have long-term renal survival. Type II MPGN typically presents as acute nephritis or recurrent macroscopic hematuria. The disease is more aggressive than Type I MPGN and is associated with a median renal survival of 5–10 years. Nephrotic syndrome is the predominant clinical feature of Type III disease. Hypertension may occur in all three variants.

Complement activation and hypocomplementemia are associated with all types of idiopathic MPGN. Reduced levels of C3, CH50, and, in some patients, C4 are found in Type I MPGN due to activation of both the classic and alternative complement pathways. In type II disease, C3 is low but C4 is normal, and C3 nephritic factor, an autoantibody directed against the C3 convertase of the alternative pathway, is detectable in the majority of patients. In Type III disease, C3 levels are reduced in approximately half the patients, C4 levels are normal, and C3 nephritic factor is not detectable.

4. Treatment

The optimal treatment of MPGN has not been defined. In children with Type I disease, alternate-day prednisone in gradually decreasing doses over several years has been associated with a very low relapse rate. Some adults with Type I disease will respond to glucocorticoids as well. The response rate in adults with MPGN Types II or III is much lower. Antiplatelet agents have been used in this disease but have not been found to be effective.

E. IgA Nephropathy

IgA nephropathy, also known as Berger's disease, is the most common form of glomerulonephritis worldwide. The course of the disease is variable, but a significant proportion of patients eventually progress to end-stage renal disease. Unfortunately, efforts to identify an effective treatment for this disease have met limited success.

1. Epidemiology and Pathogenesis

IgA nephropathy is mainly a disease of young adults but can occur over a wide range of ages. There is a male predominance, with a male: female ratio of 2:1. Geographic variations in IgA nephropathy, with higher rates in Japan, Australia, and southern Europe and lower rates in the United Kingdom and North America, may be due to differences in biopsy practice patterns and may not reflect a true difference in disease incidence.

The pathogenesis of IgA nephropathy is not understood. It is generally believed that an abnormal immune response to exogenous or endogenous antigens leads to increased production of IgA and ultimate deposition of IgA-containing immune complexes. Whether the IgA per se is responsible for the glomerular damage is not clear. A role for complement activation has been suggested, and it is likely that other inflammatory mediators also contribute to the ongoing injury.

2. Pathology

The characteristic histological feature of IgA nephropathy is mesangial IgA deposition. IgG, IgM, C3, and kappa or lambda light chains may co-localize with the IgA. Focal or diffuse mesangial hypercellularity and extracellular matrix deposition may be evident by light microscopy. In addition to the glomerular changes, tubulointerstitial fibrosis, tubular atrophy, and sclerosis of the vessels may be present. Extracapillary epithelial cell crescents may be seen, especially in the small subset of patients who develop rapidly progressive glomerulonephritis. Histological features associated with a poor prognosis include glomerular sclerosis, interstitial fibrosis, and extensive epithelial crescents.

3. Clinical and Laboratory Features

The typical patient with IgA nephropathy presents with asymptomatic microscopic hematuria with or without proteinuria. A less common presentation is episodic macroscopic hematuria occurring in association with a febrile illness, usually an upper respiratory infection. Unlike poststreptococcal glomerulonephritis (see later), hematuria in IgA nephropathy occurs within a few days of the onset of the infection. Some of these patients have loin pain, fatigue, or myalgias, but most are asymptomatic. Episodes may recur over many years.

The clinical course of IgA nephropathy is variable. For many years this was felt to be a benign disease characterized by chronic hematuria and low-grade proteinuria but stable renal function. Some patients do follow such a course, but it is now recognized that a substantial percentage will progress to end-stage renal disease. Progression typically is slow occurring over several decades; however, a rapidly progressive course can occur. Predictors of a poor long-term renal prognosis include an elevated creatinine, severe proteinuria, hypertension, older age at onset, and male gender. Those patients with recurrent episodes of gross hematuria may have a better outcome than those with persistent microscopic hematuria.

4. Treatment

A variety of agents have been used to treat IgA nephropathy, but the heterogeneity of the disease, the indolent course, and, in many cases, the lack of controls have complicated the interpretation of clinical studies and no consensus has been reached. Patients with isolated hematuria have a good prognosis and generally do not require treatment but should be monitored on a regular basis for the development of proteinuria, hypertension, or renal impairment. Proteinuric patients should be treated with an ACE inhibitor in an effort to reduce proteinuria and decrease intraglomerular capillary pressures. Aggressive control of hypertension is recommended. Dietary fish oil has been shown in some studies to retard the progression of renal impairment in IgA nephropathy and can be used along with ACE inhibitors in patients with proteinuria and normal or mildly impaired renal function. Treatment with fish oil does not appear to be beneficial once significant renal impairment is present. Glucocorticoids do not appear to be effective in this disease, except possibly in patients who develop a crescentic glomerulonephritis. Azathiaprine, cyclosporine, intravenous immunoglobulin, platelet inhibitors, anticoagulants, and mycophenolate mofetil have all been used in IgA nephropathy with varying results. In general, it appears that immunosuppressive medications may reduce proteinuria, but there has not been a convincing demonstration that they preserve renal function.

5. Secondary IgA nephropathy

IgA nephropathy can occur in association with chronic liver disease, HIV infection, dermatitis herpetiformis, psoriasis, ankylosing spondylitis, inflammatory bowel disease, and various malignancies. In most cases therapy should be directed toward the underlying disease. (See later for a discussion of Henoch-Schönlein purpura.)

III. GLOMERULAR DISEASE ASSOCIATED WITH SYSTEMIC ILLNESS

A. Infection-Associated Glomerular Disease

A summary of the features of glomerular disease associated with systemic infection is shown in Table 7.

1. Poststreptococcal Glomerulonephritis

Poststreptococcal glomerulonephritis (PSGN) is an immune complex–mediated disease that occurs in association with pharyngeal or pyodermic group A streptococcal infection. It is the most common form of acute glomerulonephritis in children.

a. Epidemiology and Pathogenesis. PSGN usually occurs in children between ages of 4 and 10 years but may be seen at any age. The disease is more common in males, with a 2:1 male-to-female ratio. PSGN may occur following either sporadic or epidemic infection with specific serological types of streptococcus known as nephritogenic strains. The rate of glomerulonephritis with such strains has been difficult to determine because cases manifested only by microscopic hematuria often go unrecognized. Early treatment of streptococcal infection does not seem to prevent the development of PSGN, although it may diminish the severity. The disease becomes apparent 10–14 days after a pharyngeal infection and 3–6 weeks after a skin infection.

The mechanisms underlying the immune complex formation in PSGN have not been determined. It is not clear, for example, whether the immune complexes form in the circulation and subsequently deposit in the kidney, or whether they initially develop in the kidney. Similarly it is not known whether the antigen is a bacterial product or an endogenous antigen recognized by antistreptococcal antibodies.

b. Pathology. Light microscopy shows a diffuse proliferative glomerulonephritis. Proliferation of mesangial and endothelial cells as well as glomerular infiltration by neutrophils and, to a lesser extent, monocytes and eosinophils, result in occlusion of the capillary loops. Irregularities in the capillary walls may be visible by light microscopy. These irregularities appear as subepithelial cell "domes" by electron microscopy and as granular deposits of IgG and C3 by immunofluorescence. Occasionally epithelial cell crescents occur, and interstitial infiltrates and edema may be present.

c. Clinical and Laboratory Features. The majority of patients with PSGN have subclinical disease with microscopic hematuria, hypocomplementemia, and a mild elevation in blood pressure. In patients with clinically evident

Table 7 Clinical and Laboratory Features of Glomerular Disease Associated with Systemic Infection

Characteristic	Poststreptococcal glomerulonephritis	Endocarditis	Hepatitis B infection	Hepatitis C infection	HIV infection
Creatinine	Elevated	Elevated	Often elevated	Often elevated	Elevated
Urinalysis	Protein, rbcs, rbc casts	Protein, rbcs, rbc casts	Protein, rbcs	Protein, rbcs, ± rbc casts	Protein, ± rbcs
Urine protein[a]	Nephrotic or subnephrotic	Nephrotic or subnephrotic	Nephrotic	Nephrotic	Nephrotic
Complements	Low	Low	Normal	Low	Normal
Serologies	ASO Ab, anti-DNase B Ab	Negative	Hepatitis B SAg	Hepatitis C Ab, cryoglobulins	HIV Ab
Associated findings	Edema, hypertension	Edema, hypertension	Edema, hypertension	Edema, hypertension	Often no edema and normal bp

Abbreviations: HIV, human immunodeficiency virus; rbcs, red blood cells; ASO, antistreptococcal O; Ab, antibody; anti-DNase B, antideoxyribonuclease B; SAg, surface antigen; bp, blood pressure.

[a] Nephrotic refers to urinary protein excretion of ≥ 3 g/day. Subnephrotic refers to urinary protein excretion of 0.2–3 g/day.

disease, the onset of symptoms is usually abrupt. Gross hematuria resulting in ''cola-colored'' or ''rusty'' urine, hypertension, oliguria, and edema due to marked sodium avidity are typical. Anuria is rare and is usually associated with epithelial crescent formation. Children may have ascites, and elderly patients may develop congestive heart failure. Encephalopathy may occur in association with PSGN and is not clearly due to hypertension.

Urinalysis shows red cells and red cell casts. Leukocytes, leukocyte casts, and renal tubular epithelial cells may be present as well. Proteinuria is present in most patients but is usually in the subnephrotic range. GFR is decreased in the majority of patients. A reduction in the C3 and CH50 complement levels is found early in the disease. Both usually return to normal levels within 6–8 weeks, and persistently low C3 levels should raise suspicion for a different disease such as MPGN, lupus nephritis, endocarditis, or occult abscess. Throat cultures or skin cultures frequently grow group A streptococci. Antibodies to extracellular streptococcal products such as streptolysin (ASO), streptokinase, hyaluronidase, and deoxyribonuclease B (anti-DNase B) provide evidence of recent infection. In most patients elevated ASO titers develop within several weeks of pharyngeal infection, and serial determinations should show rising levels during this time period. Antibiotic administration may diminish the ASO response.

The clinical presentation of PSGN may resemble that of IgA nephropathy. However, serological evidence of recent streptococcal infection, hypocomplementemia, and a duration between pharyngitis and onset of glomerulonephritis of greater than a few days all distinguish PSGN from IgA nephropathy. Renal biopsy is usually not necessary in PSGN but should be considered with atypical presentations.

d. Treatment. Although antibiotic treatment does not prevent development of PSGN, it may attenuate the course and prevent transmission of the nephritogenic organism to others. Penicillin, or erythromycin in penicillin-allergic individuals, is the preferred antibiotic. Treatment otherwise is supportive and should consist of sodium and water restriction, diuretics, and antihypertensive agents. Pulse intravenous methylprednisolone is often used in patients with crescentic glomerulonephritis and rapidly progressive disease; however, the efficacy of either glucocorticoids or cytotoxic agents has not been demonstrated in clinical studies.

The acute episode of PSGN is usually self-limited, with resolution of edema and hypertension within a few weeks. Hematuria and proteinuria may persist for several months. Most children with PSGN have a good long-term prognosis and do not develop chronic renal insufficiency. The long-term outcome is less predictable in adults. Patients with nephrotic-range proteinuria at presentation, extensive crescentic lesions by biopsy, and persistent heavy proteinuria are more likely to have chronic progressive renal impairment.

2. Endocarditis-Associated Glomerulonephritis

Renal disease is a common complication of bacterial endocarditis. The following discussion will be limited to endocarditis-associated glomerulonephritis (GN), an immune complex–mediated disease. However, other etiologies such as antibiotic-induced acute interstitial nephritis, embolization, or sepsis should be considered when evaluating a patient with renal dysfunction in this clinical setting.

a. Epidemiology and Pathogenesis. Although the incidence of endocarditis-associated GN has decreased markedly since the development of effective antibiotic therapy and prophylaxis, it may still complicate the course in as many as 20–50% of cases. Prolonged bacteremia predisposes to the development of GN but is not a requirement as cases have been reported within one week of a clinically evident *Staphylococcus aureus* infection. As in PSGN, the nature of the antigen (i.e., bacterial vs. endogenous) is not known.

b. Pathology. The renal biopsy in endocarditis-associated GN shows focal or diffuse hypercellularity due to polymorphonuclear cell infiltration and endogenous cell proliferation. Crescent formation is common. Immunofluorescence reveals C3, IgG, or IgM in a granular pattern, and corresponding subendothelial, subepithelial, intramembranous, or mesangial deposits are evident by electron microscopy.

c. Clinical and Laboratory Features. Most patients with endocarditis-associated GN are identified because of a rising serum creatinine. A nephritic urine sediment with red cells and red cell casts is typical. Nephrotic-range proteinuria is unusual. Low C3 levels are characteristic, and persistent hypocomplementemia may be indicative of antibiotic failure.

d. Treatment. Eradication of bacterial infection with antibiotic therapy and valve surgery, when necessary, usually results in improvement in renal function. Urinary sediment abnormalities may persist for several months. Immunosuppressive therapy may be appropriate if renal failure persists or progresses despite a microbiological cure.

3. Hepatitis B–Associated Glomerular Disease

Several types of glomerular disease have been associated with hepatitis B infection. The most common of these are membranous nephropathy, polyarteritis nodosa (PAN, see later), and membranoproliferative glomerulonephritis (MPGN). Because the liver disease in affected patients often is not clinically apparent, hepatitis B serologies should be obtained whenever clinical features or renal histology is consistent with these glomerular lesions.

a. Epidemiology and Pathogenesis. Although the proportion of hepatitis B–infected individuals who develop associated glomerular disease appears to be small, hepatitis B infection accounts for a substantial percentage of cases of PAN, MPGN, and, in endemic regions, childhood membranous nephropathy. Immunological mechanisms likely underlie the development of hepatitis B–associated renal diseases. Hepatitis B antigenemia is almost universally present, and surface, core, and envelope antigens together with IgG, IgM, and complement components have been demonstrated in the kidneys of affected patients.

b. Pathology. The histological features of the hepatitis B–associated glomerulopathies are similar to the corresponding idiopathic diseases and are described elsewhere in this chapter.

c. Clinical and Laboratory Features. The clinical features of hepatitis B–associated membranous nephropathy are similar to those of the idiopathic variety. Rarely, a rapidly progressive glomerulonephritis with crescentic changes by biopsy can occur. In children, spontaneous remission often occurs within 1–2 years and is associated with disappearance of the envelope antigen and development of envelope antibodies. Spontaneous remission is less common in adults, most of whom have progressive disease.

The presentation of hepatitis B–associated PAN resembles that of the idiopathic form described later in this chapter. Hepatitis B infection also can be associated with MPGN, although this histological pattern is more common in patients with hepatitis C.

d. Treatment. Except in cases of rapidly progressive glomerulonephritis, immunosuppressive treatment is generally not used in hepatitis B–associated membranous nephropathy or MPGN. Glucocorticoid treatment may stimulate viral replication, thereby aggravating both the liver disease and the glomerulopathy. Treatment with antiviral agents such as interferon α (IFN-α) has not been highly successful. Even in patients who respond initially, the high rate of recurrence of nephrotic syndrome following discontinuation of treatment limits the utility of this agent.

Aggressive treatment with glucocorticoids and cyclophosphamide appears to improve the prognosis of PAN, a disease with high morbidity and mortality. Treatment with these agents is therefore warranted despite the potential effects on viral replication. Plasmapheresis has been used in conjunction with immunosuppression as well; however, its efficacy in this disease has not been clearly demonstrated in clinical studies. Similarly, limited information exists regarding the efficacy of IFN-α or other antiviral agents in hepatitis B–associated PAN.

4. Hepatitis C–Associated Glomerular Disease

Most patients with hepatitis C–associated renal disease have MPGN, although cases of membranous nephropathy and IgA nephropathy have also been reported.

Mixed cryoglobulinemia usually accompanies hepatitis C–associated MPGN, and most cases of mixed ''essential'' cryoglobulinemia (see later) are secondary to hepatitis C infection.

a. Epidemiology and Pathogenesis. Hepatitis C is the cause of 10–20% of cases of Type I MPGN (see earlier for classification of MPGN) and the majority of cases of mixed cryoglobulinemia. Cryoglobulins are immunoglobulins that precipitate reversibly at cold temperature and are classified on the basis of their components. Type I cryoglobulins consist of a single monoclonal immunoglobulin molecule usually produced by clonal B cells in the setting of a lymphoproliferative disorder. Types II and III cryoglobulins are mixed, meaning that they contain two immunoglobulins, a polyclonal IgG and a second anti-immunoglobulin, usually IgM. The IgM component is monoclonal in Type II and polyclonal in Type III. Glomerulonephritis is associated with Type II cryoglobulins. Hepatitis C antigens are present within Type II cryoglobulins. Type III cryoglobulins occur in a variety of diseases including systemic lupus erythematosis but generally do not cause renal disease.

b. Pathology. Renal biopsy shows a Type I MPGN pattern (see earlier for pathological classification). Cryoglobulin deposits may obliterate capillary lumens and are visible by electron microscopy as large subendothelial densities with a characteristic substructure.

c. Clinical and Laboratory Features. Hepatitis C–associated MPGN is characterized by microscopic hematuria, proteinuria, peripheral edema, hypertension, and hypocomplementemia. Mild or occasionally moderate renal insufficiency may be present. An acute nephritic syndrome may occur in some cases. Extrarenal manifestations of cryoglobulinemia include purpura, arthralgia or arthritis, Raynaud's phenomenon, peripheral neuropathy, and hepatitis.

Detection of cryoglobulins in the serum requires that the blood sample be kept at 37°C prior to serum separation. Allowing the sample to cool to room temperature may result in precipitation of cryoglobulins and loss from the serum during subsequent centrifugation. Repeated testing for cryoglobulins may be necessary to demonstrate their presence.

d. Treatment. Progression to renal failure occurs rarely in cryoglobulinemic glomerulonephritis, but the morbidity from the systemic vasculitic syndrome can be high. The optimal treatment of cryoglobulinemia is not known. Acute episodes are often treated with intravenous methylprednisolone followed by oral glucocorticoids and cyclophosphamide and, in some cases, plasmapheresis to rapidly remove circulating cryoglobulins. When renal disease is less severe, antiviral agents such as IFN-α may be used. Unfortunately, the relapse rate is high following discontinuation of this therapy, and its impact on ultimate outcome is not clear.

5. HIV-Associated Nephropathy

HIV-associated nephropathy (HIVAN) has a characteristic pathology and clinical course. It is important to be aware, however, that HIV infection can also be associated with several other renal syndromes, such as IgA nephropathy, thrombotic thrombocytopenic purpura, and acute renal failure due to nephrotoxic medications, volume depletion, or sepsis.

a. Epidemiology and Pathogenesis. HIVAN is 5–10 times more common in men than in women and has a marked predilection for African Americans. Among Caucasians, other HIV-associated immune renal diseases occur with much greater frequency than HIVAN. The pathogenesis of HIVAN has not been elucidated. Components of HIV have been found in renal tissue of HIV-infected individuals, but a direct pathogenic role of the virus has not been demonstrated.

b. Pathology. The histological lesion of HIVAN is focal glomerulosclerosis with cystic dilatation of the tubules and tubulointerstitial fibrosis. Glomerular capillary tuft collapse, indistinguishable from that seen in the collapsing variant of idiopathic FSGS (see earlier), is often present. Endothelial cell tubuloreticular structures are often visible by electron microscopy in patients infected with HIV whether or not HIVAN is present. These structures are not specific to HIV infection and are also associated with systemic lupus erythematosis.

c. Clinical and Laboratory Features. Patients with HIVAN usually have nephrotic-range proteinuria. Interestingly, the proteinuria and hypoalbuminemia often are not accompanied by peripheral edema. HIVAN typically progresses rapidly to end-stage renal failure within several months following the development of renal insufficiency. Definitive diagnosis of HIVAN requires a renal biopsy; however, the presence of certain clinical and laboratory features are strongly suggestive of this disease. Urinalysis may show giant casts, and renal ultrasound shows markedly echogenic kidneys of normal or increased size. As stated above, peripheral edema is often absent despite heavy proteinuria, and hypertension usually is not present.

d. Treatment. There is no specific treatment for HIVAN. ACE inhibitors may be beneficial based on experience in other proteinuric diseases. Glucocorticoids have been associated with reductions in proteinuria and serum creatinine in small series, but their role needs to be better defined. Anecdotal evidence supports a beneficial effect of antiretroviral therapy. The life expectancy of patients with end-stage renal disease secondary to HIVAN has increased significantly with advances in antiretroviral therapy and treatment of opportunistic infections.

B. Lupus Nephritis

Systemic lupus erythematosis (SLE) is an autoimmune disease with a wide range of manifestations resulting from tissue deposition of pathogenic immune complexes. Renal involvement adversely influences the prognosis of this disease and is one of its most serious complications (Table 8).

1. Epidemiology and Pathogenesis

Although SLE is most common in young females, it can occur in males and in the elderly. The prevalence is highest in persons of African or Hispanic descent. Associations with certain HLA haplotypes suggest a genetic predisposition to the disease. Although referral bias may result in overestimation of incidence, data from tertiary care centers suggest that lupus nephritis occurs in 45–75% of SLE patients.

Glomerular deposition or in situ formation of immune complexes and subsequent recruitment of inflammatory mediators underlies the development of lupus nephritis. The autoantibody components of the immune complexes are directed against a variety of subcellular antigens including DNA, ribonucleoprotein, and other nuclear and cytoplasmic proteins.

2. Pathology

The location of the deposits and the extent of the inflammatory response provide the basis of the widely utilized World Health Organization (WHO) histological classification scheme outlined in Table 9. Because of the correlation between histological features and renal prognosis, renal biopsy plays a role in guiding treatment of lupus nephritis.

3. Clinical and Laboratory Features

Lupus nephritis rarely develops prior to other manifestations of SLE. The exception to this is Class V disease (membranous nephropathy), which may be the first manifestation of lupus. Patients with Class II disease usually have no urine sediment abnormalities and urinary protein excretion of <1 g/day. Class III disease is often but not always associated with microscopic hematuria and red cell casts. Proteinuria is usually present but typically is <3 g/day. Class IV disease is virtually always associated with hematuria, red cell casts, and heavy proteinuria, often in the nephrotic range. Hypertension and decreased GFR are often present, and rapidly progressive glomerulonephritis may develop. Class V or membranous

Table 8 Clinical and Laboratory Features of SLE, Goodpasture's Syndrome, and Glomerular Deposition Diseases

Characteristic	Systemic lupus erythematosis	Anti-GBM/ Goodpasture's syndrome	Amyloidosis	Multiple myeloma	Fibrillary/ Immunotactoid GN
Creatinine	Often elevated	Elevated	Normal or elevated	Elevated	Often elevated
Urinalysis	Protein, rbcs, rbc casts	Protein, rbcs, rbc casts	Protein, ± rbcs	± protein	Protein, rbcs, rbc casts
Urine protein[a]	Nephrotic or subnephrotic	Subnephrotic	Nephrotic	Nephrotic	Nephrotic
Complements	Low	Normal	Normal	Normal	Normal
Serologies	ANA, anti-ds DNA	Anti-GBM	M protein (in AL only)	M protein	Normal
Associated findings	Edema, ± hypertension	Normal bp	Edema	± edema	Edema, hypertension

Abbreviations: GBM, glomerular basement membrane; GN, glomerulonephritis; rbcs, red blood cells; ANA, antinuclear antibody; ds DNA, double-stranded deoxyribonucleic acid; AL, light chain amyloid; M protein, monoclonal protein; bp, blood pressure.

[a] Nephrotic refers to urinary protein excretion of ≥3 g/day. Subnephrotic refers to urinary protein excretion of 0.2–3 g/day.

Table 9 Histological Classification of Lupus Nephritis

Class I	Normal glomeruli
Class II	Isolated mesangial abnormalities
IIa	mesangial deposits
IIb	mesangial hypercellularity and deposits
Class III	Focal segmental glomerulonephritis (<50% of glomeruli)
Class IV	Diffuse glomerulonephritis (>50% of glomeruli)
Class V	Membranous glomerulonephritis

lupus is associated with nephrotic syndrome. The urine sediment is usually unremarkable, although red cells and red cell casts may be seen. The serum creatinine is usually normal.

Most patients who develop lupus nephritis do so early in the course of their disease, but it may occur at any time. Renal disease occurs more often in patients with autoantibodies directed against double-stranded DNA (anti-ds DNA), and changes in the anti-ds DNA titer may provide an indication of renal disease activity. Similarly, in many patients the concentrations of C3 and C4 complement components decrease during periods of renal disease activity. However, following these markers should not substitute for regular monitoring of the urine sediment and serum creatinine in all patients with SLE.

4. Treatment

The prognosis of lupus nephritis depends to a large extent on the histological class. Treatment is somewhat controversial. The recommendations that follow are based largely on cohort studies rather than randomized, controlled trials. Class II disease does not require specific treatment. Class III disease can be treated with glucocorticoids alone if the renal biopsy specimen shows ''less aggressive disease'' (i.e., involvement of only a small proportion of glomeruli and absence of extensive immune deposits, necrotizing features, or extracapillary proliferation). Histologically ''aggressive'' Class III disease and Class IV disease warrant treatment with a combination of glucocorticoids and a cytotoxic agent. Cyclophosphamide is the most widely used cytotoxic agent for lupus nephritis and has the best track record for inducing remission of renal disease and preventing progressive loss of renal function. Other immunosuppressive agents used in this setting or under investigation include azathioprine, mycophenolate mofetil, cyclosporine, and newer ''biological'' agents which alter the activity of cytokines. Glucocorticoids alone or in combination with cyclophosphamide are recommended for Class

V disease if nephrotic-range proteinuria is present. Because renal outcome of Class V disease is relatively good, extended treatment should not be undertaken if a clinical response is not apparent.

The potential for transformation from one histological class to another necessitates close clinical and laboratory monitoring and, in some cases, repeated renal biopsies. The transformation from nonproliferative to proliferative disease is usually accompanied by increased activity of the urinary sediment, increasing levels of urinary protein, and increased serological activity.

5. Antiphospholipid Syndrome

In addition to lupus nephritis, patients with SLE may develop renal manifestations of the antiphospholipid syndrome. This disorder, which can also be idiopathic, is discussed in Section V.

C. Anti–Glomerular Basement Membrane Disease and Goodpasture's Syndrome

Anti–glomerular basement membrane (anti-GBM) disease is a disorder in which circulating autoantibodies directed against a specific component of the glomerular basement membrane produce a rapidly progressive glomerulonephritis (Table 8). When these antibodies are also associated with pulmonary hemorrhage the disease is called Goodpasture's syndrome. Rapid diagnosis and initiation of treatment are critical in these disorders as progression to end-stage renal failure occurs quickly and pulmonary hemorrhage can be life-threatening. The combination of glomerulonephritis and pulmonary hemorrhage is not unique to Goodpasture's syndrome. Examples of other diseases that may produce pulmonary-renal syndromes include Wegener's granulomatosis, PAN, mixed cryoglobulinemia, and systemic lupus erythematosis.

1. Epidemiology and Pathogenesis

The epidemiologies of Goodpasture's syndrome and anti-GBM disease differ somewhat. Both have a male predominance and are more common in whites than in African Americans. Patients with Goodpasture's syndrome, however, tend to be young adults, while renal-limited anti-GBM disease is more common in elderly individuals.

The target antigen for the anti-GBM antibodies is the NC1 (noncollagenous 1) domain of the α-3 chain of type IV collagen. Autoantibody binding to this antigen occurs in the kidney because the fenestrated nature of the glomerular capillary endothelium exposes components of the basement membrane to the circulating blood. Because the alveolar endothelium is not fenestrated, it is likely that injury to the alveolar capillaries must occur in order for anti-GBM antibodies to produce pulmonary disease. The observation that the majority of individuals with Goodpasture's syndrome have a history of cigarette smoking or exposure to volatile solvents provides support for this hypothesis.

2. Pathology

The renal biopsy shows a necrotizing crescentic glomerulonephritis by light microscopy. The crescent formation may be focal in early disease but becomes diffuse as disease progresses. Immunofluorescence shows diffuse, linear deposition of IgG along the glomerular basement membrane. Antibody deposition along the tubular basement membrane is present in many patients as well. A linear immunofluorescence pattern is strongly suggestive of anti-GBM antibody–mediated disease but may occur in diabetic nephropathy and fibrillary glomerulonephritis. These disorders usually can be easily distinguished from anti-GBM disease because they are not associated with crescent formation.

3. Clinical and Laboratory Features

In patients with Goodpasture's syndrome, pulmonary disease is typically evident prior to clinically apparent renal disease. Pulmonary manifestations include asymptomatic radiographic infiltrates, exertional dyspnea, mild hemoptysis, and massive pulmonary hemorrhage. Anemia is common, and a viral prodrome is reported in approximately half of patients. The urinalysis in Goodpasture's syndrome or anti-GBM disease reveals a nephritic sediment with mild proteinuria, microscopic hematuria, and red cell casts. Although some patients have mild renal disease, rapidly progressive glomerulonephritis is common and often results in end-stage renal failure.

The presence of circulating anti-GBM antibodies can be demonstrated by either indirect immunofluorescence using patient serum and normal renal tissue or by direct enzyme-linked immunosorbent assay (ELISA) using purified or recombinant α-3 Type IV collagen NC1 domain. The ELISA is a more sensitive and specific test for anti-GBM antibodies and has replaced indirect immunofluorescence in most centers.

A substantial proportion of patients with anti-GBM antibodies also have anti-neutrophil cytoplasmic antibodies (ANCA) detectable in the serum. Some of these patients have evidence of systemic vasculitis, and interestingly, ANCA positivity is associated with a more favorable renal prognosis.

4. Treatment

Treatment of anti-GBM disease or Goodpasture's syndrome should be instituted rapidly to avoid irreversible renal or lung injury or death. A combination of cyclophosphamide, glucocorticoids, and plasmapheresis is the most effective treatment. Because most patients with creatinine levels greater than approximately 6.5 mg/dL do not recover renal function, many advocate conservative treatment in such patients in order to avoid the significant risk of infection associated with aggressive treatment. However, marked renal insufficiency should not preclude treatment of patients with pulmonary manifestations.

D. Glomerular Deposition Diseases

The glomerular deposition diseases, systemic amyloidosis, multiple myeloma, and fibrillary/immunotactoid glomerulopathy, constitute a diverse group of disorders characterized by the glomerular deposition of protein or protein fragments (Table 8). In several of these diseases the deposited proteins form macromolecular structures with a fibrillary appearance by electron microscopy.

1. Systemic Amyloidosis

Amyloidosis is a multisystem disease in which specific proteins form insoluble fibrils in the extracelluar matrix of a variety of tissues. By definition the fibrils have a characteristic β-pleated sheet configuration that renders them avid for Congo Red dye. The accumulation of the amyloid fibrils in tissue ultimately results in severe organ dysfunction. Because of the marked variability in the clinical presentation of amyloidosis, significant delays in diagnosis are common.

Amyloidosis is classified by the nature of the protein that forms the fibrillary deposit. In primary amyloidosis (AL) the amyloidogenic protein is an immunoglobulin light chain or light chain fragment produced by an abnormal clone of plasma cells in the bone marrow. The plasma cell burden is typically low, but approximately 10% of patients have associated multiple myeloma. Secondary amyloidosis (AA) occurs in the setting of a longstanding inflammatory condition. Serum amyloid A protein (SAA), an acute phase reactant synthesized by the liver, is the amyloidogenic protein in secondary amyloidosis. In familial amyloidosis, an inherited mutation in one of several different proteins renders it amyloidogenic. The most common protein mutated in familial amyloidosis is transthyretin.

a. Epidemiology and Pathogenesis. AL amyloidosis presents most often after the age of 50 years, but it may occur as early as the third decade. In contrast to multiple myeloma, the clinical manifestations of primary amyloidosis do not result from plasma cell proliferation, but instead are due to the pathogenic light chains produced by a relatively small number of clonal plasma cells.

Secondary amyloidosis is decreasing in incidence as a result of improvements in the treatment of chronic inflammatory conditions. SAA, the precursor for AA amyloid, is present in normal serum in trace amounts. Its concentration rises severalfold in response to a variety of inflammatory stimuli and diseases. The fact that most patients with elevated SAA levels do not develop amyloid suggests that factors other than serum concentration must play a role in the pathogenesis of AA amyloidosis.

The familial amyloidoses usually do not produce clinical symptoms until adulthood. Not surprisingly, clusters of families may be found within specific ethnic groups or geographic regions. The mechanisms by which specific mutations render the protein amyloidogenic have not been elucidated. Similarly the determinants of the tissue specificity of individual amyloidogenic proteins have not been identified.

b. Pathology. Although the amyloidogenic proteins in primary, secondary, and familial amyloidosis share virtually no structural features, the renal biopsies are indistinguishable by light or electron microscopy. Mesangial expansion with Congo Red–positive material, nodular sclerosis, and varying amounts of Congo Red positivity in the vasculature and tubulointerstitium are the characteristic histological findings. Randomly oriented fibrils approximately 10 nm in diameter are visible by electron microscopy in regions of Congo Red positivity. Immunofluorescence may demonstrate immunoglobulin light chains or AA protein in primary and secondary amyloidosis, respectively.

c. Clinical and Laboratory Features. Most patients with renal amyloid present with nephrotic syndrome. Proteinuria may be massive and edema may be refractory to diuretics because of severe hypoalbuminemia or coexisting cardiac or autonomic nervous system involvement. Progressive loss of GFR occurs at varying rates, and end-stage renal disease eventually develops in at least one third of patients. Renal insufficiency without significant proteinuria may be seen in patients with predominant tubular, interstitial, or vascular amyloid deposition. The nonrenal manifestations of systemic amyloidosis include restrictive cardiomyopathy, autonomic or peripheral neuropathy, macroglossia, nail dystrophy, heptomegaly, ecchymoses, and soft tissue or muscle involvement.

The diagnosis of amyloidosis requires demonstration of Congo Red–positive material in tissue. Abdominal fat can be obtained by relatively noninvasive means for staining and is Congo Red–positive in 85% of patients with AL amyloidosis. The type of amyloid can be determined in most cases using a combination of clinical features and laboratory tests including serum and urine immunofixation electrophroresis, immunohistochemistry of tissue biopsies, and, for some of the familial amyloidoses, gene sequencing or serum isoelectric focusing.

d. Treatment. The treatment of amyloidosis is aimed at managing organ dysfunction and preventing production and deposition of new amyloid. The approach to reducing production of amyloid obviously differs for primary, secondary, and familial forms of amyloidosis. Oral melphalan and prednisone given for 4–7 days every 6 weeks has been shown to increase the median survival in primary amyloidosis from 8 to 18 months. A more aggressive approach is the intravenous administration of marrow-ablative doses of melphalan followed by autologous peripheral blood stem cells for bone marrow reconstitution. This treatment can completely eradicate the clonal plasma cells in a significant proportion of patients, but it is associated with significant toxicity and the duration of response has not yet been determined. There is no specific treatment for secondary amyloidosis; the most effective approach is to treat the underlying inflammatory disease. Familial amyloidosis can be treated with orthotopic liver transplantation. Removal of the native liver is necessary to eliminate expression of the amyloidogenic protein.

2. Multiple Myeloma

Multiple myeloma is caused by the proliferation of an abnormal clone of plasma cells. The excessive immunoglobulin light chains produced by these cells can cause several morphologically distinct renal lesions with varying clinical manifestations. The physiochemical properties of the pathological light chains are the major determinants of the type of renal disease that occurs, and it is unusual for more than one type of myeloma-associated renal disease to be present in an individual patient.

a. Epidemiology and Pathogenesis. Multiple myeloma occurs most often between the ages of 50 and 70 years and is rare before the fourth decade. Renal failure may occur in as many as 50% of patients and is a frequent cause of death. Cast nephropathy, also called myeloma kidney, is the most common type of myeloma-associated renal disease and occurs when free light chains in the urine bind to Tamm-Horsfall glycoprotein, producing insoluble casts that obstruct the tubules and damage tubular epithelial cells.

Light chain deposition disease (LCDD) is a second form of multiple myeloma–associated renal disease. Rather than obstructing the tubules, the monoclonal light chains deposit in the mesangium and stimulate extracellular matrix production, which reduces the filtering capacity of the glomerular capillaries. Not all patients with LCDD have multiple myeloma, but it is presumed that they all have some type of B lymphocyte or plasma cell dyscrasia. The renal disease is often the predominant manifestation of non–myeloma-associated LCDD, although biopsies of other tissues will often reveal extrarenal disease. Renal amyloidosis occurs in the relatively small proportion of multiple myeloma patients who produce an amyloidogenic monoclonal light chain. Deposition of amyloid fibrils in the mesangium, glomerular basement membrane, vessels, and tubulointerstitium produce clinical and histological renal disease identical to that of primary amyloidosis.

b. Pathology. Tubular casts surrounded by mononuclear cells and macrophages is the prominent feature of the renal biopsy in cast nephropathy. Tubular epithelial cell damage, varying degrees of interstitial fibrosis, and normal-appearing glomeruli are additional findings. LCDD is characterized by nodular glomerulosclerosis. Monotypic light chain deposits along tubular basement membranes, often evident by immunofluorescence, help distinguish the glomerular lesions from those of diabetic nephropathy. The histological findings of multiple myeloma–associated amyloid are identical to those of primary amyloidosis (see earlier).

c. Clinical and Laboratory Features. Multiple myeloma should be considered in all adult patients, particularly those over age 50 years, with unexplained renal insufficiency, anemia, or hypercalcemia. Because light chains are not detected by colorimetric reagent strips, a urinalysis that is negative for protein should not be interpreted as negative for light chains. The presence of urinary light chains should be presumed when there is a discrepancy between the urine dipstick and a sulfosalicylic acid precipitation test. Quantitative urine light chain measurement and urine protein immunoelectrophoresis are confirmatory tests.

Cast nephropathy is characterized by renal insufficiency that is usually insidious in development but may be rapid in onset. The urinalysis may be normal or may show tubular epithelial cells and granular casts. Volume depletion, hypercalciuria, low urinary pH, and high intratubular sodium concentration, such as that resulting from diuretic administration, all facilitate the binding of light chains to Tamm-Horsfall protein and should be avoided if possible. Heavy proteinuria, usually nephrotic-range, due to albumin excretion is the prominent feature of both LCDD and amyloidosis.

Fanconi syndrome, a proximal tubulopathy resulting from accumulation of light chains in the lysosomes of the proximal tubular cells, can occur in isolation or in conjunction with other renal manifestations of multiple myeloma. The characteristic laboratory findings are glucosuria, metabolic acidosis, hypophosphatemia, hypouricemia, and hypokalemia. Although it can also be idiopathic or secondary to other systemic diseases, the presence of Fanconi syndrome in an adult should prompt an evaluation for a plasma cell dyscrasia.

d. Treatment. The treatment of all of the multiple myeloma–associated renal diseases should be directed at the underlying plasma cell dyscrasia. Cyclic oral melphalan and prednisone, combination chemotherapy with vincristine, doxorubucin, and dexamethasone (VAD), and autologous stem cell transplantation are the regimens most frequently employed by oncologists. Although remission of multiple myeloma can be induced, it is unfortunately rarely sustained with any of these chemotherapeutic regimens. In the setting of acute renal failure or significant renal insufficiency, VAD is the preferred regimen because of its more rapid induction of a hematological remission. Plasmapheresis effectively reduces the serum concentration of light chains and should be considered in conjunction with chemotherapy in patients with acute renal failure due to cast nephropathy. Preventing volume depletion and avoiding renal vasoconstrictors such as nonsteroidal anti-inflammatory agents and radiographic contrast are important components of the treatment of cast nephropathy.

3. Fibrillary Glomerulonephritis and Immunotactoid Glomerulopathies

Fibrillary glomerulonephritis (GN) and immunotactoid glomerulopathy are uncommon disorders characterized by the presence of nonamyloid glomerular fibrils visible by electron microscopy. Although some authorities consider fibrillary GN and immunotactoid glomerulopathy to be a single entity, others consider them to be clinically and pathologically distinct.

a. Epidemiology and Pathogenesis. Fibrillary and immunotactoid GN occur with equal frequency in males and females and appear to be more common in whites than in African Americans. The fibrils in both disorders contain immunoglobulin and complement. Whether the fibrils are comprised of immunoglobulin-antigen immune complexes or form from aggregates of pure immunoglobulin has not been determined. The stimulus to production of the immunoglobulin components of the fibrils is not known.

b. Pathology. Renal biopsy is required to make the diagnosis of fibrillary GN or immunotactoid glomerulopathy. Light microscopy findings are not specific for these disorders. Capillary wall thickening and mesangial matrix expansion are the most common features, and glomerular hypercellularity and crescent formation are present in some patients. Congo Red staining is negative, a finding that definitively differentiates these fibrils from amyloid. Immunofluorescence may be positive for IgG, IgM, and C3. A diagnosis of fibrillary GN or immunotactoid glomerulopathy requires the electron microscopic identification of fibrils deposited extracellularly in the mesangium and capillary walls. The size and arrangement of the fibrils form the basis of the distinction between fibrillary GN and immunotactoid glomerulopathy, with randomly dispersed fibrils of approximately 20 nm diameter in the former and parallel arrays of fibrils of 30–50 nm diameter in the latter.

c. Clinical and Laboratory Features. Proteinuria, usually nephrotic-range, is a uniform finding in these disorders, and most patients have microscopic hematuria. Red cell casts may be seen, and hypertension is often present. Renal insufficiency may be present at the time of diagnosis and is progressive in a large proportion of patients. Immunotactoid glomerulopathy may be associated with a systemic lymphoproliferative disease such as lymphoma, but extrarenal disease manifestations are otherwise extremely rare.

d. Treatment. There is no established treatment for these disorders. Treatment of an associated lymphoproliferative disease, if present, may result in improvement in the renal manifestations.

IV. RENAL DISEASE ASSOCIATED WITH SYSTEMIC VASCULITIS

Vasculitis is characterized by inflammation of blood vessels and consequent tissue ischemia or necrosis (Table 10). Vascular injury may be immune complex–mediated (e.g., Henoch-Schönlein purpura) or it may be pauci-immune (e.g., Wegener's granulomatosis), meaning that very few or no immune deposits are seen by tissue biopsy. The diagnosis of vasculitis should be considered in patients who have single or multiorgan dysfunction and systemic signs or symptoms such as fever, weight loss, fatigue, purpura, mononeuritis, eosinophilia, or anemia. Because many of the manifestations of vasculitis are nonspecific, diagnosis is often delayed. Mononeuritis multiplex and palpable purpura are two findings that are strongly suggestive of vasculitis; however, their occurrence is by no means universal and is, in fact, unusual in certain types of vasculitis. Classification and diagnosis of specific forms of vasculitis is discussed below.

A. Medium-Sized Vessel Vasculitis: Classic or Macroscopic Polyarteritis Nodosa

Polyarteritis nodosa (PAN), also referred to as classic PAN or macroscopic PAN, can be idiopathic or can occur in association with hepatitis B infection. It affects medium-sized and, to a lesser extent, small arteries. The kidney, bowel, liver, skeletal muscle, skin, and peripheral nervous system are frequently involved in PAN. Lung involvement is usually not present in PAN. Renal insufficiency results from glomerular hypoperfusion or cortical infarcts.

1. Epidemiology and Pathogenesis

Polyarteritis nodosa is an uncommon disease. It occurs somewhat more frequently in males than females, and although seen most often in adults between the ages of 40 and 60 years, it may occur in children and in elderly individuals.

2. Pathology

PAN is characterized pathologically by focal, necrotizing inflammatory lesions predominantly in medium-sized arteries but also in small arteries. Glomerulonephritis is not a prominent feature of PAN. The glomeruli may, however, appear small due to hypoperfusion. Immunofluorescence is negative, reflecting the pauci-immune nature of this type of vasculitis.

3. Clinical and Laboratory Features

Virtually any organ can be affected in PAN. The most frequently involved organs include the kidney, the peripheral nervous system (mononeuritis multiplex), the

Table 10 Clinical and Laboratory Features of Renal Vasculitis

Characteristic	Polyarteritis nodosa (macroscopic)	Wegener's granulomatosis	Microscopic polyangiitis	Henoch-Schönlein purpura	Cryoglobulinemia
Creatinine	Elevated	Elevated	Elevated	Normal or elevated	Elevated
Urinalysis	Protein, ± rbcs, ± rbc casts, ± granular casts	Protein, rbcs, rbc casts	Protein, rbcs, rbc casts	Protein, rbcs, rbc casts	Protein, rbcs, rbc casts
Urine protein[a]	Subnephrotic	Subnephrotic	Subnephrotic	Nephrotic or subnephrotic	Nephrotic or subnephrotic
Complements	Normal	Normal	Normal	Normal	Low
Serologies	Normal	ANCA	ANCA	Normal	Cryoglobulins, hepatitis C Ab
Associated findings	Hypertension, multisystem disease	Upper and/or lower respiratory tract disease	Multisystem disease	Rash, gastrointestinal disease	Hypertension, multisystem disease

Abbreviations: rbcs, red blood cells; ANCA, antineutrophilic cytoplasmic antibodies; Ab, antibody.

[a] Nephrotic refers to urinary protein excretion of ≥3 g/day. Subnephrotic refers to urinary protein excretion of 0.2–3 g/day.

skin (palpable purpura, livedo reticularis, or digital ischemia), joints, and gastrointestinal tract (abdominal pain, occult GI bleeding). Constitutional signs such as fever, weight loss, and malaise are common. Pulmonary or central nervous system involvement is unusual in PAN. Occasionally patients will have single organ involvement both at presentation and at follow-up.

Renal involvement occurs in approximately 70% of cases. Proteinuria is common and is usually in the subnephrotic range. Microscopic hematuria from renal infarcts and granular casts from ischemic tubular necrosis are typical features of the urine sediment. Red cell casts may be present but are not a typical feature. Hypertension mediated by the renin-angiotensin system accompanies the renal disease.

An elevated erythrocyte sedimentation rate, normochromic normocytic anemia, hypoalbuminemia, and thrombocytosis all reflect the systemic inflammatory nature of PAN, but none is sensitive or specific for the disease. Hepatitis B surface antigen is detectable in 10–50% of patients. The diagnosis of PAN is made by a combination of clinical findings and angiography and/or tissue biopsy. The characteristic arterial aneurysms often visible by renal arteriography provide strong support for the diagnosis of PAN. There is no serological test for this disease. Anti-neutrophil cytoplasmic antibodies are not present.

4. Treatment

The prognosis of PAN depends on the organ involvement and rate of progression. If untreated, the 5-year survival is less than 15%. Glucocorticoids are used as initial treatment in most patients, but cyclophosphamide should be added in those with extensive visceral involvement and evidence of disease progression. Plasmapheresis has been used in this disease as well, although the existing clinical studies do not allow evaluation of its efficacy. Antiviral agents, such as IFN-α and lamivudine, may improve the outcome of PAN associated with hepatitis B.

B. Small Vessel Vasculitis

1. Pauci-Immune Small Vessel Vasculitis: Wegener's Granulomatosis and Microscopic Polyangiitis

The term pauci-immune necrotizing vasculitis is used to describe the spectrum of glomerulonephritides associated with an absence of both immune deposits and evidence of direct antibody-mediated injury. Microscopic polyangiitis and Wegener's granulomatosis are systemic vasculitides associated with pauci-immune glomerulonephritis. When pauci-immune necrotizing and crescentic glomerulonephritis occurs without evidence of systemic vasculitis, the renal disease has been called idiopathic crescentic glomerulonephritis.

a. Epidemiology and Pathogenesis. The pathogenesis of pauci-immune vasculitis is unknown. Identification of antineutrophil cytoplasmic antibodies (ANCA) in the majority of patients together with experimental studies demonstrating ANCA-mediated leukocyte activation suggests a pathogenic role of these autoantibodies. An infectious trigger of ANCA-associated vasculitis has been suggested by the occurrence of a flu-like prodrome in many patients, by the increased frequency of nasal *Staphylococcus aureus* colonization in Wegener's patients, and by in vitro effects of cytokines on ANCA-mediated leukocyte activation.

b. Pathology. The small vessel pauci-immune vasculitides all produce similar renal histological lesions. A crescentic glomerulonephritis with focal necrosis and very little or no endocapillary proliferation is characteristic. As the name implies, immune deposits are not present, nor is there evidence of direct antibody binding to glomerular components by immunofluorescence studies. Necrotizing inflammation of renal arteries and arterioles may be seen, but because of the small sampling of vessels by renal biopsy, the absence of such findings should not rule out the diagnosis. Peri-glomerular granuloma formation occurs occasionally in patients with Wegener's granulomatosis, but granulomatous inflammation is much more common in the respiratory tract.

c. Clinical and Laboratory Features. The respiratory tract and kidney are the organs predominantly involved in Wegener's granulomatosis. Sinusitis, nasal discharge, and nasal ulcerations are common manifestations of upper airway involvement. Pulmonary infiltrates and nodular or cavitary lesions are typical chest radiographic findings associated with lower respiratory tract disease. Massive pulmonary hemorrhage can occur and is one of the life-threatening manifestations of Wegener's granulomatosis. A nephritic urinary sediment and renal insufficiency, which may progress to dialysis-requiring renal failure, are the characteristic renal manifestations. Not all patients have clinically evident renal disease at presentation, but the majority develop it at some point in the course of the disease. Additional manifestations include episcleritis, uveitis, serous otitis media, skin nodules, palpable purpura, and cranial nerve deficits. The clinical manifestations of microscopic polyangiitis are similar to those of Wegener's granulomatosis except that upper respiratory tract and otorhinolaryngeal involvement are unusual. In contrast with macroscopic PAN, the small vessel vasculitides are often not accompanied by hypertension.

Assays for ANCA are useful tools in the diagnosis of the pauci-immune small vessel vasculitides. Two different staining patterns have been identified by incubating patient serum with ethanol-fixed neutrophils. The cytoplasmic staining pattern (c-ANCA) occurs when the autoantibody is directed against the proteinase 3 (PR3) serine protease. The perinuclear staining pattern (p-ANCA) results with antibodies directed against myeloperoxidase (MPO). Antibodies directed against other intracellular proteins such as elastase, lactoferrin, and cathepsin G may also produce a p-ANCA by immunofluorescence, but these have not been closely associated with renal diseases. The specificity of ANCA testing is greatly enhanced by combining the results of immunofluorescence with those of antigen-specific enzyme-linked immunosorbent assays (ELISA) for antibodies to PR3 and MPO. Most patients with Wegener's granulomatosis and renal involvement have anti-PR3 antibodies; however, the absence of this finding does not rule out the disease as approximately 20% of patients have MPO antibodies and 10–30% have no ANCA. MPO antibodies are present in the majority of patients with microscopic polyangiitis.

d. Treatment. The mainstay of treatment for Wegener's granulomatosis and microscopic polyangiitis is cyclophosphamide. A typical regimen consists of intravenous pulse methylprednisolone administered in three doses over 3–5 days followed by oral prednisone and cyclophosphamide. Prednisone is usually tapered over 3–4 months, and the cyclophosphamide is typically continued for 6–12 months after clinical remission. There is controversy regarding the relative benefits of daily oral versus monthly intravenous dosing of cyclophosphamide. In an effort to avoid the significant toxicities of long courses of cyclophosphamide, treatment protocols utilizing methotrexate or azathioprine are used in some centers. Plasmapheresis together with cytotoxic agents has been shown to improve renal function in dialysis-dependent patients with ANCA-associated vasculitis. A long-term efficacy of this treatment modality, however, has not been demonstrated. Trimethoprim-sulfamethoxazole may be effective for upper respiratory tract disease associated with Wegener's granulomatosis but has no significant effect on renal disease.

The prognosis of pauci-immune small vessel vasculitis has improved markedly with the treatments described above. Survival is now greater than 70% at 5 years. Prompt initiation of treatment is necessary, however, in order to prevent irreversible fibrosis of lung or kidney. Because relapse is common, patients in remission need to be evaluated on a regular basis for signs of recurrent disease.

2. Immune Complex–Mediated Small Vessel Vasculitis: Henoch-Schönlein Purpura and Essential Cryoglobulinemia

a. Henoch-Schönlein Purpura. Henoch-Schönlein Purpura (HSP) is a systemic vasculitis characterized by the deposition of IgA-containing immune complexes in the kidneys, gastrointestinal tract, and skin.

EPIDEMIOLOGY AND PATHOGENESIS. HSP occurs primarily, but not exclusively, in children. The pathogenesis is thought to be similar to that of IgA nephropathy.

PATHOLOGY. The renal biopsy abnormalities are essentially identical to those found in patients with IgA nephropathy (see earlier), although cellular crescents are more often present in HSP. Biopsy of skin lesions shows leukocytoclastic vasculitis, a nonspecific change associated with other small vessel vasculitides as well. Vascular IgA deposits in the skin biopsy is an insensitive but specific finding in HSP.

CLINICAL AND LABORATORY FEATURES. The clinical manifestations of HSP include a purpuric rash, which is often most prominent on the buttocks and thighs, arthralgias most commonly affecting the knees and ankles, abdominal pain which may be accompanied by gastrointestinal bleeding or intussusception, and glomerulonephritis. The renal disease, when present, becomes clinically evident within a few days to a few weeks of the onset of systemic symptoms. Urinalysis shows hematuria (which may be macroscopic) and red cell casts. Proteinuria is usually mild but in severe cases can be in the nephrotic range. The degree of renal insufficiency is variable. Most patients have a normal or slightly elevated serum creatinine, but acute renal failure may occur.

HSP usually resolves spontaneously, and the long-term outcome is good in most patients. A small percentage of patients have persistent proteinuria and renal insufficiency, and some patients have late progression of renal insufficiency despite apparent resolution of active HSP.

TREATMENT. Most patients with HSP do not require specific treatment although glucocorticoids, cyclophosphamide, and plasmapheresis have all been used in patients with marked proteinuria or acute renal failure. The benefit of aggressive treatment has not been convincingly demonstrated.

b. Mixed Essential Cryoglobulinemia. Mixed essential cryoglobulinemia is discussed in Section III.A. Because it can produce a systemic vasculitic syndrome in addition to glomerulonephritis, cryoglobulinemia should be included in the differential diagnosis of patients with features of small vessel vasculitis.

V. THROMBOTIC MICROANGIOPATHIES

A summary of the features of thrombotic microangiopathies is shown in Table 11.

A. Hemolytic Uremic Syndrome and Thrombotic Thrombocytopenic Purpura

Hemolytic uremic syndrome (HUS) and thrombotic thromboctyopenic purpura (TTP) are related disorders with overlapping features. HUS is characterized by hemolytic anemia, thrombocytopenia, and renal injury. TTP is defined by the pentad of hemolytic anemia, thromboctypenia, fever, central nervous system (CNS) involvement, and renal insufficiency. Renal failure is usually the promi-

Table 11 Clinical and Laboratory Features of Thrombotic Microangiopathies

Characteristic	Hemolytic uremic syndrome	Thrombotic thrombocytopenic purpura	Antiphospholipid syndrome	Systemic sclerosis
Creatinine	Elevated	Normal or elevated	Normal or elevated	Elevated
Urinalysis	Protein, rbcs, ± rbc casts	Protein, rbcs, ± rbc casts	Protein, rbcs, ± rbc casts	Protein, rbcs, granular casts
Urine protein[a]	Subnephrotic	Subnephrotic	Subnephrotic or nephrotic	Nephrotic or subnephrotic
Complements	Normal	Normal	Normal	Normal
Serologies	Normal	Normal	Anticardiolipin Abs, lupus anticoagulant	Anti-Scl 70, RNP, and centromere Abs
Associated findings	Hypertension, edema, hemolysis, thrombocytopenia	± Hypertension, hemolysis, thrombocytopenia	Hypertension, hemolysis, thrombocytopenia	Hypertension, hemolysis, thrombocytopenia

Abbreviations: rbcs, red blood cells.

[a] Nephrotic refers to urinary protein excretion of ≥3 g/day. Subnephrotic refers to urinary protein excretion of 0.2–3 g/day.

nent feature of HUS, while renal involvement is often relatively mild in TTP. Conversely, the CNS findings are usually more marked in TTP. Despite these differences it is sometimes difficult to distinguish the two disorders.

1. Epidemiology and Pathogenesis

HUS occurs in both children and adults. Most childhood cases follow an episode of infectious diarrhea due to verocytoxic or shigatoxic bacteria such as *E. coli* strain O157:H7. In addition to sporadic cases, HUS can be inherited as an autosomal recessive disorder usually presenting in childhood, or as an autosomal dominant disease presenting in adults, or it can be associated with medications such as cyclosporine, mitomycin C, or quinine sulfate. TTP is less common than HUS, rarely occurs in children, and is not preceded by a diarrheal illness. Although TTP may be associated with HIV infection or ticlopidine, the majority of cases have no known cause or disease association. Vascular endothelial cell injury is a prominent feature of both HUS and TTP and likely underlies the hemolysis, thrombocytopenia, and end-organ damage.

2. Pathology

Microthrombi in the glomerular capillaries and arterioles, endothelial cell swelling, widening of the subendothelial space due to deposition of fibrin and lipid, and narrowing of the capillaries are the characteristic pathological features. Intimal thickening and ''onion-skin'' hypertrophy of the arterioles and arteries are seen during the healing phase. These findings are not specific to HUS or TTP but are seen in other disorders of the renal vascular endothelium, such as malignant hypertension, systemic sclerosis, and antiphospholipid syndrome.

3. Clinical and Laboratory Features

HUS and TTP typically present as acute illnesses requiring hospitalization. In diarrhea-associated HUS, hemolysis and thrombocytopenia occur suddenly following the prodromal illness. Bloody diarrhea is common, and severe colitis with bowel ischemia and necrosis may occur. Hematuria, severe oliguria, hypertension, and edema are the characteristic features of the renal involvement. CNS symptoms such as seizure, altered mental status, and coma are common in TTP but may occur in HUS as well. Neurological symptoms are often the first manifestation and the predominant feature of TTP. Anemia, fever, fatigue, and arthralgias follow. Hematuria and proteinuria are common, although overt renal failure is not typical of TTP.

Laboratory studies are similar in HUS and TTP. The peripheral blood smear shows fragmented red cells, burr cells, and helmet cells. Elevations in serum LDH, indirect bilirubin, and reticulocyte count, and a low haptoglobin level provide additional evidence for hemolysis. Thrombocytopenia is a universal finding in both HUS and TTP and results from platelet injury and destruction in the microvessels of affected organs. Neither the prothrombin time nor the partial thromboplastin time is prolonged. The urinalysis shows proteinuria, red cells, and occasionally red cell casts.

4. Treatment

The treatment of diarrhea-associated HUS should consist of supportive measures such as bowel rest for hemorrhagic colitis, careful control of fluid balance and electrolyte abnormalities, blood transfusions, and, if necessary, dialysis. Platelet transfusions should not be administered unless there is active bleeding. Specific therapies such as glucocorticoids, fresh frozen plasma infusion, anticoagulants, or plasmapheresis have not been shown to alter the course of the usually self-limited diarrhea-associated HUS. Fresh frozen plasma infusion or plasmapheresis is recommended for inherited forms of HUS, non–diarrhea-associated disease with severe manifestations, or recurrent disease. In contrast to diarrhea-associated HUS, intensive plasmapheresis with fresh frozen plasma does have a marked impact on the mortality of TTP and should be tried in most patients in conjunction with glucocorticoids. Plasma infusion has also been shown to be of benefit and can be used if plamapheresis is not available. Vincristine and splenectomy may play a role in the treatment of relapsing TTP.

The prognosis of both HUS and TTP are variable. Patients with diarrhea-associated HUS have the best prognosis with complete recovery in approximately two thirds of patients and end-stage renal disease in approximately 15% of patients. The hereditary forms of HUS are associated with poor renal outcome and a high mortality. Although the prognosis of TTP has improved significantly with current treatment approaches, the mortality rate is approximately 30%.

B. Antiphospholipid Syndrome

The antiphospholipid syndrome (APS) is characterized by recurrent vascular thrombosis, pregnancy loss, and thrombocytopenia in association with elevated levels of antiphospholipid antibodies. The full spectrum of APS is still being characterized. Other clinical manifestations thought to be associated with the disorder include hemolytic anemia, livido reticularis, and valvular heart disease. Thrombotic microangiopathy of the kidney occurs in some patients with APS. The disease is considered primary when it occurs alone and secondary when it occurs in the setting of systemic disease such as systemic lupus erythematosis. A fulminant form of APS, referred to as ''catastrophic APS,'' has also been described.

1. Epidemiology and Pathogenesis

APS appears to have a female predominance, but this may be the result of increased diagnosis in women experiencing recurrent pregnancy loss. Antiphospholipid antibodies are directed against either phospholipids or plasma proteins bound to anionic phospholipids. The mechanism of thrombosis in APS has not been fully elucidated. There is evidence that the antiphospholipid antibodies are involved in the pathogenesis.

2. Pathology

Renal involvement occurs in 20–30% of patients with primary APS. The pathological changes in the kidney include noninflammatory occlusion of any of the renal blood vessels. Intimal thickening, subendothelial fibrosis, and medial hyperplasia result from thrombotic lesions. Thrombi can be seen in affected glomerular capillaries with lesions resembling other thrombotic microangiopathies such as HUS, TTP, and scleroderma. Such findings on renal biopsy should prompt an investigation for the presence of antiphospholipid antibodies.

3. Clinical and Laboratory Features

The renal manifestations of APS are varied. Some patients present with mild proteinuria and normal or slightly elevated serum creatinine, while others may have nephrotic-range proteinuria, an active urine sediment, and acute renal failure. Renal vein or artery thrombosis can produce flank pain, hematuria, and reduction in GFR. The antiphospholipid antibodies include anticardiolipin antibodies and the lupus anticoagulant. The presence of antiphospholipid antibodies in and of itself is not diagnostic of the syndrome as positive tests for antiphospholipid antibodies can occur in unaffected individuals.

4. Treatment

Anticoagulation with warfarin is the mainstay of treatment. Immunosuppressive agents have not been found to reduce the titers of antiphospholipid antibodies. Plasmapheresis has been used to remove the pathogenic antibodies in patients with acute renal failure; however, the response rate appears to be low.

C. Systemic Sclerosis (Scleroderma)

Systemic sclerosis (scleroderma) is a connective tissue disorder affecting the skin and multiple internal organs. The manifestations are heterogeneous and include Raynaud's phenomenon, tightening and thickening of the skin, pulmonary fibrosis, pulmonary hypertension, esophageal dysmotility, arthralgias, myopathy, and myocardial fibrosis. Renal involvement is one of the most serious complications of the disease and can result in rapid loss of renal function and life-threatening hypertension if not treated promptly.

1. Epidemiology and Pathogenesis

Systemic sclerosis presents most often during the fourth or fifth decade and is approximately three to four times more commen in women than men. The pathogenesis of systemic sclerosis is unknown. Fibrotic arteriosclerosis and accumulation of extracellular matrix, particularly collagen, occur in all involved organs.

2. Pathology

The histological findings are similar to those of HUS, TTP, and malignant hypertension. The predominant changes are in the small renal arteries and arterioles, which show intimal proliferation, medial thinning, fibrinoid necrosis, and reduplication of the elastic lamina. Thrombosis of glomerular capillaries is evident by glomerular fibrin deposition. Glomerular hypoperfusion may produce small, sclerotic glomeruli.

3. Clinical and Laboratory Features

Renal disease in systemic sclerosis can manifest as a slowly progressive nephropathy or as scleroderma renal crisis. The slowly progressive renal disease is characterized by proteinuria (usually subnephrotic), hypertension, and gradual reduction in GFR. Scleroderma renal crisis is manifest by the sudden onset of severe hypertension, rapidly progressive renal failure, microangiopathic hemolytic anemia, and thrombocytopenia. Marked elevations in plasma renin activity due to acute vasospasm of the renal vasculature exacerbates renal ischemia and end-organ damage. Urinalysis shows proteinuria, microscopic hematuria, and granular casts. Patients with diffuse cutaneous scleroderma and rapid progression of skin involvement appear to be at greatest risk for scleroderma renal crisis. Those with limited cutaneous scleroderma (previously often referred to as CREST syndrome) rarely develop renal crisis.

4. Treatment

The prognosis of scleroderma renal crisis has improved markedly with aggressive use of ACE inhibitors. One-year mortality, as high as 80% prior to the use of ACE inhibitors, is now approximately 20%, and progression to end-stage renal disease occurs in approximately 50% of patients. Reversal of renal failure has been documented in a small percentage of patients who began treatment with ACE inhibitors after the initiation of dialysis. Chronic ACE inhibition should be used if possible not only in patients who have had scleroderma renal crisis, but in all systemic sclerosis patients with hypertension, proteinuria, or renal insufficiency. Glucocorticoids should probably be avoided in patients with scleroderma because they appear to be associated with the development of renal involvement.

SUGGESTED READINGS

Agnello V, Chung RT, Kaplan LM. A role for hepatitis C virus infection in type II cryoglobulinemia. N Engl J Med 1992; 327:1490–1495.

Austin HA, Balow JE. Natural history and treatment of lupus nephritis. Semin Nephrol 1999; 19:2–11.

Bolton WK. Goodpasture's syndrome. Kidney Int 1996; 50:1753– 1756.

Brady HR. Fibrillary glomerulopathy. Kidney Int 1998; 53:1421–1429.

Cameron, JS. Lupus nephritis. J Am Soc Nephrol 1999; 10:413–424.

Dember LM, Salant DJ. Minimal change disease. In: Brady HR, Wilcox CS, eds. Therapy in Nephrology and Hypertension. Philadelphia: W.B. Saunders Co., 1999, pp. 165–177.

Donadio JV, Grande JP. Immunoglobulin A nephropathy: a clinical perspective. J Am Soc Nephrol 1997; 8:1324–1332.

Donahoe JF. Scleroderma and the kidney. Kidney Int 1992; 41:462–477.

Eknoyan G, Riggs SA. Renal involvement in thrombotic thrombocytopenic purpura. Am J Nephrol 1986; 6:117 131.

Falk RH, Comenzo RL, Skinner M. The systemic amyloidoses. N Engl J Med 1997; 337: 898–909.

Hogan SL, Muller KE, Jennette JC, Falk RJ. A review of therapeutic studies of idiopathic membranous glomerulopathy. Am J Kidney Dis 1995; 25:862–875.

Jennette JC, Falk RJ. Small-vessel vasculitis. N Engl J Med 1997; 337:1512–1523.

Kallenberg CG, Brouwer E, Weening JJ, Tervaert JW. Anti-neutrophil cytoplasmic antibodies: current diagnostic and pathophysiological potential. Kidney Int 1994; 46: 1–15.

Kaplan BS, Meyers KE, Schulman SL. The pathogenesis and treatment of hemolytic uremic syndrome. J Am Soc Nephrol 1998; 9:1126–1133.

Kimmel PL, Bosch JP, Vassalotti JA. Treatment of human immunodeficiency virus (HIV)-associated nephropathy. Semin Nephrol 1998; 18:446–458.

Korbet SM. Primary focal segmental glomerulosclerosis. J Am Soc Nephrol 1998; 9: 1333–1340.

Lochshin MD. Antiphospholipid antibody syndrome. Rheum Dis Clin North Am 1994; 20:45–59.

Schieppati A, Mosconi L, Perna A, Mecca G, Bertani T, Garattini S, Remuzzi G. Prognosis of untreated patients with idiopathic membranous nephropathy. N Engl J Med 1993; 329:85–89.

Tejani A, Ingulli E. Poststreptococcal glomerulonephritis. Current clinical and pathologic concepts. Nephron 1990; 55:1–5.

Winearls CG. Acute myeloma kidney. Kidney Int 1995; 48:1347–1361.

20

Drug- and Toxin-Induced Renal Injury

William M. Bennett
Legacy Good Samaritan Hospital, Portland, Oregon

I. INTRODUCTION

Pharmacotherapeutic agents and industrial chemicals carry a finite potential for acute and chronic adverse effects on the kidneys. A single toxic agent may produce more than one clinical picture, depending on factors such as dose and duration of exposure as well as on host factors such as immune-response genes (Table 1). In addition to acute and chronic renal insufficiency, drugs may also produce various fluid electrolyte and acid-base disturbances. This chapter reviews clinically relevant nephrotoxic agents, the mechanisms by which they induce injury, and the management of this injury.

II. DEFINITION AND DIAGNOSIS OF TOXIC RENAL INJURY

The diagnosis of drug nephrotoxicity is often delayed until renal damage is sufficient to decrease glomerular filtration rate (GFR). Abnormalities in GFR are assessed indirectly by elevation of serum creatinine by a decrease in creatinine clearance (C_{Cr}) (see Chapter 5). These insensitive markers may fail to detect many drug-induced toxic insults. In addition, renal injury that is sufficient to reduce GFR does not always produce symptoms until well advanced. For example, excessive use of combination analgesics or nonsteroidal anti-inflammatory drugs (NSAIDs) may produce renal papillary necrosis, which is often clinically silent until the disease is far advanced. Because many nephrotoxins injure renal tubular

Table 1 Drug-Related Nephrotoxic Syndromes

Renal syndrome	Mechanism	Prototypical agents
ARF (Acute tubular necrosis)	Direct injury to renal tubular cells	Aminoglycosides, cisplatin, amphotericin B, cephaloridine, heavy metals
ARF (prerenal)	Decreased renal perfusion	NSAIDs, converting enzyme inhibitors, cyclosporine, FK506
ARF (interstitial nephritis)	Immunologic, inflammatory	Penicillins, sulfonamides, cephalosporins, dilantin, allopurinol, NSAIDs, diuretics
ARF (obstruction)	Intratubular obstruction; retroperitoneal fibrosis	Methotrexate, acyclovir, methysergide
Chronic renal failure	Chronic tubulointerstial damage	Analgesics, lead, nitrosoureas, lithium, cyclosporine
Nephrotic syndrome	Primary glomerulopathy	Gold, penicillamine, captopril, NSAIDs, heroin

cells, a compensatory response by uninjured nephrons minimizes the impact of nephron injury until a considerable amount of kidney tissue is irreparably lost. Experimental studies have used more sensitive indices of cell injury such as enzymuria and tubular proteinuria as markers of cadmium and mercury; heavy exposure correlated with the presence of these sensitive markers. However, these tests have achieved limited acceptance in clinical medicine due to lack of data correlating them with GFR or histopathological findings. Thus, in clinical practice nephrotoxicity is defined primarily as a toxin-induced reduction in GFR.

The kidneys are particularly vulnerable to drugs and toxins because high blood flow rate and tubular transport process result in exposure of renal cells to large amounts of drugs and chemicals. In addition, the kidney has metabolic pathways that generate biologically active metabolites. Due to the capacity of the kidney to concentrate urine, the concentrations of drugs and chemicals in tubular lumina of individual nephrons is usually much higher than in blood.

III. CELLULAR MECHANISMS OF RENAL DAMAGE

Some nephrotoxins, such as amphotericin B, interact directly with tubule cell membranes to produce damage, whereas others, such as the hydrophobic immunosuppressive molecules, cyclosporine, and tacrolimus, insert into kidney cell lipid membranes without apparent adverse effect. Aminoglycosides enter proximal tubule cells via interaction with a specific receptor. Binding and cellular uptake of the cationic aminoglycosides via this receptor interferes with endocytosis and recycling of anionic phospholipids. The nephrotoxicity of some cephalosporins and cisplatin are related to uptake and cell transit by known organic ion transport systems. Some nephrotoxins are taken into cells after complexing with proteins. Binding of ionic cadmium to an inducible low-molecular weight hepatic protein can be demonstrated shortly after an acute dose of this industrial pollutant is administered. The complex is transported into the proximal tubular cell, where the ionic cadmium is released, causing cell injury. With various nephrotoxins, cell calcium overload may cause damage to mitochondria and other intracellular organelles. Presumably calcium enters cells following plasma membrane injury, but it is difficult to determine whether the increased intracellular calcium is a cause or a result of cell injury.

Renal cell injury can be caused by reactive intracellular metabolites. Intracellular enzymes, including cytochrome P-450 oxidases, xanthine oxidase, and prostaglandin endoperoxide synthetase, can generate highly unstable reaction products from drugs and chemicals. Free radicals formed during oxidative reactions include superoxide and hydroxyl radicals and singlet oxygen. These react with cellular proteins and nucleic acids to produce injury by covalent binding. Metabolism of arachidonic acid by cyclooxygenase and hydroperoxidase (prostaglandin endoperoxide synthetase) can oxidize drugs such as acetaminophen, producing free radicals in the renal medulla. These or similar processes may play a role in analgesic-associated nephropathy. When reactive species are generated, plasma membranes as well as membranes of mitochondria and endoplasmic reticulum may undergo damaging lipid peroxidation, a reaction propagated by iron and hemoproteins. As with intracellular calcium, it is difficult to ascertain whether metabolic activation and free-radical production are causes or effects of injury.

Intracellular processes also work to minimize the adverse consequences of toxin-induced reactive molecules. For example, superoxide dismutase and catalase combine to enhance the conversion of superoxide to water and oxygen. Reduced glutathione reduces peroxide in a reaction catalyzed by glutathione peroxidase. Reduced glutathione is regenerated by glutathione reductase from NADPH oxidized glutathione. Ascorbic acid and vitamin E are natural free-radical scavengers.

IV. CLINICAL NEPHROTOXINS

A. Antimicrobial Nephrotoxicity

Antibiotics are the largest single class of pharmacological agents associated with drug-induced nephrotoxicity. In one prospective study, 34% of all drug-induced acute renal failure was attributable to antibiotics. The majority of cases occurred with aminoglycosides alone; the next most frequent cause was a combination of aminoglycosides with other antibiotics. However, it is important to remember that antibiotics are administered to patients who are severely ill, often with impaired renal hemodynamics and fluid imbalances,and these co-morbid factors contribute to deterioration of renal function.

B. Aminoglycosides

The most common presentation of aminoglycoside nephrotoxicity is acute renal failure (ARF). In addition, these drugs cause tubular dysfunction (Fanconi's syndrome), renal potassium or magnesium wasting, and nephrogenic diabetes insipidus. In most cases ARF is not associated with oliguria, but oliguria may occasionally occur. Up to 50% of hospitalized patients treated for more than 10 days with aminoglycosides develop a concentrating defect, followed in 2–4 days by increases in serum creatinine and blood urea nitrogen. Urinalysis reveals mild proteinuria and hyaline casts that are nondiagnostic. A variety of proximal tubule enzymes are excreted in increased amounts in treated patients but this finding is also present after a single dose in normal human volunteers. It is not clear whether enzymuria is an epiphenomenon reflecting proximal tubule uptake of aminoglycoside or actually represents subtle renal injury.

1. Pathology

Aminoglycoside nephrotoxicity is manifested by patchy proximal tubule necrosis. Tubular cell autophagocytosis is also evident by electron microscopy. Prominent cytosegrosomes containing whorled material have been identified in these structures and are termed myeloid bodies. Myeloid bodies are diagnostic of aminoglycoside nephrotoxicity only when there is associated proximal tubule cell necrosis.

2. Management

Proper dosing of aminoglycosides can minimize nephrotoxicity. For a given daily dose, frequent divided dosing is more toxic than the less frequent dosing, indicating that the serum peak level is not the factor responsible for nephrotoxicity. In addition, because bacterial growth remains inhibited for a period of time after the serum level falls below the minimum inhibitory concentration, higher but less frequent dosing is as efficacious. Thus, once-daily dosing is now recommended to reduce nephrotoxicity without losing efficacy. The peak serum level obtained 30–45 minutes after a dose of an aminoglycoside correlates best with efficacy while the trough level is the measure of renal excretion. If the trough level rises before the next dose is due, clinicians should recognize that the body has failed to excrete the administered dose and that renal functional impairment has developed.

Developing a clinical strategy to reduce the risk of aminoglycoside nephrotoxicity also requires an appreciation of clinical risk factors. Little can be done to alter factors intrinsic to the patient (age over 60, preexisting liver or renal disease), but factors such as hypotension, volume depletion, acidosis, concomitant nephrotoxic drug therapy, or hypokalemia, can be minimized by corrective therapy. Patients with cystic fibrosis or burns may require large therapeutic doses to maintain appropriate blood levels. Small children and infants tolerate large doses, by adult standards, without adverse renal effects.

C. Penicillins and Cephalosporins

The major manifestation of penicillin- and cephalosporin-associated nephropathy is acute interstitial nephritis (AIN). AIN is characteristically nonoliguric, although severe oliguria requiring dialysis occurs in approximately 15% of patients. Onset usually occurs sometime between the fifth and the fortieth day of exposure. Treatment is directed toward removal of the offending agent. With penicillin, cross-sensitivity to other penicillin-type antibiotics is well documented, although shared sensitivity with cephalosporins is uncommon. If symptomatic renal failure is present, a short course of high dose steroids will often speed the return of renal function to pretreatment levels.

With some older cephalosporins, renal dysfunction more commonly is due to ATN. Most instances of direct toxicity are associated with high doses of the drugs. At therapeutic doses, only cephaloridine and cephaloglycin demonstrate a time- and dose-dependent toxicity, and these drugs are not available in the United States. Among the third- and fourth-generation cephalosporins, the prevalence of increased serum creatinine concentration is $\geq 2\%$ (cefoperazone 2.0%, cefotaxime 1.4%, ceftazidime 0.8%, ceftriaxone 0.5%). Clinical renal insufficiency is rare. Two risk factors associated with cephalosporin nephrotoxicity are concomitant administration of an aminoglycoside antibiotic and diuretic-induced volume depletion.

D. Carbapenems

Carbapenems, which are β-lactam antibiotics, are effective antibacterials but undergo rapid inactivation by renal dehydropeptidase-1 to an inactive metabolite. In animal studies, the intracellular accumulation of this metabolite is nephrotoxic. To overcome this problem, the active antibiotics are combined with cilastain, a specific inhibitor of dehydropeptidase-1, which provides therapeutic blood levels while reducing the risk of metabolite-induced acute tubular damage. Clinical nephrotoxicity is rare.

E. Vancomycin

Vancomycin has enjoyed increased use in managing infections with gram-positive organisms. With early preparations of vancomycin, up to 25% of patients experienced azotemia, but this problem was apparently due to impurities. With better purification in the preparations currently available, ARF is not a clinically significant problem. As with other antibiotics, combination with aminoglycosides potentiates nephrotoxicity and ototoxicity.

F. Sulfonamides

ARF associated with earlier forms of sulfonamides was traceable to intraluminal precipitation of these agents due to limited water solubility. With the introduction of more highly water-soluble agents, the chief, albeit rare, manifestation of sulfonamide nephropathy is acute interstitial nephritis.

G. Rifampin

Rifampin is used as part of multiple-drug regimens for a variety of infections. There is an association between intermittent or interrupted therapy and the development of acute renal dysfunction. As a result, rifampin therapy should be limited to situations in which uninterrupted drug intake can be guaranteed. In addition, weekly monitoring of urinary protein and sediment is recommended. If a systemic syndrome accompanies acute renal dysfunction with rifampin, steroids may speed recovery along with drug discontinuation.

H. Tetracycline

Tetracycline antibiotics cause an increase in blood urea nitrogen concentration in patients with preexisting renal impairment due to their antianabolic effect (increasing urea production) rather than through any direct effect on the kidney. Historically, outdated lots of tetracycline caused a proximal tubular syndrome consisting of aminoaciduria, glycosuria, and metabolic acidosis. The condition has been prevented by modern quality-control measures in manufacturing. Demeclocycline, which has been used to treat severe hyponatremia in certain cases of congestive heart failure or cirrhosis, can cause deterioration of renal function. If a patient with renal insufficiency does require tetracycline, the drug of choice is doxycycline, due to its minimal antianabolic properties.

I. Amphotericin B

Amphotericin B has a dose-related nephrotoxicity that manifests itself at cumulative doses over 1 g. The most frequent clinical presentation is nonoliguric ARF with tubular defects in both concentrating ability and acidification. Amphotericin nephrotoxicity causes proteinuria and pyuria early in its course, with granular casts found in the sediment. If the drug is continued, renal failure develops, frequently associated with hypokalemia and renal tubular acidosis. Repetitive exposure to amphotericin B can be associated with the development of chronic renal dysfunction. Amphotericin toxicity is related to two pharmacological actions. The first is disruption of tubular cell membrane integrity, accounting for defects in urinary concentration and acidification. The second is vasoconstriction, reducing GFR. Several strategies have been used to modify amphotericin B toxicity. Volume expansion with saline has been the most successful, as has reducing the total dose required by combining amphotericin with newer antifungal drugs. Another promising approach is the use of the methylester of amphotericin B, rendered less nephrotoxic by incorporating the drug in liposomes or other lipid vehicles. While these formulations show less nephrotoxicity, they are not completely protective and are very expensive.

J. Acyclovir

Acyclovir is an antiviral agent whose solubility is extremely limited. Administration in high doses (500 mg/m^2 intravenously) has been associated with the development of a dose-dependent ARF. The ARF is caused by precipitation of the drug in the renal tubules; nephrotoxicity is associated with peak serum drug levels over 20 ng/mL. Pretreatment volume expansion and slow infusion of the drug (over 1–2 hr) have greatly reduced the incidence of ARF. However, despite such precautions, cases of acyclovir-induced ARF still occur, reinforcing the importance of maximizing volume status when administering this drug intravenously. Oral dosing can also cause nephrotoxicity, especially in hot, humid environments or with volume depletion. Ganciclovir is more soluble, and there is little evidence of nephrotoxicity.

K. Pentamidine

Pentamidine has gained widespread acceptance for the management of pneumocystis infections in patients with AIDS. Approximately 25% of patients treated with this agent will demonstrate nephrotoxicity. Renal failure is thought to be due to direct tubular damage. Besides maintenance of intravascular volume, there is no proven antidote. Inhaled pentamidine has also been associated with acute nephrotoxicity.

L. Foscarnet

Foscarnet is used in the treatment of resistant cytomegalovirus infections. Therapy is complicated by dose-related nephrotoxicity manifesting itself as acute renal failure, associated with hyperphosphatemia. Tubular syndromes associated with potassium and magnesium wasting may also occur. The pathogenesis of nephrotoxicity is unclear, but tubular damage is likely. Volume expansion, as with most nephrotoxins, provides some protection.

V. CONTRAST MEDIA-ASSOCIATED NEPHROPATHY

Contrast-associated nephropathy is defined as an acute reduction in GFR following exposure to radiographic contrast agents. The incidence varies from 0 to 22%. This wide variation is most likely due to differences in the time over which surveillance is carried out. Many reports limit observations to less than 48 hours after exposure, despite the fact that serum creatinine often rises to peak levels 3–5 days after exposure.

The key risk factors for contrast nephropathy are preexisting renal disease and diabetes mellitus. Other factors include volume depletion, dysproteinemia, and peripheral vascular disease. For diabetic patients, concurrent renal insufficiency markedly increases the risk. For example, for patients with baseline serum creatinine values between 1.5 and 4.5 mg/dL, the risk is two times greater for diabetic patients than for others; at baseline serum creatinine values over 4.5 mg/dL the incidence approaches 100%, while the incidence in nondiabetic controls is only 60%.

The decline in GFR is always temporally linked to performance of a contrast study, with the serum creatinine peaking within 3–5 days of the study. Oliguria occurs in up to 30% of cases. The urinary sediment has little diagnostic value. Fractional excretion of sodium is often low, but this measurement has little diagnostic or prognostic value. Contrast nephropathy is principally a diagnosis of exclusion and is rarely the sole cause of acute renal dysfunction. In patients who are at high risk, monitoring serum creatinine values after the contrast study is crucial in detecting nephrotoxicity.

The single most important clinical axiom about preventing contrast nephropathy is to always use the least invasive diagnostic procedure available. If the patient falls into a high-risk group for contrast nephropathy, one should carefully consider whether the information from the contrast study will contribute enough to management decisions to incur the risk.

Because of the association between hypertonicity and reduced renal blood flow, new low-osmolality, nonionic contrast media have been introduced. The incidence of contrast nephropathy is reduced by using nonionic agents, but only in high-risk patients, namely diabetic patients with previous renal insufficiency. Thus, these costlier nonionic drugs are justified only in these patients. Various preventative strategies have been tried, but none is superior to saline loading with

100–150 mL/hr starting 8–12 hours before the procedure and continuing for 3–4 hours afterwards.

VI. ANGIOTENSIN-CONVERTING ENZYME INHIBITORS/ ANGIOTENSIN RECEPTOR BLOCKERS AND RENAL DYSFUNCTION

Angiotensin-converting enzyme (ACE) inhibitors, and likely angiotensin receptor blockers as well, have demonstrated efficacy in slowing the progression of renal disease and should be used in patients with renal insufficiency (see Chapter 16). Nonetheless, in certain settings these drugs cause a reversible ARF through their effects on glomerular capillary hemodynamics. Reversible acute renal insufficiency has been observed with ACE inhibitors used to treat both hypertension and congestive heart failure. Severe acute renal failure may occur in patients with bilateral renal artery stenosis or renal artery stenosis in a solitary kidney. Similar cases are reported in patients with stenosis of the main renal artery to a renal transplant. Under all these circumstances, glomerular filtration pressure is dependent on angiotensin II–induced efferent arteriolar vasoconstriction. With a decline in efferent resistance induced by interference with the synthesis or action of this hormone, glomerular filtration pressure falls and acute renal dysfunction ensues. When acute renal dysfunction follows initiation of therapy with ACE inhibitors or angiotensin receptor blockers, underlying renal artery stenosis should be suspected. This complication is particularly likely in patients on diuretics or rigid sodium restriction.

Rapid recovery of renal function when the drug is stopped is evidence for a hemodynamic effect and against ischemic injury. In some patients with advanced parenchymal renal disease or renal transplants, however, renal dysfunction may be irreversible. Renal function (i.e., serum creatinine concentration) should be checked 1–2 weeks after initiating therapy in all patients at risk (older patients with diffuse vascular disease, patients with solitary functioning kidneys, patients on concomitant diuretics, and renal transplant patients). In patients with severe congestive heart failure, filtration fraction falls when the synthesis or action of angiotensin II is inhibited, and azotemia can result despite a decline in renal vascular resistance. This is a hemodynamic effect that can be reversed by judicious sodium repletion. Patients with diabetes and renal insufficiency or those on β-blockers should be monitored carefully for hyperkalemia if converting enzyme inhibitors or angiotensin II receptor blockers are used. Fever and eosinophilia have been reported due to ACE inhibitors without overt renal involvement. Thus, the relationship between these drugs and AIN remains unclear. Reversible membranous nephropathy has also been reported.

VII. NEPHROPATHY INDUCED BY CANCER CHEMOTHERAPEUTIC AGENTS

A. Platinum

The major limitation to platinum use in chemotherapeutic regimens is dose-dependent nephrotoxicity, particularly with cisplatin. Newer platinum analogs, such as carboplatin, are effective antineoplastic agents with reduced nephrotoxicity. Cisplatin nephrotoxicity is due to inhibition of tubular cell DNA synthesis. The concentration of platinum in the renal cortex is approximately six times that in other parts of the body, due to transport into the cell via the basolateral membrane of proximal tubular cells. Once in the cell, it is distributed through all subcellular components, producing cell damage.

Cisplatin nephropathy involves alteration of three distinct aspects of renal function. The most notable change is polyuria. Immediate polyuria, which develops during the first 24–48 hours following dosing, can be reversed by ADH and is suspected to be mediated by enhanced synthesis of prostaglandin E_2. A second phase of polyuria usually occurs between 72 and 96 hours after administration and is independent of either ADH or prostaglandin production. This late polyuria is associated with a reduction in GFR, the second manifestation of cisplatin nephrotoxicity. The third effect of cisplatin on the kidney is to increase magnesium excretion. More than 50% of all patients treated with cisplatin develop significant hypomagnesemia (serum values commonly <1 mEq/L). The most likely cause of this defect is a failure of tubular magnesium reabsorption.

Administration of cisplatin as a slow intravenous infusion is less likely to cause nephropathy. In addition, pretreatment with saline reduces toxicity. It is important that saline infusion and diuresis be maintained at between 100 and 200 mL/hr and be sustained for at least 6 hours after administration of the drug.

B. Nitrosoureas

Nitrosoureas such as methyl-CCNU and streptozotocin cause diffuse tubulointerstitial damage and tubular atrophy. With CCNU, delayed renal toxicity can occur in patients who have received more than 1400 mg/m^2. The appearance of a significant elevation of either blood urea nitrogen or serum creatinine concentration may be delayed up to 2 years after receiving the drug. In some patients, once renal insufficiency develops, a progressively downhill course ensues. Streptozotocin has been recognized as a significant nephrotoxin since its introduction. Up to two thirds of the patients receiving the compound develop either Fanconi's syndrome (aminoaciduria, glycosuria, renal phosphate wasting) or heavy proteinuria. Rarely, ARF can occur. Renal toxicity appears to have a threshold effect; significant abnormalities are rare at doses of 1 g/m^2/week or less.

C. Methotrexate

Methotrexate has a dose-dependent nephrotoxicity. With the advent of high-dose methotrexate therapy, the incidence of nephrotoxicity has risen. Acute renal failure is believed to be associated with precipitation of the 7-hydroxyl metabolite, which is less soluble than the parent compound. The combination of volume expansion and alkalinization of the urine minimizes renal dysfunction.

D. Other Chemotherapeutic Agents

Mithramycin is associated with a 33% prevalence of ARF. Acute renal failure appears to be dose dependent and is associated with necrosis in both the proximal and distal tubules. Mitomycin C therapy causes proteinuria, hematuria, or both. In some cases, severe microangiopathic hemolytic anemia develops. The histological changes in these instances resemble those of the hemolytic uremic syndrome. Glomerular changes, including mesangiolysis with fibrin thrombi, have also been noted.

Adriamycin has been studied extensively because of its ability to induce nephrosis in experimental animals. Due to the dose limiting cardiac toxicity in humans, adriamycin rarely manifests itself as a renal toxin.

VIII. IMMUNOSUPPRESSIVE DRUGS

A. Cyclosporine

Cyclosporine A is one of the primary immunosuppressive agents for recipients of renal and extrarenal allografts and is now being used to treat a variety of autoimmune disorders as well. The most frequent and potentially limiting consequence of cyclosporine treatment is nephrotoxicity (Table 2).

Table 2 Clinical Nephrological Manifestations of Cyclosporine Toxicity

Prolonged delayed graft function
Reversible episodes of acute renal dysfunction
Chronic cyclosporine-associated nephropathy
Reversible chronic depression of GFR
Progressive renal insufficiency
Hemolytic-uremic syndrome: thrombotic microangiopathy
Hypertension de novo or aggravating preexisting hypertension
Electrolyte disturbances: hyperkalemia, metabolic acidosis, hyperuricemia
Hypomagnesemia

Cyclosporine is metabolized by hepatic cytochrome P-450 mixed-function oxidase enzymes. Drugs that inhibit the cytochrome P-450 enzymes inhibit cyclosporine metabolism, sustaining high concentrations of this drug and potentiating nephrotoxicity, hypertension, and other side effects. Conversely, drugs that induce these enzymes reduce cyclosporine levels and lead to reductions in the drug's immunosuppressive action.

To highlight the importance of such interactions, ketoconazole, erythromycin, verapamil, and diltiazem have actually been used to reduce daily cyclosporine doses and thereby the cost of treatment. Inhibition of cyclosporine metabolism allows a ''therapeutic'' blood concentration with as little as 25% of the usual dose. Because hepatic metabolism is crucial for cyclosporine biotransformation, patients with liver dysfunction require downward adjustment of cyclosporine doses.

1. Acute Nephrotoxicity

Cyclosporine produces intense renal vasoconstriction. Previously unexposed vessels are sensitive to even small doses of the drug. This vasoconstriction reduces GFR and raises arterial blood pressure. Some degree of renal vasoconstriction is evident in virtually every patient who receives cyclosporine-based immunosuppressive therapy, regardless of peak and trough blood levels of the drug. Many renal transplant patients treated with cyclosporine develop one or more episodes of acute renal insufficiency (defined as a 25% increase in serum creatinine above baseline). These episodes rapidly improve when the cyclosporine dose is reduced. Although trough cyclosporine levels are often high in patients with acute cyclosporine nephrotoxicity, a normal or low level does not exclude the diagnosis. In some circumstances, cyclosporine may act synergistically with rejection to produce renal dysfunction. Because these episodes are sometimes difficult to distinguish from acute rejection, biopsy of the renal allograft is occasionally necessary to exclude treatable rejection.

Rejection can be diagnosed with confidence if a diffuse interstitial infiltrate, arteritis, or tubulitis is present. Cyclosporine nephrotoxicity is manifested by arteriolar hyalinosis, but this characteristic finding is only occasionally present. If the transplant biopsy fails to show acute rejection, particularly if arteriolar hyalinosis is present, dose reductions are indicated in an attempt to avoid chronic tubulointerstitial fibrosis.

2. Chronic Nephropathy

Progressive renal insufficiency is well documented in organ transplant recipients who receive cyclosporine for over 12 months. Long-term cyclosporine-treated renal transplant recipients, as a group, also have lower GFRs than comparable patients treated with azathioprine. Chronic renal dysfunction occurs in liver transplant recipients and in patients receiving long-term cyclosporine therapy for autoimmune disease. Approximately 5% of patients with successful heart transplants require dialysis for end-stage renal disease due to chronic cyclosporine nephrotoxicity.

While excessive doses of cyclosporine may play a role in initiating chronic nephrotoxicity, the condition may progress despite dose reduction. In some patients, discontinuation of cyclosporine results in rapid improvement in renal function. Biopsy findings in recipients of kidneys and other solid organs as well as autoimmune disease show afferent arteriolopathy, striped and chronic tubulointerstitial fibrosis, and focal glomerulosclerosis (Table 3). Cumulative

Table 3 Renal Histopathology in Cyclosporine-Treated Allograft Recipients

Clinical condition	Findings	Comments
Acute renal dysfunction	Proximal tubule cell vacuolization; microcalcification in tubule cells	Nonspecific, probably a maker of cyclosporine treatment as tubule function is preserved; cell necrosis absent
	Glomerular capillary thrombi	Associated with poor graft outcome; can be noted in grafts without cyclosporine and in grafts with stable function
	Obliterative arteriopathy in interlobar and arcuate vessels of varying severity; patchy cell necrosis	May produce microangiopathic hemolytic anemia and thrombocytopenia; results in graft loss; found in approximately 10% of cases
Initial oligoanuria with ARF	Arteriole wall hyalinosis	Present with prolonged renal failure; may be permanent; infrequently found
	Diffuse interstitial fibrosis	Renal failure may be partially reversible; seen primarily in nonbeating heart cadaver donors
	Normal posttransplant biopsy results	Most frequent finding in first 3–4 weeks posttransplant
Chronic renal dysfunction	Striped pattern of tubulointerstitial fibrosis, glomerulosclerosis	Irreversible changes; associated frequently with hypertension
	Hyalinosis and sclerosis of arterioles and small arteries	May be observed in normotensive patients

cyclosporine dose, frequent episodes of acute renal dysfunction, prolonged high trough levels, arterial hypertension, and concomitant immunological assault on the kidney combine to produce chronic cyclosporine nephrotoxicity in renal transplantation. The chronic nephrotoxicity of cyclosporine can be dissociated from the drug's acute vasoconstrictive action, but the mechanism is unclear. It may involve activation of the renin angiotensin system.

3. Hemolytic-Uremic Syndrome/Thrombotic Microangiopathy

In some patients treated with cyclosporine, fulminant ARF and thrombocytopenia develop. This syndrome occurs primarily in bone marrow transplant recipients but can also occur in other settings. In renal transplantation, this type of vasculopathy carries a poor prognosis for the allograft. Histological examination of the kidneys reveals arteriolar lesions similar to those of the hemolytic-uremic syndrome with thrombotic microangiopathy and occasionally afferent arteriolar thrombosis.

B. Tacrolimus

Tacrolimus is a potent immunosuppressive agent now used in about one third of solid organ transplants in place of cyclosporine. Although it binds to a different intracellular target molecule, tacrolimus is similar to cyclosporine in that it inhibits interleukin-2 gene transcription early in the T-cell activation cascade. It produces both acute and chronic nephrotoxicity that is indistinguishable from that produced by cyclosporine. Tacrolimus may produce less increase in peripheral vascular resistance than cyclosporine, but this appears to be offset by tacrolimus-associated increases in renal vascular resistance.

IX. NEPHROTOXICITY DUE TO NONSTEROIDAL ANTI-INFLAMMATORY DRUGS

NSAIDs are widely prescribed and effective analgesic and anti-inflammatory drugs. Many drugs of this class are now available without prescription. It has been estimated that 30–40 million people use NSAIDs on any given day in the United States. With this common use has come the realization that a number of adverse renal syndromes occur, particularly in patients with risk factors such as congestive heart failure, cirrhosis, preexisting renal disease, age greater than 65 years, diuretic therapy, or reduction of actual or ''effective'' extracellular fluid volume (Table 4).

Table 4 Renal Syndromes Due to NSAIDs

ARF
Renal dysfunction due to enhanced renal vasoconstriction
AIN with heavy proteinuria
ARF, flank pain, and hematuria
Acute cortical necrosis
Renal papillary necrosis/CRF
Worsening hypertension
Sodium and water retention
Hyperkalemia due to hyporeninemic hypoaldosteronism

A. Vasoconstrictive ARF

The most common type of NSAID nephrotoxicity is due to inhibition of renal prostaglandins synthesis. Although local production of prostaglandins does not ordinarily play an important role in maintaining renal function, synthesis of these locally acting vasodilators is critical for maintaining GFR under conditions of generalized vasoconstriction, (e.g., volume depletion, congestive heart failure). When this local adaptation is inhibited by NSAIDs, unopposed renal vasoconstriction leads to an abrupt fall in GFR. This adverse effect is rapidly reversible when the drug is discontinued. All of the available chemical classes of NSAIDs cause this syndrome by virtue of their inhibition of cyclooxygenase, a key enzyme for prostaglandin synthesis. Vasoconstrictive renal dysfunction due to NSAIDs is characterized by an abrupt rise in blood urea nitrogen and creatinine and sodium retention. Some or all of the above-mentioned risk factors are usually present. As opposed to ischemic ARF, fractional sodium excretion is low despite the presence of azotemia, and the urine sediment shows no abnormalities.

B. Papillary Necrosis

Renal papillary necrosis has been linked to NSAIDs by virtue of the ability of these drugs to produce medullary ischemia. Many patients have underlying renal disease or are taking other analgesic drugs. Similar to compound analgesics, long-term exposure to NSAIDs can lead to chronic renal insufficiency, which develops slowly over 4–5 years. Population studies show an increased risk for renal failure in patients receiving continuous therapy with NSAIDs, but the specific etiology is unclear.

C. Interstitial Nephritis

Rarely, interstitial nephritis occurs in patients taking NSAIDs. The most common presentation of this interstitial nephritis is the combination of nephrotic syndrome and renal insufficiency. In contrast to antibiotic-induced AIN, fever, skin rash, and eosinophilia are present in less than 20% of cases. Nephrotic syndrome can sometime occur without acute renal dysfunction, and ARF can occur without heavy proteinuria. Typically, the patient has been taking the NSAID for months prior to the development of edema or renal failure. When such patients undergo renal biopsy, glomeruli most frequently show minimal glomerular changes with epithelial cell foot process fusion. The interstitial infiltrate is composed predominantly of thymic-derived lymphocytes. Recovery from renal failure is the rule, although improvement may take months. Remission of minimal-change pathology occurs when the offending drug is withdrawn, but relapse without further drug exposure has been described. Steroid therapy is frequently used, although there is no proof of its efficacy. The minimal-change lesion can progress to focal glomerular sclerosis even when the offending drug is stopped. Although a rare complications of NSAIDs, this is one of the more common causes of interstitial nephritis.

D. Sodium and Water Retention

Sodium retention caused by NSAIDs is seldom clinically relevant unless underlying cardiac, liver, or renal disease is present. In such patients, NSAIDs-induced prostaglandin inhibition causes resistance to diuretics and worsening edema. Prostaglandin inhibition also leads to heightened sensitivity of the kidney to vasopressin with a tendency to water retention and hyponatremia. The sodium retention caused by NSAIDs can also exacerbate hypertension or blunt the effects of antihypertensive therapy.

E. Hyperkalemia

Hyperkalemia due to inhibition of the renin-angiotensin system can be a serious problem with NSAIDs. Diabetics and patients on beta blockers or converting enzyme inhibitors are at particular risk. The increase in serum potassium with NSAIDs is greater in patients with underlying renal failure.

F. Anaphylaxis

Anaphylactic reactions with circulatory shock have been reported within 1 hour of NSAID ingestion. A variety of chemical types of cyclooxygenase inhibitors have been implicated. A history of previous brief drug exposure is noted in many, but not all, cases. Acute cortical necrosis has also been associated with over-the-counter ibuprofen without other apparent risk factors for vasoconstrictive ARF.

X. ANALGESIC NEPHROPATHY

Chronic renal damage due to excessive and prolonged use of analgesic mixtures remains a prominent cause of end-stage renal disease in some European countries. In the United States, its prevalence, significance, and economic impact are unknown. Because analgesic-associated nephropathy is a preventable cause of ESRD, it is important to recognize it early and discontinue the offending agents.

A. Clinical Presentation

Clinical signs and symptoms are nonspecific and include loss of urinary concentrating capacity, sodium wasting, hypocalcemia, and defective urinary acidification. A rise in serum creatinine heralds the development of renal insufficiency. Associated complications include hypertension, recurrent urinary tract infections, and anemia. Early in the course, histological evidence of analgesic-induced injury is confined to the medullary portion of the kidney. With continuing exposure, cortical involvement ensues with the renal biopsy, yielding a diagnosis of chronic interstitial nephritis without specific cause. The diagnostic finding of most use clinically is papillary necrosis.

B. Epidemiology

As its name indicates, analgesic nephropathy (AN) is directly related to the regular long-term consumption of substantial amounts of analgesics. In early literature, AN was generally referred to as ''phenacetin nephritis'' due to the belief that phenacetin was the offending agent. In some countries that have banned phenacetin without limiting access to analgesics, however, there has been no corresponding decline in the incidence of AN (Table 5). The incidence of AN varies widely and can be correlated with the sales and consumption of analgesic mixtures. In Europe, there is an inverse correlation between the prevalence of analgesic nephropathy and the incidence of ESRD of unknown cause. This is likely true in the United States as well because specific causes for ESRD are rarely sought in patients with advanced chronic renal insufficiency. Local pockets of analgesic nephropathy are known to occur in the southeastern United States. This phenomenon of local areas of high prevalence is also seen in other countries. National sales figures of combined analgesics, including those available for over-the-counter sales, correlate with the incidence of ESRD due to analgesic-induced disease in European countries (Table 6). Similar national or regional data are not available in the United States, although sales are high and advertising intense.

Table 5 Case-Control Studies Demonstrating an Association between analgesic intake and renal failure

Study location	Cases, No. and Dx[a]	Controls, No. and type	Definition of minimal abuse	Principal results—OR[b] (95% CI)
United States, 1983	257 ESRF patients	1047 hospitalized patients	Almost daily for 30 days	1.1 (0.8–1.5)
Australia, 1982	80 RPN women	80 healthy women	3 units/week for one year	17.2 (8.5–34.7)
United States, 1989	554 CRF patients	516 population based	Daily for one	2.8 (1.8–4.2)
Germany, 1989	517 ESRF patients	517 outpatients	15 units/month for one year	2.4 (1.8–3.4)
Spain, 1990	340 ESRF patients	673 hospitalized patients	15 units/month for 30 days	2.9 (1.8–4.7)

[a] ESRF = End-stage renal failure; RPN = renal papillary necrosis; CRF = chronic renal failure.
[b] Odds ratios (OR) with 95% confidence interval (CI), estimating the risk for the development of renal impairment after analgesic abuse (Randhawa et al., 1993).
Source: Adapted from deMatos et al., 1997.

Table 6 Analgesic Nephropathy in European Countries

	% Incidence[a]					% Prevalence 1990†		
Country	1986	1987	1988	1989	1986–1989	Dialysis	Grafted	Total
Switzerland	17.8	18.6	18.0	18.4	18.2	21.7	13.5	16.5
Belgium	11.1	10.0	12.9	10.5	11.2	15.5	3.0	9.8
Austria	6.0	10.2	8.0	7.5	8.0	8.2	4.0	6.4
FR Germany	5.7	5.0	5.7	5.1	5.4	6.2	2.6	4.8
DD Germany	4.7	2.5	5.0	5.7	4.5	4.4	1.1	3.3
Czechoslovakia	5.4	5.7	3.7	4.6	4.8	4.2	3.2	4.1
Denmark	6.3	5.8	3.2	1.1	4.3	3.8	3.0	3.9
Netherlands	5.0	3.4	3.1	2.9	3.5	3.7	2.0	2.9
Portugal	2.2	2.8	2.9	3.1	2.8	3.0	0.7	2.5
Yugoslavia	1.6	1.5	1.7	1.6	1.6	1.8	1.1	1.5

[a] Incidence data on total number of new end-stage renal failure patients entering chronic renal replacement therapy.

[b] Total prevalence data on all patients alive December 31, 1990, including dialysis patients, grafted patients, and patients whose treatment is unknown (N. H. Selwood, 1990, personal communication).

XI. LEAD NEPHROTOXICITY

Lead use and clinical lead poisoning dates back to ancient times and has continued throughout history. Gout, which was felt to be more common in the rich and intellectual classes of eighteenth-century Europe, was probably due in large part to addition of lead to wine. The causal link between lead exposure and chronic nephropathy was first recognized in the late nineteenth century. Clinical and epidemiological observations in Europe, Australia, and the United States have now made it clear that environmental or occupational lead exposure can lead to chronic renal failure and excess renal death. Government regulation now limits most occupational lead exposure, but isolated cases still are reported among, e.g., painters, art restorers, welders, and plumbers. Currently the major sources of lead arise from environmental pollution due primarily to leaded gasoline, steel production, and coal processing.

A. Diagnosis

The diagnosis of excess lead exposure is difficult. Blood lead concentrations reflect recent but not cumulative exposure. Furthermore, 90% of blood lead is associated with red cells, requiring a correction for anemia. Mobilization and urinary excretion of greater than 650 μg of lead following two 1-g doses of the chelating agent EDTA gives the best current assessment of total body lead burden. The value of the test is maximized when lead excretion after EDTA is compared to a 24-hour baseline excretion value. With this dose of EDTA there has been no nephrotoxicity. Renal failure per se does not interfere with the body content of mobilizable lead. Basal and post-EDTA collection periods should be extended to 4 days in patients with impaired GFR. Excess body burdens of lead have been documented in some patients with renal dysfunction that was thought to be secondary to gout and hypertensive nephrosclerosis. Data from patients with mild renal insufficiency given EDTA as a diagnostic test or from dialysis patients with bone lead determined from an iliac crest biopsy suggest that lead nephropathy still exists and is underdiagnosed.

B. Pathogenesis

The pathogenesis of lead nephropathy is unclear. Nuclear inclusion bodies in proximal tubule epithelium probably include a lead-binding protein that sequesters intracellular lead. Children with acute lead intoxication develop reversible proximal tubule dysfunction and Fanconi's syndrome, generally without progression to renal failure. With chronic lead exposure, the renal pathological features are nonspecific. Specifically, lead inclusion bodies are not observed. Instead, shrunken kidneys, interstitial fibrosis, tubular atrophy, and nephrosclerosis are seen. Vascular lesions can be extensive even without clinical hypertension.

1. Clinical Presentations

Clinical presentation is usually subtle, with an unremarkable urinary sediment, minimal proteinuria, hyperuricemia, and hypertension being the only features. Recurrent gouty arthritis affects half the patients. Any woman with symptomatic gout and renal dysfunction should prompt consideration of lead nephropathy, because there is an overwhelming male predominance of idiopathic gout. Age-adjusted blood lead levels have been shown to correlate directly with diastolic blood pressure. An increased prevalence of hypertension due to lead could add to other renal insults. Chronic lead exposure in humans suppresses plasma renin concentration and blunts the renin response to sodium deprivation.

2. Treatment

When excess body burden of lead is documented, low-dose chelation treatment with 1 g of EDTA in procaine given intramuscularly three times per week may be useful, depending on the extent of preexisting chronic renal damage. Normalization of the EDTA lead mobilization test defines the endpoint of therapy, although actual documentation of improved renal function is limited. Other chelating compounds such as 2,3-dimercaptopropane sulfonate and 2,3-dimercaptosuccinic acid can be administered orally and are tolerated well.

XII. CADMIUM NEPHROTOXICITY

Cadmium is widely used in industry and when absorbed into the body has a biological half-life exceeding 10 years. Once in the body, cadmium accumulates in the liver and kidneys. In proximal tubule cells, it is bound to a cystine-rich protein metallothionein. This protein synthesized in the liver transfers bound cadmium to the kidneys via the bloodstream. The cadmium-metallothionein complex is nephrotoxic after pinocytosis and accumulation in the lysosomes of proximal tubule cells. Most renal disease from cadmium in humans is a result of prolonged low-dose exposure in the workplace or environment. Blood cadmium concentrations fall rapidly after exposure, as cadmium is bound in the liver. Urinary excretion does not increase until a renal cortical threshold cadmium concentration of 100–300 ng/g cortex is exceeded. This renal cortical threshold corresponds roughly to a total body cadmium content of 160–170 mg. Urinary cadmium excretion of >20 μg/L or 10 μg/g creatinine denotes excessive body cadmium even if blood levels are normal. The threshold renal concentration correlates roughly with proximal tubule dysfunction.

Clinically, proximal tubule dysfunction due to cadmium is characterized by aminoaciduria, glycosuria, renal tubular acidosis, and excretion of low molecular weight proteins such as β_2-microglobulin. Nephrolithiasis and metabolic bone disease with fractures resulting from urinary mineral losses usually dominate the clinical picture. Overt chronic renal failure is unusual despite proximal tubule dysfunction. In a Japanese village, cadmium-polluted rice and water led to widespread painful bone disease with fractures, associated with Fanconi's syndrome. This cadmium-related syndrome was known as ''itai itai'' (''ouch ouch''), describing the painful fractures. Postmenopausal women who had superimposed age- and diet-related problems with bone mineralization were most severely affected, with some developing overt renal failure. Interstitial nephritis is the histological picture most often observed in the limited pathological material available. In most cases, cadmium-related tubule dysfunction is irreversible even when the patient is protected from further exposure.

XIII. RENAL CONSEQUENCES OF ILLICIT DRUG USE

A substantial portion of patients who use illicit drugs develop proteinuria and renal failure due to focal glomerular sclerosis. As many as 10% of patients entering some ESRD programs have methamphetamine, heroin, or cocaine-associated nephropathy. Illicit drugs are often prepared as powder diluted with lactose, mannitol, sucrose, or quinine and injected intravenously subcutaneously. Sharing of needles and paraphernalia is common and leads to viral infections (e.g., hepatitis, HIV) that are also associated with renal disease. Although these infections are also associated with renal failure, it is clear that the drugs (and/or impurities in the diluting solutions) are also responsible. ATN due to rhabdomyolysis and coma often follows heroin or methadone overdose. A necrotizing angiitis occurs in heroin addicts that is indistinguishable from idiopathic polyarteritis nodosa. Severe hypertension, proteinuria, and hematuria with renal dysfunction are part of a multisystem illness. Renal angiography demonstrates aneurysmal dilatations of medium-sized renal vessels. The mortality rate is high, and acute and chronic vasculitis is noted throughout the body. Multiple drug use is common and methamphetamines have also been implicated in the vasculitis syndrome.

More common in heroin or cocaine addicts is nephrotic syndrome progressing over a few months to severe renal failure. Renal biopsy most frequently shows focal and segmental glomerular sclerosis, which can progress rapidly to a more global sclerosis. Various degrees of tubular atrophy and interstitial fibrosis are observed. Focal renal deposition of IgM and C3 are common, suggesting an immune-mediated pathogenesis. Diffuse deposition of IgG is also reported. Renal function may stabilize if narcotic withdrawal can be achieved.

Amyloidosis can cause nephropathy in heroin addicts who develop suppurative skin infections from unsterile subcutaneous injections. Nephrotic syndrome from amyloidosis frequently progresses to renal failure despite discontinuation of heroin and treatment of any infection.

XIV. RENAL DISEASE DUE TO PENICILLAMINE

Penicillamine has been used to treat Wilson's disease, cystinuria, severe rheumatoid arthritis, and scleroderma with some success. Proteinuria and nephrotic syndrome are the most common manifestations of renal disease secondary to penicillamine. Fewer percent of patients with rheumatoid arthritis treated with penicillamine over 3 years, develop proteinuria with the incidence peaking during the second 6 months of treatment. Proteinuria appears to occur in patients who receive higher doses. Proteinuria disappears with drug withdrawal, usually within 6–12 months.

The most common histopathological change in proteinuric patients is membranous nephropathy. Discrete deposits of immunoglobulins in the glomerular basement membrane and circulating antibodies to penicillamine have been demonstrated. Other clinical and pathological renal manifestations of penicillamine include rapidly progressive glomerulonephritis with crescents, AIN, minimal-change nephrotic syndrome with IgM deposition, and a systemic lupus-like picture. Pulse methylprednisolone therapy and plasma exchange have been reported to favorably influence these aggressive manifestations of penicillamine nephropathy.

XV. GOLD NEPHROPATHY

Gold salts are used therapeutically for rheumatoid arthritis, and their association with the nephrotic syndrome is well documented. The prevalence of proteinuria in gold-treated persons is approximately 3%; however, most have 24-hour protein excretion values of <3 g. The majority of patients demonstrate a membranous pattern of glomerular immune complex deposition, but minimal-change pathology and mesangial and subendothelial electron dense deposits have also been described. If gold is withdrawn, proteinuria disappears within 6–12 months in most patients. Renal insufficiency is distinctly unusual; however, reversible renal failure and severe nephrotic syndrome have been described. Oral gold salts are less likely than parenteral preparations to be associated with proteinuria.

The pathogenesis of gold-induced nephropathy is unclear. Tubular proteinuria, β_2-microglobulinuria, and excretion in the urine of renal tubule epithelial cell antigens are common in gold-treated patients. However, these changes correlate poorly with the total dose of gold. Renal tubule epithelial cell antigen can be demonstrated by indirect immunofluorescence in glomerular deposits. Renal toxicity during gold or penicillamine treatment for rheumatoid arthritis is strongly associated with HLA-DR3 and HLA-B8 histocompatibility antigens, suggesting a genetic link to this disease and its treatment.

XVI. HEAVY METALS AND THE KIDNEY

Although mercury salts produce experimental ARF, their role in human disease is limited to industrial or accidental exposures. Mercury, largely from vapors, remains an occupational hazard in mining and in manufacturing alloys, mirrors, and batteries. Mercury in its elemental form is virtually harmless when ingested, but biotransformation to organic and inorganic salts may occur in industrial and agricultural processes. The various chemical forms of mercury accumulate in proximal tubule cells. Toxicity is determined by intracellular reactions with sulfhydryl groups, lysosomes, and phospholipid membranes. The diagnosis of mercury-induced renal disease depends on a known exposure plus renal dysfunction, as many workers have enhanced urinary mercury excretion, apparently without adverse effects on the kidney.

Accidental or suicidal ingestion of as little as 0.5 g of mercuric chloride leads to oliguric acute renal failure with proximal tubule necrosis. The clinical picture is dominated in the first few days by gastrointestinal hemorrhage and erosive gastritis. Prognosis for renal recovery is excellent with modern supportive care. Administration of intravenous BAL (2,3-dimercaptopropanol) prior to oliguria in the first 24–48 hours may limit the extent of renal-disease.

Mercury may also be a triggering agent for immune reactions leading to proteinuria and nephrotic syndrome. Membranous glomerulopathy is most often noted on renal biopsy, but minimal glomerular changes and antiglomerular basement membrane antibody deposition are also described. Immune-mediated glomerulonephritis probably occurs as a genetically determined idiosyncratic response. Methyl mercury poisoning by industrial effluent in Japan produced neurological disease in several hundred adults who ingested contaminated fish. Minor proximal tubule dysfunction without azotemia was the only renal consequence observed.

Uranyl nitrate is also used in the study of ARF in animals. In humans, exposure is limited to low-level industrial sources. Renal excretion of amino acids and β_2-microglobulin were increased in uranium workers compared to unexposed age-matched controls. Similar tubular dysfunction has resulted from exposure to chromium and bismuth. Arsenic and arsine gas (AsH_3) poisoning may cause ARF, in association with massive hemolysis and circulatory collapse. Arsenic contamination of moonshine whiskey can produce irreversible patchy cortical necrosis. Thallium, copper, nickel, antimony, and silver can all produce acute toxic renal syndromes, but reports are extremely rare.

XVII. NEPHROPATHIES ASSOCIATED WITH OTHER ENVIRONMENTAL TOXICANTS

Although some types of renal injury are associated with environmental or industrial exposure, a firm causal relationship between prolonged exposure and disease is unclear. Organic solvents and glomerulonephritis have been associated in epidemiological case-control and cross-sectional studies. However, many of these were methodologically flawed. Only a few studies make a strong case for a causal relationship.

SUGGESTED READINGS

Bennett WM, deMattos A, Meyer M, Andoh T, Barry JM. Chronic cyclosporine nephropathy: the Achilles' heel of immunosuppressive therapy. Kidney Int 1996; 50:1089–1100.

Bennett WM, Henrich WL, Stoff JS. The renal effects of non-steroidal anti-inflammatory drugs: summary and recommendations. Am J Kidney Dis 1996; 28:556–562.

Bennett WM. Clinical aspects of nephrotoxicity. In: Goldstein R, ed. Oxford, England: Pergamon, 1997, pp. 1–19.

Bennett WM. Immunosuppressive drug nephrotoxicity. In: Tilney NL, Strom TB, Paul LC, eds. Transplantation Biology: Cellular and Molecular Aspects. Philadelphia: Lippincott-Raven, 1996, pp. 587–600.

Bennett WM. Mechanisms of aminoglycoside nephrotoxicity. Clin Exp Pharmacol Physiol 1989; 16:1–6.

Branch RA. Prevention of amphotericin B-induced renal impairment: a review of the use of sodium supplementation. Arch Intern Med 1988; 148:2389–2394.

deMattos AM, Olyaei AJ, Bennett WM. Mechanisms and risks of immunosuppressive therapy. In: Neilson EG, Couser WG, eds. Immunologic Renal Diseases. Philadelphia: Lippincott-Raven, 1997, pp. 861–885.

Elseviers MM, Bosteels V, Cambier P, De Paepe M, Godon JP, Lins R, Lornoy W, Mathys E, Moeremans C, Roose R, Theelen B, Van Caesbroeck D, Verbanck J, De Broe ME. Diagnostic criteria of analgesic nephropathy in patients with end-stage renal failure: results of the Belgian study. Nephrol Dial Transplant 1992; 7:479–486.

Gilbert DN. Once daily aminoglycoside dosing. Antimicrob Agents Chemother 1992; 36: 121–124.

Giroux L, Bettez P, Giroux L. Mitomycin-C nephrotoxicity: a clinico-pathologic study of 17 cases. Am J Kidney Dis 1985; 6:28–39.

Henrich WL, Agodoa LE, Barrett B, Bennett WM, Blantz RC, Buckalew VM, D'Agati VD, DeBroe ME, Duggin GG, Eknoyan G, Elseviers MM, Gomez A, Matzke GR, Porter GA, Sabatini S, Stoff JS, Striker GE, Winchester JF. Analgesics and the Kidney: Summary and Recommendations to the Scientific Advisory Board of the National Kidney Foundation from an Ad Hoc Committee of the National Kidney Foundation. Am J Kidney Dis 1996; 27:162–165.

Perico N, Ruggenenti P, Gaspari P, Moscini L, Benigni A, Amuchastequi CS, Gasparini F, Remuzzi G. Daily renal hypoperfusion induced by cyclosporine in patients with renal transplantation. Transplantation 1992; 54:56–60.

Randhawa PS, Shapiro R, Jordan ML, Starzl TE, Demetris AJ. The histopathological changes associated with allograft rejection and drug toxicity in renal transplant recipients maintained on FK506. Am J Surg Pathol 1993; 17:60–68.

Rudnick MR, Berns JS, Cohen RM. Contrast media-associated nephrotoxicity. Curr Opin Nephrol Hypertens 1996; 5:127–133.

Schacht RG, Feiner HD, Gallo GR, Lieberman A, Baldwin DS. Nephrotoxicity of nitrosoureas. Cancer 1981; 48:1328–1334.

Shuler C, Bennett WM. Antimicrobial nephrotoxicity. In: Massry S, Glassock RJ, eds. Textbook of Nephrology. Baltimore: Williams and Wilkins, 1995, pp. 930–935.

Swan SK, Bennett WM. Nephrotoxic Acute Renal Failure. In: Lazarus M, Brenner B, eds. Acute Renal Failure. New York: Churchill Livingstone, 1993, pp. 357–392.

21

Management of Kidney Stones

Melanie P. Derman
Beth Israel Deaconess, Boston, Massachusetts

David A. Bushinsky
University of Rochester Medical Center, Rochester, New York

I. KIDNEY STONE FORMATION

The kidney has the dual task of excreting relatively insoluble waste and conserving water. The waste must be excreted without forming a solid phase, a kidney stone, which would interfere with kidney function and cause considerable morbidity. Stones can form when the concentrations of the ions that form the solid phase increase to where they become insoluble in the urine. When these concentrations are achieved, the urine is "supersaturated" with respect to a solid phase and the ions may precipitate and form a kidney stone. This small stone may be washed out of the renal tubule and excreted into the urine. Alternatively, the crystal may adhere to the urothelium and increase in size, leading to a clinically significant kidney stone. There are several urinary proteins, including Tamm-Horsfall protein and nephrocalcin, that help to protect against stone formation by inhibiting formation of a solid phase in a supersaturated solution. The goal of management of patients who have formed a kidney stone is to decrease urinary supersaturation so that stones do not recur. At present we cannot regulate inhibitor proteins.

II. GENERAL CONSIDERATIONS

Up to 10% of Americans experience at least one kidney stone in their lifetime. Seventy percent of kidney stones consist primarily of calcium (calcium oxalate or phosphate). The remainder consist of uric acid (~10%), struvite (~20%), and cystine (<1%). With the exception of uric acid stones, all are radio-opaque. Because the pathophysiology and therapy of these stones differ, it is important to have all stones analyzed for content in order to direct appropriate therapy.

A. Clinical Presentation

The typical presentation of acute nephrolithiasis is renal colic. The patient complains of sudden severe flank pain that migrates anteriorly and then to the groin as the stone moves along the urinary tract to the bladder. The patient may also complain of nausea, vomiting, and exhibit gross hematuria. Dysuria and urgency may be experienced as the stone approaches the uterovesicular junction. In contrast, some kidney stones develop painlessly and are only detected on routine radiographs. Patients with infection stones often present without pain but with recurrent or refractory urinary tract infections

B. Acute Management

In a reliable and young patient, the initial evaluation of renal colic can be limited to a careful history, physical examination, urinalysis and serum electrolytes, blood urea nitrogen, and creatinine. The urinalysis typically demonstrates microscopic hematuria, although this finding is often absent in the setting of complete urinary obstruction. Evidence of urinary tract infection in patients with renal colic, that is, with a urinalysis showing more than 3 white blood cells per high-powered field or prominent bacteria, should prompt a urine culture and more aggressive intervention. In such cases one should undertake an imaging procedure (see below for options) for evidence of obstruction, because infection in the setting of obstruction can lead to rapid destruction of the renal parenchyma.

Imaging in the acute setting is appropriate if there is evidence of renal dysfunction or concern for infection. Although a plain abdominal radiograph is often obtained in the emergency room evaluation of renal colic, this study is neither sensitive nor specific when used alone. An intravenous pyelogram (IVP) or renal ultrasound may be more appropriate. An IVP allows evaluation of the entire urinary tract with one image, whereas ultrasound avoids the risks of radiocontrast dye and radiation. More recently clinicians have begun using a helical CT scan without radiocontrast dye. This latter technique has been found to be a rapid and cost-effective method for establishing the diagnosis of nephrolithiasis in the acute setting.

Initial treatment should emphasize pain control and either oral or intravenous hydration. Reliable patients who can achieve adequate pain control with oral analgesics can be managed at home with strict instructions to seek medical attention if (1) pain worsens, (2) pain does not resolve in 72 hours, or (3) a fever develops. Furthermore, patients should be instructed to strain their urine for 72 hours following the resolution of pain. Finally, follow-up should be arranged within several weeks to address the cause of the stone. In contrast, patients who have evidence of altered renal function or infection require immediate intervention either by urological approach to remove the obstructing stone or by interventional radiology to provide temporary relief of obstruction via percutaneous nephrostomy. In addition, stones that have a diameter of >7 mm are unlikely to pass without intervention and should have prompt urological referral.

In patients who cannot achieve pain control with oral analgesics, parenteral analgesia is required. Historically, analgesia was achieved with narcotics (e.g., morphine sulfate or meperidine). Parenteral nonsteroidal anti-inflammatory drugs, however, are also effective and have become increasingly popular because sedation can be avoided. There is a risk of producing renal dysfunction with these drugs, particularly if used in patients with volume depletion or those who receive intravenous radiocontrast dye (see Table 1).

C. Evaluation of the Patient with a Single Stone

The National Institutes of Health consensus conference on prevention and treatment of kidney stones recommended that all patients who have formed a single stone have a basic evaluation to identify easily remediable causes of nephrolithiasis (Table 2). All stones should be analyzed to guide subsequent treatment.

The evaluation begins with a history and physical examination. The history includes a careful review of the patient's stone episodes beginning with a detailed account of the first stone passage and every occurrence thereafter. The account

Table 1 Acute Management of the Nephrolithiasis Patient

Diagnosis	History Physical examination CBC Serum chemistry Urinalysis
Radiological imaging possibilities	Ultrasound IVP Noncontrast helical CT
Analgesia	Narcotic NSAIDS
Follow-up	

Table 2 Evaluation of Patient with a History of a Single Kidney Stone

- Stone history
  - Age at onset
  - Associated symptoms
  - Number
  - Type
  - Previous therapy
- Past medical history
  - Detailed general history
  - Inquire specifically about;
    - hypercalcemic disorders
    - malabsorptive disorders
    - renal insufficiency
    - urinary tract infections
- Medications
  - Prescribed
  - Over the counter
  - Herbal/Unconventional remedies
- Family history
- Social history
  - Occupation
  - Exercise
- Oral intake
  - Diet
  - Fluids
- Physical examination
- Laboratory data
  - Stone analysis
  - Urinalysis
    - Crystals
    - Cells
    - Evidence of infection (send for culture)
  - Screen for cystine
    - Cyanide nitroprusside test
  - Blood chemistry
    - Electrolytes
    - Creatinine
    - Calcium (if elevated, check PTH)
    - Phosphorus
    - Uric acid
- Imaging
  - Kidney, ureter, and bladder or plain film of abdomen
- Possibilities
  - Intravenous pyelogram
  - Ultrasound

should include presenting and associated symptoms and whether the stone passed spontaneously or required surgical intervention. Inquiry into the past medical history should also probe for evidence of hypercalcemic disorders such as hyperparathyroidism or granulomatous diseases, malabsorptive disorders, renal insufficiency, and urinary tract infections. All medications, including vitamins or unconventional remedies, should be listed. A family history of nephrolithiasis is an important finding because several types of stone disease are hereditary. Idiopathic hypercalciuria appears to be inherited, and the gene defects that result in cystinuria and primary hyperoxaluria have been identified.

Occupation and recreation can also play an important role in stone formation. Patients whose jobs involve physical labor or whose nonwork activity includes regular exercise may have large insensible fluid losses without adequate replenishment. Those who drive long distances may avoid fluid intake to minimize the need for micturition. Even patients who believe they are ingesting adequate fluid may actually drink little water. Ingestion of large amounts of cola, tea, or other caffeinated beverages may contribute to nephrolithiasis. Although some carbonated beverages contain citric acid, an inhibitor of calcium oxalate crystallization, most colas contain phosphoric acid, and absorbed phosphate may increase calcium and uric acid excretion. Traditional black tea is high in oxalate and the diuretic effect of caffeinated beverages can contribute to volume depletion and cause a subsequent decrease in urinary volume. Physical examination is often normal but may identify contributing factors such as tophacious gout or an immobilizing illness.

Laboratory evaluation should begin with a urinalysis. An elevated specific gravity suggests inadequate fluid intake, which clearly contributes to increasing urinary supersaturation and stone formation. A urinary pH of <6 is typical for patients with uric acid stones, whereas an elevated urinary pH creates a favorable milieu for the precipitation of calcium phosphate and should raise the concern for renal tubular acidosis or infection with urease-producing bacteria. Proteinuria is not characteristic of nephrolithiasis and may indicate intrinsic renal disease. Examination of the urine sediment may demonstrate hematuria if there is active stone disease or evidence of infection if more than 3 white blood cells per high-powered field or prominent bacteria are present. Crystalluria is diagnostically important if either cystine or triple phosphate crystals are seen. However, other crystals, such as uric acid or calcium oxalate, can be present in normal urine and are not indicative of a tendency to form stones. A urine culture should be performed if there is pyuria or bacteruria, and an aliquot of urine should be sent for cystine screening.

Serum should be sent for electrolytes, blood urea nitrogen, creatinine, calcium (which should be checked on at least two occasions), phosphate, uric acid, and albumin concentrations. This laboratory evaluation should identify patients with abnormal renal function, evidence of renal tubular acidosis, hypokalemia, dehydration (hypernatremia), hypercalcemia, and hyperuricemia. Finally, the stone ''burden,'' that is, the presence of already formed stones in the kidney, should be assessed. If no imaging study was performed during the acute event, an IVP may be the most appropriate since this will also identify anatomical defects that may contribute to the disorder. If an IVP or ultrasound has already been done and stones are known to be calcium containing, a simple flat plate of the abdomen will suffice. Once the initial work-up has been performed, all leads must be followed. For example, if the serum calcium concentration is abnormally elevated, then the etiology of hypercalcemia must be identified (see Chapter 14).

D. General Measures

Regardless of the cause of the stone, most patients will benefit from the following measures:

1. Increased oral fluid intake: patients should be instructed to drink 8 glasses of water a day to achieve a daily urine volume of 2 L and thereby reduce urinary supersaturation.
2. Reduced protein intake: patients should be instructed to reduce dietary protein intake if it exceeds 1 g/kg/day (aim for 0.8–1 g/kg/day) to decrease the daily acid load, decrease uric acid production, and reduce urine calcium excretion.
3. Limit sodium intake: patients should be instructed to decrease Na^+ intake to 2–3 g/day because excess Na^+ causes volume expansion, which leads to decreased proximal sodium and calcium reabsorption and to increased calcium excretion in the urine.

Age- and gender-appropriate dietary intake of calcium should be maintained to maintain bone mineral stores and, in some cases, to reduce calcium stone formation (see later).

E. Evaluation of the Patient with More Than One Stone

Patients who have developed a second kidney stone, evidence of progression of stone disease, or stones in childhood should undergo careful evaluation of urine composition in addition to the basic workup described above. Urine composition should be determined by several 24-hour urine collections. Collections should be timed several weeks after the passage or removal of a stone at a time when patients are consuming their regular diet. Patients should be instructed to pass the first morning void in the toilet and then include the second urine and all urine thereafter including the first void of the following morning in the collection. If the laboratory uses boric acid as the preservative, the urine can be evaluated as a single collection for volume, calcium, oxalate, sodium, phosphorus, uric acid,

Table 3 Optimal Values for 24-Hour Urine

	Men	Women
Volume	>2–2.5 L	>2–2.5 Liter
Calcium	<300 mg	<250 mg
Oxalate	<40 mg	<40 mg
Uric acid	<800 mg	<750 mg
Citrate	>320 mg	>320 mg
Sodium	<200 mEq (<4600 mg)	<200 mEq (<4600 mg)
Phosphorus	<1100 mg	<1100 mg
pH	>5.5 and <7	>5.5 and <7
Creatinine	>15 mg/kg/d	>10 mg/kg/d

N.B. always check the units used to assess adequacy of the collection

citrate, and cystine (see Table 3 for optimal values). If possible, the laboratory should calculate supersaturation with respect to solid phases. While most in-hospital laboratories do not perform all of the analyses necessary to do these calculations, several central laboratories offer this service. The goal of the supersaturation calculations is to determine if the patient's urine is supersatuated to a solid phase. Therapy can then be directed at lowering urinary supersaturion. For additional accuracy, two separate collections, separated by a few days or more, are recommended. Therapy should be tailored to the specific abnormalities found in the 24-hour urines (see later) in addition to the stone composition.

III. CALCIUM STONES

Calcium-containing stones account for approximately 70% of all kidney stones. Of these, approximately 35% are calcium oxalate, 10% are pure calcium phosphate, and the rest are mixed. Risk factors range from intrarenal abnormalities to a variety of metabolic disorders including hypercalciuria, hypocitraturia, hyperoxaluria, and hyperuricosuria.

A. Hypercalciuria

An abnormally high urinary calcium excretion (hypercalciuria) is found in up to half of all patients with calcium-containing kidney stones. Hypercalciuria may be the result of hypercalcemia or renal tubular acidosis. More commonly, however, the precise cause of the hypercalciuria is not known. The presence of hypercalciuria without a clear cause or associated abnormalities is termed idiopathic hypercalciuria (IH). IH is defined as hypercalciuria (calcium excretion > 300 mg/24 hr in men and > 250 mg/24 hr in women) with normal serum calcium and serum phosphate concentrations and no other apparent metabolic disorder. IH appears to be familial, is more common in men than women, and often results in stone formation in the third decade.

The excessive urine calcium excretion in patients with IH may be due to a defect at one of several sites in the body where calcium flux is tightly regulated. These sites include intestinal calcium absorption, bone calcium formation and resorption, and renal calcium reabsorption. Each of these potential sites of dysregulation could be analyzed, but such an investigative workup is not recommended because separation of the possible causes of hypercalciuria has little utility in the management of IH. Misdiagnosis could lead to inappropriate and potentially harmful treatment.

Thiazide diuretics are the mainstay of treatment in patients with IH and are recommended along with general measures to decrease stone formation. Thiazides increase calcium reabsorption in the distal tubule. In addition, the mild volume depletion induced by thiazide treatment stimulates proximal sodium reabsorption and subsequent passive calcium reabsorption. Chlorthalidone, a long-acting thiazide drug, is recommended, using an initial dose of 25 mg/day. If hypokalemia develops, it should be treated with either a potassium supplement such as potassium citrate or a potassium-sparing diuretic such as amiloride. Triamterene should be avoided because this drug can precipitate in the urine and cause kidney stones. As indicated earlier, limitation of calcium intake is not advised. Dietary calcium restriction is paradoxically associated with an increase in nephrolithiasis, presumably by promoting oxalate absorption in the small intestine. In addition, dietary calcium restriction may further reduce bone mineral density, which is already decreased in many patients with nephrolithiasis.

B. Hypercalcemia

Hypercalcemia results in hypercalciuria because it increases the filtered load of calcium, leading to excess calcium excretion. Hypercalciuria occurs regardless of whether or not parathyroid hormone excess (due either to primary hyperparathyroidism or mediated by PTH-related peptide) is the cause of the hypercalcemia. Although parathyroid hormone increases renal tubular calcium reabsorption, it also increases bone resorption and stimulates the synthesis of 1,25-dihydroxycholecalciferol [$1,25(OH)_2D_3$], the active form of vitamin D, leading to an increase in both bone release and gut absorption of calcium. These effects both cause hypercalcemia, and the resultant increase in filtered calcium is not counterbalanced by a sufficient increase in PTH-mediated tubular calcium reabsorption to avoid the development of hypercalciuria. Excess $1,25(OH)_2D_3$, whether from exogenous or endogenous sources (i.e., granulomatous disorders), can also lead to hypercalcemia by increasing intestinal reabsorption of calcium and bone calcium resorption. Therapy is directed at the underlying disorder and may range from parathyroidectomy for primary hyperparathyroidism to steroids for active sarcoid disease.

C. Distal Renal Tubular Acidosis (Type 1)

Distal renal tubular acidosis is caused by a defect in collecting duct hydrogen ion secretion, leading to retention of endogenously produced acid (see Chapter 11 for a full discussion of its pathogenesis). This disorder is associated with intrarenal calcium deposition and calcium-containing renal stones. Stone formation is explained by the following factors:

1. Defective urinary acidification, characterized by an inability to reduce urine pH to <5.5 (when advanced, <6.0)
2. Chronic metabolic acidosis, reducing renal production of citrate, as well as enhancing tubular citrate reabsorption, leading to hypocitraturia
3. Retention of endogenously produced acid, leading to bone resorption and increased filtered calcium and phosphorus.

Each of these mechanisms contributes to increasing supersaturation with respect to calcium phosphate stones, the most common stone type in patients with distal renal tubular acidosis. Treatment with supplemental alkali reduces urinary calcium excretion and limits production of new stones; however, large doses of base (1–3 mEq/lg/day) may be required to correct the acidosis.

D. Hypocitraturia

Patients who form kidney stones are often found to have decreased citrate excretion (hypocitraturia). This finding is not surprising because citrate is an important inhibitor of crystallization, binding calcium to form a highly soluble complex. When levels of citrate are low in the urine (<320 mg), the patient is more prone to nephrolithiasis. Hypocitratuia can occur in any clinical setting where there is chronic metabolic acidosis (diarrhea, RTA, or renal insufficiency), increased exogenous acid load (high dietary protein intake), or hypokalemia (intracellular acidosis). Although administration of any alkali or alkali precursor will increase urinary citrate excretion, citrate itself is usually recommended, in doses of 30–75 mEq divided over the course of the day. Potassium citrate, rather than sodium citrate, should be used because sodium administration enhances urine calcium excretion (see earlier).

E. Hyperoxaluria

Excess oxalate excretion (>40 mg/day) can also contribute to nephrolithiasis. Oxalate from dietary sources is absorbed in the gastrointestinal tract. Oxalate is also produced endogenously from the metabolism of purines, glycine, and other amino acids. Intestinal oxalate absorption is increased by excessive intake of foods rich in this organic anion (e.g., rhubarb, spinach, cocoa, peppers, wheat germ, and certain nuts). Ascorbic acid and the toxin ethylene glycol (antifreeze) are metabolized to oxalic acid, and both lead to hyperoxaluria. The most common cause of hyperoxaluria, however, is from gastrointestinal malabsorption or ''enteric hyperoxaluria.'' Enteric hyperoxaluria occurs with small bowel malabsorption from inflammatory bowel disease, chronic biliary or pancreatic disease, and postoperative consequences of jejunoileal bypass for obesity or ileal resection. Oxalate absorption is increased in these settings because calcium, which normally binds to oxalate and limits its absorption, is bound instead to fatty acids that are not being absorbed. At the same time, the colonic mucosa is exposed to bile salts and fatty acids, both of which act as detergents and increase the permeability of the colon to small molecules such as oxalate.

Enteric hyperoxaluria can be readily treated with several maneuvers to decrease fatty acid and bile salt malabsorption, including a low-fat diet and cholestyramine and calcium supplementation, which provides more calcium to bind oxalate in the gut. Diets low in oxalate and high in fluid are important. Other defects such as metabolic acidosis, hypokalemia, and hypomagnesiemia should also be addressed.

In contrast to these secondary forms of hyperoxaluria, primary hyperoxaluria is a challenge to treat. This disease is an autosomal recessive disorder characterized by extreme hyperoxaluria and nephrolithiasis in childhood leading to progressive interstitial nephritis and renal insufficiency. Deposition of calcium oxalate also occurs outside of the kidney in the bone marrow and blood vessels. Two abnormalities have been described in primary hyperoxaluria. One is in the enzyme alanine: glyoxalate aminotransferase (AGT) in the liver and the other is in glycerate dehydrogenase in peripheral leukocytes. Both defects result in an increase in the production of oxalate from precursors. Medical treatment must begin before significant renal disease develops. The treatment consists of pyridoxine, magnesium supplements, and oral orthophosphate. Pyridoxine, a co-enzyme for the conversion of glyoxate to glycine, helps to shunt precursors away from forming oxalate. Magnesium supplements complex with oxalate in the urine to form a soluble complex. Oral orthophosphate acts to increase citrate and phosphate concentrations in the urine and to increase urine pH and decrease urinary calcium and oxalate excretion.

F. Hyperuricosuria

Patients who form calcium stones have a higher incidence of hyperuricosuria by comparison with non–stone formers. In general, the hyperuricosuria is related to excess purine intake. The mechanism that links uric acid to calcium oxalate crystallization is not clear but may be related to ''heterogeneous nucleation'' of calcium oxalate onto preformed uric acid crystals. Another possibility is that the excess uric acid interferes with the natural inhibitors of stone formation. Here, a low-purine diet and the use of a low dose of allopurinol may be helpful.

G. Idiopathic

Even after the most extensive of evaluations, some patients will have no discernible risk factor for nephrolithiasis. In this setting, ideally, stone analysis will guide treatment. However, if stone analysis is not available and stones continue to form in spite of the general advice outlined earlier, then the clinician may have to make an educated guess and proceed with therapy. Particularly in these patients, determination of urinary supersaturation is advisable with subsequent referral to a center skilled in the management of patients with nephrolithiasis.

IV. URIC ACID STONES

Uric acid, the degradation product of purines, is excreted in the urine. It is a weak acid with a pK of 5.35; at this pH approximately 50% exists in the poorly soluble undissociated form (uric acid), and the remaining 50% exists as the more soluble monosodium urate. As the urine pH rises, the fraction that is uric acid falls and the fraction that is urate increases. Because the solubility of undissociated uric acid is only approximately 100 mg/L, a small fraction of the typical daily excretory load of 300–500 mg/day, one would expect uric acid nephrolithiasis to be quite common. Yet uric acid stones account for only a small fraction of kidney stones. The disparity in the frequency of uric acid stones and the striking odds in favor of their formation and propagation highlights the role of renal defenses, almost certainly including inhibitory proteins, against nephrolithiasis. One of these defenses is the ''alkaline tide'' that occurs after meals. This transient increase in bicarbonate concentration is caused by the secretion of bicarbonate into the blood by parietal cells as they secrete protons in the lumen of the stomach. The result is a transient rise in urine pH with meals that may minimize the risk of uric acid nephrolithiasis by dissolving stones previously formed in the renal tubular lumen.

Uric acid stones are more frequent when at least one of the following abnormalities is present: increased production and excretion of uric acid, persistent low urine pH and/or low urine volume. Hyperuricosuria typically is the result of excess dietary purine ingestion, which results both in excess urinary uric acid excretion ($\geq$600 mg) and a low urine pH, the latter as a result of the accompanying increase in metabolic acid production. Abnormalities in the salvage pathway for purine synthesis may shunt precursors into uric acid and myeloproliferative disorders, which result in rapid turnover of purines and can predispose to uric acid stones. Persistently low urine pH is most common with diets high in animal protein or with diarrhea. Finally, a low urine volume is a risk factor for the formation of all types of kidney stones.

A low-purine diet should be instituted if hyperuricosuria is present. Allopurinol can be initiated, especially if serum uric acid is elevated. The urine pH can be raised above 6.5 with potassium citrate at an initial dose of 30 mEq twice a day. As urinary pH rises there is an increasing percentage of soluble urate. However, more extreme alkalization will increase the risk of calcium phosphate precipitation. Some patients may require acetazolamide before bedtime to avoid acidic urine during the night. Increased intake of fluid should be encouraged. During subsequent visits, 24-hour urine should be reassessed to confirm the improvement in urine output, pH, and decreased uric acid load.

V. STRUVITE STONES

Struvite stones are associated with urinary tract infections. These stones, also termed triple phosphate stones, consist of magnesium ammonium phosphate ($MgNH_4PO_4$) and carbonate apatite [$Ca_{10}(PO_4)_6CO_3$]. In order to develop a struvite calculus, infection with bacteria that elaborates the enzyme urease must be present. Urease is responsible for the hydrolysis of urea to ammonia and carbon dioxide. The former is further hydrolyzed to ammonium (NH_4^+), alkalinizing the urine and promoting precipitation of phosphate ions as $MgNH_4PO_4$. The carbon dioxide is rapidly hydrolyzed to carbonate, which also precipitates with phosphate. *Proteus vulgaris* is the most common bacterial organism that secretes urease, but *Staphylococcus aureus*, *Klebsiella pneumonia*, and *Pseudomonas aeruginosa* also secrete urease. *Esherichia coli* does not produce urease. Struvite stones occur in patients who have an increase in susceptibility to frequent urinary tract infections—women, the elderly, patients with indwelling catheters or stents, and those with anatomical abnormalities.

The goal of therapy is to render the patient both stone and infection free without compromising renal function. This difficult task requires a joint medical and surgical approach. Antimicrobial agents are the mainstay of medical therapy because struvite stones cannot form in a sterilized urine. The choice of antibiotic should be tailored to the results of urinary culture and given chronically to suppress infection. Unfortunately, antibiotics cannot eradicate infection because these agents are unable to penetrate the interstices of the struvite stones where bacteria reside. Antibiotics are therefore inadequate as monotherapy for the struvite stone. Urease inhibitors are another logical approach to the struvite stone. The most commonly used is acetohydroxyaminic acid (typical dose, 250 mg every 8 hours). This medication decreases urine pH and the generation of NH_4^+, which may lead to stone dissolution. Unfortunately, severe adverse effects including hemolytic anemia, deep venous thrombosis, gastrointestinal and neurological symptoms limit use of this medication. In addition, acetohydroxyaminic acid is not recommended in patients with renal dysfunction because the drug is partially excreted by the kidney.

Surgical therapy remains the primary method for removing struvite calculi. Options range from open surgery to percutaneous nephrostolithotomy. The most appropriate modality is best determined by evaluation of the stone's size in the context of the particular patient. Although the density of struvite stones make them quite amenable to extracorporeal shock wave lithotripsy (ESWL), there are several limitations including the large size of struvite stones (stones >2 cm are generally not amenable to ESWL), the risk of peri-procedure sepsis, the potential for obstruction by the stone fragments and the high incidence of recurrence. Instead, most are best treated with percutaneous nephrostolithotomy (i.e., percutaneous stone removal with endoscopic techniques).

VI. CYSTINE STONES

Cystine stones account for less than 1% of kidney stones. These stones are caused by an autosomal recessive trait resulting in defective transport of dibasic amino acids (ornithine, lysine, cystine, and arginine) in the renal proximal tubule and the jejunum. The only clinical manifestation of the disorder is the precipitation of cystine (HOOC-CHNH$_2$-CH$_2$-SH) in the urinary tract leading to the formation of cystine stones. Despite a similar defect in the jejunum, there is no evidence of malnutrition in these patients.

Normally, amino acids are freely filtered by the glomerulus and then nearly completely reabsorbed in the proximal tubule. This absorption is achieved by cotransport with sodium and driven by energy generated from the Na-K-ATPase. In patients with cystinuria, the fractional excretion of urinary cystine is more than 100%, indicating that there is both filtration and secretion of the cystine.

Clinical presentation occurs typically in the second or third decade and is similar to that of other kidney stones. The diagnosis should be suspected in patients with a strong family history of kidney stones, those with recurrent stones, or those who present at a relatively young age. The urine will often (but not always) have flat hexagonal crystals that are characteristic of cystinuria. Excretion should be quantified by collecting a 24-hour urine for cystine. This test is of both diagnostic and therapeutic significance. Levels over 250 mg/g creatinine indicate a homozygous disorder.

Because the solubility of cystine is 240–480 mg/L, one can estimate the necessary daily urine volume to maintain solubility of excreted cystine. Usually, a minimum urine volume of 2.5 L daily is required, and this volume should be distributed evenly throughout the day. Alkalinization of the urine will increase cystine solubility but only slightly until the pH is greater than 7.5. Because it is difficult to maintain a urinary pH at this level and there is an increased risk of precipitation of calcium salts onto the cystine matrix, alkalinization should be viewed as an adjunct to therapy. Potassium citrate at bedtime can assist with the nighttime propensity to acidic urine. Sodium citrate or sodium bicarbonate are less advisable because the sodium load increases cystine excretion. Chelating agents have also been used with success in cystinuria. D-Penicillamine increases the solubility of cystine by undergoing thiol-disulfide exchange to form a cysteine-penicillamine complex, which is significantly more soluble. Just as the urine volume can be titrated to the concentration of cystine, so too can be dose of penicillamine: for every 250 mg, urinary cystine will be reduced by 75–100 mg/day. This therapy, however, is limited by significant side effects, which occur in two thirds of all patients and include fever, rash, arthralgias, pancytopenia, and nephrotic syndrome. Another agent that works in a similar fashion is mercaptopropionylglycine (Thiola). Unfortunately, this agent has a side effect profile similar to that of D-penicillamine, although these reactions are less frequent. The surface of cystine stones is relatively resistant to fragmentation by shock waves, and therefore patients may require more invasive approaches than extracorporeal shock wave lithotripsy.

VII. SURGICAL INTERVENTION

Several new technologies have expanded the urologist's repertoire and provided less invasive means for approaching nephrolithiasis. These include ESWL, ultrasonic lithotripsy, and laser lithotripsy. ESWL is the safest and least invasive mode. This technique works based on the principle that human tissue has an acoustic impedance similar to that of water. Therefore, shock waves generated in water can pass through normal human tissue unimpeded and without causing significant damage. By contrast, if a substance with a significantly different acoustic interface such as a kidney stone is encountered, it will be destroyed. With the first-generation machines, the patient was partially submerged and the shock wave was generated under water by an electrohydraulic energy source. Newer lithotriptors have electromagnetic energy sources and do not require water immersion. Complications from this procedure include those related to the stone fragments, which can themselves cause colic or obstruction, and those related to the shock waves, including skin damage, perinephric hematoma, and diastolic hypertension.

Ultrasonic lithotripsy utilizes high-frequency sound waves with minimal depth penetration; the probe must be applied directly to the stone endoscopically. Laser lithotripsy delivers high peak energy through a small-diameter fiber. Both techniques allow flexible endoscopic approach with a ureteroscope. In addition, they are extremely well tolerated and can be employed on an ambulatory basis.

Indications for intervention have changed dramatically with the advent of new technologies; stones that were previously followed may now be treated with lithotripsy to avoid morbidity in the future. In general, ureteral calculi <4 mm generally pass without intervention, whereas those >7 mm do not. Infection is an emergency indication for intervention, whereas intractable pain, stone growth, or failure to resolve are relative indications.

Renal pelvic calculi generally require intervention because they are usually too large to pass through the ureter and if untreated tend to grow and cause further damage. ESWL can be attempted, but if the stone is >2 cm, a percutaneous technique may be more appropriate because fragments can be removed directly. By contrast, calyceal stones often do not need intervention unless there is associated pain or infection. Importantly, lithotripsy cannot replace the value of medical prevention. Several weeks after any intervention, the cause should be carefully pursued and treated.

SUGGESTED READINGS

Bushinsky DA. Renal lithiasis. In: Kelly WF, ed. Kelly's Textbook of Medicine. New York: J.B. Lippincott Co., 1996, pp. 1024–1028.

Bushinsky DA. Genetic hypercalciuric stone forming rats. Semin Nephrol 1996; 16:448–457.

Bushinsky DA, Monk RD. Calcium. Lancet 1998; 352:306–311.

Coe FL, Parks JH. New insights into the pathophysiology and treatment of nephrolithiasis: new research venues. J Bone Miner Res 1997; 12:522–533.

Consensus Conference. Prevention and treatment of kidney stones. JAMA 1988; 260:977–981.

Curhan GC, Willett WC, Rimm EB, Stampfer MJ. A prospective study of dietary calcium and other nutrients and the risk of symptomatic kidney stones. N Engl J Med 1993; 328:833–838.

Lieske JC, Coe FL. Urinary inhibitors and renal stone formation. In: Coe FL, Favus MJ, Pak CYC, Parks JH, Preminger GM, eds. Kidney Stones: Medical and Surgical Management. Philadelphia: Lippincott-Raven, 1996, p. 65.

Monk RD, Bushinsky DA. Pathogenesis of Idiopathic Hypercalciuria. In: Coe F, Favus M, Pak C, Parks J, Preminger G, eds. Kidney Stones: Medical and Surgical Management. New York: Raven Press, 1996, pp. 759–772.

Monk RD, Bushinsky D. Treatment of calcium, phosphorus, and magnesium disorders. In: Halperin M, ed. Therapy in Nephrology and Hypertension: A Companion to Brenner and Rector's The Kidney. Philadelphia: W.B. Saunders Company, 1999, pp. 303–315.

Parks JH, Coe FL. Pathogenesis and treatment of calcium stones. Semin Nephrol 1996; 16:398–411.

22

Treatment of Urinary Tract Infections

Christopher J. Grace, W. Kemper Alston, and Mary B. Ramundo
University of Vermont, Burlington, Vermont

I. GENERAL PRINCIPLES

The medical management of urinary tract infections (UTI) can be broadly categorized as preventive, prophylactic, and therapeutic. Management begins with categorizing the infection as upper or lower tract, complicated or uncomplicated, acute or chronic, symptomatic or not, and initial or recurrent (see Chapter 10 for these definitions and a general approach). Conditions that may mimic UTIs, such as urethritis and vaginitis, should be excluded by history and, if needed, pelvic exam. In addition, the immune status of the host and the presence of indwelling catheters must be considered.

A. Prophylactic Therapy

Prophylactic or preventive antibiotic therapy may reduce the risk of symptomatic infection in patients at high risk for UTI. Examples include children with urological abnormalities, patients with spinal cord injuries, preoperative patients for urological or gynecological surgery, recipients of kidney transplants, pregnant women, and patients with chronic indwelling bladder or nephrostomy catheters. These patients should have a urine culture performed before any urological surgery. Patients with positive cultures should be treated and the urine sterilized prior to urological manipulation. It is difficult to prevent colonization in patients with chronic indwelling urinary catheters. Prophylactic use of systemic antibiotics, methenamine, or bladder irrigation with povidine iodine or chlorhexadine are minimally effective, select for resistant bacteria, favor superinfection with yeast, increase costs, and expose the patient to drug toxicity. The best approach is to remove the catheter if at all possible. Substituting indwelling catheters with condom catheters in men, intermittent catheterization, or suprapubic catheterization has decreased the incidence of colonization and subsequent infection.

Prophylactic measures may prevent the recurrence of established infections. Patients who may benefit from prophylactic measures include women with frequent UTIs (more than three in 6 months), patients with infected renal stones that cannot be removed, and men with chronic prostatitis. Approaches include nonspecific interventions and specific antibiotic agents. Unproven but commonly used nonspecific interventions include increased fluid intake to dilute the bacteriuria, voiding after sexual intercourse, and urine acidification. None of these interventions are routinely advocated. Both the use of topical estrogen creams vaginally and ingestion of cranberry juice (300 cc per day) have reduced the incidence of UTIs in elderly women. Neither of these latter modalities have been proven efficacious in premenopausal women. Contraceptive diaphragms used with spermacidal jellies have been associated with increased UTIs in women and should be avoided in women with frequent recurrences. Other more experimental approaches include the use of lactobacillus vaginal suppositories and vaccines.

B. Antibiotic Therapy

Therapeutic management involves the use of antibiotic agents to treat patients with symptomatic urinary tract infections. Patients with asymptomatic infections or bladder colonization do not routinely need antibiotic therapy, except for the preventative as above. The selection of a particular antibiotic depends on its phamacokinetics, toxicity, cost, spectrum of activity, and effects on normal vaginal and gut flora. The duration of therapy (1, 3, 7, or 14 days or more) will depend on the clinical diagnosis, age of the patient, and complexity of the clinical syndrome. These issues are discussed further below.

The goal of therapy is to eradicate pathogens from the urinary system and remove uropathogenic bacteria from the bowel and vagina while leaving intact the normal protective microflora of these areas. *Lactobacillus* and anaerobic species, the major normal flora involved, are not urinary pathogens. Their presence helps prevent colonization with *Escherechia coli*, *Klebsiella* spp., *Proteus* spp., and *Staphylococcus saprophyticus*, the usual UTI pathogens. Agents such as amoxacillin and cephalosporins that kill normal bowel and vaginal flora increase potential pathogen growth and may increase the risk of recurrent infection. Some agents such as the combination drug trimethoprim/sulfamethoxazole inhibit bacterial adherence to urinary epithelium, lessening the risk of colonization and future infection. Bacterial resistance is a growing problem. More than 30% of the common UTI pathogens are currently resistant to amoxacillin. There is growing concern that bacterial resistance to trimethoprim/sulfamethoxazole and the fluoroquinolones will emerge. If urine cultures are taken prior to empiric therapy, the antibiotics can be tailored to culture results.

II. ORAL ANTIBIOTIC THERAPY FOR UTIs

The patient with uncomplicated cystitis should experience improvement in dysuria and frequency within 24–48 hours of starting oral antibiotic treatment. For patients with severe dysuria, urinary analgesics such as phenazopyridine HCl (pyridium, 200 mg orally TID) may be used for the first 1–2 days in addition to antibiotic therapy. Complications of these agents include orange-red discoloration of the urine and, less commonly, methemoglobinuria, hemolytic anemia, and renal/hepatic failure.

Presented below are the commonly used outpatient antibiotic agents for UTIs. Amoxacillin and first-generation cephalosporins are no longer recommended because of rising levels of bacterial resistance (see Table 1).

A. Trimethoprim/Sulfamethoxazole (Bactrim, Septra, Co-trimoxazole)

Trimethoprim/Sulfamethoxazole (TMP-SMZ) is a synergistic antibiotic combination that inhibits bacterial folic acid synthesis. It is bactericidal against the majority of UTI pathogens, with the important exception of *Pseudomonas*. It is well absorbed orally and attains high levels in the urinary system. It also reduces vaginal gram-negative rod (GNR) colonization and bacterial adherence, thus decreasing the risk of recurrent UTI. It is relatively inexpensive. Sulfonamides should not be used during the third trimester of pregnancy because of kernicterus in the newborn. Since these agents inhibit folate metabolism and data regarding teratogenicity are not conclusive, these drugs should be used with caution throughout pregnancy.

B. Trimethoprim

When used alone, trimethoprim has excellent activity against most of the UTI pathogens. It is well absorbed orally and attains high urinary tract levels. It has fewer side effects than TMP-SMZ. It has no antipseudomonal activity. Trimethoprim attains high levels in the prostate gland and is commonly used either alone or with sulfamethoxazole for the treatment of acute and chronic bacterial prostatitis.

C. Nitrofurantoin

This bactericidal drug most likely exerts its effect by interfering with bacterial DNA synthesis. Oral absorption is good, but systemic levels of antibiotic are not

Table 1 Oral Antibiotics Commonly Used for Urinary Tract Infections

Drug	Absorption	3-day cost	GNR	*Staphylococcus saprophyticus*	*Pseudomonas aeruginosa*	Common toxicities
TMP-SMX 1 DS orally BID	Good	$	+++	+++	None	Rash, N, V, DI
Trimethoprim 200 mg orally BID	Good	$	++	++	None	<TMP-SMX
Nitrofurantoin Nitrofurantoin 100 mg orally QID Macrobid 100 mg orally BID	Good	$$	++	+++	None	N, H/A
Fosfomycin 3 g orally once daily	Good	$$$$	+++	+++	None	D, H/A
Fluoroquinolones ciprofloxacin, 250 mg orally BID ofloxacin, 200 mg orally BID enoxacin, 400 mg orally once daily norfloxacin, 400 mg orally BID levofloxacin, 250 mg orally BID lomefloxacin, 400 mg orally once daily trovofloxacin, 100 mg orally once daily	Good	$$$-$$$$	+++	++	+++	N, V
Third-generation cephalosporins Cefixime, 400 mg orally once daily Cefpodoxime, 200 mg orally BID	Good	$$$	+++	++	None	Rash, N, D

+ = poor activity, ++ = good activity, +++ = excellent activity, N = nausea, D = diarrhea, H/A = headache, GNR = nonpseudomonas aerobic gram-negative rod, < = less frequent than, DI = drug interactions, BID = twice daily, $ = <$10, $$ = $10–20, $$$ = $20–40, $$$$ = >$40, TMP-SMX = trimethoprim sulfamethoxazole.

adequate for treating infections except for uncomplicated cystitis and pyelonephritis. Prostate concentrations are not adequate for treatment. The macrocrystalline forms (Macrobid, Macrodantoin) are better tolerated than the microcrystalline form. Twice-daily dosing of Macrobid has been found to be as efficacious as four-times-daily Macrodantoin. Highly resistant *Klebsiella* spp. and *Proteus* spp. are widespread, but the great majority of *E. coli*, the most common uropathogen, are sensitive. If nitrofurantoin is used to treat uncomplicated cystitis, a 7-day course should be given. It has no antipseudomonal activity.

D. Fosfomycin Tromethamine

This drug is a bactericidal phosphonic acid derivative that inhibits cell wall synthesis. It has excellent activity against the majority of uropathogens except *Pseudomonas*. It is well absorbed and well tolerated. Its long half-life makes once-daily dosing possible, but it is very expensive.

E. Fluoroquinolones

This class of drugs includes ciprofloxacin, norfloxacin, ofloxacin, lomefloxacin, levofloxacin, enoxacin, and trovafloxacin. The fluoroquinolones are bactericidal agents that inhibit DNA gyrase. They are well absorbed and attain high urinary tract concentrations. They have excellent activity against the major uropathogens, including *P. aeruginosa*. Norfloxacin does not attain adequate systemic levels and should only be used for cystitis or uncomplicated pyelonephritis. The fluoroquinolones are relatively expensive and should be reserved for use in patients unable to take less expensive agents or those infected with *P. aeruginosa*. They should not be used during pregnancy or to treat women who are breast-feeding.

F. Third-Generation Oral Cephalosporins (Cefixime, Cefpodoxyl Proxetil)

The oral third-generation cephalosporins are well absorbed, well tolerated, and effective. They have no antipseudomonal activity and are expensive. They should be reserved for patients intolerant of less expensive agents.

III. ANTIBIOTIC THERAPY FOR PYELONEPHRITIS: GENERAL CONSIDERATIONS

Antibiotic treatment of acute pyelonephritis is based on the same bacteriology as that causing cystitis, although enterococci can cause infections in the complicated patient. A Gram stain of unspun urine can be helpful in excluding these gram-positive cocci in chains (see Chapter 10). An oral agent (see Table 1) can be used initially if the patient is clinically stable, can maintain oral hydration, and has adequate pain control. In most cases, however, parenteral agents are necessary until the patient's status has improved and can be discharged from the hospital. Selection of the appropriate intravenous antibiotics depends on the spectrum of the drug required (e.g., activity against *Pseudomonas* and *Enterococcus*), toxicity, cost, and ease of administration. Infection with *Pseudomonas* should be suspected in patients with recent hospitalization or frequent use of antibiotics that favor the growth of resistant organisms. Empiric antibiotics should be changed to narrower agents based upon results of the urine and blood cultures.

A. Ceftriaxone

This third-generation cephalosporin has excellent activity against the majority of GNRs that cause pyelonephritis and is relatively inexpensive, easy to use (1 g daily IV or IM), and well tolerated. It does not have activity against *Pseudomonas* or *Enterococcus*.

B. Ceftazidime

This third-generation cephalosporin has a similar spectrum as ceftriaxone with additional activity against *Pseudomonas*. It is more expensive and must be administered three times daily (1–2 g IV every 8 hours), with normal renal function. Its empiric use should be limited to those patients strongly suspected of having *Pseudomonas* infection.

C. Aztreonam

This monobactam antibiotic is a pure aerobic GNR agent and must be given three times daily, similar to ceftazidime. Its empiric use should be limited to those patients strongly suspected of having *Pseudomonas* infection or patients with allergies to cephalosporins and penicillins.

D. Piperacillin and Piperacillin-Tazobactam

Both these agents are ureidopenicillins with a broad spectrum of activity against aerobic GNR including *Pseudomonas* and *Enterococcus*. The beta-lactamase inhibitor tazobactam improves activity against *Staphylococcus* and anaerobic and aerobic GNR. These drugs are expensive and must be dosed four times a day. They should be reserved for patients with mixed infections caused by *Pseudomonas* and *Enterococcus* or complicated patients with hospital acquired infections.

Normal dosing is piperacillin 4 g IV every 6 hours and piperacillin-tazobactam 3.375 g every 6 hours.

E. Ampicillin-Sulbactam

This beta-lactam/beta-lactamase inhibitor combination has activity against many GNR and *Enterococcus*. It has no *Pseudomonas* activity. It is expensive and must be administered (1.5 g) IV three times daily.

F. Trimethoprim/Sulfamethoxazole

TMP-SMX can be used parenterally as well as orally. The daily dose is 10 mg/kg of the trimethoprim component intravenously divided into three or four doses. In some areas of the country there is increasing resistance to TMP-SMX and empiric use requires caution in nosocomial infections and severely ill patients.

G. Flouroquinolones

These agents are generally well tolerated, safe, and have excellent aerobic GNR activity. As in the case of cystitis, these agents should be reserved for suspected *Pseudomonas* infection or when the patient is unable to tolerate cephalosporins, aminoglycosides, or TMP-SMX. Standard dosing is ciprofloxacin 200–400 mg IV every 12 hours, levofloxacin 250–500 mg IV once daily, and ofloxacin 200–400 mg IV every 12 hours. Fluoroquinalones are well absorbed orally and are less expensive in this form. Intravenous dosing should be reserved for patients unable to take oral medications.

H. Aminoglycosides (Gentamicin, Tobramycin, Amikacin)

Aminoglycosides have excellent activity against aerobic GNR. Gentamicin is inexpensive and may be dosed once daily (7 mg/kg/day). Tobramycin and amikacin may be considered for patients infected with gentamicin-resistant bacteria. Because of the significant risk for nephrotoxicity, including acute renal failure and tubular dysfunction and ototoxicity, it may be prudent to avoid these agents, especially in the elderly and patients with renal insufficiency and diabetes. With bactericidal activity against aerobic GNRs and synergistic activity against the *Enterococcus* when combined with ampicillin, aminoglycosides are still used for severe UTIs with bacteremia or sepsis and for complicated enterococcal infections.

IV. SPECIFIC TREATMENTS

A. Uncomplicated UTI (Cystitis)

Women with dysuria and pyuria in whom urethritis and vaginitis have been ruled out should be treated with antibiotics. Because the organisms involved in cystitis in healthy individuals are predictable, these infections can be treated without obtaining a urine culture. Single-dose therapy is less effective, and most experts favor a 3-day regimen of antibiotics. Any of the agents discussed in the prior section on cystitis can be used, but trimethoprim/sulfamethoxazole is the drug of choice if the prevalence of resistant *E. coli* is low (Fig. 1). The cephalosporins and nitrofurantoin may be less effective than the others in 3-day regimens. With most antibiotics, regimens of 7 days or longer offer no additional therapeutic benefit and are associated with increased cost and increased adverse effects. Because of cost and concern with emergence of resistance, fluoroquinolones are not considered the agents of choice in uncomplicated cystitis. If symptoms resolve with a 3-day course of therapy, no follow-up culture is necessary. If short-course therapy fails or symptoms recur, a urine culture should be obtained. In contrast to women, men with uncomplicated UTI should be treated for 7 days.

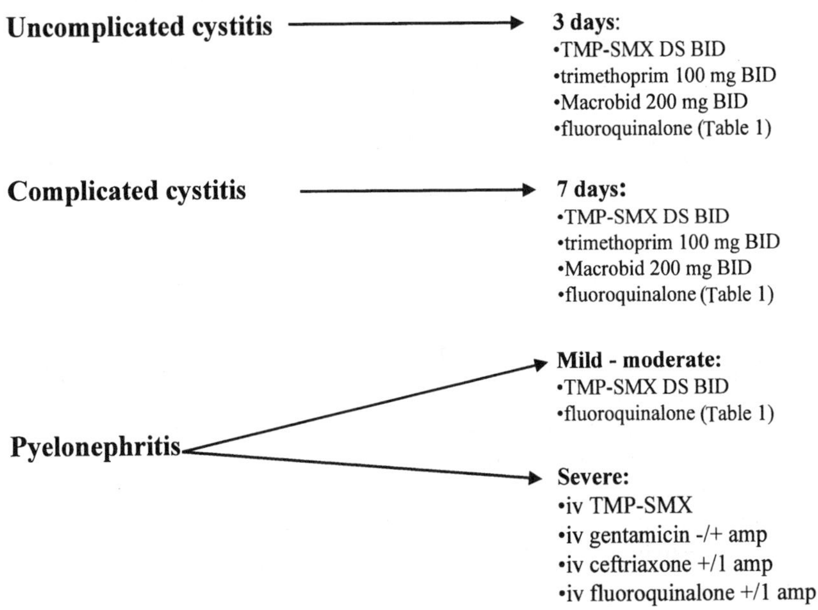

Figure 1 Treatment of adult patients with UTIs.

B. Recurrent UTI

Recurrent UTI can be due either to relapse, i.e., recrudescence of partially treated infection, reinfection, or new infection with a different organism (Fig. 2). The distinction is important in terms of evaluation and treatment. Reinfection is the most common cause and usually occurs more than 2 weeks after completion of therapy. Recurrent UTIs occur in approximately 20% of women; behavioral and genetic factors may play a role. Women with more than three episodes of UTIs in a 6-month period are candidates for prophylactic therapy. Recurrent cystitis in otherwise healthy individuals can be managed by the use of postcoital prophylaxis, therapy initiated by the patient at the onset of symptoms, or continuous (daily) antibiotic prophylaxis. Continuous antibiotic prophylaxis should not be used in patients with chronic indwelling catheters.

The distinction between upper and lower tract disease is difficult to make on a clinical basis. There are no readily available laboratory tests to distinguish upper from lower tract disease. Approximately 10–20% of women treated for cystitis have upper tract disease. Relapse of infection following short course ther-

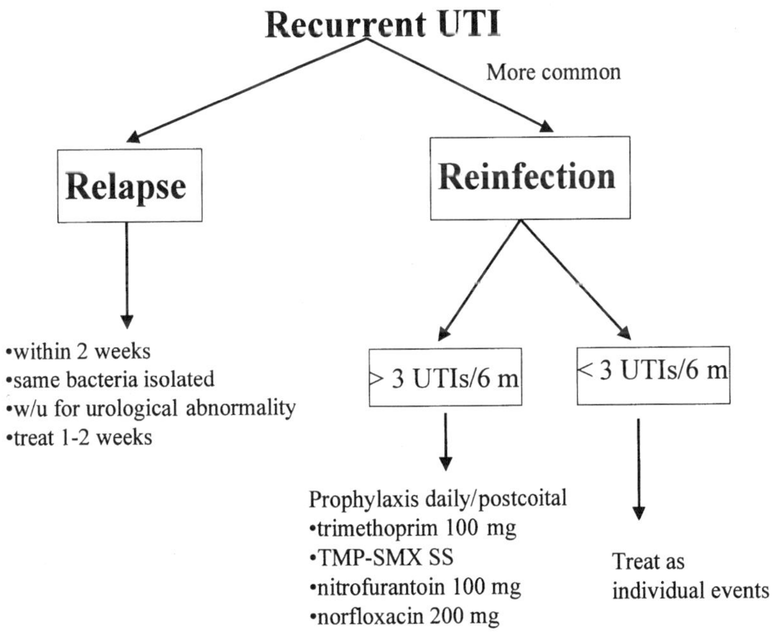

Figure 2 Recurrent urinary tract infections in women.

apy is associated with occult upper tract infection, and relapse usually occurs within 2 weeks of treatment. In males relapse may occur because of occult prostatitis. Patients with relapse of infection should have a urine culture obtained and should receive a more prolonged course of therapy (7–14 days). Follow-up urine culture should be performed 1–4 weeks after completion of therapy. Recurrent or persistent UTI in pregnancy is an indication for chronic suppressive therapy. Because of the high incidence of recurrent UTI in patients following renal transplant, daily trimethoprim/sulfamethoxazole is used for chronic prophylaxis in some transplant programs. In addition, this agent provides protection against opportunistic infections such as *Pneumocystis carinii* pneumonia and *Nocardia*.

C. Pyelonephritis

There are limited clinical trials dealing with treatment of pyelonephritis. The clinical spectrum of pyelonephritis ranges from a cystitis-like illness to septicemia. A urine culture should be obtained in all persons with suspected pyelonephritis. Blood cultures should also be obtained prior to antibiotics and will be positive in approximately 15% of patients. In the absence of systemic toxicity or vomiting, patients can be treated on an outpatient basis. Indications for hospitalization include inability to take oral medications, uncertain diagnosis, severe systemic toxicity, and pregnancy. There is no evidence that bacteremia per se is associated with a worse prognosis or warrants a longer course of treatment. Any of the parenteral regimens discussed previously can be used. If the infection was acquired in the hospital, empiric therapy should include coverage for *Pseudomonas*. An aminoglycoside such as gentamicin can be clinically effective but carries the risk of acute renal failure. Ultrasound should be considered in patients with persistent signs or symptoms of infection after 72 hours of therapy. Routine urological evaluation is neither necessary nor useful in patients with pyelonephritis.

Treatment should be continued for a full 14 days. Repeat urine culture should be obtained 2 weeks after completion of treatment. The failure rate for treatment of pyelonephritis has been reported to be as high as 30% in some studies. Asymptomatic pyelonephritis occurs in alcoholics, persons with diabetes mellitus, and in persons with a kidney transplant. Treatment of pyelonephritis during pregnancy is the same as for nonpregnant women, although the drugs of choice may differ. Pregnant women with an episode of pyelonephritis should be treated for a full 2 weeks followed by chronic suppressive therapy and monthly urine cultures until delivery.

D. Complicated UTI

A complicated UTI is defined as one occurring in persons with structural or functional abnormalities of the urinary tract, with a history of urological manipulation, with significant medical co-morbidity, such as diabetes or with infection by resistant or unusual organisms. UTI during pregnancy is considered complicated because of the structural and functional changes that occur in the urinary tract, all of which increase the risk of infection. The pathogens involved in complicated infections are varied and can have unusual patterns of sensitivity to antibiotics. A urine culture should be obtained in all of these settings before embarking on antibiotic therapy.

The wide variety of underlying conditions and the broad spectrum of causative agents make it difficult to provide general recommendations for treatment. Fluoroquinolones are a good choice for empiric treatment in the outpatient setting. In hospitalized patients, third-generation cephalosporins, piperacillin-tazobactam, aztreonam, or a combination of ampicillin and gentamicin are potential regimens. Antibiotic therapy should be modified as needed once urine culture results are available. Complicated UTI should be treated with a longer course of therapy (7–14 days). Follow-up urine cultures should be obtained after completion of therapy.

E. Asymptomatic Bacteriuria

1. In Elderly Patients

Asymptomatic bacteriuria is very common in the elderly (age > 65 years), affecting at least 10–20% with less female preponderance than in young adults. Prostatic obstruction, uterine prolapse, incontinence, frequent catheterization, instrumentation, and hospitalization all contribute to this syndrome. Pyuria may or may not be present. As age and disability increase and hospitalization becomes more common, the rates of both bacteriuria and antibiotic resistance among the organisms isolated increases. Asymptomatic bacteriuria in this population is generally benign, and this fact combined with high relapse rates after antibiotic therapy argue against either routine screening or treatment. As is true for younger patients, special host factors such as neutropenia, anatomical abnormalities, and organ transplantation may warrant therapy on an individual basis. Treatment of symptomatic UTIs in the elderly should be guided by the same principles used in younger patients, with special attention given to drug interactions, age-related toxicity, and pharmacokinetics. For younger adults there is no urgency to treat asymptomatic bacteruria. A follow-up urinalysis and culture may help establish if the infection is persistent and is in fact due to a single organism. Treatment can then be considered if a uropathogen is present.

2. During Pregnancy

Asymptomatic bacteriuria during pregnancy has special significance. The prevalence is approximately 5% and is frequently followed by symptomatic upper

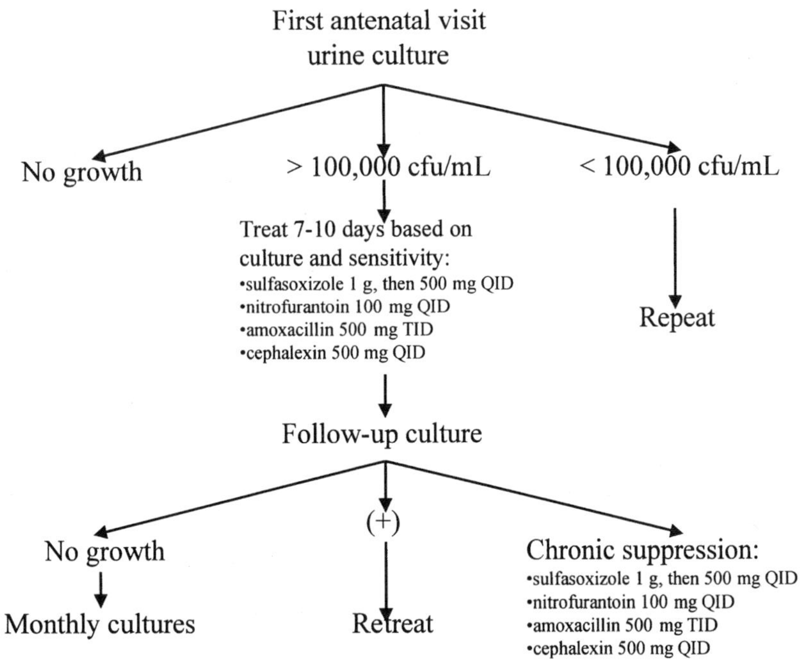

Figure 3 Asymptomatic bacteruria in pregnant women.

tract infection, due to the anatomical changes that normally occur during pregnancy. As many as one third of pregnant women with asymptomatic bacteriuria will develop pyelonephritis. Urinary tract infections in this population have been linked to prematurity and low birthweight infants. Routine screening with quantitative urine culture should be carried out at the first prenatal visit (see Fig. 3). All cases of significant bacteriuria ($\geq 10^5$/mL) should be treated with the goal of maintaining sterile urine. Samples with lower colony counts or nonpathogenic organisms should be repeated, especially if obtained by clean-catch. Antibiotics that may be used in this setting include amoxicillin, amoxicillin–clavulanic acid, nitrofurantoin, and oral cephalosporins. Sulfa-based drugs should not be used during the third trimester. Quinolones and tetracyclines should not be used during pregnancy. Treatment duration should be 7 days, although shorter courses may be adequate in some cases. A follow-up culture should be obtained 1–2 weeks after the completion of therapy. Monthly cultures can then be performed during subsequent visits to screen for relapse or reinfection.

3. In Surgical Patients

Patients with asymptomatic bacteriuria at the time of genitourinary instrumentation or surgery are at significant risk of developing bacteremia and should be treated. A 3-day course of amoxicillin, trimethoprim-sulfamethoxazole, or nitrofurantoin is recommended. Patients with asymptomatic bacteriuria undergoing renal transplantation should also be treated preoperatively.

F. Prostatitis

Acute bacterial prostatitis responds well to antibiotics. Trimethoprim-sulfamethoxazole, fluoroquinolones, amoxicillin, and cephalosporins have all been used with success. Severe cases may require hospital admission for intravenous antibiotics, hydration, stool softeners, and suprapubic catheter placement if obstruction is present. A minimum 4-week course of antibiotic therapy is advocated to reduce the risk of chronic infection. Prostatic abscess may rarely complicate acute prostatitis and should be considered when bacteremia, persistent pain, or fluctuance on digital rectal exam occurs. Chronic bacterial prostatitis is frequently treated with long courses (2–3 months) of fluoroquinolones or trimethoprim-sulfa, both of which penetrate the gland well in the animal model, have broad-spectrum activity, and are relatively nontoxic.

G. Abscess

Abscesses may occur either within the renal parenchyma or in perirenal tissue as a complication of ascending UTI or as a result of haematogenous spread from a remote or bloodstream infection. Although surgical intervention with nephrectomy was a common therapeutic approach, it is now clear that many cortical and corticomedullary abscesses respond well to antibiotic therapy alone. Staphylococcal abscesses can be treated with nafcillin, first-generation cephalosporins, or vancomycin depending on the sensitivity pattern and the patient's allergies. Gram-negative bacilli such as *E. coli*, *Klebsiella* spp., and *Proteus* spp. can be treated with extended-spectrum penicillins or third-generation cephalosporins, with or without an aminoglycoside. The duration of therapy is normally one month, either entirely intravenous (*S. aureus*) or switching to oral antibiotics when the patient has responded with clearing of their symptoms. Perinephric abscesses are an uncommon complication of pyelonephritis and are in general more severe and require drainage in addition to systemic antibiotics. Open surgical drainage, with or without nephrectomy, remains an option but has been replaced in many cases by computed tomography or ultrasound guided aspiration and drainage. Beta-lactam antibiotics are given empirically or as indicated by blood and urine cultures. Duration of therapy needs to be individualized depending on the organism, host factors, and clinical response.

H. Catheter-Associated Infection

Bacteriuria is virtually always present when urinary catheters are used for more than 2 or 3 days. Therefore, it is not surprising that catheter-associated UTIs are the most common cause of nosocomial infection. Ideally, catheters should be removed whenever possible to reduce the risk of infection and to eliminate catheter-associated bacteriuria when present. Because bacteriuria always recurs if the catheter is left in place, treatment should be reserved for those who are symptomatic or are having the catheter removed or changed. Seven to ten days of treatment is usually sufficient. In hospitalized patients with fever, intravenous antibiotic therapy should be administered until the results of urine and blood cultures are known. Because a biofilm on the catheter may contribute to the persistence of organisms, contaminated catheters should be removed or changed whenever possible. The temptation to treat all positive urine cultures in chronically catheterized asymptomatic patients should be resisted. With repeated courses of antibiotics more unusual and resistant pathogens will be selected.

I. Fungal Infections

Urinary tract infections with *Candida* spp. are increasingly common in those with urinary catheters, diabetes, pregnancy, and immunosuppression, especially in the setting of recent antibacterial use. Most cases represent asymptomatic colonization, but severe fungal UTIs and even disseminated infection may complicate candiduria. Symptomatic patients and those with significant pyuria should have any catheters removed or at least changed. This will lead to resolution in the majority of cases. Those that persist or are at risk of upper tract disease or dissemination should be treated with fluconazole 100 mg orally daily for 3 days. An older alternative that is more cumbersome and provides only topical coverage is intermittent or continuous bladder irrigation with amphotericin B.

SUGGESTED READINGS

Andriole, VT, ed. Urinary Tract Infections. Philadelphia: W.B. Saunders, 1997.

Avon J, Monane M, Gurwitz JH, et al. Reduction of bacteriuria and pyuria after ingestion of cranberry juice. JAMA 1994; 271:751–754.

Elmer GW, Surawicz, CM, McFarland LV. Biotherapeutic agents. A neglected modality for the treatment and prevention of selected intestinal and vaginal infections. JAMA 1996; 275:870–876.

Kim ED, Schaeffer AJ. Antimicrobial therapy for urinary tract infections. Semin Nephrol 1994; 14:551–569.

Kunin CM. Chemoprophylaxis and suppressive therapy in the management of urinary tract infections. Br Soc Antimicrob Chemother 1994; 33:51–62.

Millar LK, Cox SM. Urinary tract infections complicating pregnancy. Infect Dis Clin North Am 1997; 11:13–26.

Pinson AG, Philbrick JT, Lindbeck HG, et al. Oral antibiotic therapy for acute pyelonephritis. J Gen Intem Med 1992; 7:544–553.

Raz Raul, Stamm WE. A controlled trial of intravaginal estriol in postmenopausal women with recurrent urinary tract infections. N Engl J Med 1993; 329:753–756.

23
Obstructive Nephropathy

E. Darracott Vaughan Jr. and Diane Felsen
Weill Medical College of Cornell University, New York, New York

Frederick A. Gulmi
Brookdale University Hospital and Medical Center, and State University of New York, Brooklyn, New York

I. INTRODUCTION

Obstruction to the urinary tract, usually partial, is one of the most common renal or urological diseases seen by the primary care physician. The clinical manifestations are variable and depend on whether the obstruction is acute or chronic, unilateral or bilateral, or intrinsic or extrinsic to the urinary tract. Fortunately, most obstruction to the urinary tract does not result in irreversible renal damage if diagnosed and corrected appropriately. Chronic obstructive nephropathy nonetheless remains a significant cause of end-stage renal disease; therefore, recognition of its many manifestations is critical in order to minimize renal damage and prevent this costly outcome.

This chapter encompasses the definitions concerning obstruction to the urinary tract and a review of clinical manifestations, and places emphasis on the diagnostic modalities that are currently used for identification of patients with this problem. A brief discussion of the pathophysiology of obstructive nephropathy is necessary, because both the patient's symptoms and a number of diagnostic tests are based on renal abnormalities that occur with obstruction, including increased renovascular resistance and tubular damage that leads to a defect in urinary concentrating ability. The reader is directed towards more extensive reviews of the subject for more comprehensive information (see Suggested Readings).

II. DEFINITIONS AND TERMINOLOGY

There are numerous terms used to describe patients with obstruction of the urinary tract. The title of this chapter indicates that obstruction can cause damage to the renal parenchyma, leading to a decrease in glomerular function and inducing nephron loss and interstitial fibrosis. The term *obstructive uropathy* indicates structural impedance to the flow of urine but not necessarily nephron damage. The term *hydronephrosis* is derived from the Greek *hydro* (water), *nephros* (kidney), and *osis* (condition) and therefore is defined as dilatation of the renal pelvis and calyces. An important point is that dilatation of the renal pelvis and calyces can occur without obstruction, particularly in some congenital abnormalities involving the urinary tract, and thus this term is nonspecific.

III. INCIDENCE

The incidence and prevalence of obstructive uropathy are difficult to determine because prostatic obstruction can be unrecognized, stone disease with transient obstruction is extremely common and often not reported, and obstruction can be a component of other systemic diseases and may not be the primary problem. However, ureteral obstruction with subsequent hydronephrosis is a common clinical occurrence. The incidence of hydronephrosis in a general autopsy series that includes a large number of individuals ranging from birth to age 80 is approximately 3%. In women, obstruction is more likely to occur at a younger age as the result of pregnancy or uterine cancer. In men, prostate disease has, in the past, been a major cause of hydronephrosis. At the present time, with earlier diagnosis and treatment of men with benign prostatic hypertrophy and prostatic cancer, this is a less common finding. In young adults, stone disease is the most common cause of obstruction.

In children, obstruction is a major problem mainly due to congenital abnormalities. Congenital obstructive uropathy accounted for almost 6% of the total cases of end-stage renal disease as of 1998. As will be discussed later, obstructive uropathy is now fortunately being identified more frequently in utero because of the wide use of maternal ultrasound. Immediate intervention following birth will hopefully decrease this number in the future. In 1985 in the United States, almost 400,000 hospital discharges were coded as obstructive uropathy and approximately 166 per 100,000 had an admission diagnosis of obstruction. More recent information has shown that obstructive nephropathy accounted for 2% of the patients treated under Medicare for ESRD and interestingly the vast majority (74%) were males.

IV. ETIOLOGY

The causes of urinary obstruction are manifold, as are the clinical presentations. A comprehensive list of the causes of ureteral obstruction is shown in Table 1. A common breakdown of the causes of obstruction is by age, gender, level of obstruction, whether the obstruction is intrinsic or extrinsic, and whether the ob-

Table 1 Causes of Urinary Obstruction

Level of obstruction	Pathological processes
All	Calculi
	Papillary tissue
	Trauma
	Blood clots
	Fungus balls
Tubule	Uric acid
	Polycystic kidneys (adult and childhood types)
	Protein in multiple myeloma
	Acute tubular necrosis (?)
Renal infundibulum	Tuberculosis
	Peripelvic cyst
	Primary urothelial tumor
	Polycystic kidney
	Renal neoplasm
	Renal cyst
	Aberrant vessel
	Hydatid cyst
Renal pelvis	Wilms' tumor
	Ectopic kidney
	Tuberculosis
	Fibrous bands at ureteropelvic junction (UPJ)
	Ureteropelvic stricture (acquired or congenital)
	Aberrant vessel at UPJ
Ureter	
Retroperitoneal disease	Lymphoma
	Metastatic or primary carcinoma
	Aortic aneurysm
	Retroperitoneal fibrosis
	Hemangioma
	Retroperitoneal hemorrhage
	Ovarian vein
	Retroperitoneal abscess
	Uroma posttrauma
	Lymphocele

Table 1 Continued

Level of obstruction	Pathological processes
Congenital disease	Stricture
	Ureterocele
	Retrocaval ureter
	Ectopic kidney
	Ureterovesical reflux
	Diverticulum
	Ectopic position of orifice
	Adynamic ureteral segment
	Ureteral valve
	Mesenteric cyst
Primary Genitourinary Disease:	Carcinoma of the ureter and bladder
	Ureteral polyp
	Neurogenic bladder
	Ureteritis cystica
	Gumma of ureter
	Tuberculosis
	Schistosomiasis haematobia
Miscellaneous Causes:	Abdominal and pelvic neoplasm
	Granulomatous bowel disease
	Acquired traumatic ureteral stricture (postinstrumentation)
	Congenital absence of the abdominal musculature (''prune belly'')
	Endometriosis
	Pregnancy
	Obstetrical trauma
	Antituberculous therapy
	Nephrosis
	Radiation therapy
	Renal artery aneurysm
Bladder and posterior urethra	Benign prostatic hypertrophy
	Foreign body
	Hypertrophy of verumontanum (?)
	Müllerian remnant cyst
	Contraction of the bladder neck (acquired or congenital)
	Posterior or median bar
	External sphincter spasm (?)
	Hydrocolpos
	Carcinoma of prostate
	Carcinoma of the bladder
	Sarcoma of the bladder or prostate

Table 1 Continued

Level of obstruction	Pathological processes
	Sarcoma of the seminal vesicles
	Neurogenic bladder
	Inflammatory diseases of the prostate
	Hematocolpos
	Prostatic abscess
Urethra	Valves (posterior and anterior)
	Diverticulum
	Phimosis
	Meatal stenosis
	Stricture (acquired—infections or traumatic)
	Stricture (congenital)
	Condyloma acuminata of the urethra
	Paraurethral abscess
	Foreign body
	Polyp
	Meatal atresia
	Hypospadias
	Carcinoma of the urethra
	Carcinoma of the penis
	Epispadias
	Ectopic ureter

Source: Wright FS, Howards SS. Obstructive injury. In: Brenner BM, Rector FC, eds. The Kidney. 2d ed. Philadelphia: W.B. Saunders, 1981, pp. 2008–2044.

struction is primarily due to intrinsic disease within the urinary tract or extrinsic disease.

V. CLINICAL MANIFESTATIONS

A. Symptoms

Urinary tract obstruction can result in a wide range of symptoms from none to the classic picture of renal colic. In general, acute obstruction is manifested by colicky pain, whereas chronic obstruction may present with signs or symptoms of renal insufficiency. An example of the latter is the disease entity ''silent'' prostatism, whereby patients do not realize they have progressive obstructive nephropathy until they present with hypertension, extracellular fluid (ECF) volume overload, and renal failure.

Acute obstruction is usually associated with flank pain that may radiate to the groin or genital region of the ipsilateral thigh. Patients with acute urinary tract obstruction commonly experience nausea, vomiting, and chills. If the renal unit is infected, high fevers may ensue. This event is a medical emergency requiring acute decompression of the urinary tract to prevent sepsis and rapid deterioration of renal function. Acute bilateral obstruction is rare, but when it occurs the patient can present with a sudden onset of anuria. This can occur with bilateral renal calculi, uric acid nephropathy secondary to cellular breakdown during chemotherapy or following ureteral ligation during a surgical procedure. More commonly, when the obstruction is bilateral and chronic, patients present with nonspecific complaints, such as an increase in abdominal girth, ankle edema, malaise, anorexia, headache, weight gain, fatigue, and shortness of breath. They may also have symptoms of uremia, such as mental status changes, tremors, and gastrointestinal bleeding. Unfortunately, chronic unilateral obstruction may go totally unnoticed, and total renal destruction may occur before the disease is identified.

One manifestation of obstruction, which should be sought for in taking a history, is the relationship of flank pain to fluid intake. Patients may develop pain when they drink, particularly alcoholic beverages or beverages with caffeine. An example of intermittent obstruction due to a ureteral pelvic junction lesion is shown in Figure 1. The diagnosis was not made until the patient was studied when

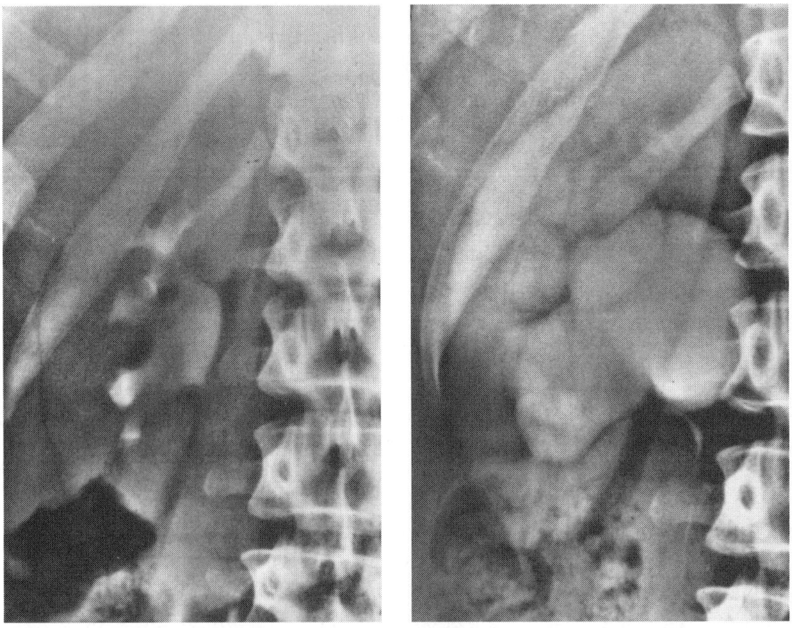

(a) (b)

Figure 1 An example of intermittent obstruction during diuresis: (a) a normal pyelogram when the patient was not hydrated; (b) significant ureteral pelvic junction obstruction with hydration and an episode of pain.

symptoms were present. Thus, obstructive uropathy should not be eliminated in a differential diagnosis of abdominal pain until appropriate imaging studies are carried out while the patient is having a painful episode.

The hydronephrotic kidney is susceptible to injury, and, therefore, if a patient complains of flank pain, or has a gross or microscopic hematuria following minimum trauma, the physician should consider an underlying abnormality such as hydronephrosis.

The common manifestations of obstructive disease due to prostatic enlargement or stricture disease are well known in male patients with symptoms of outlet obstruction. These patients complain of decreased force and caliber of urinary stream, intermittency, postvoiding dribbling, frequency, or nocturia. It is a recommendation that primary care physicians use the World Health Organization Symptom Score in their evaluation of patients with benign prostatic hypertrophy (Fig. 2). The Agency for Health Care Policy recommends treatment when the symptom score is greater than 7 and the quality of life score is 3 or more.

A paradoxical manifestation of obstruction of the urinary tract is polyuria and polydipsia. As will be discussed later, obstruction leads to tubular damage, distortion of the medullary interstitium, and impairment of urinary concentrating ability. Patients may present with polyuria and polydipsia as their sole manifestation of obstructive nephropathy. Finally, all patients who present with azotemia should be evaluated for what has been termed postrenal azotemia, which is simply another term for obstructive nephropathy.

B. Clinical Signs

The clinical signs of obstructive uropathy are nonspecific and depend on the underlying problem. The patient with acute renal colic is characteristically unable to remain in a stationary position, writhing on the table and complaining of severe pain. The patient with chronic unilateral obstruction and massive hydronephrosis may present with a smooth movable renal mass lesion, although this is unusual. More commonly, patients with intravesical obstruction will present with a palpable bladder and may also have signs of volume overload such as pedal edema, pulmonary congestion, and hypertension. Finally, signs of renal failure (see Chapter 3) may be present.

During the physical examination, the examiner should always examine the penis carefully, including the meatus and the foreskin, because severe obstruction can occur with both meatal stenosis and phimosis. A careful pelvic and rectal examination should be undertaken to look for signs of prostatic enlargement, rectal carcinomas, or potential extrinsic disease, such as intra-abdominal carcinoma with a rectal shelf. During the rectal examination, evaluation of anal sphincter tone should be carried out to help identify occult neurological disease. In women, a pelvic examination can identify any pelvic masses, e.g., carcinoma of the cervix, that may produce ureteral obstruction.

	Not at all	Less than 1 time in 5	Less than half the time	About half the time	More than half the time	Almost always
1. INCOMPLETE EMPTYING Over the past month or so, how often have you had a sensation of not emptying your bladder completely after you finished urinating?	0	1	2	3	4	5
2. FREQUENCY Over the past month or so, how often have you had to urinate again less than two hours after you finished urinating?	0	1	2	3	4	5
3. INTERMITTENCY Over the past month or so, how often have you found you stopped and started again several times when you urinated?	0	1	2	3	4	5
4. URGENCY Over the past month or so, how often have you found it difficult to postpone urination?	0	1	2	3	4	5
5. WEAK STREAM Over the past month or so, how often have you had a weak urinary stream?	0	1	2	3	4	5
6. STRAINING Over the past month or so, how often have you had to push or strain to begin urination?	0	1	2	3	4	5
	None	1 time	2 times	3 times	4 times	5 or more times
7. NOCTURIA Over the past month or so, how many times did you most typically get up to urinate from the time you went to bed at night until the time you got up in the morning?	0	1	2	3	4	5

Quality of life due to urinary symptoms	Delighted	Pleased	Mostly satisfied	Mixed–about equally satisfied and dissatisfied	Mostly dissatisfied	Unhappy	Terrible
If you were to spend the rest of your life with your urinary condition just the way it is now, how would you feel about that?	0	1	2	3	4	5	6

Figure 2 International Prostate Symptom Scoring (IPSS) Questionnaire.

C. Obstruction with infection

We cannot overemphasize the importance of diagnosing coexisting obstruction and infection. The presence of infection in an obstructed urinary tract is a potentially life-threatening situation and a true emergency. Appropriate imaging studies (excretory urogram, renal ultrasound, or CT scanning; see later) must be performed immediately and the obstruction relieved either by a percutaneous nephrostomy or a ureteral stent.

The rationale for immediate relief of obstruction is based on the physiology of fluid reabsorption during obstruction. After the onset of obstruction, there is an increase in intrapelvic pressure, resulting in pyelolymphatic and pyelovenous backflow, as well as possible forniceal rupture and extravasation. As a result, infected urine can flow directly into the vascular system during obstruction, resulting in life-threatening sepsis. In addition, animal studies have shown that the coexistence of obstruction and infection markedly accelerates nephron damage and limits recoverability following relief of obstruction.

VI. MECHANISM OF OBSTRUCTIVE RENAL INJURY

The pathophysiological events that occur in response to obstruction of the urinary tract are summarized in Table 2. In this section we focus on key events that form the basis of some of the diagnostic tests used to identify patients with obstructive

Table 2 Pathological Changes in Obstructive Uropathy

Increased renal vascular resistance
Afferent arteriole
Glomerular tuft
Efferent arteriole
Tubular damage
Concentrating defect
Sodium loss
Acidification defect
Infiltrating cells
Macrophages
T lymphocytes
Mast cells
Interstitial fibrosis
Fibroblasts
Ureteral changes

nephropathy. Acute obstruction to the ureter results in a characteristic triphasic relationship between renal blood flow and ureteral pressure (Fig. 3). The first phase is characterized by a rise in both ureteral pressure and renal blood flow, apparently mediated by vasodilatory prostaglandins and perhaps also by the nitric oxide system. Following this transient increase in pressure and blood flow, vasoconstriction of the afferent arteriole occurs with continued obstruction, resulting in a decrease in renal blood flow (phase 2) and eventually in ureteral pressure (phase 3). With continued obstruction, glomerular filtration is minimal, and over

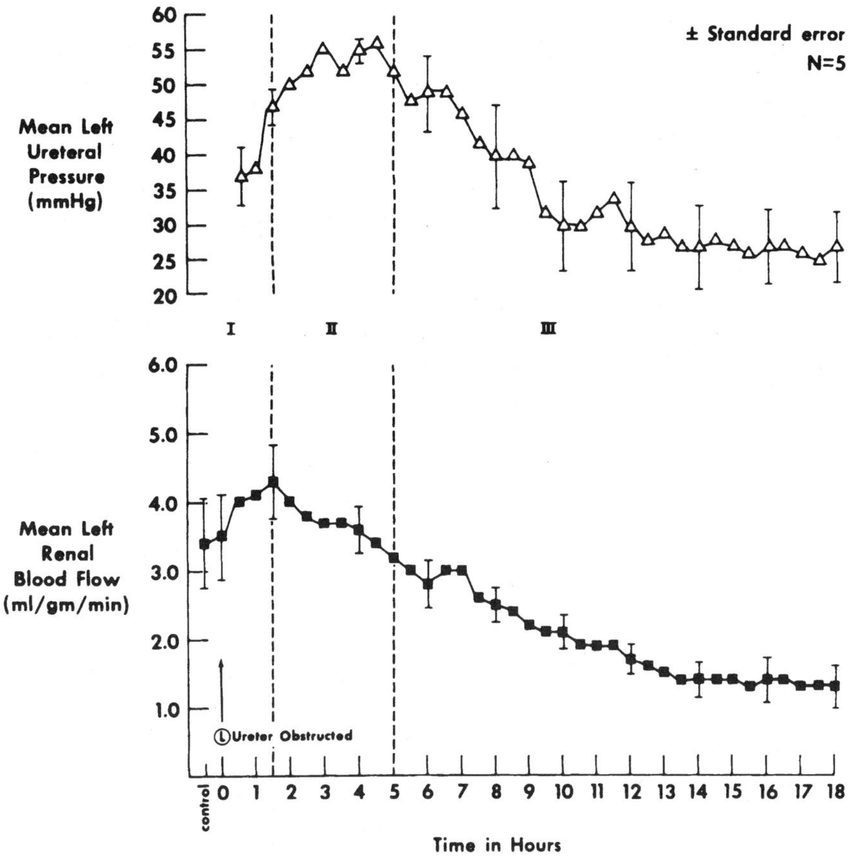

Figure 3 Typical triphasic response to unilateral ureteral occlusion. Phase I, initial transient vasodilatation. Phase II, the beginning of a decrease in renal blood flow. Phase III, typical decrease in renal blood flow signifying afferent increased resistance with a fall in ureteral pressure. (From Moody and Vaughan, 1975.)

time there is progressive renal destruction leading to irreversible renal tubular and glomerular changes. The time period for irreversibility of renal damage due to obstruction is not well documented in humans, but it appears to be longer than in dogs, where irreversibility occurs within 8 weeks.

The mechanism of the vasoconstriction that occurs in response to obstruction remains unclear despite exhaustive study. Several candidate factors are shown in Figure 4. There is evidence suggesting that angiotensin II and the vasoconstrictor prostaglandin thromboxane play at least a partial role in this reduction in renal blood flow. An alternative hypothesis is that there is exhaustion of the vasodilatory nitric oxide system, a notion supported by the fact that administration of arginine to the obstructed kidney returns renal blood flow towards normal. In children, evidence supports a major role for the intrarenal renin-angiotensin-aldosterone system as a mediator of the vasoconstriction. Regardless of the factors responsible, preglomerular vasoconstriction plays a major role in nephron damage. No pharmacological intervention has been proven to be effective in either reducing obstructive injury or enhancing recovery following release of obstruction.

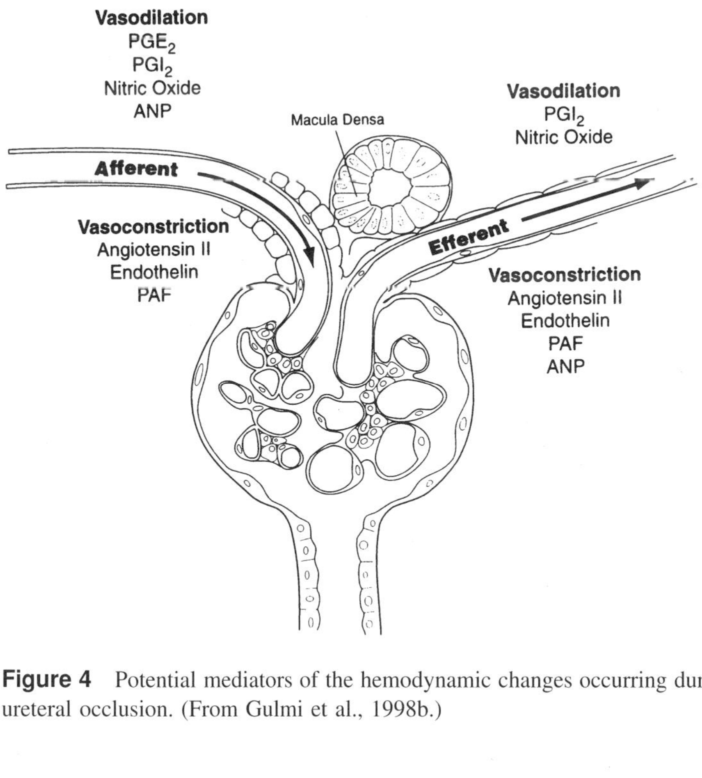

Figure 4 Potential mediators of the hemodynamic changes occurring during unilateral ureteral occlusion. (From Gulmi et al., 1998b.)

The presence of intrarenal vasoconstriction is the basis for one of the more useful tests in diagnosing obstructive nephropathy. Renal ultrasound has been used for some years to show hydronephrosis from an anatomical viewpoint (Fig. 5). Now doppler sonography is used in conjunction with ultrasonography to determine whether renal vascular resistance (an index of decreased renal blood flow; see below) is present. If resistance is elevated in an obstructed kidney, this finding suggests that the hydronephrosis has led to the physiological changes that we know experimentally lead to renal injury.

The second mechanism of damage in obstructive nephropathy is stimulation of fibroblasts and collagen production in the tubulointerstitial compartment of the kidney, leading to interstitial fibrosis. The recognition that interstitial fibrosis contributes to the damage in obstructive nephropathy offers the possibility of medical intervention with new antifibrotic agents in order to enhance recovery.

When only one ureter is obstructed, compensatory mechanisms in the other kidney minimize any change in overall renal function and normal homeostasis is maintained. By contrast, when bilateral high-grade obstruction is present or obstruction to a solitary kidney occurs, there will be systemic manifestations as

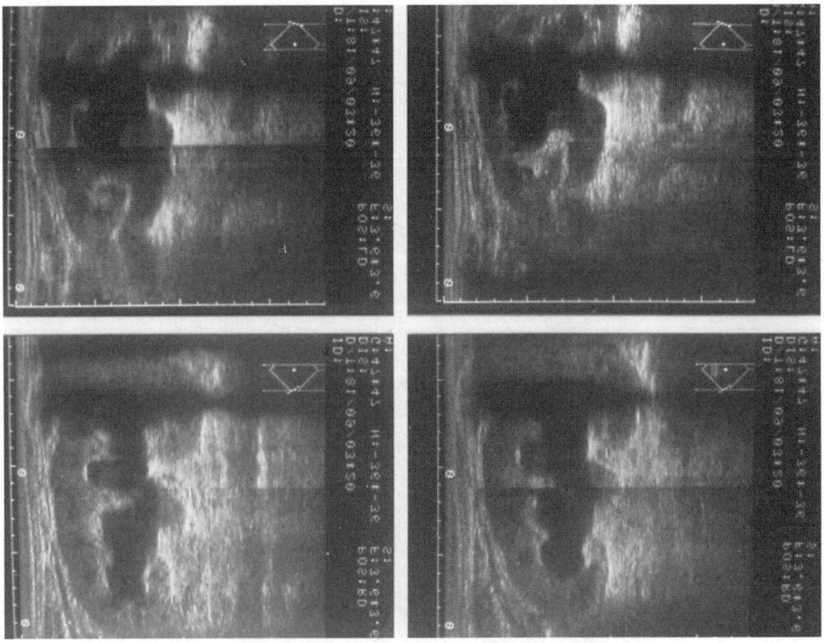

Figure 5 Ultrasound of a hydronephrotic kidney showing the dilated pyelocalyceal system and upper ureter in a case of hydronephrosis due to stone disease.

GFR falls and the patient retains Na^+ and water and becomes azotemic. In this setting, renal blood flow and GFR falls, but ureteral pressure is higher and there is less afferent vasoconstriction than with unilateral obstruction. This difference may play a role in the postobstructive diuresis that occurs after release of bilateral obstruction (see later). In contrast to unilateral obstruction, atrial natriuretic peptide (ANP) secretion is stimulated with bilateral obstruction, which enhances sodium excretion and maintains GFR. Administration of ANP may potentially enhance recovery of renal function following obstruction. Obstruction to the urinary tract impacts upon almost every parameter of renal function if the duration and severity of the obstruction are sufficient.

One entity commonly seen in clinical practice is ureteropelvic junction obstruction. Study of function after prolonged obstruction of one kidney, compared to its unobstructed partner in patients with this disorder, has given a snapshot of obstructive injury (Fig. 6). In Figure 6 renal function in a patient one week after release of a chronic ureteropelvic junction obstruction is shown. There is a reduction in GFR and in proximal tubular function as shown by T_{mPAH}, concentrating

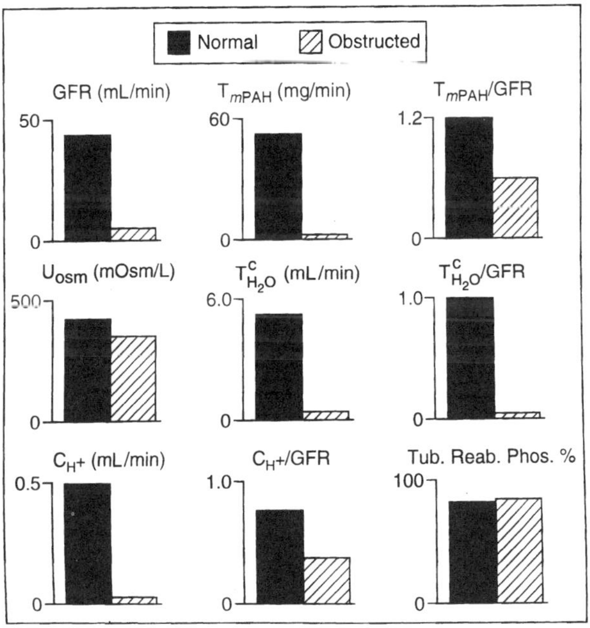

Figure 6 Differential renal function a week after correction of a ureteral pelvic junction obstruction (mannitol + ADH stimulation). The decrement in function of the obstructed kidney is shown in the hatched bars. (From Gillenwater et al., 1975.)

ability (T^c_{H2O}), and distal acidification. The ability to dilute the urine and proximal tubular reabsorption of phosphorus are normal. There is a disproportionate amount of tubular damage relative to glomerular damage when these two parameters are expressed in the form of a ratio. However, it is interesting that the glomerular damage is often quite severe, and therefore a postobstructive diuresis due to a defect in concentrating ability does not occur, except in the rare incidence where there is preservation of GFR on the obstructed side.

VII. DIAGNOSIS

A. Intravenous urography

The characteristic finding in obstructive uropathy is the presence of hydronephrosis with marked renal atrophy and a large collecting system. The traditional test to identify obstruction has been the intravenous urogram. As previously stated, the urogram shows anatomical hydronephrosis, but the simple finding of hydronephrosis does not necessarily mean there is renal damage. Examples of this phenomenon are shown in Figure 7. Figure 7a shows an intravenous urogram demonstrating massive ureteropelvic junction obstruction in an elderly woman who had the study performed because of microscopic hematuria. Despite this gross anatomical abnormality, she had a normal serum creatinine concentration (0.8 mg/dL), no clinical symptoms, and only hydronephrosis without renal damage. By contrast, Figure 7b shows an infant with bilateral ureteropelvic junction obstruction, hydrocalyces, thinning of the renal parenchyma, and a marked decrease in renal function requiring bilateral correction of the anatomical obstruction.

An additional point deserving emphasis is that obstruction can be intermittent, as shown in Figure 1. In Figure 1a, when the patient was not having pain, the kidney appeared perfectly normal, with fine cupping of the calyces and a normal renal parenchyma. However, when an intravenous urogram was performed during an episode of pain (Fig. 1b), ureteropelvic junction obstruction was obviously present, with marked fullness of the renal pelvis and swelling of the calyceal chambers.

B. Ultrasonography

Because of concern about the nephrotoxicity of intravenous contrast material, the first test ordered in patients presenting with acute obstruction is often a renal sonogram (Fig. 5). Renal ultrasonography is an excellent first study, but there is a small but finite possibility of obtaining a false-negative result in patients with a high degree of obstruction and little renal function, and of obtaining a false-positive result where there is a capacious collecting system but no true obstruction. Most centers now have the capability of using duplex doppler imaging dur-

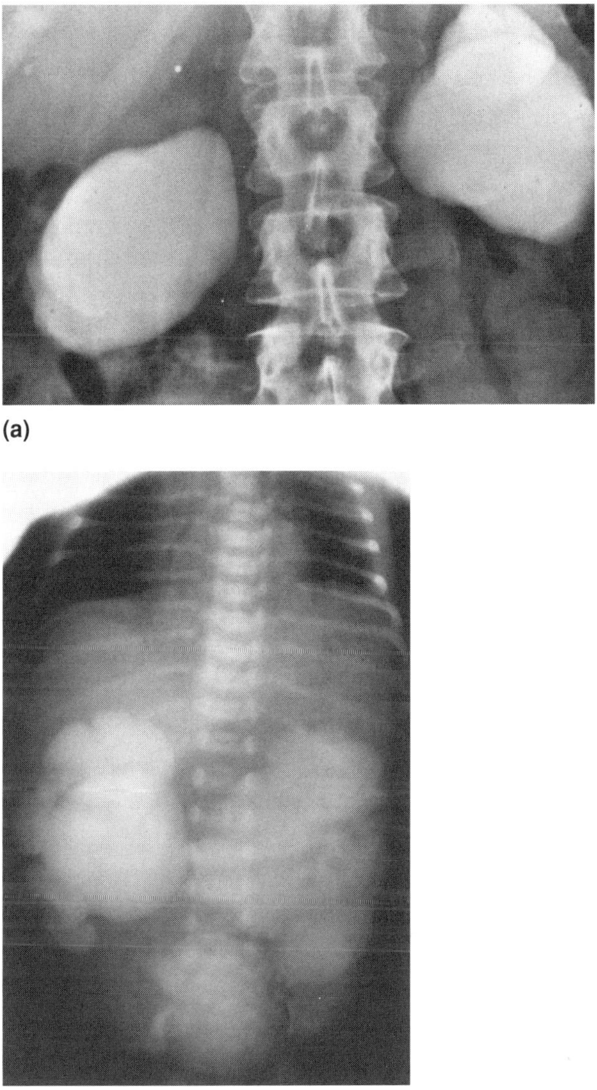

(a)

(b)

Figure 7 Examples of ureteral pelvic junction obstruction: (a) chronic obstruction in a patient without loss of renal function; (b) ureteral pelvic junction obstruction in an infant requiring surgical intervention.

ing ultrasonography, a technique that allows assessment of renal blood flow and vascular resistance. Flow velocities are measured and a ratio, termed the resistive index, is calculated as follows:

$$\text{Resistive index} = \frac{\text{Peak systolic velocity} - \text{lowest systolic velocity}}{\text{Peak systolic velocity}}$$

A value of 0.7 has been taken as the upper limit of normal. In obstructive nephropathy, the index is higher than normal, and it drops after relief of the obstruction. However, there is a great deal of variability in the test, and the radiologist performing the test needs to be well trained and sophisticated in interpretation and needs to pay attention to detail in performing the test.

C. Cystography

In children, additional valuable information can be obtained by cystography either with contrast or with radioactive material. In a child with intravesical obstruction due to posterior urethral valves or neurogenic bladder disease, obstructive nephropathy is often due to reflux of urine into the upper systems rather than obstruction. Fortunately, most mothers now receive ultrasound studies during pregnancy, and, therefore, many children are diagnosed with obstruction of the urinary tract before birth. Many of these ''obstructed'' systems return to a normal anatomical state without intervention; in contrast, some patients need immediate surgical intervention.

D. CT Scanning

Computerized axial tomography gives a great deal of information concerning not only the urinary system, but also other structures in the retroperitoneum and abdomen. This test is particularly useful when extrinsic obstruction of the urinary tract is suspected to make the diagnosis and to give the surgeon an aid as to the location and cause of the obstruction.

E. Diuretic Renogram

As stated throughout this chapter, there can often be anatomic hydronephrosis without true obstruction. The test used to separate these entities is the diuretic renogram (Fig. 8). The utility of this test is based on the notion that the excretion rate of an isotope-labeled compound taken up by the kidney is directly related to the volume of urine flowing through the collecting system. If the anatomical observation is truly obstructive, then impaired excretion or ''washout'' of the isotope is seen (Groups II and IIIb, Fig. 8). By contrast, there will be appropriate

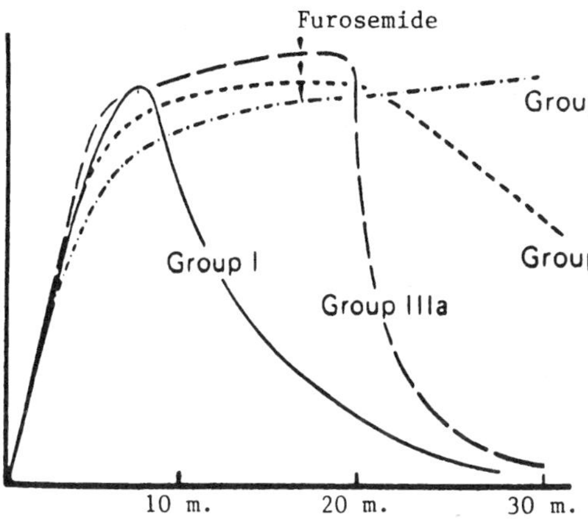

Figure 8 Different patterns found with a furosemide (lasix) renogram. Normal responses are shown in Group I. Progressive accumulation in Group II confirms obstruction. Rapid emptying after furosemide in Group IIIa indicates dilatation without obstruction. The partial excretory response of Group IIIb indicates either partial obstruction or renal dysfunction. (From Gulmi et al., 1998b.)

washout of the isotope if the dilated collecting system is simply due to an anatomical variation such as a megaureter (Group IIIa, Fig. 8). The most commonly used radiopharmaceutical agents are ^{99m}Tc mercaptoacetyltriglycine (MAG3) or the glomerular tracer ^{99m}Tc diethylenetriaminepentaacetic acid (DTPA). An advantage of the diuretic strategy is that it minimizes the radiation dose and obviates the need for potentially nephrotoxic radiocontrast material. Although there is still some controversy as to the exact technique, the radiopharmaceutical agent is generally administered first, followed by imaging. Twenty minutes later a diuretic, usually furosemide, is given intravenously and then the $t^{1}/_{2}$ for the clearance of tracer from the collecting system is measured.

Although not a perfect test, the diuretic renogram is widely used. Another use of the renogram is simply to determine the percent of function remaining in an obstructed kidney. From a surgical point of view, if there is minimum function (usually less than 10%) in an obstructed kidney, then the approach will be nephrectomy rather than attempting some form of reconstruction.

F. Whitaker Test

The Whitaker test is sometimes used by urologists to make a definitive diagnosis of obstruction, although it is not routinely necessary. This test measures renal pelvic pressure via a nephrostomy tube during infusion into the collecting system of fluid, at rates varying between 2 and 10 mL/min. A catheter is placed in the bladder to avoid bladder distention and renal pressures are monitored. The unobstructed system should have the capability of passing the infusion at 10 mL/min with a pressure of <15 cm of water.

G. Summary

At present, if urinary tract obstruction is suspected by either history or physical examination, the best initial screening test is the renal ultrasound. If anatomical changes suggestive of obstruction are found on this exam, the patient should be referred to a urologist for further workup and intervention if necessary. If the patient continues to have symptoms in spite of a negative ultrasound, an intravenous urogram at the time of symptoms, or a diuretic renogram at the time that the patient is having symptoms, intermittent obstruction may exist.

Sonography is also the first screening test to evaluate the cause of an elevated serum creatinine concentration to evaluate whether bilateral obstructive disease is responsible. In addition to demonstrating dilated upper tracts, this technique can also uncover an enlarged bladder due to urethral obstruction.

VIII. TREATMENT

Treatment of an obstruction to urine flow depends on its cause. Thus, placement of a urethral catheter gives marked relief to the unfortunate elderly male with acute urinary retention due to benign prostatic hypertrophy. Similarly, the passage of small ureteral calculus results in relief in the patient with unilateral obstruction due to stone disease. By contrast, multiple congenital anomalies of the urinary tract can lead to an obstruction that requires sophisticated diagnostic techniques and urological surgical expertise for correction. For the best care, patients should be referred to a urologist in a timely fashion for the treatment of obstructive uropathy, regardless of the specific cause. Often in the setting of acute unilateral obstruction resulting in severe pain, the initial treatment is the passage of a ureteral catheter or the placement of a percutaneous nephrostomy tube by an interventional radiologist.

IX. POSTOBSTRUCTIVE DIURESIS

After relief of obstruction, patients may exhibit a phenomenon referred to as a postobstructive diuresis, characterized by marked polyuria. One of the hallmarks of obstruction is impairment of urinary concentrating ability. In addition, when a patient has a severe bilateral obstruction, there may be retention of Na^+ and water as well as accumulation of factors that promote Na^+ excretion, such as atrial natriuretic factor (ANP). The diuresis that occurs after relief of obstruction may simply be a normal physiological response to fluid overload caused by retained urea, Na^+ and water, or it could represent a pathological event, i.e., injury to the kidney that leads to impairment of concentrating ability or Na^+ reabsorption. In most instances, the diuresis is a normal response to fluid overload, perhaps enhanced by high circulating levels of ANP. The patient most likely to develop a postobstructive diuresis can often be identified by history, physical examination, and laboratory evaluation. Patients at high risk have signs of volume overload with hypertension or perhaps congestive heart failure, peripheral edema, history of weight gain, and laboratory evidence of azotemia. By contrast, patients who present in urinary retention with normal laboratory findings, a short history, and no evidence of fluid overload will rarely develop a significant a postobstructive diuresis.

The optimal management is to anticipate the possibility of polyuria by monitoring the urine output carefully after relief of obstruction. If the urinary output exceeds 200 mL/hr for 2 hours, then urine output should be measured hourly and the patient's vital signs monitored (Fig. 9). To replace losses, an intravenous infusion should be initiated utilizing 5% dextrose in 0.45% saline in most instances and the rate adjusted to approximately half of the hourly urinary output. If the patient is awake and alert, then normal thirst and volume sensors will

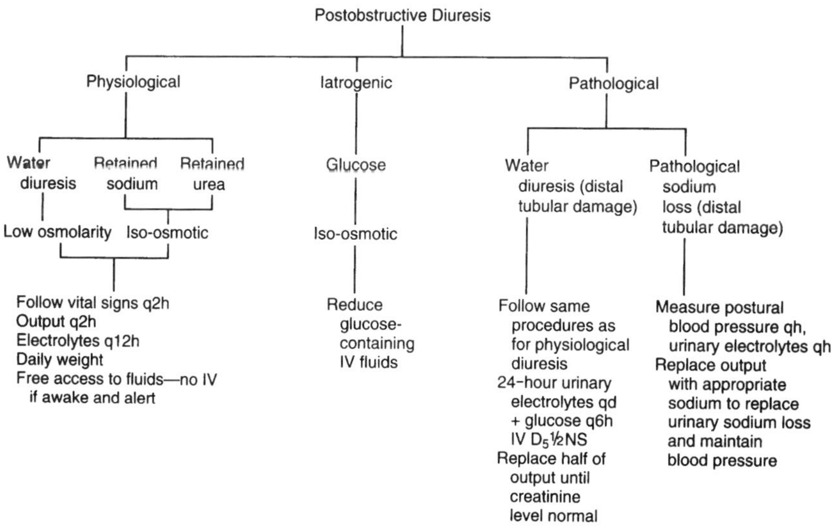

Figure 9 Findings of history and physical examination placing patients at high or low risk for postobstructive diuresis.

stimulate oral intake and close surveillance is less urgent. By contrast, very close monitoring and intravenous replacement is mandatory in the comatose or confused patient. The best way to evaluate water and electrolyte loss is to measure urine volume and Na^+ and K^+ excretion over a timed interval, e.g., 12 or 24 hours. Intravenous replacement of fluids should be used to maintain normal serum electrolytes while allowing the patient to lose appropriate Na^+ and volume, not to drive further diuresis.

The vast majority of patients will only have a physiological loss of Na^+ and water after relief of obstruction, after which the diuresis will remit. In another subset of patients, there will be a transient pathological Na^+ and water loss, but the patient can maintain homeostasis by eating and drinking. Rarely, patients exhibit a severe salt-wasting syndrome. These patients can become volume depleted rapidly and develop postural hypotension or hyponatremia. In such instances, nephrology consultation is necessary and close monitoring of salt replacement is mandatory.

X. HYDRONEPHROSIS AND HYPERTENSION

The incidence of hypertension among patients with ureteral obstruction varies according to whether the renal obstruction is unilateral and bilateral. The most common cause of hypertension and obstruction is a patient with acute stone disease, and the hypertension may well be due to the pain of the episode. However, hypertension and hydronephrosis can be related in a causal fashion through two mechanisms. In some cases of unilateral obstruction, the fall in renal blood flow to the obstructed kidney stimulates renin secretion, resulting in angiotensin II–mediated hypertension. In this setting, the investigator needs to assess the renin-angiotensin system in a systematic fashion to make the diagnosis (see Chapter 9). The peripheral plasma renin should be elevated due to increased renin secretion from the hydronephrotic kidney, and the renin measurement from the contralateral renal vein should be suppressed. In this setting, correction of the obstruction or nephrectomy will relieve the hypertension. In most cases of unilateral renal hydronephrosis, however, the hypertension and the hydronephrosis are simply coincidental and intervention should not be attempted with the thought that the hypertension will be cured.

In contrast to the rare instance of vasoconstrictor hypertension that occurs with unilateral obstruction, hypertension due to Na^+ and water retention (ECF volume expansion) is quite common in patients with chronic bilateral obstruction. We have found reversible hypertension in 88% of patients who presented with chronic obstruction and who demonstrated a postobstructive diuresis. Thus, the hypertension in these patients remits spontaneously with relief of obstruction and the excretion of excess Na^+ and water.

XI. SUMMARY

Obstructive nephropathy is one of the most common renal diseases encountered in primary care medicine. Fortunately, with a high index of suspicion and a careful history and physical examination, most cases can be diagnosed and treated promptly, avoiding significant renal damage. Despite vigilant medical care, silent obstruction also remains a common entity, occurring in either one or both urinary collecting systems. This entity should not be forgotten, particularly in the patient who has signs of impaired renal function without evidence of intrinsic renal disease. Renal ultrasonography is a simple and useful screening tool to identify most patients with obstructive uropathy.

SUGGESTED READINGS

Bell ET. Renal Diseases. Philadelphia: Lea & Febiger, 1946.

Curhan GC, Zeidel ML. Urinary tract obstruction. In: Brenner BM, ed. *The Kidney*. 5th ed. Philadelphia: W.B. Saunders Co. 1996, pp. 1936–1958.

Fung LCT, Steckler RE, Khoury AE, et al. Intrarenal resistive index correlates with renal pelvis pressure. J Urol 152:607–611, 1994.

Gillenwater JY, Westervelt FB, Jr, Vaughan ED, Jr, Howards SS. Renal function after release of chronic unilateral hydronephrosis in man. Kidney Int 7:179–186, 1975.

Gulmi FA, Felsen D, Vaughan ED, Jr. Management of post-obstructive diuresis. A.U.A. Update Series, Vol. XVII, Lesson 23, 1998a, pp. 178–183. Published by the Am. Urological Assoc.

Gulmi FA, Felsen D, Vaughan ED, J. Pathophysiology of urinary tract obstruction. 9 In: Walsh PC, Retik AB, Stamey TA, Vaughan Jr ED, eds. Campbell's Urology. 7th ed. Philadelphia: W.B. Saunders Co. 1998b, pp. 342–385.

Gulmi FA, Matthews GJ, Marion D, et al. Volume expansion enhances the recovery of renal function and prolongs the diuresis and natriuresis after release of bilateral ureteral obstruction: a possible role for atrial natriuretic peptide. J Urol 153:1276–1283, 1995.

Gulmi FA, Mooppan UMM, Chou S, Kim H. Atrial natriuretic peptide in patients with obstructive uropathy. J Urol 142:268–272, 1989.

Klahr S. Obstructive nephropathy. Kidney Int 54:286–300, 1998.

McConnell JD, Barry MJ, Bruskewitz RC, et al. Benign prostatic hyperplasia: diagnosis and treatment. Agency for Health Care Policy and Research. Clin Pract Guide/ Quick Ref Guide Clin 8:1–17, 1994.

Moody TE, Vaughan ED Jr, Gillenwater JY. Relationship between renal blood flow and ureteral pressure during 18 hours of total unilateral ureteral occlusion. Invest Urol 13:246–251, 1975.

Muldowney FR, Duffy GJ, Kelly DG, Duff FA, Harrington C, Freaney R. Sodium diuresis after release of obstructive uropathy. N Engl J Med 274:1294–1298, 1966.

National Kidney and Urologic Diseases Advisory Board. 1990 Long-Range Plan. Window on the 21st Century. Bethesda, MD: U.S. Department of Health and Human Services, 1990.

Palmer JM, DiSandro M. Diuretic enhanced duplex doppler sonography in 33 children presenting with hydronephrosis: a study of test sensitivity, specificity and precision. J Urol 154:1885–1888, 1995.

Peters CA. Obstruction of the fetal urinary tract. J Am Soc Nephrol 8:653–663, 1997.

Schlossberg SM, Vaughan ED, J. The mechanism of unilateral postobstructive diuresis. J Urol 131:534–536, 1984.

Schulsinger DA, Gross SS, Vaughan ED, Jr. Role of the NO system in urinary tract obstruction. In: Goligorsky MS, Gross SS, eds. Nitric Oxide and the Kidney—Physiology and Pathophysiology. New York: Chapman & Hall, 1997, pp. 443.

Stenberg A, Bohman SO, Morsing P. Back-leak of pelvic urine to the bloodstream. Acta Physiol Scand 134:223–234, 1988.

USRDS. 1998 Annual Data Report. Am J Kidney Dis 32(suppl 1):S98–S108, 1998.

USRDS: Annual Data Report. II Incidence and Prevalence. ESRD. Am J Kidney Dis 18(suppl 2):S34–S47, 1996.

Vaughan ED, Jr, Gillenwater JY. Recovery following complete chronic ureteral occlusion: functional radiographic and pathologic alterations. J Urol 106:27–35, 1971.

Vaughan ED, Jr, Sosa RE. Hypertension and hydronephrosis. In: Laragh JH, Brenner BM, eds. Hypertension: Pathophysiology, Diagnosis and Management, Vol. 2. 2nd ed. New York: Raven Press, 1995, pp. 2103–2110.

Vaughan ED, Jr, Sosa RE. Renovascular hypertension. In: Walsh PC, Retik AB, Stamey TA, Vaughan ED, eds. Campbell's Urology. 7th ed. Philadelphia: W.B. Saunders Co., 1998, pp. 423–459.

Whitaker RH. Perfusion pressure flow studies. In: O'Reilly PH, George NJR, Weiss RM, eds. Diagnostic Techniques in Urology. Philadelphia: W.B. Saunders Co., 1990, pp. 135–141.

Wright EJ, McCaffrey TA, Robertson AP, et al. Chronic unilateral ureteral obstruction associated with interstitial fibrosis and tubular expression of transforming growth factor-β. Lab Invest 74:528–537, 1996.

24
Inherited Renal Diseases

William D. Kaehny
University of Colorado School of Medicine and VA Medical Center, Denver, Colorado

I. INTRODUCTION

Major advances in genetics and molecular biology over the last decade have opened new vistas by defining the defects and precise inheritance of many inherited renal diseases. As a result of these advances, we have now identified the abnormal genes responsible for these diseases, identified the proteins produced by these genes, and in many instances shown how these abnormal gene products influence cell and organ function. Incorporation of this new information into our clinical diagnosis and management is an ongoing process. The task of the clinician is to be able to recognize the clinical manifestations of inherited diseases early on so that patients and their families can gain access to the latest information regarding the pattern of genetic transmission and interventions that can help them. As indicated below, there are a large number of hereditary renal diseases involving the glomeruli, tubules, and interstitium. Discussing each of these diseases in detail is beyond the scope of this chapter. Here we review some basic genetics, discuss the relationship between genetic defects and renal function, and then look at some of the more common hereditary renal diseases in greater detail.

II. INHERITED DISEASES AFFECTING THE KIDNEYS

Table 1 contains a listing of inherited renal diseases. To help think about these disorders in an orderly fashion, they are divided in the table into broad categories based on whether their predominant effect is on the glomeruli or the tubules. The tubular disorders are further subdivided into diseases that are dominated by cysts, stones, or functional abnormalities. Most inherited renal diseases are not mani-

Table 1 Inherited Disorders Affecting the Kidneys

- Disorders with major impact on the glomeruli
  - Alport's syndrome
  - Benign familiar hematuria (thin GBM disease)
  - Cystinosis
  - Fabry's disease
  - Lecithin-cholesterol acyltransferase (LCAT) deficiency
  - Lipodystrophy
  - Nail-patella syndrome
  - Sickle cell disease
  - Familial Mediterranean fever
  - Finnish congenital nephrotic syndrome
- Disorders with major impact on the tubules
  - Cystic disorders
    - Autosomal dominant polycystic kidney disease
    - Autosomal recessive polycystic kidney disease
    - Juvenile nephronophthisis
    - Medullary cystic disease
    - Medullary sponge kidney
    - Tuberous sclerosis
    - von Hippel-Lindau disease
  - Stone Disorders
    - Cystinuria
    - Familial distal renal tubular acidosis
    - Isolated hyperuricemia
    - Primary hyperoxaluria
    - X-linked recessive nephrolithiasis (Dent's disease)
  - Functional Disorders
    - Bartter's syndrome
    - Congenital nephrogenic diabetes insipidus
    - Familial proximal renal tubular acidosis
    - Fanconi syndrome
    - Gitelman's syndrome
    - Hartnup disorder
    - Iminoglycinuria
    - Liddle's syndrome
    - Oncogenic osteomalacia
    - X-linked hypophosphatemia
    - Vitamin D–dependent rickets (types 1 and 2)

fested at birth (congenital); some congenital renal diseases are inherited, but some are not.

A. Genetics of Inherited Renal Diseases

1. Very Basic Genetics

Humans pass on heredity by defining the nature of the proteins in their children. Proteins exist in three varieties—structural, membrane, and enzyme proteins. Absence of or alterations in the structure of any of these proteins (e.g., truncations, deletions, alterations in one or more amino acids) cause a loss of normal protein function, and abnormal or reduced protein function results in the manifestations or phenotype of a genetic disorder.

How are proteins inherited? Each protein is coded for in the genetic material passed on, the phosphorylated sugar-base deoxyribonucleic acid, DNA. Although a DNA molecule may be extremely large, it is composed entirely of repeated variations in only four—nucleotides, thymidine, guanidine, cytosine, and adenine—arranged in a linear sequence along its length. A sequence of three of these nucleotides (e.g., thymidine, adenine, adenine, abbreviated as TAA) is termed a triplet. Each triplet codes for a specific amino acid. The DNA triplets are packaged into linear segments in a chromosome, defining the specific amino acid sequence that determines the structure of a specific protein. The segment that codes for a specific protein is called a gene. Each chromosome of the 23 pairs in humans contains 2000–5000 genes. The total package of genetic material is called the genome.

How does a gene produce a protein? The DNA is activated and transcribes its message onto a messenger ribonucleic acid, RNA. This mRNA in turn leaves the cell nucleus and enters cytoplasmic ribosomes, where it translates the message into the desired arrangement of amino acids that constitutes a specific protein.

2. Genetic Mutations

The simplest genetic mutation is one that occurs in a single gene, encoding a single protein. Such mutations are termed monogenic or Mendelian disorders, and most of the new advances in inherited diseases are confined to such mutations. When the phenotype or disease expression does not follow the monogenic Mendelian pattern of inheritance described below, it may be due to polygenic (multiple altered genes) inheritance, mitochondrial inheritance (purely maternal via oocyte cytoplasmic mitochondria), genomic imprinting (one parental allele silent), or uniparental disomy (both alleles from same parent). The polygenic disorders most likely include many of the more common diseases (e.g., diabetes and hypertension) and are the target of ongoing research.

In this chapter we are most interested in single-gene or Mendelian disorders in which one abnormal gene is the determinant of the abnormal phenotype. They are the causes of the disorders presented in Tables 2 and 3. Mutations or changes in a gene may be of various types, but all result in a change in the structure of the protein product. Products that are abnormal, reduced, or absent result in the diseases presented in the tables.

The mode of inheritance of monogenic mutations follows Mendel's principles, and his terms are used to characterize them. Autosomal dominant inheritance means that an abnormal gene on one of the 22 paired nonsex chromosomes results in an abnormal protein, which in turn produces a detectable clinical phenotype. Autosomal recessive inheritance means that both of the paired genes (alleles) must be abnormal to produce a clinically detectable abnormality. When both alleles are identical for the gene in question, the individual is termed homozygous for that gene. If only one allele is abnormal, the individuals are termed heterozygous and are carriers without clinical abnormalities. In such heterozygotes, only half the normal protein may be produced, but this amount is sufficient for normal cell and organ function. Sex-linked disorders are caused by a monogenic mutation on the X chromosome.

The pattern of appearance of the abnormal phenotype in monogenic mutations is dependent on whether the mutation is dominant, recessive, or X-linked. An autosomal dominant disorder has its abnormal phenotype manifest in roughly half the children when one of the parents also has the disorder. An autosomal recessive disorder, by contrast, is fully manifested in only those affected with a double dose (homozygotes), not in the carriers of only one mutant allele (heterozygotes). Thus the carrier parents usually are unaffected, and, on average, one quarter of their children are affected. This pattern of inheritance may be hard to detect if the family is small.

X-linked defects are caused by mutations in one or both X chromosomes. They are always expressed phenotypically in male offspring, who have only one X chromosome. Women may have recessive or dominant phenotypes. Phenotypic expression in women with a recessive monogenic mutation requires that the genes be altered on both X chromosomes. Dominant trait expression requires only one mutant allele. Because one X chromosome in each cell is normally inactivated in women, phenotypic expression of both dominant and recessive monogenic mutations may vary from cell to cell. Because the X chromosome is not transmitted from father to son, fathers cannot transmit X-linked mutations to their sons.

Diseases that are transmitted by these classic Mendelian principles are the best studied and characterized but in most instances are rare. Exceptions in the area of renal diseases are the adult form of polycystic kidney disease (ADPKD) and Alport's syndrome, which are discussed in greater detail below. As mentioned earlier, more complex patterns of heredity occur with many common renal diseases, and the linkage of a clinical phenotype with a specific genetic mutation is often challenging.

Table 2 Mendelian Classification of Selected Inherited Renal Diseases

Disease	Pattern[a]	Chromosome[b]	Altered protein
Glomerular disorders			
Alport's syndrome	XL	Xq21.3	α 5 chain, type IV collagen
	AR	2q35-6	α 3 chain, type IV collagen
	AD	2q35-37, 13q34	Various chains, type IV collagen
Benign familial hematuria	AD, AR	Unknown	α 5 chain, type IV collagen
Fabry's syndrome	XL	Xq22.1	α-Galactosidase
LCAT[a] deficiency	AR	16q	Lecithin-cholesterol acyltransferase
Nail-patella syndrome	AD	9q34	Unknown
Sickle cell	AR	11	β Globin
Finnish congenital nephrotic syndrome	AR	19q13.1	Nephrin
Tubular disorders			
Autosomal dominant polycystic kidney disease	AD	16q13.3, 4q21-23	Polycystin-1 Polycystin-2
Autosomal recessive polycystic kidney disease	AR	6p	Unknown
Cystinuria	AR	2p16	Dibasic amino acid transporter
Dent's disease	XL	Xp11.22	Chloride channel
Juvenile nephronophthisis	AR	2q13	Nephrocystin
Medullary cystic disease	AD	Unknown	Unknown
Medullary sponge	Not inherited	—	—
kidney	AD	Unknown	Unknown
Nephrogenic diabetes insipidus	XL	Xq28	Vasopressin V2 receptor
	AR	12q13	Aquaporin-2 water channel
	AD	Unknown	Unknown
Tuberous sclerosis	AD	9q34	Unknown
	AD	16p13.3	Tuberin
von Hippel-Lindau disease	AD	3p25–26	g7 protein

[a] XL = X-linked; AD = autosomal dominant; AR = autosomal recessive, LCAT, lecithin-cholesterol acyltransferase.

[b] p refers to short arm, q to long arm of chromosome.

Table 3 Clinical Manifestations of Selected Inherited Renal Diseases

	Hematuria	Major Proteinuria	Stones	Hypertension	Hearing/ Vision	Renal failure
Alport's syndrome	X	X			X	X
ADPKD	X		X	X		X
ARPKD	X			X		X
Benign familial hematuria	X					
Fabry's disease		X			X	X
LCAT deficiency		X			X	X
Juvenile nephronophthisis						X
Medullary cystic disease						X
Medullary sponge disease	X		X			
Nail-patella syndrome	X	X		X		
Tuberous sclerosis						X
von Hippel-Lindau disease					X	X

ADPKD = Autosomal dominant polycystic kidney disease; ARPKD = autosomal recessive polycystic kidney disease; LCAT = lecithin-cholesterol acyltransferase.

3. Family History

When a hereditary renal disease is suspected, a complete family history is key. The physician should have all patients record a simple table of grandparents, parents, sibs, and children with name, gender, age if alive or at death, and all known diseases for each individual. In addition, the simple question ''Do any diseases or problems run in the family?'' should be included in the workup. Ethnic background is useful for some inherited renal diseases. The hereditary amyloidoses, including familial Mediterranean fever and Finnish congenital nephrotic syndrome, are examples (see Table 1).

4. Mendelian Inheritance of Renal Diseases

The linkage between a specific inherited renal disease and a monogenic mutation is complicated by the fact that many inherited renal diseases manifest several different patterns of inheritance (indicating that the disease can be caused by mutations at several different sites in the genome). Examples are Alport's syndrome, which has X-linked, autosomal dominant and autosomal recessive patterns of inheritance, and benign familial hematuria, which has autosomal dominant and autosomal recessive forms (see Table 2). Another variation is that the pattern of inheritance and disease manifestation can be identical but be caused by mutations in different genes, affecting different proteins. The most prominent example of this variation is ADPKD, which is caused by mutations in either the PKD1 gene on chromosome 16 or the PKD2 gene on chromosome 4. These genes code for very different proteins, but they cause the same type of cystic degeneration in the kidney. As research continues into the genetics of this common disease, additional genetic mutations that can cause the same disease are being uncovered.

B. Clinical Manifestations and Diagnosis of Inherited Renal Disease

The clinical manifestations of inherited renal disease are as broad as those for renal diseases in general. They include stones, gross and microscopic hematuria, back pain, dysuria, hypertension, edema, proteinuria, pyuria, azotemia, and electrolyte disorders. Nonetheless, the presence of one of these diseases is often first suspected by the characteristic constellation of findings that are manifested. Table 3 presents a summary of the signs and symptoms characteristic of the more common inherited diseases. Although they may have a characteristic group of symptoms and signs, none are sufficient to make a firm diagnosis. In most cases the clinical presentation needs the support of a positive family history or laboratory or biopsy findings to make the diagnosis. As discussed further below, critical to management is the ability to make a specific diagnosis. Misdiagnosis can have significant consequences not only for the patients but also for their families and their planning for future generations. The use of genetic mapping to identify specific mutations within families remains a research tool at present and is not routinely used for diagnosis and management. However, it is likely that this approach will become the mainstay for making specific diagnoses in the future, avoiding the risk of invasive diagnostic techniques such as renal biopsy.

C. Management of Inherited Renal Diseases

The specific management of inherited renal diseases is as varied as the diseases themselves (see Table 1), and a full discussion is beyond the scope of this chapter. With most of the rarer diseases, consultation should be sought for both diagnosis and management. This section covers some general principles and is followed by a more detailed presentation of several of the more common inherited renal diseases.

1. Genetic Counseling

One of the most important aspects of management for both the patients and their families is education about the mode of transmission and in particular the probability that future offspring will manifest the disease. Such education is relatively straightforward for autosomal dominant disorders such as ADPKD but is more complex with many disorders. In such instances referral for genetic counseling is recommended.

2. Natural History and Nonspecific Treatment

Until gene therapy or protein-replacement therapy becomes available, the clinician needs to emphasize education about the natural history of these diseases and focus on their treatable aspects. In this regard it is critical to make the correct diagnosis. For example, the young patient with gross or microscopic hematuria may have Alport's syndrome or thin basement membrane disease, disorders with markedly different prognoses (see later).

When hereditary renal diseases cause renal injury that can progress to renal failure, one should use the general approach discussed in Chapter 16. First and foremost is the need to control hypertension vigorously. In most instances, we recommend an angiotensin converting enzyme (ACE) inhibitor or angiotensin II receptor blocker. Next is the need to avoid use of nephrotoxic treatments and to adjust the doses of all medications for the level of renal function. Third is the need to treat urinary tract infections aggressively and to avoid urinary tract instrumentation.

III. MAJOR INHERITED RENAL DISEASES

A. Autosomal Dominant Polycystic Kidney Disease

1. Genetics and Pathology

ADPKD is a common cause of end-stage renal disease in the United States, accounting for about 10% of dialysis and transplant patients. ADPKD is an autosomal dominant disorder. Mutations of the PKD1 gene on chromosome 16 account for approximately 90% of the cases, and PKD2 mutations on chromosome 4 account for most of the remaining 10%. These genes code for the proteins polycystin 1 and 2, which both form heteromers in cell membranes with extensions into the cytoplasm. The functions of these complex proteins are not entirely established, but they may interact with each other to regulate cell-cell communication. A mutation in either polycystin produces the same disease. A PKD3 mutation has recently been identified, but its nature is not defined at this time.

The genetic mutations in ADPKD result in the formation of multiple cysts in both kidneys, and these cysts ultimately cause hypertension and slowly progressive renal failure. The cysts start as tubular diverticuli but then become disconnected from the tubules as they get larger. The cysts grow by secretion of fluid and cellular proliferation. The enlarged cysts compress and attenuate adjacent blood vessels. Tissue ischemia, inflammatory cell influx, tubulointerstitial inflammation, and fibrosis develop. The kidneys often enlarge to 12–16 inches in length and are readily palpable in most adult patients. At the end-stage of disease, the kidneys remain enlarged but consist mainly of fluid-filled cysts and scar tissue.

2. Clinical Manifestations

The three most common early manifestations of ADPKD are pain, gross hematuria, and hypertension. This triad of symptoms and signs is obviously not sufficiently specific to make a diagnosis, but if the kidneys are palpably enlarged, then ADPKD is highly likely. Other symptoms and signs that might bring a patient with ADPKD to the attention of a physician include stones (uric acid or calcium oxalate stones) and pyelonephritis. Although the kidney is the most affected organ in ADPKD, cystic degeneration is a systemic possibility. These patients commonly have liver and pancreatic cysts, although these only rarely compromise organ function. Extensive colonic diverticulae are also common. Five to ten percent of patients with ADPKD have cerebral aneurysms and may present with acute cerebral hemorrhage. Uremic symptoms occur late in the course of the disease. Most patients with ADPKD do not progress to renal failure until after the age of 50. Patients with the PKD2 mutation may not reach renal failure until they reach the age of 70.

3. Diagnosis

Despite the autosomal dominant pattern of heredity and the ease of diagnosis, a family history is present in only 60% of patients. The reason for this is that family size may be small, and parents and grandparents may have died from other causes before the disease would have become clinically apparent. In addition, asymptomatic siblings are often reluctant to undergo screening tests (see below). The presence of a clear family history and the usual constellation of findings—pain, hematuria, hypertension, and palpable, distorted kidneys—establishes the diagnosis. Renal ultrasound confirms the diagnosis by showing multiple cysts in both kidneys and showing cysts in the liver in about 50% of patients. The ultrasound findings are sufficiently pathognomonic to make the diagnosis in adults even in the absence of a family history, and ultrasound is currently the main tool for uncovering this diagnosis.

The diagnosis may not be as clear with ultrasonography in children, young adults, and occasionally in older individuals. In these cases, sensitive and accurate imaging can demonstrate definite renal cysts. Computed tomography is more sensitive than ultrasonography but is reserved for difficult cases. Simple cysts and cystic renal cell carcinoma are rare in people under 30 years. Therefore two or more cysts in one kidney and a positive family history are diagnostic of ADPKD. After age 30, the diagnosis requires two or more cysts in each kidney, and after 60 years at least four per kidney should be seen to avoid confusion with multiple, simple cysts, obstructive nephropathy, and chronic renal failure states.

On rare occasions, the clinician and ADPKD family may wish to determine the gene carrier state of a fetus, infant, child, or problematic adult. Gene linkage is more than 99% accurate but requires two informative family members with unequivocal ADPKD. The clinical need for diagnosis must be weighed against the effects on the occupational and insurance future of the individual. At present there are no definite therapeutic benefits to early diagnosis.

4. Complications of ADPKD

(a) Hypertension. Hypertension occurs early on in the course of ADPKD and is a well-established risk factor for increasing the rate of progression to renal failure. By the time advanced renal insufficiency occurs (serum creatinine concentration > 3.0 mg/dL), 80% of patients with ADPKD have hypertension. An activated renin-angiotensin system and increased extracellular fluid volume both appear to contribute. Left ventricular cardiac muscle mass seems more sensitive to hypertrophy when blood pressure is elevated in ADPKD than in other renal diseases. Although the effect of blood pressure control on disease progression in ADPKD is less well established than in other renal diseases (see Chapter 16), a strong benefit seems likely. In addition to protecting the kidney, control of blood pressure will reduce the likelihood of cerebral hemorrhage in patients with aneurysms. Target blood pressure should be less than 140/90, and even lower levels should be sought if they can be achieved without producing symptoms. At present ACE inhibitors are the first-line drugs of choice, although serum creatinine should be monitored carefully because sudden renal failure has been reported in patients with ADPKD who have enlarged kidneys and renal insufficiency. The acute renal failure is reversible if the drug is discontinued promptly. Diuretics should be avoided unless edema develops.

(b) Pain and Bleeding. Dull, persistent, nagging pain in the back, flank, or abdomen occurs in up to 60% of patients and is more common in women with ADPKD. Relief of pain is difficult in view of the need to avoid nonsteroidal and long-term narcotic analgesics. Cyst puncture by a skilled radiologist can provide temporary relief but is not recommended because the symptoms almost always recur in a short period of time. Surgical cyst decompression is a major undertaking and should be reserved as a ''last resort'' procedure. In the hands of an experienced surgeon, this procedure may provide remarkable relief without com-

promise of renal function. However, in many patients the symptoms may recur postoperatively. Many patients suffer only acute episodes of severe localized pain. The most common cause for these attacks is bleeding into a cyst, although a renal stone or infection is also common (see below). Careful questioning, search for fever, urinalysis, cultures, and perhaps computed tomography will direct a plan. Most importantly, needless exploratory laparotomies should be avoided in these patients.

(c) Infection. Infections may be localized to a single cyst or generalized (pyelonephritis). The distinction between pyelonephritis and cyst infection may be difficult. Cyst infections more often have localized kidney surface tenderness. If fever, leukocytosis, and tenderness persist, computed tomography may be useful to demonstrate a cyst with a thickened edematous wall. Cephalosporins, semisynthetic penicillins, and aminoglycosides remain the first-line agents to treat intrarenal infections, but failure to improve is an indication for switching to a quinoline antibiotic, because these agents penetrate cysts better (see Chapter 22). Percutaneous drainage is rarely necessary.

(d) Stones. Kidney stones occur at least twice as commonly in ADPKD patients as in the general population. Most commonly the stones contain uric acid or calcium oxalate. Individuals with ADPKD should undergo the same evaluation as any stone former. Low urinary citrate levels are common and suggest that treatment with potassium citrate may be successful. Lithotripsy seems to be safe although the long-term effect is uncertain.

(e) Extrarenal Complications. Although more than a dozen extrarenal manifestations have been reported in ADPKD, only four are of notable importance—intracranial aneurysms, mitral valve prolapse, liver cysts, and colonic diverticulosis. Intracranial aneurysms occur in about 5–10% of patients with ADPKD, with a higher prevalence in members of families with aneurysms. At present, screening of asymptomatic patients for aneurysm appears to be unproductive because of the cost and morbidity from subsequent treatment. On the other hand, a new severe headache in a patient with ADPKD warrants magnetic resonance angiography.

Mitral valve prolapse occurs in about 25% of patients. Symptoms such as palpitations and atypical chest pain may develop as a result of this valve abnormality. Liver cysts increase with age. More than 75% of patients with ADPKD over age 60 years have them. Most of these cysts are asymptomatic. If symptoms develop, the most common is pain. Cyst aspiration and sclerosis or surgical unroofing may relieve disabling pain. Occasionally a hepatic cyst becomes infected. Cyst drainage should be combined with antibiotics. Rarely hepatic cysts enlarge enough to embarrass hepatic function and varices can develop. In rare instances hepatic removal and transplantation is necessary.

5. Treatment of ADPKD

The principles that govern management of patients with chronic renal disease apply generally to ADPKD. As indicated above, they include aggressive treatment of hypertension and renal infection. More specific treatment is still untested. Low-protein diets do not appear to retard the progression of ADPKD. Cyst drainage may relieve symptoms but does not alter the natural history. Therapy of animals with cystic renal disease shows benefits with a number of maneuvers. These include amiloride to reduce secretion into cysts and consequent growth, taxol to induce microtubule function, potassium citrate to reduce ammonia production and avoid potassium depletion, and growth factor inhibitors to prevent cyst growth. We await studies in humans to determine the utility of these interventions as well as the development of gene replacement therapy.

B. Alport's Syndrome

1. Definition

Alport's syndrome is defined classically as hereditary nephritis and sensorineural deafness, transmitted as an X-linked trait. However, the term has evolved to encompass all forms of hereditary nephritis, some of which are not associated with deafness and some of which are not due to mutations on the X chromosome.

2. Genetics

Alport's syndrome is a disease affecting the renal glomeruli that becomes apparent in childhood. It accounts for only 3 of 1000 adults with end-stage renal disease but for 2.5% of children with ESRD. Alport's syndrome is often associated with sensorineural deafness and occasionally with ocular abnormalities. It is a monogenic disorder with several different modes of transmission: X-linked (80%), autosomal recessive (15%), and autosomal dominant (5%). All of the abnormal genes result in the production of an abnormal type IV collagen, a critical component of epithelial basement membranes. The presence of the defective collagen in renal glomerular and tubular basement membranes and variably in cochlear and ocular basement membranes determines the phenotypic manifestations in each family. In families with X-linked transmission, the expression of the disease is variable in females due to the random inactivation of the X chromosome from cell to cell.

3. Pathology

The basement membrane abnormalities are detectable only by electron microscopy. The glomerular basement membrane has a characteristic appearance, with intermittent thickened and thinned areas. In addition the membrane is lamellated and split in places by mesangial cell interposition. In the patient with hematuria, deafness, and a suggestive family history, this lesion is pathognomonic of Alport's syndrome. However, the pathological findings are neither specific for Alport's syndrome nor universally present. Abnormalities seen with light microscopy are completely nonspecific. The glomeruli become expanded with mesangial proliferation and then progressively become focally and globally sclerotic. Interstitial fibrosis and tubular atrophy increase progressively.

4. Clinical Manifestations

In the most common form of this disease (X-linked transmission), persistent microscopic hematuria is the critical and invariable feature in males. If a boy reaches age 10 years without developing hematuria, he does not have the syndrome. As many as 90% of females who are carriers (one affected X chromosome) have intermittent hematuria. Gross hematuria is common, especially during acute viral illnesses of childhood.

Other markers of progressive glomerular disease, including hypertension, proteinuria, and an elevated serum creatinine concentration, develop gradually over time. Occasionally nephrotic syndrome occurs. End-stage renal failure develops in all males at variable ages (usually before age 35), but strikingly with the same pattern in each family. Only about 15% of females develop chronic renal insufficiency with a few progressing to end-stage renal disease in old age. By contrast, autosomal recessive disease causes renal failure in the teen or young adult years in both genders.

Deafness occurs in 55% of males and 45% of females much later than renal disease, in the teens or later. Formal testing may pick up the high-frequency losses earlier. Interestingly, renal failure seems to stabilize the hearing loss. Eye involvement is usually manifested as distortion of the lens by anterior lenticonus, a finding virtually unique to patients with Alport's syndrome. All patients with this eye abnormality have deafness and develop renal failure before age 30.

5. Diagnosis

In a child or young adult presenting with isolated hematuria, or hematuria and proteinuria, the most important step in the diagnosis is to pursue the presence of a family history of renal disease. Search for a familial pattern of disease may even entail screening family members for microscopic hematuria. Hematuria in a child or adult with a family history of progressive kidney disease virtually assures the diagnosis of Alport's syndrome, particularly if hearing loss is associated. Confirmation of the diagnosis requires a renal biopsy with electron microscopy, but such a procedure is not always necessary, particularly if the diagnosis has been established in another family member. Renal biopsy is indicated when a family history of hematuria but no renal failure is obtained, to exclude another inherited renal disease—thin glomerular basement membrane disease (see below). In the absence of a family history, it is difficult to make the diagnosis, as the biopsy findings are not pathognomonic. Genetic linkage studies are possible when a specific mutation has been identified in a particular family, but such an analysis is difficult and at present is only a research tool.

6. Treatment

No specific treatment is available. The same general measures discussed earlier should be applied. When renal failure develops, renal transplantation is the treatment of choice and is very successful. In a small fraction of patients, anti-GBM disease develops in the kidney transplant due to development of antibodies against a basement membrane protein present in the donor kidney but absent in the patient because of their genetic mutation.

IV. OTHER SPECIFIC INHERITED RENAL DISEASES

Selected aspects of a few of the many diseases listed in Table 1 are reviewed below. The key features are summarized in Tables 2–6.

A. Inherited Diseases Affecting the Glomeruli

1. Thin Glomerular Basement Membrane Disease

This disease is transmitted in an autosomal dominant (or more rarely recessive) pattern and is manifest as microscopic hematuria. The hematuria is typically per-

Table 4 Features of Selected Inherited Renal Diseases Affecting Glomeruli

Disorder	Inheritance patterns[a]	Clinical manifestations
Alport's syndrome	XL, AR, AD	Hematuria, deafness, ocular lens deformity, late hypertension, ESRD
Benign familial hematuria	AD, AR	Thin GBM disease, rarely causes renal failure
Fabry's disease	XL	Youth limb pain crises, angiokeratomas, stroke, MI, proteinuria
LCAT deficiency	AR	Late renal failure
Nail-patella syndrome	AD	Proteinuria, hematuria, hypertension, may have late renal failure
Sickle cell disease	AR	Episodes of hematuria, proteinuria, nephrotic DI, distal RTA, progressive renal failure

[a] Mendelian inheritance patterns: AD, autosomal dominant; AR, autosomal recessive; XL, X-linked. LCAT; see Table 2.

Table 5 Features of Selected Inherited Renal Cystic Disorders

Disorder	Inheritance patterns[a]	Clinical manifestations
ADPKD	AD	Pain, hematuria, hypertension
ARPKD	AR	Abdominal masses, hypertension, liver fibrosis
Juvenile nephronophthisis	AR	Childhood polyuria, insidious renal failure
Medullary cystic disease	AD	Adulthood polyuria, insidious renal failure
Medullary sponge kidney	Noninherited, AD	Stones, distal RTA
Tuberous sclerosis	AD	Brain hemangiomas with seizures, renal angiomyolipomas and cysts, hypertension
von Hippel-Lindau disease	AD	Adult CNS hemangioblastomas, renal carcinoma

[a] Mendelian inheritance patterns: AD, autosomal dominant; AR, autosomal recessive; XL, X-linked. ADPKD, ARPKD; see Table 3.

sistent and can be punctuated with episodes of gross hematuria. In contrast to Alport's syndrome, the disease is benign and is not typically associated with proteinuria or renal insufficiency. The diagnosis is made by electron microscopy of renal biopsy specimens, which show a uniform thinning of the glomerular basement membrane and no other abnormalities. Thin basement membrane disease has been linked in some instances to the same genes implicated in Alport's syndrome, and it has been postulated that it represents the heterozygote state of an autosomal recessive form of Alport's syndrome. However, this remains unproven.

2. Sickle Cell Disease

Sickle cell disease is an autosomal recessive disease caused by a mutation of the β globin gene on chromosome 11. Sickling of red cells occurs when oxygen tension is reduced, and low oxygen tensions are normally present in the renal medulla. Sickling in the renal medullary vasa recta produces ischemia of the renal medulla, resulting in hematuria, proteinuria, papillary necrosis, hyperkalemic distal renal tubular acidosis, and nephrogenic diabetes insipidus. Chronic renal failure develops due to progressive occlusive loss of glomerular capillaries and hyperfiltration injury in the remaining capillary beds. Sickle cell trait is a cause of hematuria but not progressive renal disease.

Table 6 Brief Survey of Some Inherited Renal Tubular Functional Disorders

Disorder	Inheritance patterns[a]	Clinical manifestations
Renal glucosuria	AD, AR	Glucosuria at normal blood sugar
Fanconi syndrome	AD, AR, XL	Multiple tubule defects including phosphaturia, glucosuria, aminoaciduria, bicarbonaturia due to many different causes
Bartter's syndrome	AR	Hypokalemic metabolic alkalosis with high renin-aldosterone, but no hypertension
Gitelman's syndrome	AR	Like mild Bartter's with hypomagnesemia
Liddle's syndrome	AD	Hypokalemic metabolic alkalosis with low renin-aldosterone, but hypertension
Nephrogenic diabetes insipidus	XL, AR, AD	Polyuria, hypernatremia
Cystinuria	AR	Multiple cystine stones
Dent's disease	XL	Same as X-linked recessive hypophosphatemic rickets and nephrolithiasis

[a] Mendelian inheritance patterns: AD, autosomal dominant; AR, autosomal recessive; XL, X-linked.

B. Inherited Diseases with Major Impact on the Tubules

1. Cystic Disorders

(a) Autosomal Recessive Polycystic Kidney Disease. ARPKD is a rare disease due to mutation of chromosome 6. As the name indicates, it is transmitted as a recessive trait. Thus both parents must carry the gene and not manifest the disease, and each of their children has a one in four chance of having the disease. The disease typically presents at birth with large abdominal masses that are cystic kidneys. Hepatic fibrosis is the second major feature and causes portal hypertension (see Table 5). Hypertension is severe and needs vigorous management. Over half the patients do not survive the first few hours or days of life. Almost 80% of patients who survive the first year of life, however, are alive at age 15. These individuals present with the combined problem of renal and hepatic failure and are a special challenge.

(b) Medullary Sponge Kidney. This misnamed congenital disease of the kidneys consists of cystic dilatation of the medullary collecting ducts. Some cases are familial, but most appear to be sporadic. The pattern of inheritance has not

been worked out. The disorder is manifested by hematuria, recurrent calcium kidney stones, and hypokalemic distal renal tubular acidosis (see Table 5). The diagnosis is made by finding of medullary nephrocalcinosis in association with linear striations of contrast medium in the renal papillae on intravenous pyelography. Recurrent stone formation is a therapeutic challenge (see Chapter 21), but the disorder only rarely progresses to renal failure.

(c) Medullary Cystic Disease. This disorder is subdivided into two patterns of heredity. The first is inherited as an autosomal recessive trait, and this form is termed juvenile nephronophthisis. The second is inherited as an autosomal dominant trait and is termed medullary cystic disease. The juvenile form, as implied by the name, presents as renal insufficiency in childhood (age 4–10 years). The gene mutation occurs on chromosome 1. Medullary cystic disease, the autosomal dominant form, is due to a mutation on chromosome 2 and may not cause renal insufficiency for decades. The renal pathology in the two disorders is identical and consists of multiple minute cysts at the corticomedullary junction. These cysts are not usually visualized by intravenous pyelography or renal ultrasound, but may be seen with CT scanning. The clinical presentation is that of polyuria, renal salt wasting, anemia, and slowly progressive renal insufficiency. Because of the two patterns of heredity, one should be cautious in genetic counseling and not conclude that the recessive form is present without a clear family history.

2. Stone Disorders

Inherited diseases manifested primarily by renal stone formation are a group of rare disorders. Only two are discussed below (see Tables 1 and 4–6).

(a) Cystinuria. Cystinuria is a rare autosomal recessive disorder (estimated incidence 1 in 15,000) caused by a monogenic mutation that results in the production of a defective epithelial transporter for cystine and the dibasic amino acids ornithine, lysine, and arginine. The disorder is genetically heterogeneous, with at least three types described. With all types the homozygote excretes excessive amounts of cystine in the urine, resulting in cystine stone formation. The diagnosis is made by finding the characteristic hexagonal crystals in the urine and confirmed by a 24-hour urine measurement of cystine excretion. Treatment is mainly aimed at restricting the methionine content of the diet. Renal failure rarely develops, but when it does, transplantation not only cures the renal failure but also the disease itself because the transplanted kidney has a normal cystine transporter.

(b) Dent's Disease (X-Linked Hypophosphatemic Rickets and Nephrolithiasis). Dent's disease is a rare X-linked recessive disorder, which recently has been found to be caused by a defective chloride ion channel. As such it is

one of a new group of hereditary monogenic mutations, called ''channelopathies,'' i.e., diseases caused by defective ion channels in the renal tubules. These disorders are providing new insights into the role of ion channels in epithelial cell function and transport. Dent's disease is clinically manifest by hypercalciuria and renal stone formation and also low molecular weight proteinuria. The linkage between the defect in the chloride channel and the hypercalciuria remains to be determined.

3. Disorders of Tubular Function

A wide variety of rare inherited diseases affect one or more tubular transport functions. These result in clinical diseases as diverse as nephrogenic diabetes insipidus (see Chapter 1) and iminoglycinuria. The latter is a totally benign disease manifested only by abnormal excretion of imino acids and glycine. Both metabolic acidosis (familial proximal and distal renal tubular acidosis, and Fanconi syndrome) and metabolic alkalosis (Bartter's, Gitelman's and Liddle's syndromes) are caused by monogenic mutations. Gitelman's and Bartter's syndromes are due to defects in early distal and loop of Henle sodium transporters, respectively, and both are transmitted in an autosomal recessive pattern. They cause metabolic alkalosis without hypertension. Liddle's syndrome is another example of a channelopathy, unique in that the defective channel cannot be downregulated. The channel involved is the epithelial sodium channel in collecting duct, and its lack of responsiveness to a decrease in aldosterone secretion results in hypokalemic metabolic alkalosis and hypertension (see Chapters 11 and 13).

SUGGESTED READINGS

Fick GM, Gabow PA. Hereditary and acquired cystic disease of the kidney. Kidney Int 1994; 46:951–964.

Gabow PA. Autosomal dominant polycystic kidney disease. N Engl J Med 1993; 329: 332–342.

Guay-Woodford LM. Overview: the genetics of renal disease. Sem Nephrol 1999; 19: 312–318.

Kashtan CE. Alport syndrome and thin glomerular basement membrane disease. J Am Soc Nephrol 1998; 9:1736–1750.

Kashtan CE. Alport syndrome. An inherited disorder of renal, ocular, and cochlear basement membrane. Medicine 1999; 78:338–360.

Korf BR. Genetic testing for patients with renal disease: procedures, pitfalls, and ethical considerations. Sem Nephrol 1999; 19:319–326.

Scheinman SJ, Guay-Woodford LM, Thakker RV, Warnock DG. Genetic disorders of renal electrolyte transport. N Engl J Med 1999; 340:1177–1187.

Torres VE. New insights into polycystic kidney disease and its treatment. Curr Opin Nephrol Hypertens 1998; 7:159–169.

25

Hypertension and Kidney Disease in Pregnancy

Susan Hou
Loyola University Medical Center, Maywood, Illinois

Claudia Peano
Rush-Presbyterian-St. Luke's Medical Center, Chicago, Illinois

I. INTRODUCTION

The kidney and ureters undergo profound anatomical and functional changes during pregnancy. As a result, evaluation of renal function and blood pressure must be modified for the pregnant patient based on an understanding of the unique physiology and pathophysiology of pregnancy. Hypertensive disorders of pregnancy are among the most common severe illnesses affecting pregnant women. In women with preexisting renal disease, management of both the pregnancy and the underlying renal disease is immensely complicated. However, advances in medical and obstetric care have made successful pregnancy without further renal damage the usual outcome for women with renal disease and have allowed this outcome to be a reasonable hope even for women with more severe renal dysfunction.

II. PHYSIOLOGICAL CHANGES IN NORMAL PREGNANCY

A. Anatomical Changes in the Kidneys and Ureters

Renal length is increased by 1–1.5 cm as a result of glomerular and tubular hypertrophy. A physiological dilatation of the ureters occurs, giving rise to hydronephrosis, with urinary stasis of up to 300 mL in the ureters. Ureteral dilatation occurs as early as 12 weeks gestation because of an increase in estrogen and progesterone levels. Prostaglandin E_2 production also increases, an effect that inhibits ureteral peristalsis and causes the urinary stasis mentioned above. Dilatation is later aggravated by obstruction to flow as a result of the expansion of the uterus. Hydronephrosis, graded as severe on ultrasound, may be seen in normal pregnancy. Stasis of urine in the dilated, poorly functioning, and partially obstructed ureters predisposes pregnant women to urinary tract infections (see Chapter 10) and limits the accuracy of timed urine collections for clearance measurements. If such measurements are undertaken, a brisk diuresis should be induced during the collection period. The increase in renal size usually reverses during the first week postpartum, but hydronephrosis may persist for 12 weeks postpartum.

B. Changes in Renal Function

Dramatic changes in renal function occur during pregnancy (Table 1). Renal plasma flow increases to 50–70% above the nonpregnant normal level during the first two trimesters and remains 40% above normal in the third trimester. There is an increase in glomerular filtration rate (GFR) that begins by the fourth week of gestation, peaks at 150% of normal at 13 weeks, and continues almost until term. Dilatation of both afferent and efferent arterioles occurs in pregnant rats, indicating that increased glomerular blood flow is the major reason for the increase in GFR. There is little change in pressure across the glomerular basement membrane. Blood urea nitrogen averages 9 mg/dL and serum creatinine concentration 0.5 mg/dL during pregnancy, a reflection of the higher GFR.

Table 1 Renal Changes in Normal Pregnancy

Anatomical
1 cm increase in kidney length
Dilatation of the collecting system
Physiological
40% ↑ in renal blood flow
50% ↑ in glomerular filtration rate: normal BUN 9 mg/dl, creatinine 0.5 mg/dl
Respiratory alkalosis: normal PCO_2 27–32 mmHg, [HCO_3] 18–21 mEq/L
↓ Serum osmolality: normal 276–278
↓ Uric acid: normal 3–4 mg/dl
↓ Tubular reabsorption of glucose
↓ Afferent and efferent arteriolar resistance
↓ BP Normal: <125/75 2nd trimester, <125/85 3rd trimester
↑ Renin, ↑ angiotensin, ↑ aldosterone
↑ Prostacyclin and thromboxane

Uric acid clearance increases from 6–12 to 12–20 mL/min in pregnancy because of the increase in GFR and a decrease in tubular reabsorption. Uric acid in pregnancy is normally 3–4 mg/dL. An increase in serum uric acid is a sensitive indicator of preeclampsia.

C. Changes in Fluid and Electrolyte and Acid Base Balance

1. Salt and Water

Pregnant women normally retain 900 mEq of sodium and 6–8 L of water, 75% of which is in the maternal intravascular and interstitial space. Plasma aldosterone increases early in the first trimester and reaches a 7- to 10-fold elevation by term. Plasma renin activity increases fourfold early in pregnancy and then plateaus. Angiotensin II levels double early in pregnancy and rise to three to four times normal by term.

2. Osmolality

Serum osmolality is reduced by approximately 10 mOsm/kg H_2O during pregnancy, and serum [Na^+] is reduced by 5 mEq/L. The minimum osmolality at which ADH release is stimulated decreases from 285 to 277 mOsm/kg H_2O. Although ADH is released at a lower serum osmolality, the rate of metabolic breakdown of ADH is also more rapid because of vasopressinase produced by the placenta and released into the maternal circulation. Women with mild central diabetes insipidus suffer a worsening of their disease during pregnancy because they cannot increase vasopressin production.

3. Acid-Base Metabolism

Pregnancy is accompanied by a chronic respiratory alkalosis caused by stimulation of ventilation by progesterone. PCO_2 falls progressively to 27–32 mmHg in the third trimester. As a part of the normal renal response to sustained hypocapnia, serum bicarbonate concentration falls to 18–21 mEq/L.

4. Hemodynamic Changes

Diastolic blood pressure decreases by 7–10 mmHg during the first trimester and returns to prepregnancy levels in the third trimester. Changes in systolic blood pressure are less marked because vasodilatation is offset by increased cardiac output. The drop in blood pressure in pregnancy occurs despite sodium retention and increased levels of renin, angiotensin, and aldosterone (see earlier) because of a resistance to the hypertensive effects of both endogenous and exogenously administered angiotensin. This resistance has been attributed to production of prostacyclin by placental endothelial cells as well as other vasodilators, the relative importance of which is an area of intense study.

III. HYPERTENSIVE DISORDERS

Hypertension complicates between 2 and 10% of pregnancies in the United States and is the single most important cause of maternal morbidity. Blood pressure should be evaluated by comparison with blood pressure prior to or during the first 4 weeks of pregnancy. Diastolic blood pressure drops almost immediately during gestation and reaches its lowest point between 16 and 20 weeks gestation. In a previously normotensive woman, a rise in systolic blood pressure of 30 mmHg or a rise in diastolic blood pressure of 15 mmHg on two measurements taken 6 hours apart is considered hypertension. A blood pressure of greater than 140/90 is always considered elevated. Morbidity is increased if the blood pressure is ≥120/75 in the second trimester or ≥120/82 in the third trimester. Thus, in the absence of previous measurements, even these levels should prompt increased vigilance.

A. Classification

The hypertensive disorders of pregnancy are subdivided into preeclampsia, chronic hypertension, chronic hypertension with superimposed preeclampsia, and gestational hypertension. The last is a retrospective diagnosis, defined as hypertension that occurs late in pregnancy without proteinuria and that resolves postpartum. It may recur in subsequent pregnancies and is predictive of hypertension in later life. The remaining subdivisions are defined below.

1. Preeclampsia

Preeclampsia is characterized by the triad of edema, hypertension, and proteinuria occurring after 20 weeks gestation. Eclampsia is the above syndrome with seizures. Risk factors for preeclampsia include extremes of age, first pregnancies, chronic hypertension, diabetes, renal disease, twin pregnancies, and hydatidiform mole. Severe preeclampsia is a multisystem disease (Table 2). The most common abnormalities are microangiopathic hemolytic anemia (H), elevated liver enzymes (EL), and low platelets (LP), giving rise to the acronym HELLP. Preeclampsia and eclampsia can develop immediately postpartum, as well as during pregnancy. Twenty percent of HELLP syndrome and 4–10% of eclampsia, in fact, occur postpartum.

(a) Symptoms. Symptoms of severe preeclampsia include headache, visual disturbances and right upper quadrant pain, but 60% of women who progress to eclampsia have no premonitory symptoms. The hemolytic anemia seen in se-

Table 2 Manifestations of Severe Preeclampsia

Condition	Frequency in the HELLP syndrome (%)
Hemolytic anemia	100
Elevated transaminases	100
Thrombocytopenia	100
Disseminated intravascular coagulation	21
Abruptio placentae	16
Ascites	8
Acute renal failure	8
Pulmonary edema	6
Retinal detachment	4

vere preeclampsia is characterized by schistocytes on peripheral smear. The platelet count may drop below 20,000 as a result of platelet activation and consumption. Consumption of clotting factors occurs even in the absence of changes in prothrombin time and partial thromboplastin time. In approximately 20% of patients with the HELLP syndrome, frank disseminated intravascular coagulation (DIC) is seen. The liver disease of preeclampsia presents with right upper quadrant pain and elevated bilirubin and transaminases. Preeclampsia is one of a handful of conditions that can result in transaminase levels of >1000 units/dL. The most severe manifestation of hepatic involvement is hepatic rupture, which may result in exsanguination.

(b) Hemodynamic Effects. Glomerular filtration rate generally falls in preeclampsia, but because it is normally increased in pregnancy, it may remain within the nonpregnant normal range. In severe preeclampsia, acute renal failure can occur with acute tubular necrosis and rarely cortical necrosis (see Sec. V). Although pulmonary edema may occur in severe preeclampsia, information about hemodynamic changes in preeclampsia is conflicting. In preeclampsia, peripheral resistance is markedly increased and intravascular volume markedly decreased despite sodium retention. Measurements of pulmonary capillary wedge pressure in most preeclamptic women tend to be low-normal but are increased in patients with heart failure. Eclampsia occurs in <1% of patients with preeclampsia in large centers with extensive experience in managing such patients.

(c) Pathophysiology. Preeclampsia is an endothelial cell disorder that develops in response to placental ischemia. Placental ischemia appears to be caused in turn by inadequate trophoblastic migration into the uterine spiral arter-

ies. Endothelial cell dysfunction leads to increased production of vasoconstrictors, activation of the clotting system, and increased vascular permeability. During normal pregnancy, production of both the vasodilator prostacyclin and the vasoconstrictor thromboxane by endothelial cells is increased, and the balance favors the effects of prostacyclin. In preeclampsia, the ratio of thromboxane and prostacyclin production shifts in favor of thromboxane with resultant vasoconstriction. Other vasoactive substances such as endothelin and nitric oxide may play a role, and their contribution to the hemodynamic changes in preeclampsia is currently under investigation. Much of the end organ disease seen in preeclampsia can be attributed to hypoperfusion resulting from vasoconstriction. Activation of platelets and the intrinsic coagulation pathway also plays a role, producing fibrin deposition and hemorrhage in various organs. Seizures and other neurological manifestations of preeclampsia are the result of a combination of mechanisms including hypoperfusion, bleeding, and cerebral edema. The decreased GFR appears to be caused by a combination of hypoperfusion and capillary occlusion by swollen endothelial cells.

(d) Prevention. Two interventions, low-dose aspirin and calcium supplementation, have been extensively investigated to determine whether they prevent preeclampsia. Despite initial promise, the effects of these two treatments have been disappointing.

ASPIRIN PROPHYLAXIS. The discovery of the changes in prostacyclin and thromboxane ratios mentioned above in preeclamptic pregnancies led to efforts to prevent preeclampsia in high-risk women by giving low-dose aspirin. Five prospective randomized studies including over 23,000 women have been carried out to assess the benefits of aspirin with all but one showing no benefit. Subsidiary analyses looking at some groups of high-risk women are underway, but at present aspirin appears to be of little value in preventing preeclampsia.

CALCIUM SUPPLEMENTATION. Although a beneficial effect of calcium supplementation was reported in one study, the results have not been confirmed in a larger study undertaken by the U.S. Institute of Health and Human Development. The latter, a prospective, randomized, double-blind, placebo-controlled study of women, found no difference in the frequency of preeclampsia in 2295 women taking 2g of calcium daily and in a similar number of women taking placebo.

(e) Treatment. The definitive treatment for preeclampsia is delivery of the baby. Until delivery can be effected, the manifestations of preeclampsia must be managed medically. Only when preeclampsia occurs very early in gestation and is mild is an attempt to prolong the pregnancy warranted. A women with suspected preeclampsia should be hospitalized because of the difficulty in pre-

dicting seizures. There is no reason to delay delivery if the pregnancy has reached 36 weeks gestation.

Regardless of the stage of gestation, immediate delivery should be undertaken if there is any manifestation of the HELLP syndrome, any neurological symptoms, a rising serum creatinine concentration, a blood pressure >160/110 mmHg after 24 hours of hospitalization, and impending or actual seizures. Attempts have been made to prolong pregnancy in severe preeclampsia remote from term (<28 weeks gestation) and even following a seizure, but we consider this approach too dangerous for the pregnant woman to be recommended.

SEIZURE PROPHYLAXIS. Seizure prophylaxis is required while preparations for delivery are made. Magnesium sulfate, phenytoin, and benzodiazapines have all been used for seizure prophylaxis. In a prospective randomized study including over 2000 preeclamptic women who were assigned to treatment with either magnesium or phenytoin, there were 10 instances of eclampsia in phenytoin-treated women and none in magnesium-treated women. Magnesium sulfate has also been tested against phenytoin and diazepam for prevention of recurrent seizures in women with eclampsia and has been found to be superior to both. Magnesium sulfate is excreted by the kidneys, and oliguric women or women with preexisting renal insufficiency should be monitored carefully and treated with lower doses. Magnesium is a calcium channel blocker, and its use with other calcium channel blockers may result in profound hypotension.

MANAGEMENT OF FLUID VOLUME STATUS. The combination of sodium retention and intravascular volume contraction has led to treatment of preeclampsia either with diuretics or with volume expansion. Neither intervention is indicated as initial therapy. Diuretics aggravate hypoperfusion of vital organs and should be reserved for women with congestive heart failure. Volume expansion increases the risk of pulmonary edema. Hemodynamic monitoring by Swan-Ganz catheter is advised before using either of these interventions.

TREATMENT OF HYPERTENSION. Treatment of hypertension does not reverse preeclampsia and may even disguise progression but is nonetheless essential to prevent the most severe complications of preeclampsia, including cerebral hemorrhage. Treatment is usually started when the diastolic blood pressure is 105 mmHg but should be instituted earlier in women with very low blood pressures early in pregnancy. The drugs used to treat both chronic hypertension and hypertensive emergencies in pregnant women are discussed below. The goal of blood pressure reduction is a diastolic blood pressure of 90–100 mmHg.

2. Chronic Hypertension

Essential hypertension more often affects mothers in the later childbearing years. Almost half of women with essential hypertension have a fall in blood pressure into the normal range during the second trimester, with a return in the third trimester. This drop makes it difficult to determine whether a woman seen for the first time in the second trimester with normal blood pressure has essential hypertension or preeclampsia when the blood pressure rises in the third trimester.

Women with chronic hypertension have an increased risk of preeclampsia, perinatal mortality, small-for-gestational-age babies, premature delivery, and, in some series, gestational diabetes. Women with severe essential hypertension (BP > 170/110 mmHg) are at the greatest risk for preeclampsia and are also at risk for cerebral hemorrhage and abruptio placentae. The frequency of superimposed preeclampsia in this group is high: 52% in one group of 44 such women. Perinatal mortality, prematurity, and intrauterine growth restriction are markedly increased in such pregnancies. The frequency of superimposed preeclampsia in women with mild hypertension ranges from 5 to 18%. Maternal and fetal morbidity are increased even with mild hypertension, but the efficacy of pharmacological treatment in preventing complications and the level of blood pressure at which treatment should be instituted is a matter of debate. Most experts agree that safe medications are available for the treatment of hypertension during pregnancy and that treatment should be initiated when the blood pressure exceeds 140/90 mmHg.

3. Antihypertensive Medications

The effects of various antihypertensive medications in pregnancy are reviewed in Table 3. The FDA designation is included but does not adequately reflect the risks and safety of the various drugs.

(a) Angiotensin-Converting Enzyme Inhibitors. Angiotensin-converting enzyme (ACE) inhibitors are contraindicated in pregnancy. Exposure to ACE inhibitors in the second and third trimester has been associated with congenital anomalies in the newborn, including renal tubular dysplasia, hypocalveria, hypoplastic lungs, and limb contractures. Renal tubular dysplasia has been attributed to fetal hypotension and decreased renal perfusion. ACE inhibitors are associated with decreased fetal urine output and oligohydramnios. Amniotic fluid is required for normal pulmonary development, and oligohydramnios is responsible for the instances of hypoplastic lungs. Many of the neonatal deaths in infants exposed to ACE inhibitors are the result of respiratory failure. Oligohydramnios also accounts for limb contractures. Several instances of patent ductus have been described. This effect is thought to be the result of the effects of ACE inhibitors on prostaglandin metabolism. There is less experience with angiotensin II receptor blockers, but the problems caused by decreased angiotensin effect are very likely to be similar.

In contrast to risks associated with second and third trimester exposure, no ill effects have been reported with first trimester exposure. Women with inadver-

Table 3 Antihypertensive Drugs Used in Pregnancy

Drug (FDA Category)[a]	Comments
ACE inhibitors (D)	Contraindicated; second and third trimester use associated with pulmonary hypoplasia, hypocalvaria, renal dysplasia, neonatal anuria, contractures
α Methyl dopa (C)	Safe; 40-year use; careful developmental testing of children at ages 4 and 7
β Blockers (C)	Probably safe; fetal bradycardia, hypoglycemia, respiratory depression at birth, intrauterine growth restriction
Labetolol (C)	Limited first trimester experience; less bradycardia and growth restriction than β blockers.
Clonidine (C)	Probably safe; limited first trimester exposure
Ca^{2+} channel blockers (C)	Profound ↓ BP with when used with magnesium; limited experience; reserve for severe hypertension
Hydralazine (C)	Safe. Long experience with use in pregnancy; no birth defects
Minoxidil (C)	Very limited experience; hypertrichosis and congenital anomalies in infant
Prazocin (C)	Limited experience; no problems noted
Thiazide	Congenital anomalies with chlorthalidone; ↓ intravascular volume, neonatal thrombocytopenia
Thiazides (D)	Hemolytic anemia, electrolyte abnormalities
Nitroprusside (C)	Fetal cyanide toxicity
Diazoxide (C)	Fatal maternal hypotension reported; limit dose to 30 mg boluses; ↓ uterine contraction; neonatal hyperglycemia

[a]The following are FDA designations for the risk of drugs used during pregnancy: A, controlled studies fail to demonstrate risk to the fetus even in the first trimester and the possibility of fetal harm appears remote; B, either animal reproduction studies have not demonstrated a fetal risk with are no controlled studies in pregnant women, or animal reproduction studies *have* shown an adverse effect (other than decrease in fertility) that was not confirmed in controlled studies in women; C, Either studies in animals have revealed adverse effects on the fetus (teratogenic or embryocidal effects or others) and there are no controlled studies in women, or studies in women and animals are not available. Drugs should be given only if the potential benefit justifies the potential risk to the fetus; D, There is positive evidence of human fetal risk, but the benefits from use in pregnant women may justify the risk; X, Studies in animals or human being have demonstrated fetal abnormalities and the risk of using the drug in pregnant women clearly outweighs any possible benefit. The drug is contraindicated in women who are or may become pregnant.

tent first trimester exposure need not be advised to terminate the pregnancy. A more important issue is whether women with nephropathy taking ACE inhibitors for their renoprotective effect need to discontinue them in planning for pregnancy. For women with normal renal function where conception can be expected to occur within a year, stopping ACE inhibitors in planning pregnancy is warranted. However, for women with moderately impaired renal function who may not conceive for years, discontinuation of ACE inhibitors may not be necessary as long as pregnancy is recognized promptly when it occurs.

(b) Diuretics. Diuretics are contraindicated in preeclampsia because they aggravate intravascular volume contraction. In women treated for essential hypertension with diuretics, there is subnormal expansion of intravascular volume during pregnancy but no increased perinatal mortality. For essential hypertension, other drugs are preferred, but diuretics may be useful in hypertension associated with renal insufficiency and in some demonstrated salt-sensitive hypertension. There are some reports of neonatal thrombocytopenia, hemolytic anemia, jaundice, and electrolyte abnormalities with thiazides, but most of the concern about their use centers on their effects on intravascular volume.

(c) Methyldopa. Methyldopa has been used in pregnant women for over 40 years and is still the drug of first choice for essential hypertension. Careful developmental studies have been done at 4 and 7 years of age in children exposed to the drug in utero, and no problems have been found. One study of 242 women with diastolic blood pressures of 90–110 mmHg randomized to treatment with methyldopa versus placebo showed decreased fetal loss in the methyldopa-treated group.

(d) β Blockers and Labetolol. β Blockers have been associated with neonatal bradycardia, hypoglycemia, and respiratory depression. There are mixed data concerning whether β blockers are associated with intrauterine growth restriction. There is one report of small-for-gestational-age infants born to mothers treated with β blockers for diseases such as paroxysmal arrhythmias, which are not usually associated with growth restriction. There are also data from animal models suggesting a decreased ability of the fetus to withstand anoxic stress. Despite these reservations, this group of drugs is widely used with few problems. Fetal bradycardia may make it difficult to interpret antenatal monitoring, which depends on changes in fetal heart rate. Labetolol is not associated with fetal bradycardia and growth restriction, and it is widely used in preference to β blockers. Nonetheless, data on first trimester effects of the drug are still limited, and controlled studies have not shown it to be superior to other antihypertensive agents.

(e) Calcium Channel Blockers. Nifedipine and verapamil have been used in pregnancy both for control of severe hypertension and for tocolysis. They have not been associated with congenital anomalies. The experience with diltia-

zem is more limited. There have been reports of profound hypotension when magnesium was given to women taking nifedipine since magnesium is also a calcium channel blocker. Because the experience with calcium channel blockers is limited, most experts use them only for refractory hypertension.

Other drugs for treatment of chronic hypertension are summarized in Table 3.

4. Drugs for Hypertensive Emergencies

(a) Hydralazine. Intravenous hydralazine, in doses of 5–10 mg every 20–30 minutes, is the drug of first choice for hypertensive crisis in pregnancy because it is safe and effective. However, many studies comparing hydralazine with other drugs, most often intravenous labetolol, have found no advantage of one drug regimen over another. A single study has shown a higher frequency of malignant ventricular arrhythmias in eclamptic women treated with hydralazine than in women treated with labetolol.

(b) Labetolol. Intravenous labetolol given either as a 20 mg loading dose followed by 20–60 mg every 30 minutes or a 1–2 mg/min drip is the second most commonly used regimen for treating hypertensive emergencies in pregnant women. There are occasional reports of fetal bradycardia, and the newborn should be monitored for hypotension.

(c) Diazoxide. There is rarely a reason to use diazoxide in pregnancy. It is associated with decreased uterine contractions, neonatal hyperglycemia, and, in doses of 150–300 mg, with maternal death. Its only advantage is a long duration of action, which may make it useful when the patient must be transported with minimal monitoring capability or when other drugs have failed. It should be used only in 30 mg boluses every 1–2 minutes until the desired blood pressure is reached.

(d) Nitroprusside. Nitroprusside carries the risk of fetal cyanide toxicity, and it should be used with caution, especially in women with renal insufficiency.

(e) Nifedipine. Because of its interaction with magnesium and the general movement away from using short-acting nifedipine for hypertensive emergencies in nonpregnant patients, nifedipine should not be used in hypertensive emergencies of pregnancies.

5. Chronic Hypertension with Superimposed Preeclampsia

Ten percent of women with mild hypertension and up to 50% of women with severe hypertension develop superimposed preeclampsia. The diagnosis depends on an increase in blood pressure over baseline levels and the development of proteinuria. Because a modest increase in blood pressure in hypertensive women commonly occurs in the third trimester, proteinuria is a key finding for the diagnosis. The absolute level of blood pressure is frequently higher in these women than in isolated preeclampsia, and the risk of abruptio placentae and cerebral hemorrhage is increased.

B. Secondary Hypertension in Pregnancy

1. Pheochromocytoma

Pheochromocytoma is exceedingly rare but is associated with a 50% maternal mortality rate if undiagnosed. The maternal mortality rate is 11% even if the diagnosis is made antepartum. Catecholamines do not cross the placenta and the fetus is not exposed to high levels, but there may be placental hypoperfusion secondary to vasoconstriction. Hypertension can be precipitated by labor. Urine and plasma norepinephrine and epinephrine are unchanged in normal and preeclamptic pregnancy, and the usual biochemical screening can be used. The treatment of choice is generally surgery following 2 weeks of treatment with α blockers.

2. Cocaine

Cocaine use is a common cause of secondary hypertension in young women and may have a clinical presentation similar to that of pheochromocytoma. Serum and urine screening usually makes the diagnosis, and α blockers are required for treatment. Cocaine use is associated with an increased risk of abruptio placentae.

3. Hyperaldosteronism

Medical therapy is used in the treatment of hyperaldosteronism during pregnancy. Even if an adenoma is found, surgery is rarely needed. Spironolactone is an antiandrogen and may cause abnormal genital development in male fetuses. Amiloride can be used in pregnancy to treat primary hyperaldosteronism, but it is not as effective as spironolactone.

C. Long-Term Prognosis of Hypertensive Disorders

In subsequent pregnancies in women who survive eclampsia, hypertension recurs in one third, severe preeclampsia in approximately 5%, and eclampsia in 2%. The risk of recurrence of the HELLP syndrome is approximately 20%. Nulliparous survivors of eclampsia have a long-term cardiovascular mortality similar to the general population (23–42 years follow-up). The cardiovascular mortality for the multiparous survivors of eclampsia is increased. This group is thought to have a high incidence of underlying chronic hypertension.

IV. PREECLAMPSIA VERSUS PRIMARY RENAL DISEASE

In some situations it is difficult to distinguish between primary renal disease and preeclampsia, because both can present with hypertension and proteinuria. Because the definitive treatment for preeclampsia is delivery, certainty about the diagnosis has therapeutic implications. Practically, it is rarely possible to take advantage of a brief window of opportunity when proteinuria is heavy enough to raise the question of another renal disease and before the blood pressure is too high to do the biopsy safely.

In many women, pregnancy is the first occasion for a urinalysis in adult life, and the discovery of proteinuria at the first prenatal visit may reflect preexisting renal disease. The distinction between preeclampsia and primary renal disease is made on the basis of the same diagnostic features that differentiate the two diseases when the onset of proteinuria is known to have occurred during pregnancy.

Preeclampsia is the most common cause of proteinuria in pregnant women, and most women are managed as if they have preeclampsia unless there is some atypical feature that points to another renal disease. The likelihood of another renal disease is very high if the onset of proteinuria occurs before 20 weeks gestation, if there is no hypertension, if the urine sediment shows evidence of glomerular inflammation (cellular casts), or if serum complements are depressed. Only 25% of multigravidas with proteinuria have uncomplicated preeclampsia, and intrinsic renal disease should be considered in these women. Almost all renal diseases are manifested by proteinuria. The key issues with regard to intrinsic renal disease are discussed in the following section.

V. ACUTE RENAL FAILURE

The most common cause of an acute decline in renal function associated with proteinuria is preeclampsia. A rarer cause is hemolytic uremic syndrome, which has characteristic findings (see later). If the cause of renal failure is not apparent, particularly if accompanied by an abnormal urinary sediment, a renal biopsy should be obtained in a timely fashion to make a diagnosis and guide treatment. Acute glomerulonephritis, for example, can occur in pregnant women, and a biopsy is needed to determine whether treatment is indicated or likely to be effective.

Acute renal failure (ARF) in pregnancy usually results from obstetric complications (often in the setting of preeclampsia) and is largely a preventable problem. With this in mind, pregnancy-related ARF can be viewed more as a public health problem than a nephrological problem. Historically, ARF in pregnancy once represented 20–40% of all cases of ARF and was responsible for 50% of cases in women. In 1958, the estimated incidence of ARF in pregnancy was as high as 1 in 1400. Today, in industrialized countries the approximate incidence is 1 in 20,000. In pregnancy, ARF has a bimodal distribution. In early pregnancy ARF occurs in association with septic abortion, while in the third trimester ARF occurs in in association with late obstetric complications such as preeclampsia, abruptio placentae, postpartum hemorrhage, amniotic fluid embolism, and retained dead fetus.

A. Acute Renal Failure in Preeclampsia

Decreased GFR and renal blood flow and decreased sodium excretion are characteristic of preeclampsia, but frank renal failure is unusual. Acute renal failure in preeclamptic women occurs most often when another obstetric complication such as abruptio placentae is present or when preeclampsia has progressed to the HELLP syndrome. In the largest series of patients with HELLP, 8% suffered acute renal failure. When acute renal failure follows preeclampsia, there is substantial risk of maternal mortality, almost 10% in one series. Pulmonary edema occurs in over 50% of women with acute renal failure, emphasizing the need for judicious fluid administration in women with preeclampsia. Women without essential hypertension or underlying renal disease who survive acute renal failure in the setting of preeclampsia have normal renal function at long-term follow-up. When ARF occurs in women with underlying chronic renal disease and renal insufficiency, as many as 80% are dialysis dependent at follow-up.

B. Acute Fatty Liver of Pregnancy

Acute fatty liver of pregnancy is an obstetric emergency. If left untreated, it can progress to fulminant hepatic failure, which is life threatening for both the mother and fetus. The disease most often presents in the third trimester with complaints of headache, fatigue, malaise, nausea, and abdominal pain. Late signs include jaundice, bleeding, seizures, and hepatic encephalopathy that may progress to frank coma. Liver biopsy shows microvesicular fatty infiltration of hepatocytes in a centrilobular distribution. The maternal mortality rate for the disease is approximately 20%, with the lowest mortality rate reported being 6.6%. Acute fatty liver is frequently accompanied by preeclampsia and there may be a link between the two syndromes. The etiology of the syndrome is unknown, but recent investigations have found a familial metabolic defect in fatty acid metabolism.

Some degree of acute renal failure occurs in up to 90% of women with acute fatty liver of pregnancy. Clinically, the acute renal failure in this syndrome may resemble hepatorenal syndrome with low fractional excretion of sodium and benign sediment. Treatment includes delivery of the baby and supportive care. Acute renal failure usually resolves postpartum, as does the liver failure. The availability of orthotopic liver transplant offers a life-saving treatment to women who do not recover.

C. Bilateral Cortical Necrosis

In a majority of instances, ARF secondary to preeclampsia or peripartum hemorrhage follows a course typical of acute tubular necrosis with recovery. When ARF occurs as a result of another major obstetric complication, however, a substantial minority of patients develops bilateral cortical necrosis. If cortical necrosis occurs, recovery of renal function is only partial at best, and even if some recovery occurs, most patients eventually progress to end-stage renal disease. Obstetric patients account for over 50% of cases of cortical necrosis. Cortical necrosis can be diagnosed by CT scan or angiography. The diagnosis is made primarily for prognostic purposes.

D. Postpartum Hemolytic Uremic Syndrome

Hemolytic uremic syndrome (HUS) is characterized by a microangiopathic hemolytic anemia, thrombocytopenia, and renal failure. HUS usually occurs between one day and 3 months postpartum but may occur prior to delivery as well. Thrombotic thrombocytopenic purpura (TTP), a closely related syndrome that has extrarenal manifestations, also occurs during and less often following pregnancy. Renal failure in both HUS and TTP is often severe enough to require temporary dialysis, and patients usually suffer residual renal damage, some severe enough to require chronic dialysis or transplant. The treatment for HUS/TTP is plasma exchange. Prior to the advent of plasmapheresis, the maternal mortality rate was 90%. With this treatment, maternal survival has increased to 70–80%. Plasma exchange during pregnancy does not appear to have adverse effects on the fetus. Plasma exchange is thought to work by removing factors that promote platelet aggregation and replacing inhibitory factors that may be lacking in the serum of patients with HUS/TTP. Recurrence of HUS has been described in subsequent pregnancies.

It is sometimes difficult to distinguish HUS/TTP from the HELLP syndrome. Thrombocytopenia, microangiopathic hemolytic anemia, renal insufficiency, proteinuria, and hypertension occur in both syndromes. Some distinguishing features include isolated elevation of LDH in HUS/TTP as opposed to elevation of transaminases in HELLP. Elevations of prothrombin time and partial thromboplastin time are unusual in HUS/TTP and suggest preeclampsia. Preeclampsia generally improves following delivery, although there may be transient worsening for 48 hours. HUS/TTP is not improved by termination of pregnancy. The distinction is important since preeclampsia resolves with supportive care following delivery and HUS/TTP is generally irreversible without plasma exchange.

HUS/TTP is thought to be produced by endothelial injury and enhancement of platelet aggregation. Abnormally large multimers of von Willebrand factor are present in TTP, and these cause aggregation of activated platelets. Calpain, a cysteine protease capable of causing aggregation of normal platelets and of enhancing platelet binding by von Willebrand factor, has been found in some patients with active TTP. Decreased fibrinolysis may play a role. Plasminogen activator inhibitor type 1, the major inhibitor of plasminogen activator, is increased in some cases of postdiarrheal HUS. Decreased synthesis and increased degradation of prostacyclin has been suggested on the basis of studies using plasma from individuals with TTP. There may also be some genetic predisposition to HUS/TTP

While advances in treatment have dramatically increased patient survival in obstetric HUS/TTP, it still poses a significant threat to both mother and child, particularly if not diagnosed and treated promptly. Patients with pregnancy-associated HUS/TTP should be aware of the possibility of recurrence in future pregnancies and with estrogen-containing oral contraceptives.

VI. INTRINSIC RENAL DISEASE: GENERAL CONSIDERATIONS

A. Hypertension

Hypertension is a common complication of pregnancy in women with underlying renal disease even with normal renal function. The diagnosis of superimposed preeclampsia can be difficult because all manifestations of preeclampsia can occur from the renal disease itself. The approach to the control of blood pressure in women with preexisting renal disease is similar to the approach in women with women who are not pregnant (see Chapter 16). We recommend teaching women with underlying renal disease to measure their blood pressure at home between obstetric visits, because blood pressure can increase abruptly.

B. Proteinuria

Proteinuria generally increases in women with preexisting renal disease who become pregnant, but pregnancy does not precipitate a relapse in women whose nephrotic syndrome is in remission. The increase in proteinuria is in part due to the increase in GFR (and therefore in filtered protein) that occurs. Heavy proteinuria early in pregnancy has been associated with an increased rate of fetal loss, prematurity, and growth restriction, an observation that provides support for steroid treatment of susceptible lesions (see later). Nephrotic-range proteinuria occurring later in pregnancy does not adversely affect fetal outcome. Some patients develop massive edema, occasionally leading to skin breakdown and bladder outlet obstruction.

Steroid therapy should be confined to patients with severe nephrotic syndrome, who have a steroid-responsive cause for proteinuria. If the diagnosis is unclear, a renal biopsy should be done prior to initiating steroid therapy. High-dose steroids have been used in pregnancy for a wide variety of conditions and increase the risk of hypertension and glucose intolerance as well as adrenal suppression in the infant. Their use should be confined to minimal change disease or focal sclerosis (see Chapter 19) where there is a substantial chance of response. In patients with focal sclerosis, treatment should be continued only in women who have an early response (within 6 weeks).

If heavy proteinuria is caused by a renal disease that is not responsive to steroid therapy, management can be difficult. In this setting diuretics have a fairly low risk and may be helpful in the absence of preeclampsia. Unfortunately, patients with nephrotic syndrome frequently require diuretic doses that are much higher than those previously studied for safety in pregnant women. Pregnancy may aggravate the hypercoagulability associated with nephrotic syndrome. Women with previously documented renal vein thrombosis should be fully anticoagulated with heparin throughout pregnancy. Although there are no clear data, it is reasonable to give low-dose heparin (5000 units subcutaneously bid) to women with membranous nephropathy and profound hypoalbuminemia (albumin < 2 g/dL). Treatment of elevated cholesterol should be deferred until after delivery because HMG Co-A reductase inhibitors have been associated with congenital anomalies.

C. Effect of Pregnancy on Preexisting Renal Disease

The effect of pregnancy on the progression of underlying renal disease is determined in large part by the degree of renal impairment at the time of conception rather than by the nature of the renal disease. If a woman with renal disease conceives when her renal function is normal or near normal, progression is not usually accelerated, although her pregnancy is still likely to be complicated by hypertension and increased proteinuria. The largest study of pregnancy in women with glomerulonephritis and preserved renal function included 171 women who became pregnant and 189 women who did not after the onset of glomerulonephritis. There was no difference in the frequency of end-stage renal disease, with a mean follow-up of 15 years.

In contrast, there is an accelerated rate of decline in renal function in women who become pregnant with even mild renal insufficiency. There is disagreement about the level of renal function at which pregnancy becomes a factor in the acceleration of the disease, but the most widely used marker is a serum creatinine concentration of 1.4 mg/dl. The largest study of pregnancy in women with renal insufficiency included 82 pregnancies in 67 women with primary renal disease who had serum creatinine concentrations ranging from 1.4 to 5.5 mg/dl prior to conception or in the first trimester. Renal function deteriorated in 20% during pregnancy and in an additional 23% in the first 6 weeks postpartum. At 6 months postpartum, 8% had recovered renal function and an additional 10% had deteriorated. The likelihood of an accelerated decline in renal function was greater in women whose first measured serum creatinine concentration was greater than 2 mg/dL. Eight women progressed to end-stage renal disease within a year of pregnancy, including 7 women who experienced a decline in renal function during pregnancy.

With the obstetric and neonatal care currently available, fetal survival in the setting of chronic renal disease is high. The fetal prognosis even for women who conceive with impaired renal function has improved over the last two decades, with infant survival ranging from 70 to 100%. Prematurity and intrauterine growth restriction, however, are still common. Over 70% of infants are born prematurely, and the frequency of growth restriction ranges from 43 to 57%. Although initial reports suggested that diabetic nephropathy was not adversely affected by pregnancy, the level of renal function prior to conception determines the risk of accelerated progression in this disease as well.

VII. LUPUS NEPHRITIS

Lupus can usually be distinguished from preeclampsia by finding an abnormal urine sediment (red cell casts) or positive serologies for lupus. Both lupus and preeclampsia can be multisystem diseases, however, and there is some overlap in their extrarenal manifestations. Thrombocytopenia and hemolytic anemia are common manifestations of both. In preeclampsia, hemolytic anemia is distinguished by microangiopathic changes on peripheral smear. Both lupus and preeclampsia may be characterized by hypertension, rapidly progressive renal failure, and seizures. The pulmonary hemorrhage of lupus may appear similar on chest x-ray to pulmonary edema in preeclampsia. Clinical findings that can separate the two are the findings of pericarditis, joint pain, and skin rash, which are not characteristic of preeclampsia, or markedly elevated transaminases, which are not common in lupus. Thrombocytopenia that occurs before hypertension and proteinuria raises the likelihood that lupus is responsible. When the diagnosis of lupus is made during pregnancy, renal biopsy is warranted. Lupus that develops during pregnancy frequently has the histology of diffuse proliferative glomerulonephritis and may require the initiation of aggressive therapy during pregnancy. High-dose steroids can be used in pregnancy, but cyclophosphamide is teratogenic in the first trimester.

A. Course of Lupus Nephritis During Pregnancy

The bulk of the data from over 19 reports of 276 women with lupus nephritis supports the widely held impression that pregnancy has an adverse effect on the course of the disease. There is a risk of renal failure and even death in women with lupus nephritis who become pregnant. Of 276 women who had a diagnosis of lupus nephritis, 133 (48%) became worse during pregnancy. Thirty exacerbations were characterized by acute renal failure, and of these, 18 progressed to end-stage renal disease or resulted in maternal death. An additional 8 had a permanent decline in renal function that did not lead rapidly to end-stage renal disease. Nephrotic syndrome developed in at least 44 women. In studies where renal histology was known, the frequency of exacerbations was higher for women with membranous nephropathy than with diffuse proliferative glomerulonephritis even though membranous lupus is generally thought to have a more indolent course. Women with lupus nephritis were also at risk for severe extrarenal manifestations of lupus including cerebritis, pericarditis, and mesenteric vasculitis. The risk of exacerbation is lower in women whose disease has been in remission for more than 6 months prior to conception.

B. Effects of Lupus on the Fetus

Several characteristic problems occur in the infants of women with lupus. Women with anticardiolipin antibody have an increased risk of fetal loss. Lupus-associated autoantibodies are usually IgG proteins and cross the placenta. Neonatal lupus may be associated with skin rashes, thrombocytopenia, and hemolytic anemia. These manifestations resolve over 6 months as maternal antibody disappears. Antibodies to SSA are deposited in the conducting system of the fetal heart, and this is associated with irreversible congenital heart block. Some infants die in childhood from related myocardial fibrosis and heart failure, and others require long-term pacemakers.

VIII. RENAL INFECTIONS

Asymptomatic bacteriuria, defined as $>10^5$ colony-forming units of a single organism cultured from a clean-catch midstream urine specimen, occurs in 5–10% of pregnancies. Although this frequency is no higher than for normal nonpregnant women, up to 30% of pregnant women with asymptomatic bacteriuria will develop pyelonephritis if untreated. Screening by urine culture should be done at the first prenatal visit. Urine dipstick for nitrites and leukocyte esterase has not proven to be sensitive enough for screening, and the urine sediment may contain an increased number of white blood cells during pregnancy even in the absence of infection.

Pregnant women with a positive urine culture should be treated for 7–10 days using an antibiotic chosen on the basis of sensitivity of the organism and safety in pregnancy. Surveillance cultures should be done a week after the completion of treatment and every 4–6 weeks thereafter to monitor for relapse. A second positive culture warrants another course of treatment, and a relapse within a week of the initial antibiotic therapy should be treated with a different drug. For patients who relapse a second time, the usual course of antibiotics is followed by suppressive therapy for the rest of the pregnancy. Women with two or more relapses should undergo urologic evaluation when they are 12 or more weeks postpartum to allow pregnancy-induced changes in the urinary tract to return to normal. Patients who have a negative urine culture at initial evaluation and no other risk factors for urinary tract infection do not need additional testing unless they become symptomatic. The risk of acquiring asymptomatic bacteriuria during pregnancy peaks near term at 2%.

Pyelonephritis in pregnancy is a severe infection associated with bacteremia, hypotension, premature labor, and, in 2% of patients, respiratory failure. Pyelonephritis occurring during pregnancy is often associated with a decline in GFR that returns to baseline after recovery. Pregnant women with pyelonephritis should be hospitalized and treated aggressively with antibiotics and fluid resuscitation. Women who fail to improve with 3 days of antibiotic therapy should undergo ultrasound evaluation to rule out nephrolithiasis. Ultrasound may be difficult to interpret because of hydronephrosis, and if suspicion is high additional radiographic tests may be needed. A discussion of the safety of various antibiotics during pregnancy is discussed in Chapter 22.

IX. PREGNANCY IN RENAL TRANSPLANT RECIPIENTS

Over 6000 pregnancies have been reported in women of childbearing age who have received a renal transplant. Transplant recipients are advised to wait 2 years after transplant before contemplating pregnancy. Pregnancy should be undertaken only if blood pressure is controlled and renal function is stable with a serum creatinine of <2.0 mg/dl.

A. Effect of Pregnancy on Graft Function

In three of four case-control studies, pregnancy was not found to have an adverse effect on graft function. The limitation of studies done to date is the paucity of pregnant patients with serum creatinine concentrations greater than 1.4 mg/dl.

B. Infection

Urinary tract infections are the most common bacterial infections in pregnant transplant recipients, occurring in 40% of pregnancies. Monthly urine cultures should be obtained and prompt treatment initiated for asymptomatic bacteriuria. The infections of particular concern for pregnant immunocompromised women are listeria, herpesvirus, cytomegalovirus, and toxoplasmosis. Transplant recipients should be evaluated for previous infection with the latter three organisms prior to pregnancy or at the first prenatal visit.

C. Immunosuppressive Drugs in Pregnancy

1. Prednisone

Prednisone can be used in pregnancy. Maternal-to-cord blood ratios of prednisolone are approximately 10:1. When large doses are given, there may be enough fetal exposure to cause adrenal insufficiency in the newborn.

2. Azathioprine

This drug has been associated with small-for-gestational-age babies and neutropenia but no increase in congenital anomalies. The drug has an adverse effect on fertility in the second generation in animal models, but there are no data on fertility in humans exposed to the drug in utero.

3. Cyclosporine

During pregnancy, the space of distribution of cyclosporine may increase and the dose may need to be adjusted to assure levels in the therapeutic range. The most striking finding in transplant recipients treated with cyclosporine compared to those treated with other immunosuppressive regimens is an increase in small-for-gestational-age babies. The American Registry for Pregnancy in Transplant Recipients noted a low birthweight (<2500 g) in 49.5% and a very low birthweight (<1500 g) in 17.8% of 107 infants born to mothers treated with cyclosporine during pregnancy. The frequencies of low and very low birthweight in 207 infants born to mothers treated with prednisone and azathioprine were 39.1% and 7.7% respectively. The difference in gestational age was not significant (35.6 vs. 36.2 weeks).

There is a higher frequency of maternal comorbid conditions in women treated with cyclosporine; 52% are hypertensive prior to conception as compared to 18% treated with other regimens. More women treated with cyclosporine have prepregnancy serum creatinine levels of >1.5 mg/dL (24 vs. 14%). Whether hypertension and renal insufficiency prior to pregnancy are responsible for the growth restriction seen in individuals treated with cyclosporine is unclear.

Experience with tacrolimus in pregnancy is extremely limited, but the drug has been associated with neonatal hyperkalemia and oliguria. Experience with pregnancy in women taking mycophenolate mofetil is even more limited.

X. PREGNANCY IN WOMEN RECEIVING DIALYSIS

Fertility is decreased in patients with end-stage renal disease receiving dialysis therapy. The American Registry for Pregnancy in Dialysis Patients reports a frequency of conception of 0.5% per year in women under the age of 44. For unclear reasons, conception is two to three times more common in hemodialysis patients than in peritoneal dialysis patients. In pregnancies that occur in women receiving dialysis at the time of conception, the likelihood of a surviving infant is less than 50%. In women who begin dialysis during gestation, fetal survival is higher—approximately 70%. Both hemodialysis and peritoneal dialysis have been used during pregnancy. There is no advantage to one modality over the other either in fetal survival or in degree of prematurity.

SUGGESTED READINGS

Armenti VT, Ahlswede KM, Ahlswede BA, Cater JR, Jarrell BE, Moritz MJ, Burke JF. Variables affecting 197 pregnancies in cyclosporine treated renal transplant recipients. Transplantation 59:476–479, 1995.

Barceló P, Lopez-Lilo J Cabero L, Del Rio G. Successful pregnancy in primary glomerular disease. Kidney Int 30:914–919, 1986.

Baylis C, Reckelhoff JF. Renal hemodynamics in normal and hypertensive pregnancies. Am J Kidney Dis 17:98–104, 1991.

Chesley LC, Annitto JE, Cosgrove RA. The remote prognosis of eclamptic women: sixth periodic report. Am J Obstet Gynecol 124:446–459, 1976.

Cockburn J, Moar VA, Ounsted MK, Good FJ, Redman CWG. Final report of study on hypertension during pregnancy: the effects of specific treatment on growth and development of the children. Lancet 1:647–649, 1982.

Davison JM. Pregnancy in renal allograft recipients: prognosis and management. Clin Obstet Gynaecol (Bailliere's) 8:501–525, 1994.

Douglas KA, Redman CWG. Eclampsia in the United Kingdom. Br Med J 309:1395–1400, 1994.

First MR, Combs CA, Weislttel P, Miodovnik M. Lack of effect of pregnancy on renal allograft survival or function. Transplantation 59:472–476, 1995.

Ghandour FZ, Knauss TC, Hricik DE. Immunosuppressive drugs in pregnancy. Adv Ren Replace Ther 5:31–37, 1998.

Hanssens M, Keirse MJNC, Vankelecom F, Van Assche FA. Fetal and neonatal effects of angiotensin converting enzyme inhibitors during pregnancy. Obstet Gynecol 78: 128–135, 1991.

Hayslett JP, Lynn RI. Effects of pregnancy in patients with lupus nephropathy. Kidney Int 18:207–220, 1980.

Joint National Committee on Detection, Evaluation and Treatment of Hypertension: National high blood pressure education program working group report on high blood pressure in pregnancy. Am J Obstet Gynecol 163:1689–1712, 1990.

Jones DC, Hayslett JP. Outcome of pregnancy in women with moderate or severe renal insufficiency. N Engl J Med 335:226–232, 1996.

Jungers P, Chaveau D. Pregnancy in renal disease. Kidney Int 52:871–885, 1997.

Lindheimer MD. Preeclampsia-eclampsia 1996: preventable? Have disputes on treatment been resolved? Curr Opin Nephrol Hypertension 5:452–458, 1996.

Lucas MJ, Leveno KJ, Cunningham FG. A comparison of magnesium sulfate with phenytoin for prevention of eclampsia. N Engl J Med 333:201–205, 1995.

McCrae KR, Cines DB. Thrombotic microangiopathy during pregnancy. Sem Hematol 34:148–158, 1997.

Okundaye IB, Abrinko P, Hou SH. A registry for pregnancy in dialysis patients. Am J Kidney Dis 31:766–773, 1998.

Phippard AF, Fischer WE, Horvath JS, Child AG, Korda AR, Henderson-Smart D, Duggin GG, Tiller DJ. Early blood pressure control improves pregnancy outcome in primigravid women with mild hypertension. Med J Aust 154:378–382, 1991.

Purdy LP, Hantsch CE, Molitch ME, Metzger BE, Phelps RL, Dooley SL, Hou SH. Effect of pregnancy on renal function in women with moderate to severe diabetic renal insufficiency. Diabetes Care 19:1067–1074, 1996.

Sibai BM, Ramadan MK. Acute renal failure in pregnancies complicated by hemolysis, elevated liver enzymes and low platelets. Am J Obstet Gynecol 168:1682–1690, 1993.

Sibai BM, Ramadan MK, Usta I, Salama M, Mercer BM, Freidman SA. Maternal morbidity in 442 pregnancies with the syndrome of hemolysis, elevated liver enzymes and low platelets (HELLP syndrome). Am J Obstet Gynecol 169:1000–1006, 1993.

26

Management of Cardiovascular Complications in Patients with Chronic Renal Insufficiency

Deepak Malhotra
Medical College of Ohio, Toledo, Ohio

William L. Henrich
University of Maryland School of Medicine, Baltimore, Maryland

I. INTRODUCTION

Chronic renal insufficiency (CRI) is a complex syndrome with devastating consequences in which virtually every organ system in the body is affected. Ideally, medical management of these patients incorporates therapeutic strategies designed to preserve renal function as well as attenuate the extrarenal manifestations of chronic renal disease. These principles are discussed in Chapter 16 and illustrated in Figure 1. In this figure, the reciprocal of the serum creatinine plotted against time is used to estimate the point in time that the patient will require treatment for end-stage renal disease (ESRD). The goal of optimal management of patients with CRI is to reduce the rate of decline in renal function. An equally important goal is therapy for factors that contribute to cardiac disease and vascular disease in CRI. In this chapter we focus on therapies designed to reduce the severity of cardiac and vascular disease in patients with renal insufficiency.

The mortality rate in patients with CRI is much higher than in the general population, and cardiac and vascular disease are the most common causes of mortality in these individuals. Patients with end-stage renal failure are approximately three times as likely to have an atherosclerotic cardiovascular event (stroke or myocardial infarction) than the general population. This increased mortality due to cardiovascular disease is noted in both younger (less than 44 years

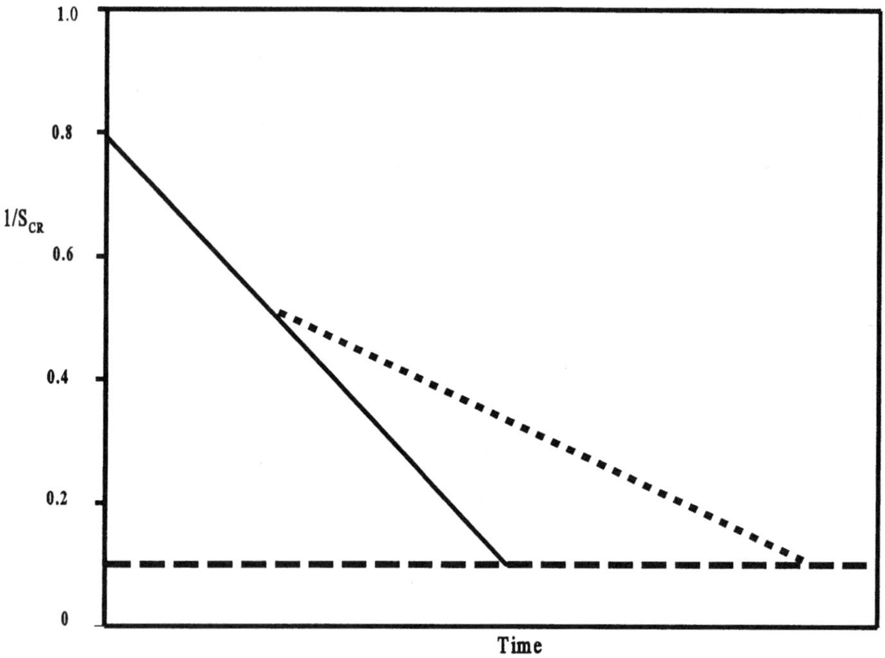

Figure 1 Altering the course of chronic renal failure. The solid line represents the decrease in renal function as a function of time in an individual with CRF. The dotted line depicts attenuation of the rate of renal function loss with various maneuvers such as good BP control. The dashed line represents the degree of renal function in which renal replacement therapy should be started.

of age) as well as older individuals with ESRD. The high incidence of cardiac disease in younger patients suggests that the derangements causing accelerated atherosclerosis probably begin early in the course of renal insufficiency and are not simply a coincidental feature of aging. Therefore, if progress in reducing the high incidence of morbidity and mortality in renal failure is to be made, interventions to slow or reverse the development of cardiac and vascular disease in patients with renal insufficiency should be undertaken early in the course of the disease. These interventions include dietary manipulations, behavioral techniques to reduce risk, and pharmacological therapies.

II. CARDIAC ABNORMALITIES

The cardiac disorders that occur in individuals with CRI are grouped into two main categories, left ventricular hypertrophy (LVH) and coronary artery disease

(CAD). Often the two disorders coexist. Either can result in congestive heart failure, increasing morbidity and mortality and complicating the management of renal failure. LVH has several associated consequences including the development of diastolic dysfunction, an abnormality that may predispose to episodes of sudden ("flash") pulmonary edema and may reduce the ability to decrease extracellular fluid (ECF) volume during hemodialysis. CAD eventually may result in myocardial infarction and fibrosis and thus contribute to left ventricular (LV) systolic dysfunction and a predisposition to pulmonary edema.

A. Left Ventricular Hypertrophy

The association between LVH and renal disease was first noted by Bright in 1836. He proposed that a greater force was required to pump the blood through the capillaries in patients with renal disease. Interestingly, this observation was made approximately 75 years prior to the development of a blood pressure–measuring device. It is estimated that 75% of individuals beginning dialysis have abnormal echocardiograms. The most common abnormality is concentric LVH. The abnormalities in cardiac structure are associated with physiological abnormalities such as diastolic or systolic dysfunction in many patients. The major contributors to the development of LVH are hypertension and anemia, although other factors have been implicated as well. Hypertension contributes not only to the development of cardiac dysfunction but also to an accelerated loss of kidney function.

1. Hypertension

The kidney is directly involved in blood pressure homeostasis, and its contribution is largely accomplished through control of extracellular fluid volume. It is, therefore, not unexpected that a decrease in renal function is associated with hypertension (see Chapter 17). Hypertension in patients with renal insufficiency is associated with abnormalities in the renin-angiotensin-aldosterone axis as well as with the sympathetic nervous system and may involve other vasoconstrictive peptides as well. Evidence is accumulating that abnormalities in vascular endothelial function that lead to an imbalance between vasodilators (e.g., prostaglandins, kallikrein, nitric oxide) and vasoconstrictors (e.g., endothelin) may favor the development of hypertension in patients with renal disease. Many endogenous vasoconstrictors are also growth factors and promoters of fibrosis. In particular, angiotensin II is known to be a potent growth factor, and aldosterone may independently promote fibrosis. These substances have been implicated in the development of the characteristic cardiac abnormalities induced by hypertension.

The frequency of hypertension in individuals with CRI varies with the etiology of the underlying kidney disease (see Table 1) and severity of renal insufficiency. For instance, in membranous nephropathy, 18% of individuals will have

Table 1 Reported Incidence of Hypertension in Renal Disease

Chronic glomerulonephritis	61%
Postinfectious glomerulonephritis	45–82%
Hemolytic uremic syndrome	60%
Vasculitis	25%
Systemic lupus erythematosus with renal involvement	15–60%
Membranous nephropathy	25–30%
Membranoproliferative glomerulonephritis	30–42%
Focal and segmental glomerulosclerosis	29–63%
IgA nephropathy	8–37%
Reflux nephropathy	17–41%
Polycystic kidney disease	40–90%
Diabetes mellitus	10–80%

hypertension if the glomerular filtration rate (GFR) is greater than 80 mL/min, whereas with ESRD the prevalence of hypertension is estimated at 85%. Hypertension often precedes the development of overt renal insufficiency in diabetic nephropathy, autosomal dominant polycystic kidney disease, and reflux nephropathy.

Control of hypertension is a major focus of therapy because it is the major contributor to LVH. A presistently elevated systolic blood pressure leads both to the development of LVH and impairment in diastolic relaxation. If this is prolonged, LV decompensation gradually develops and heart failure ensues. Successful treatment of hypertension can reverse LVH. Angiotensin-converting enzyme (ACE) inhibitors, calcium channel blockers, β blockers, and central acting adrenolytic agents have all been shown to reduce LVH in a relatively short time (4–8 weeks). Diuretics and direct smooth muscle dilators also can reverse or reduce LVH but require a longer time interval in order to elicit this effect. A recent meta-analysis probed the ability of a variety of antihypertensive drugs to reverse LVH in individuals with essential hypertension and concluded that ACE inhibitors are superior in this regard to β blockers and diuretics. The calcium channel blockers also decreased LVH, albeit to a smaller extent than ACE inhibitors.

Not only can blood pressure control reduce or reverse LVH, it also attenuates the progression of renal insufficiency of any etiology (see Chapters 16–18). In individuals with type 2 diabetes mellitus, the rate of decline of renal function is significantly slowed in individuals who are treated with an ACE inhibitor or a nondihydropyridine calcium channel blocker (e.g., verapamil and diltiazem) but is not affected in individuals who are treated with a β blocker. To date there appears to be no advantage to the dihydropyridine calcium channel blockers, and there is some concern that at least the short-acting agents in this class may increase the risk of myocardial infarction. In patients without diabetes who have renal insufficiency, ACE inhibitors have been shown to have the greatest efficacy in slowing the progression of renal disease as well (see Chapters 16 and 17).

The majority of individuals with chronic renal insufficiency will require pharmacological therapy of their elevated BP. However, it should be stressed that nonpharmacological measures should also be utilized. These include limitation of alcohol intake (e.g., not to exceed 1 or 2 alcoholic beverages per day) and dietary salt intake. Other dietary manipulations can also facilitate a decrease in BP. In particular, diets high in fruits, vegetables, and low-fat dairy foods with reduced total saturated and total fat have been found to reduce both the systolic and diastolic blood pressure in individuals with mild hypertension. Aerobic exercise is also beneficial in the control of hypertension.

2. Anemia

Anemia is present in nearly all individuals with chronic renal insufficiency. It results in decreased myocardial oxygen delivery, reduced peripheral resistance, and a reflex increase in cardiac output. These factors all contribute to the development of LVH. The anemia in CRI is primarily the result of deficient erythropoietin production by the kidney. However, a search for other causes of the anemia (particularly iron deficiency) should be undertaken. Erythropoietin replacement therapy is ineffective if iron stores are inadequate. Current recommendations are that iron supplementation should be started first, and then erythropoietin therapy added to raise the hematocrit to a level between 33 and 36% (hemoglobin between 11 and 12 g/dL). Correction of the anemia to a hematocrit greater than 30% has been shown to decrease LVH by about 18%. This decrease occurs within 6 months of starting erythropoietin. It should be noted that the decrease in LVH is not the result of a decrease in blood pressure; in fact, there is actually a trend toward an increase in blood pressure in patients treated with erythropoietin.

3. Hyperparathyroidism

Secondary hyperparathyroidism is almost an inevitable consequence of chronic renal insufficiency (see Chapter 16). Hyperplasia of the parathyroid gland with excessive parathyroid hormone release is due to a variety of factors. These factors include a low ionized serum calcium concentration and a decrease in 1,25-dihydroxycholecalciferol (calcitriol) production. The precise role of parathyroid hormone in the development of LVH is unsettled; however, several studies suggest it may play a permissive role. To minimize any risk for LVH and to protect against the development of renal osteodystrophy, individuals with chronic renal insufficiency should receive appropriate treatment to prevent runaway hyperparathyroidism. Such treatment includes adequate amounts of phosphate binders (such as calcium acetate, calcium carbonate, or sevelamer hydrochloride) to control hyperphosphatemia, calcium supplements as needed, and calcitriol supplementation early in the course of renal insufficiency (see Chapter 16 for specific recommendations).

B. Coronary Artery Disease

As noted earlier, CAD is a common problem noted in individuals with CRI. The major risk factors for CAD include diabetes mellitus, hypertension, cigarette smoking, family history, and lipid abnormalities. Because diabetes mellitus accounts for approximately 40% of the ESRD in the United States, it is perhaps not surprising that CAD is as prevalent as it is. Both hypertension and lipid abnormalities are also very common in individuals with CRI and ESRD. Several studies have shown that successful treatment of hypertension decreases the incidence of myocardial infarction. The pharmacological and nonpharmacological therapies for hypertension are discussed above and in Chapters 16 and 17. Management of the dyslipidemia is discussed below.

1. Dyslipidemia

Approximately 50–60% of patients with kidney disease have lipid abnormalities. Patients with the nephrotic syndrome have elevations in low-density lipoprotein (LDL), intermediate-density lipoprotein (IDL), and lipoprotein(a) [LP(a)]. All three of these abnormalities are associated with premature CAD. Many individuals with DM and microalbuminuria have increased levels of LDL, LP(a), and decreased levels of high-density lipoprotein (HDL). In nonnephrotic patients with renal insufficiency, an increased level of triglycerides is the most commonly observed abnormality. Whether elevated triglyceride concentrations are a cause of atherogenesis via association with small dense LDL particles and a decrease in the HDL particles is under investigation. Of the lipid abnormalities observed in patients with CRI, a decrease in HDL concentration and an unfavorable LDL: HDL ratio may assign the greatest cardiovascular risk. The cause of these lipid abnormalities is unclear. In animal models of CRI, it has been reported that lipoprotein lipase (LPL) is downregulated, and this may be ameliorated by correcting secondary hyperparathyroidism.

Laboratory studies in the rat have suggested that elevated lipid levels also contribute to the progression of renal disease. In an animal model of reduced kidney mass, the use of a hydroxymethylglutaryl-coenzyme A (HMG-CoA) reductase inhibitor or clofibric acid is associated with a decrease in serum lipid levels, a decrease in albuminuria, and attenuation of glomerular sclerosis. In a model of experimental nephrotic syndrome induced by puromycin aminonucleoside, HMG-CoA reductase inhibitors are also able to preserve kidney function.

Hyperlipidemia in patients with chronic renal insufficiency can be treated effectively with lipid-lowering agents. In patients with nephrotic syndrome, ACE inhibitors and HMG-CoA reductase inhibitors reduce cholesterol and LDL concentrations. In individuals with CRI and the nephrotic syndrome, the HMG-CoA reductase inhibitors and fibric acid analogs both decrease cholesterol concentration; HMG-CoA reductase inhibitors also reduce LDL concentration. Fibric acid analogs are the only agents that consistently reduce triglyceride concentrations. The effect of lipid-lowering drugs on the rate of progression of renal insufficiency has not been examined in humans. Currently, there is not an effective method to treat elevations in LP(a) concentrations.

2. Increased Oxidant Stress

Fatty acids as well as other molecules may be chemically altered by oxidation secondary to the release of free oxygen radicals, initiating an inflammatory response. An increase in the potential for such lipid peroxidation (termed increased oxidant stress) may be present in individuals with CRI or ESRD, and this inflammatory process may contribute to increased atherogenesis. The factors responsible for such an increase in oxidant stress are undefined, but may include the presence of metabolic acidosis. The intake of free radical scavengers such as β carotene or vitamin E in individuals without renal disease is associated with reductions in the risk of fatal myocardial infarctions. In humans with type 2 diabetes, vitamin E supplementation favors an increase in vitamin E incorporation into the LDL particle and LDL subfractions. This reduces the susceptibility of LDL to oxidation except in the small dense LDL fraction. It has also been hypothesized that individuals with type 2 diabetes have a decrease in vasodilation due to inactivation of nitric oxide by oxygen-derived free radicals. These patients have a decreased vasodilator response to intra-arterial methacholine as compared to normal control subjects. The vasodilator response to methacholine is augmented after administration of vitamin C (which acts as an antioxidant). The use of antioxidant therapy has not been studied extensively in individuals with CRI, but studies are emerging that suggest that such therapy may be useful in maintaining vascular reactivity in patients with CRI, particularly those with diabetes mellitus.

3. Homocysteine

Homocysteine is an amino acid derived from the demethylation of methionine. Increased levels of homocysteine are associated with an increased risk for atherosclerotic vascular disease. Homocysteine concentrations are consistently elevated in individuals with CRI to levels that are two to three times normal. This elevation is probably related to a decrease in the elimination of homocysteine. Supplementation with folic acid (5 mg/day) decreases homocysteine levels by about 30%

by increasing the remethylation process. While clinical trials to examine the long-term safety and efficacy of using high-dose folic acid are needed, measurement of homocysteine early in the course of renal failure is rational. Therapy with folic acid (5–10 mg/day) appears to be safe in short-term studies.

4. Nutrition

Malnutrition also contributes to cardiac disease in individuals with renal insufficiency. A decrease in the albumin concentration is a common feature in many diseases that lead to CRI and is, of course, a component of the nephrotic syndrome. As noted above, the nephrotic syndrome is independently associated with abnormalities in serum lipid levels. Hypoalbuminemia may contribute to cardiac disease because albumin is an antioxidant. Although a first reaction to hypoalbuminemia is to consider increasing dietary protein intake, such an approach is not useful and may actually be deleterious because it may increase the rate of progression to renal failure (see Chapter 16). Interestingly, restriction of dietary protein attenuates renal protein losses and may slow the progression of renal disease. However, such an intervention should be undertaken with caution because it may exacerbate malnutrition. As renal insufficiency progresses, dietary intake often falls because of anorexia and distaste for foods high in protein content. In prescribing the appropriate diet for a given patient, clinicians must pay close attention to assuring that malnutrition does not occur as renal failure progresses. This is a particular challenge in older subjects and individuals on fixed incomes, and such individuals now comprise the majority of patients with CRI. Patients in whom the serum albumin and serum transferrin concentrations decline should be referred to a skilled dietition to ensure that their diet contains adequate, but not excessive, protein.

The Diabetes Control and Complication Trial (DCCT) prospectively assessed the incidence of diabetic complications as a function of blood sugar control in individuals with type 1 diabetes mellitus. Rigorous control of blood sugar levels is clearly associated with attenuation of the progression of renal insufficiency early on in the course of the disease. Similar results have now been demonstrated in individuals with type 2 diabetes. It is, therefore, recommended that blood sugar be strictly controlled in diabetics with renal disease via appropriate diet, exercise, and insulin, with a goal hemoglobin A-1c level of $\leq$8%.

III. SUMMARY

Individuals with ESRD have increased morbidity and mortality due to hypertensive and atherosclerotic cardiovascular and cerebrovascular disease. The alterations in the chemical milieu that promote hypertension and atherosclerosis begin early in the course of renal insufficiency. Particular effort should be devoted to therapies that will benefit cardiac function in the short and long term. In this regard, hypertension, anemia, and lipid abnormalities require constant and persistent attention. It should be also emphasized that, among the positive benefits of these efforts, early referral of the patient for placement of an arteriovenous fistula and an early start on dialysis is particularly important in reducing subsequent morbidity and mortality.

SUGGESTED READINGS

Bennett WM, Aronoff GR, Golper TA, Morrison G, Brater DC, Singer I. Drug Prescribing in Renal Failure Dosing Guidelines for Adults. 3d ed. Philadelphia: American College of Physicians, 1994.

The Diabetes Control and Complications Trial Research Group. The effect of intensive treatment of diabetes on the development and progression of long-term complications in insulin-dependent diabetes mellitus. N Engl J Med 329:977–986, 1993.

Jungers P, Massy ZA, Nguyen Koha T, et al. Incidence and risk factors of atherosclerotic cardiovascular accidents in predialysis chronic renal failure patients: a prospective study. Nephrol Dial Transplant 12:2597–2602, 1997.

Klahr S, Levey AS, Beck GJ, et al. The effects of dietary protein restriction and blood-pressure control on the progression of chronic renal disease. Modification of Diet in Renal Disease Study Group. N Engl J Med 330:877–884, 1994.

Levey AS, Adler S, Caggiula AW, et al. Effects of dietary protein restriction on the progression of advanced renal disease in the modification of diet in renal disease study. Am J Kidney Dis 27:652–663, 1996.

Maschio G, Alberti D, Janin G, et al. Effect of the angiotensin-converting-enzyme inhibitor benazepril on the progression of chronic renal insufficiency. The Angiotensin-Converting-Enzyme Inhibition in Progressive Renal Insufficiency Study Group. N Engl J Med 334:939–945, 1996.

Massy ZA, Ma JZ, Louis TA, et al. Lipid-lowering therapy in patients with renal disease. Kidney Int 48:188–198, 1995.

Pedrini MT, Levey AS, Lau J, et al. The effect of dietary protein restriction on the progression of diabetic and nondiabetic renal diseases: a meta-analysis. Ann Intern Med 124:627–632, 1996.

U.S. Renal Data System. USRDS 1998 Annual Data Report. Bethesda, MD: National Institutes of Health, National Institute of Diabetes and Digestive and Kidney Diseases, 1998.

27
Medical Management of Renal Transplant Patients

John D. Scandling
Stanford University, Stanford, California

I. INTRODUCTION

Kidney transplantation is the preferred treatment for patients with end-stage renal disease (ESRD). Transplantation offers better quality of life and greater life expectancy than dialysis. Despite these advantages only 15–20% of the U.S. ESRD population is awaiting cadaver donor kidney transplantation. Age and comorbid disease preclude transplantation in many, but some ESRD patients do not consider transplantation for economic (anticipated eventual loss of public health insurance after successful transplantation) or personal reasons. Transplant candidates and recipients therefore are a highly select group, both in terms of health status and motivation. Many are employed, full-time students or homemakers. Their average age at transplantation is 40–45 years, 20 years younger than the average age of an U.S. patient at onset of ESRD.

The transplant population is now aging, however, along with the rest of the ESRD population. A third of transplant recipients are now over 50 years of age at the time of transplantation. Many have diabetes mellitus, as diabetic nephropathy is the leading cause of ESRD in the United States. Furthermore, relaxation of former contraindications to transplantation due to comorbidity has led to transplantation of patients with greater medical complexity. Socioeconomic factors frequently compound the complexities of transplant care, as many ESRD patients are from disadvantaged or immigrant groups.

The challenges notwithstanding, care of the transplant patient is rewarding because most recipients do realize the promise of transplantation. Patient and graft (the transplanted kidney) survival have improved markedly over the last decade, largely due to advances in immunosuppressive therapy. Nowadays, over 90% of recipients have a functioning graft one year after transplantation, with good prospect for long-term graft function (approximately 50% will still have a functioning graft 10 years after transplantation). Furthermore, the morbidity of immunosuppressive therapy has been reduced, as transplant physicians have become more skilled at management of immunosuppression and its complications. New immunosuppressive agents have reduced the occurrence of acute rejection of the transplant kidney and enabled tailoring of immunosuppressive regimens to reduce drug toxicities and side effects.

Long-term care of the transplant patient has traditionally been the responsibility of transplant physicians in transplant centers. As patients have returned to their communities or moved, knowledgeable local nephrologists have also assumed this responsibility. Over recent years, changes in medical insurance have restricted access of transplant patients to transplant center physicians and local nephrologists, increasing the frequency of appearance of these patients in the offices of primary care physicians. Now compounding this issue is the soon-to-be-realized shortage of practicing nephrologists in the United States. The aim of this chapter is to aid the primary care physician in the long-term medical management of the renal transplant patient.

It must be remembered that kidney transplantation, despite its high profile, remains a relatively infrequent occurrence. There are now only about 12,000 kidney transplants performed yearly in the United States. Care of renal transplant patients represent a small fraction of the practice of the typical practicing U.S. nephrologist (15% in a recent survey of members of the American Society of Nephrology) and a rare encounter in the practice of a primary care physician. Therefore, the local nephrologist and primary care physician, as well as the transplant recipient, must have ready access to a transplant physician in a transplant center for consultation as necessary.

II. FACTORS AFFECTING RENAL GRAFT SURVIVAL AND FUNCTION

A. Donor, Recipient, and Early Posttransplant Variables

The source of the donor organ and age of the donor are the predominant donor factors affecting graft survival and function. On average, kidneys transplanted from living related or unrelated donors provide longer survival and better function than cadaver donor kidneys. The optimal cadaver donor age is 12–30 years of age, but the majority of cadaver donors fall outside this ideal range. Renal graft survival and function can be compromised when the donor age is very young (<5 years) or very old (>60 years). The major recipient factors affecting graft survival and function are sensitization to human leukocyte antigen (HLA) loci as manifest by high levels of preformed panel-reactive antibodies (PRA), prior transplantation, and African-American ethnicity. These factors predispose recipients to acute renal graft rejection, which can jeopardize renal graft survival acutely or lead to chronic rejection and limit the life of the graft. Chronic rejection, which may be a consequence of chronic cyclosporine nephrotoxicity and hypertensive nephropathy as well as HLA incompatibility, is the major cause of renal graft loss over time. Patients can develop antibodies to HLA loci as a result of exposure through pregnancy, blood transfusion, and prior transplantation. African Americans, who represent 30% of the U.S. ESRD population, have a significantly higher rate of renal graft loss to acute rejection than whites, even when they are recipients of very well-matched renal grafts from siblings. The major posttransplant events affecting eventual renal graft survival and function are delayed graft function (usually a consequence of postischemic acute tubular necrosis), early acute rejection of the graft, and poor initial function, which may reflect these two early events or the quality of the donor organ.

B. Immunosuppressive Therapy

Renal graft function is also affected by immunosuppressive therapy. The two major immunosuppressive agents currently used for kidney transplantation, cyclosporine and tacrolimus (FK506), are paradoxically nephrotoxic (see later). Unfortunately, toxicity does not necessarily correlate with blood levels of the drugs. Acute nephrotoxicity, due to drug-induced vasoconstriction, is usually reversible, but chronic toxicity, associated with interstitial fibrosis in the graft, is not. It is debated whether the chronic form of the nephrotoxicity contributes to renal graft loss, but it is well established to cause renal failure in heart and liver transplant recipients (up to 10% of these recipients within 10 years of transplantation). The average best serum creatinine in a renal transplant patient receiving either of these agents is in the 1.5–2.0 mg/dL range, higher than in the precyclosporine era.

III. THE COURSE OF RENAL GRAFT FUNCTION

Most if not all recipients reach their best renal graft function by 1–2 months following transplantation. The level of graft function achieved at that point reflects the source (living vs. cadaver donor) and quality of the donor organ and its early function. Recipients of grafts with excellent early function, evidenced by a serum creatinine concentration <1.6 mg/dL within 1–2 weeks following transplantation, can expect longer survival of the renal graft than recipients of grafts with worse early function. Nearly half of recipients with poor early graft function (i.e., those with serum creatinine >3.5 mg/dL) at the time of initial hospital discharge will lose their grafts within 3–6 months after transplantation.

Renal graft function usually remains stable for years, until chronic rejection sets in. Chronic rejection is typified by a slowly rising serum creatinine concentration, hypertension, and proteinuria. It is a rather indistinct syndrome, as this triad can also represent chronic cyclosporine or tacrolimus nephrotoxicity, chronic hypertensive nephropathy, or recurrence of the original renal disease. On occasion, chronic rejection is manifest as nephrotic syndrome; indeed, the most common cause of the nephrotic syndrome in a renal transplant recipient is chronic rejection.

The etiology and pathophysiology of chronic rejection are not well understood. Both immunological and nonimmunological factors appear to play a role. There may be a link between acute and chronic rejection, because transplant recipients who experience acute rejection, particularly repeated episodes, are more likely to lose their grafts to chronic rejection than those who have had no bouts of acute rejection. Once a graft begins to succumb to chronic rejection, its demise is not imminent. Progression to end-stage graft failure typically takes months to years, and not infrequently the progression stalls and the graft dysfunction stabilizes at some level for a number of years.

IV. EARLY SIGNS OF RENAL GRAFT DYSFUNCTION

As with dysfunction in native kidneys, dysfunction in the transplant kidney is usually insidious. In the absence of acute oliguria, there are virtually no symptoms of renal graft dysfunction and no signs other than biochemical abnormalities. For this reason, renal transplant recipients should always have regular monitoring of the serum creatinine (as well as other serum chemistries and blood counts) and urinalysis, in addition to history and physical examination, for the life of the renal graft. A suggested schedule for routine laboratory testing in a transplant recipient more than one year posttransplant is shown in Table 1.

A. Serum Creatinine

Acute and chronic renal graft dysfunction are usually manifest only as an increase in serum creatinine concentration. Acute graft dysfunction is unusual beyond the first 3–6 months after transplantation, as the risk of acute rejection wanes (but never disappears) and maintenance cyclosporine or tacrolimus doses have been achieved, lessening the risk of acute toxicity. When it does occur, late acute graft dysfunction may still represent acute rejection as a consequence of suboptimal maintenance immunosuppression or noncompliance with the immunosuppressive regimen. Late acute graft dysfunction can also be caused by acute cyclosporine

Table 1 Schedule for Routine Laboratory Testing After the First Transplant Year

Quarterly	Half-yearly	Yearly
Creatinine	CBC	Lipid profile
Cyclosporine or tacrolimus (12-hour trough)	Electrolytes	
	Magnesium	
	Glucose	
	BUN	
	Albumin	
	Calcium	
	Phosphorus	
	Uric acid	
	Liver enzymes	
	Urinalysis	

or tacrolimus nephrotoxicity, frequently as a consequence of unappreciated drug interactions (see later), or by any of the myriad causes of acute renal failure (see Chapter 15)

Acute renal graft dysfunction, manifest by an abrupt 20–25% or greater rise in serum creatinine concentration, requires immediate evaluation by a transplant nephrologist in a transplant center. Review of recent medications should turn up any offending agents that might predispose to acute cyclosporine or tacrolimus nephrotoxicity through inhibition of cyclosporine or tacrolimus metabolism. Ultrasound study of the transplant kidney should be undertaken to exclude the possibility of obstructive uropathy. Percutaneous core needle biopsy will confirm the clinical suspicion of acute rejection. The skills necessary for the prompt and thorough evaluation of acute renal graft dysfunction reside only in transplant centers. Slowly progressive renal graft dysfunction, manifest as a more gradual increase in serum creatinine concentration (typically over months rather than weeks), should also be evaluated by a transplant nephrologist.

B. Urinalysis

The urinalysis should be normal in a long-term renal transplant recipient with stable, excellent graft function. The new onset of hematuria and/or proteinuria usually represents the development of chronic rejection or recurrence of the original renal disease in the transplant kidney. The hematuria or proteinuria may be isolated or accompanied by progressive graft dysfunction. A transplant recipient with these findings should be referred to a transplant nephrologist in a transplant center for evaluation.

C. Blood Pressure

Most renal transplant recipients have hypertension, the most common complication of transplantation (see later). Worsening or difficult-to-control hypertension may be a sign of transplant renal artery stenosis, a condition with an incidence of less than 5–10% and onset usually between 3 months and 2 years after transplantation. A bruit over the renal graft is not always present and is a nonspecific finding. Frequently there is concomitantly worsening graft function due to renal ischemia. When transplant renal artery stenosis is suspected, the patient should be referred to a transplant nephrologist in a transplant center for evaluation.

V. MAXIMIZING RENAL GRAFT SURVIVAL

The chief cause of renal graft loss is chronic rejection. Chronic rejection may begin within months of transplantation but is usually not clinically evident for a number of years, when it is manifest as slowly progressive graft dysfunction, proteinuria, and hypertension. The course of the progressive failure of a renal graft with chronic rejection is highly variable. There is no specific treatment for chronic rejection. Although not proven, vigorous control of the blood pressure (to levels of 130/85 or lower) is likely to slow the course of graft failure. Any new treatment for blood pressure should be reviewed for possible interaction with cyclosporine and tacrolimus. These patients are most commonly treated with dihydropyridine calcium channel blockers that do not affect immunosuppressive blood levels (see later) or β blockers. Treatment with an angiotensin-converting enzyme (ACE) inhibitor is of unproven benefit and may be problematic because it can acutely lower glomerular filtration rate (GFR) in the setting of advanced renal insufficiency in patients receiving cyclosporine or tacrolimus immunosuppressive therapy. Dietary protein restriction is also of unproven benefit in patients with chronic rejection.

Increasing or altering maintenance immunosuppression once chronic rejection is established is not beneficial and is potentially hazardous, as the risk of infection may increase. Maintenance immunosuppression is usually continued at its current dosage, with adjustments made as necessary for the level of renal dysfunction.

As the renal graft fails, preparations for a return to chronic dialysis and possible repeat transplantation must be made. Because few patients actually undergo repeat transplantation before the graft fails, it is best to anticipate a return to dialysis. Vascular access may need to be constructed, or a peritoneal dialysis catheter may need to be placed. The medical complications of renal failure recur and require treatment. The patient is best managed by a nephrologist through this difficult period.

Once the renal graft has failed and chronic dialysis has begun, immunosuppression is discontinued (prednisone is usually withdrawn over a period of weeks). Removal of the transplant kidney is almost always necessary in those patients who lose their grafts in the first year after transplantation, as they develop symptoms and signs of acute rejection (malaise, fever, graft pain) after withdrawal of immunosuppression. Transplant nephrectomy is less often necessary in those patients who lose their grafts after the first year.

VI. IMMUNOSUPPRESSIVE DRUGS IN CURRENT USE AND THEIR MAJOR SIDE EFFECTS

The immunosuppressive drugs currently in use are shown in Table 2. They are subdivided into ''old'' and ''new,'' but both types of programs remain in use. The older maintenance treatments are in use mainly in patients that were transplanted more than 5–10 years ago.

Patients at high risk for acute rejection typically receive ''induction'' immunosuppression during the early weeks after transplantation. Agents used for induction therapy have been the polyclonal antilymphocyte antibody preparations antilymphocyte globulin (ALG) and antithymocyte globulin (ATG or ATGam)

Table 2 Immunosuppression, Old and New

Old	New
Induction	Induction
Antilymphocyte globulin (ALG)	Antithymocyte globulin (ATG)
Antithymocyte globulin (ATG)	Muromonab-CD3 (OKT3)
Muromonab-CD3 (OKT3)	Daclizumab (Zenapax)
	Basiliximab (Simulect)
Maintenance	Maintenance
Cyclosporine (Sandimmune)	Cyclosporine (Neoral)
	Tacrolimus, a.k.a. FK506 (Prograf)
Azathioprine (Imuran)	Mycophenolate mofetil (CellCept)
Corticosteroid	Corticosteroid
Acute rejection	Acute rejection
Corticosteroid	Corticosteroid
Muromonab-CD3 (OKT3)	Muromonab-CD3 (OKT3)
Antithymocyte globulin (ATG)	Antithymocyte globulin (ATG)
	''Rescue'' therapy for resistant rejection
	Tacrolimus, a.k.a. FK506 (Prograf)
	Mycophenolate mofetil (CellCept)

and the monoclonal antibody muromonab-CD3 (Orthoclone OKT3). These agents, primarily OKT3, are also used for treatment of the small percentage of acute rejections that are resistant to corticosteroids. For induction therapy, these agents may be replaced by two new monoclonal antibodies released in the United States in 1998: the interleukin-2 (IL-2) T-cell receptor blockers daclizumab (Zenapax) and basiliximab (Simulect). Both are chimeric mouse/human antibodies; daclizumab is more ''humanized'' as it is 90% human. These agents have proven effective in preventing acute rejection in the early weeks after transplantation and do not cause the ''cytokine release syndrome'' typical of OKT3.

The drugs in current use for maintenance immunosuppression are from three classes: calcineurin inhibitors, antiproliferative agents, and corticosteroids. Patients are usually on one drug from each class; thus they receive ''triple'' therapy. Investigative protocols, drug toxicity, and recipient factors may result in patients being on dual (calcineurin inhibitor and prednisone or calcineurin inhibitor and antiproliferative agent) or monotherapy (calcineurin inhibitor alone).

A. Calcineurin Inhibitors

Cyclosporine and tacrolimus induce immunosuppression by inhibiting T lymphocytes through inhibition of calcineurin, an intracellular enzyme that is central for T-cell activation via production of interleukin 2 (IL-2). Despite their nephrotoxicity, they are the cornerstones of maintenance immunosuppression.

1. Cyclosporine (Sandimmune, Neoral)

Cyclosporine (Sandimmune) was released for use in renal transplantation in the United States in late 1983. A newer formulation of cyclosporine with improved bioavailability (Neoral) was released in the United States in the summer of 1995 and has largely replaced the Sandimmune formulation. Sandimmune and Neoral are *not* bioequivalent. There are both liquid and capsule formulations of Sandimmune and Neoral. SangCya, a generic liquid formulation bioequivalent to Neoral, was released in the United States in late 1998. Cyclosporine remains the primary maintenance immunosuppressive drug in renal transplantation. Nephrotoxicity and neurotoxicity are the major toxicities of cyclosporine, but the cosmetic side effects are sometimes the most troublesome to patients.

Nephrotoxicity, a consequence of vasoconstriction of the renal microvasculature, may be acute (usually reversible) or chronic (usually irreversible as the chronic renal ischemia leads to interstitial fibrosis—see Chapter 20). In most instances nephrotoxicity is related to dose (and blood level), although as noted earlier it can occur in some patients even when the dose and blood level are well controlled. It is manifest by a rise in serum creatinine concentration. Other renal effects include hyperkalemia due to impaired renal potassium excretion, hypomagnesemia due to impaired renal magnesium conservation, hyperchloremic metabolic acidosis due to impaired renal net acid excretion, and hyperuricemia due to impaired uric acid excretion.

Neurotoxicity is typically manifest by tremor and paresthesias, is dose-related, and produces symptoms typically an hour or so after the oral dose. Rarely, more serious neurotoxicity can occur, including seizures and coma.

The cosmetic side effects are a consequence of hyperplasia of the skin and its appendages. Hypertrichosis (hirsutism) and gingival hyperplasia (sometimes aggravated by nifedipine) are the most disturbing and may lead to patients discontinuing the drug. With the availability of tacrolimus, we now have alternative therapy for these individuals.

Hypertension, hyperlipidemia, and glucose intolerance are other major side effects of cyclosporine and usually require pharmacological treatment when they occur. As many as 10–15% of transplant recipients are intolerant of cyclosporine due to gastrointestinal distress, primarily nausea and vomiting.

2. Tacrolimus

Tacrolimus, also known as FK506 (Prograf), was approved for use in kidney transplantation in the United States in 1997, but it had been used for this indication since 1994 when it was released for use in liver transplantation. As many as 20–25% of renal transplant patients in the United States are now receiving tacrolimus as their primary immunosuppressive agent. Tacrolimus is a more potent drug than cyclosporine and has been used as "rescue" therapy in patients on cyclosporine with intractable acute rejection. Because of its potency, tacrolimus is also "steroid sparing" in liver transplant patients and so may hold promise for steroid withdrawal in renal transplant patients as well.

As with cyclosporine, the major toxicity of tacrolimus is nephrotoxicity (see Chapter 20) and neurotoxicity, with neurotoxicity being more problematic than with cyclosporine. The neurotoxicity is dose-related and manifest as headache and nightmares in addition to tremor and paresthesias. The intravenous formulation of tacrolimus seems to be more nephrotoxic than the intravenous formulation of cyclosporine and is rarely used.

Tacrolimus does not cause hair or gum growth. Many patients are switched to tacrolimus from cyclosporine for this reason. Tacrolimus infrequently causes hair loss, and when this occurs it is usually mild. Tacrolimus may also cause diarrhea. Hypertension and hyperlipidemia are less frequent with tacrolimus than with cyclosporine, but glucose intolerance and posttransplant diabetes mellitus may be more frequent, particularly in two major U.S. minorities—African Americans and Latinos. Tacrolimus appears to cause a dose-related reduction in insulin production. This complication may become less of a problem as newer protocols use lower dosages (and target lower blood levels).

B. Antiproliferative Agents

Azathioprine and mycophenolate mofetil inhibit proliferation of T cells through inhibition of purine nucleotide (DNA) synthesis.

1. Azathioprine (Imuran)

Azathioprine has been used in renal transplantation since 1961 and was the mainstay of maintenance immunosuppression until the advent of cyclosporine. It is still used as a component of ''triple'' therapy but has been largely supplanted by mycophenolate mofetil. The major toxicity of azathioprine is bone marrow suppression, manifest as leukopenia, thrombocytopenia, or macrocytic anemia. Dose reduction or temporary drug cessation is necessary. Azathioprine may also cause hair loss.

The dosage of azathioprine should be reduced in chronic renal insufficiency. It must also be reduced by 50% or more when allopurinol is added to the medication regimen for control of gout, a not uncommon complication after transplantation. Allopurinol inhibits xanthine oxidase, the enzyme responsible for the metabolism of azathioprine.

2. Mycophenolate Mofetil (CellCept)

Mycophenolate mofetil was released for use in kidney transplantation in the United States in 1995. It has largely replaced azathioprine as adjunctive therapy with cyclosporine or tacrolimus, because, in combination with either of these primary agents and steroid, it reduces the risk of acute rejection in the early months after transplantation.

The major toxicities of mycophenolate mofetil are gastrointestinal and bone marrow suppression. Dyspepsia, nausea, vomiting, or diarrhea are common and usually occur shortly after beginning this drug if they are going to develop. Bone marrow suppression usually develops 8–12 weeks after initiation of treatment and is manifest as leukopenia, thrombocytopenia, or anemia. Dose reduction or temporary drug cessation is necessary with either toxicity.

Mycophenolate mofetil may also cause hair loss but not as dramatically as azathioprine. Mycophenolate mofetil is to be avoided in pregnancy, as it has been shown to be teratogenic in experimental animals. It must be discontinued at least 6 weeks prior to conception.

C. Corticosteroids

Prednisone has been an element of maintenance immunosuppression protocols since the early 1960s, when it was first demonstrated to reverse acute renal allograft rejection. Through the years there have been a number of clinical trials aimed at steroid withdrawal after transplantation due to the complications of chronic steroid therapy. The majority of patients nowadays are subjected to a much lower cumulative steroid dose than were patients in the past. Nonetheless, steroid withdrawal remains attractive because of the improvements in hypertension, glucose intolerance, and hyperlipidemia that accompany cessation of steroid therapy. Although steroid withdrawal is undertaken by some transplant programs, most currently do not recommend stopping this agent for fear of precipitating acute or chronic rejection.

D. New Agents

Sirolimus, or rapamycin, is a new agent that was released in the United States in late 1999. Sirolimus binds the same immunophilin as tacrolimus, but it has a mechanism of action distinct from the calcineurin inhibitors. It does not appear to be nephrotoxic by itself but may add to the nephrotoxicity of the calcineurin inhibitors when used in combination with them. In combination with cyclosporine and steroid, sirolimus has been shown to prevent acute rejection in the early months after transplantation. Its major side effect is marked hyperlipidemia in some patients, which may limit its use. It may also cause arthralgia and diarrhea, anemia, and thrombocytopenia. The eventual place of sirolimus in the immunosuppression armamentarium remains to be defined.

VII. DRUG INTERACTIONS

Drug interactions are a major concern after renal transplantation because of potential effects on cyclosporine or tacrolimus metabolism, renal graft function, and serum potassium.

A. Effects of Drugs on Cyclosporine and Tacrolimus Metabolism

Both cyclosporine and tacrolimus are metabolized in the liver by the cytochrome P450 system. Many drugs induce or inhibit this enzyme system and as a result affect cyclosporine and tacrolimus metabolism when administered concomitantly. These drugs are best avoided. If their use is necessary, mon-

Table 3 Drugs Likely to Increase Cyclosporine and Tacrolimus Blood Levels

Calcium channel blockers
Diltiazem
Verapamil
Dihydropyridines
Amlodipine
Nicardipine
Macrolide antibiotics
Clarithromycin
Erythromycin
Antifungal agents
Ketoconazole
Others
Danazol

itoring of cyclosporine or tacrolimus blood levels and dosage adjustments are necessary to prevent either underimmunosuppression or toxicity. Drugs that may affect cyclosporine and tacrolimus blood concentrations are listed in Tables 3–5.

Cisapride should be avoided in patients on tacrolimus because of the risk of serious cardiac arrhythmia (torsades de pointes associated with QT prolongation). Tacrolimus is a macrolide (as is sirolimus) and may inhibit cisapride metabolism (also through the cytochrome P450 system), leading to high cisapride blood levels, which can prolong the QT interval.

Table 4 Drugs That May Increase Cyclosporine and Tacrolimus Blood Levels

Antifungal agents
Fluconazole
Itraconazole
Others
Amiodarone
Cimetidine
Imipenem

Table 5 Drugs Likely to Decrease Cyclosporine and Tacrolimus Blood Levels

Anticonvulsants
Carbamazepine
Phenobarbital
Phenytoin
Antibiotics
Isoniazid
Rifampin
Others
Troglitazone

B. Effects of Drugs on Renal Graft Function

Drugs may also adversely affect renal graft function through direct renal cell toxicity or through effects on renal hemodynamics. These drugs, shown in Table 6, are best avoided or used with caution.

C. Effects on Serum Potassium Concentration

Hyperkalemia can occur in renal transplant recipients as a consequence of the effects of cyclosporine and tacrolimus on the renin-angiotensin-aldosterone axis and as a consequence of renal graft dysfunction. Drugs that can cause hyperkalemia, shown in Table 7, are best avoided or used with caution.

In our transplant program we distribute a laminated wallet card to all of our transplant recipients, listing drugs that should be avoided or used with caution. They are advised to carry the card and show it to any treating physician. The card also contains instructions on how to contact the transplant center.

Table 6 Drugs That May Adversely Affect Renal Function

Nephrotoxic potential
Aminoglycosides
Amphotericin
Cisplatin
Affect renal hemodynamics
ACE inhibitors
NSAIDs (avoid)

Table 7 Drugs That Can Cause Hyperkalemia

Diuretics
Amiloride
Spironolactone
Triamterene
Others
ACE inhibitors
NSAIDs (avoid)
Potassium supplements

VIII. LONG-TERM EFFECTS OF IMMUNOSUPPRESSIVE THERAPY

The major causes of death in renal transplant patients are cardiovascular disease and infection, both of which are exacerbated by immunosuppressive therapy. Because the incidence of irreversible acute rejection has decreased dramatically, death due to cardiovascular disease is also a leading cause of renal graft loss. Death due to infection is not as common as it was two or three decades ago, because infection prophylaxis and treatment have improved. Chronic immunosuppression also increases the risk of malignancy.

A. Cardiovascular Disease

Immunosuppressive drugs contribute to the development of cardiovascular disease through their effects on cardiac risk factors. Corticosteroids and the calcineurin inhibitors cyclosporine and tacrolimus all increase blood pressure. Both classes of drugs cause hyperlipidemia, cyclosporine moreso than tacrolimus within the calcineurin-inhibitor class. Both classes of drugs also may cause diabetes mellitus, tacrolimus moreso than cyclosporine within the calcineurin-inhibitor class. Weight gain to the point of obesity, a serious problem for many transplant recipients, may aggravate cardiac risk factors and their management.

B. Hypertension

Hypertension is extremely common after transplantation. Virtually all cadaver kidney transplant recipients have hypertension. A recipient with a well-matched living-related transplant kidney and excellent graft function is the most likely to be free of hypertension. Hypertension following transplantation may be caused by persistent renin production by the native kidneys, donor kidney factors such as nephrosclerosis, acute or chronic rejection, or, more rarely, transplant renal artery stenosis. As mentioned earlier, the immunosuppressive drugs themselves also cause hypertension. Cyclosporine is thought to induce hypertension through vasoconstriction and increased sympathetic nervous system activity. Cyclosporine-induced renal vasoconstriction causes sodium retention and renin suppression. Corticosteroid also causes sodium retention. Tacrolimus is similar to cyclosporine in its vasoconstrictor property. The most common causes of posttransplant hypertension are the calcineurin-inhibitor immunosuppressive agents and chronic rejection.

Calcium channel blockers are the first-line therapy for posttransplant hypertension because they may ameliorate calcineurin inhibitor–induced vasoconstriction. Nifedipine and other members of the dihydropyridine class that do not raise cyclosporine and tacrolimus levels (see Table 3) are preferred and are usually the most effective. These agents are generally well tolerated but can produce significant dependent edema and may aggravate gingival hyperplasia induced by cyclosporine. These side effects may necessitate their discontinuation.

β Blockers and diuretics are second-line therapy. Care must be exercised with diuretic use because graft function is quite volume-sensitive in the presence of the calcineurin inhibitors. As a result, overly aggressive diuresis can cause an acute reduction in graft filtration rate. α-Adrenergic blockers are usually not very effective. ACE inhibitors and angiotensin II receptor blockers are particularly effective in the setting of native kidney-mediated hypertension. They must be used with care, with monitoring of serum creatinine during the first few weeks of treatment, because graft filtration rate may fall precipitously with these agents as well. In addition, these agents can cause anemia, possibly by inhibiting erythropoeitin production by the allograft.

C. Hyperlipidemia

Hypercholesterolemia is the predominant lipid disorder after transplantation. Its prevalence may well be greater than 50%. Hyperlipidemia is due in large part to the choice of immunosuppression (cyclosporine, corticosteroid), choice of antihypertensive regimen (beta-blocker, diuretic), diabetes mellitus, and weight gain. While steroid withdrawal may yield gratifying improvements in hyperlipidemia, as well as in blood glucose and hypertension, there is no evidence that it results in a reduction in cardiovascular events in transplant recipients. Nor has pharmacological therapy of hyperlipidemia been shown to reduce cardiovascular events in this population.

The lack of efficacy notwithstanding, most transplant centers now treat hypercholesterolemia aggressively, particularly in recipients with additional cardiovascular risk factors (diabetes mellitus, current smoking, hypertension, or a family history of premature coronary heart disease). Treatment is begun when the LDL cholesterol is >160 mg/dL or, if there are two additional risk factors for cardiovascular disease, when the LDL cholesterol is >130 mg/dL. The goal of therapy is the same as in the general population: LDL cholesterol < 130 mg/dL, or < 100 mg/dL if coronary heart disease or other atherosclerotic disease is present. Short of dramatic dietary change and considerable weight loss, pharmacological therapy is virtually always necessary.

The HMG CoA reductase inhibitors are the drugs of choice; the other classes of antihyperlipidemic agents are problematic and best avoided in transplant recipients. The HMG CoA reductase inhibitors must be used with care as they can cause liver and muscle injury, particularly in combination with cyclosporine (which may inhibit their metabolism) in the setting of renal insufficiency. The HMG CoA reductase inhibitors (inhibitors of 3-hydroxy-3-methylglutaryl-coenzyme A) are best introduced at half the usual starting dosage and gradually increased as necessary, with clinical monitoring and monitoring of liver enzymes and creatine kinase. Dosages are best kept to a maximum of 20–40 mg daily to minimize the risk of liver and muscle injury.

D. Diabetes Mellitus

Posttransplant diabetes mellitus may develop in as many as 10–20% of recipients. Corticosteroids and the calcineurin inhibitors play an important role in the pathogenesis. The onset is rapid, with 50% of those affected manifesting the disease within 3 months of transplantation. Older recipients (age >40 years), African Americans, and Latinos are at greater risk. Posttransplant diabetes mellitus has a deleterious effect on long-term recipient and graft survival, perhaps due to a higher frequency of infectious complications.

As in the general population, diet and exercise are important in management. Many of the affected recipients require insulin. Of the oral agents, glipizide is preferable because its metabolism is not affected by renal dysfunction. Metformin can cause lactic acidosis in the setting of renal dysfunction and is best avoided. Troglitazone may decrease cyclosporine levels. Steroid withdrawal and calcineurin-inhibitor dose reduction may improve glucose intolerance, but these changes in maintenance immunosuppression are best managed by the transplant center.

E. Weight Gain

Most recipients gain weight. Weight gain is commonly attributed to corticosteroid effects, but the steroid is not solely responsible. The dysgeusia (altered sense of taste) of renal failure resolves and eating becomes a pleasure. Many recipients gain weight to the point of obesity, even when aggressively counseled. Weight gain can aggravate glucose intolerance, hyperlipidemia, and hypertension and complicate would healing and transplant kidney biopsy. Some recipients develop sleep apnea following weight gain. Transplant recipients should begin dietary control and a routine of daily mild to moderate exercise (continuous walking or swimming for 20–30 minutes) within weeks of transplantation.

F. Infection

Transplant candidates should be immunized prior to transplantation. All patients with chronic renal disease should receive the hepatitis B vaccine, pneumococcal vaccine, and yearly influenza vaccine. Vaccination against tetanus should be updated. Yearly tuberculin skin testing with control should be done.

Virtually all transplant centers now employ antimicrobial prophylaxis in the early months following transplantation, when immunosuppression is greatest. Nystatin or clotrimazole are prescribed during the first month to prevent thrush. Acyclovir or ganciclovir are given for herpes simplex virus and cytomegalovirus prophylaxis, usually for 3 months. Trimethoprim/Sulfamethoxazole is commonly prescribed as a urinary aseptic and for pneumocystis carinii prophylaxis for 6–12 months, sometimes indefinitely. Recipients with a history a positive tuberculin skin test are treated with a 6- to 12-month course of isoniazid if not previously treated.

By 6 months after transplantation, most recipients have good renal graft function and are on a stable regimen of maintenance immunosuppression. In this population, infection is uncommon and, when it does occur, is usually community acquired. A stable long-term recipient with a serious or recurrent infection, e.g., recurrent urinary tract infection, should be referred to a transplant center for evaluation.

A minority of long-term recipients is at risk for serious infection (see Table 8). These patients are plagued by chronic viral infection or have poor graft function due to rejection and have been exposed to excessive immunosuppression. Typical chronic viral infections include hepatitis C virus, papilloma virus, and, to a much lesser degree, hepatitis B virus, cytomegalovirus (CMV), and Epstein-Barr virus (EBV). Excessively immunosuppressed recipients are at risk for infection with opportunistic organisms such as *Cryptococcus* and *Nocardia* in addition to those seen earlier after transplantation—CMV, *Pneumocystis*, *Listeria*, *Aspergillus*, and *Candida*. Certain infections may reactivate during chronic immunosuppression. Reactivation of tuberculosis, toxoplasmosis, coccidioidomycosis, and histoplasmosis is unusual but does occur. Reactivation of viral infection due to herpes simplex or herpes zoster is more common. Serious late infection and reactivation infection are best managed in a transplant center.

Transplant recipients should also be immunized, because maintenance im-

Table 8 Possible Late Infections[a] in the Renal Transplant Recipient

Viral	Bacterial	Fungal	Parasitic
Common		Common	
Herpes simplex		*Candida*	
Herpes zoster		Dermatophytosis	
Papillomavirus		Onychomycosis	
Hepatitis C			
Uncommon	Uncommon	Uncommon	Uncommon
Hepatitis B	*Listeria*	*Pneumocystis*	*Strongyloides*
Cytomegalovirus	*Nocardia*	*Cryptococcus*	Toxoplasmosis
Epstein-Barr virus	Tuberculosis	*Aspergillus*	
		Coccidioimycosis	
		Histoplasmosis	

[a] After 6 months.

munosuppression does not necessarily impair the response to a vaccine. Yearly influenza vaccine and pneumococcal vaccine every 2–3 years are recommended. Hepatitis B vaccine is recommended if not previously administered.

Live virus vaccines, including oral polio, measles, mumps, and rubella vaccine (MMR), yellow fever vaccine, and varicella-zoster vaccine (VZV), as well as the two bacteria vaccines, oral typhoid and BCG, are to be avoided.

Antibiotic prophylaxis is usually recommended for dental, genitourinary, gastrointestinal, and surgical procedures, following the American Heart Association recommendations for the prevention of bacterial endocarditis. Clindamycin is preferable to erythromycin in those recipients with penicillin allergy, because of the effect of erythromycin on the metabolism of the calcineurin inhibitors.

Treatment is available for acute viral exposures in susceptible recipients. Measles exposure can be treated with standard immune globulin, and chickenpox exposure can be treated with varicella-zoster immunoglobulin within 72 hours. Recipients exposed to influenza A can be treated with immediate vaccination and amantadine.

G. Malignancy

Malignancy is a well-known complication of chronic immunosuppression (see Table 9). Estimates of the occurrence of de novo cancer in kidney transplant recipients are variable, because the risk of skin malignancy, the most common posttransplant malignancy, is influenced by climate. The risk of developing cancer increases with the duration of immunosuppression.

Skin cancers account for up to 50% of the posttransplant malignancies.

Table 9 Malignancy in Renal Transplant Recipients

Increased incidence	Decreased incidence(?)
Skin	Lung
squamous cell carcinoma	Breast
basal cell carcinoma?	Prostate
malignant melanoma	Colon
Lymphoma	
Non-Hodgkin's lymphoma	
PTLD (see text)	
Cervix	
Kaposi's sarcoma	
Kidney	
native	
transplant	
Vulva and perineum	
Hepatobiliary	

Squamous cell carcinoma is the most common. Squamous cell cancer may rarely develop from warts, a problem in a significant minority of recipients. It is not clear if the risk of basal cell carcinoma, the most common skin cancer in the general population, is increased. The risk of malignant melanoma is increased. Limiting sun exposure and the use of sunscreen is recommended, particularly in fair-skinned recipients. Annual skin examination by a dermatologist is recommended in susceptible individuals.

Non-Hodgkin's lymphoma is the second most common malignancy. The majority are B-cell lymphomas. The term posttransplant lymphoproliferative disorder (PTLD) is now used to encompass all posttransplant lymphoid hyperplasia, including malignancy. Primary EBV infection or reactivation of EBV in the recipient have been implicated in the development of PTLD. The risk of developing PTLD is 1–2% in renal transplant recipients. Recipients at risk for primary EBV infection and those who receive heavy immunosuppression are at greatest risk. PTLD may involve the renal graft alone. Extranodal, including central nervous system, involvement is common. Treatment includes discontinuation or reduction of immunosuppression, antiviral therapy, and surgery, local radiation, and chemotherapy as necessary. PTLD carries a high mortality rate.

Other cancers seen at increased frequency include in situ cancer of the cervix, Kaposi's sarcoma, cancer of the kidney (transplant and native), cancer of the vulva and perineum, and hepatobiliary cancers. Cancer of the lung, breast, prostate, and colon are seen at no greater frequency than in the general population. In addition to the recommendations for malignancy screening in the general population, yearly gynecological examination and Pap smear are recommended in female recipients.

H. Bone and Mineral Metabolism

The effect of transplantation on bone metabolism is primarily beneficial. Renal osteodystrophy heals and secondary hyperparathyroidism resolves over time. However, bone loss is common after transplantation and is a consequence of a steroid-induced decrease in bone formation. Bone demineralization is greatest during the first 12–18 months following transplantation, when steroid exposure is greatest, and may then improve. As many as 20–30% of long-term recipients may have osteoporosis, as measured by lumbar spine bone mineral density determination by dual x-ray absorptiometry. Bone fracture is a late complication, occurring in up to 10% of recipients an average of 8 years after transplantation. Fractures occur in both vertebral and peripheral bone. Steroid-induced bone loss can be treated. Treatments that are effective include calcium and vitamin D supplementation and antiresorptive therapy with hormonal replacement therapy and bisphosphonates.

The incidence of osteonecrosis (avascular necrosis) following transplantation has declined since the introduction of cyclosporine. The decline is attributed to the steroid-sparing effect of cyclosporine-based immunosuppression. Avascular necrosis most commonly affects the hip but may also involve the knee, shoulder, elbow, and ankle. Pain with activity is the presenting symptom. Magnetic resonance imaging is the most sensitive technique for early detection.

As many as 10–20% of recipients develop hypercalcemia within the first 2 years after transplantation due to persistent secondary hyperparathyroidism. In the past, 5% or more of recipients have required parathyroidectomy to control symptomatic hypercalcemia. Such an intervention is necessary when the total serum calcium is persistently greater than 12–12.5 mg/dL.

I. Hyperuricemia and Gout

Hyperuricemia following kidney transplantation is due to reduced renal clearance of uric acid, and this laboratory abnormality should not be treated. Attacks of gout must be treated with care. Nonsteroidal anti-inflammatory drugs (NSAIDs) are best avoided. Colchicine may be used for treatment of acute episodes and may suffice for chronic prophylaxis. If allopurinol therapy is necessary in patients receiving azathioprine, the dosage of azathioprine must be reduced when allopurinol is begun (see earlier). It is safe to use allopurinol with mycophenolate mofetil.

J. Erythrocytosis

Posttransplant erythrocytosis occurs in 10–15% of recipients, men more commonly than women, and usually develops within the first or second year after transplantation. It may remit spontaneously, but most patients require treatment to maintain the hematocrit at <50%. The erythrocytosis may be controlled by serial phlebotomy, but a preferable treatment is to prescribe an ACE inhibitor or an angiotensin II receptor antagonist. These agents may reduce red cell production by inhibiting erythropoietin production by the graft. As discussed earlier, close monitoring of renal function is necessary when starting one of these agents.

K. Reproductive Function

Libido, menstrual function, and ovulation return in premenopausal women after transplantation. They are fertile and may become pregnant. It is best to postpone pregnancy until after the first or second posttransplant year. Oral conceptives are commonly used. Intrauterine devices should be avoided. (See Chapter 25 for a complete discussion of the special issues relating to pregnancy in transplant recipients.) Impotence is common in men with ESRD. Following transplantation libido improves and potency usually returns. However, impotence may persist due to a variety of reasons, including the use of cyclosporine, which may impair testosterone production, antihypertensive medications, vascular disease, or autonomic neuropathy. If the cause of persistent impotence is unclear, the patient should have a urological evaluation. Certainly such an evaluation should be undertaken before prescribing drugs such as sildenafil (Viagra). It is not yet known if sildenafil interferes with the metabolism of the calcineurin inhibitors.

SUGGESTED READINGS

Armenti VT, Moritz MJ, Davison JM. Medical management of the pregnant transplant recipient. Adv Renal Replace Ther 1998; 5:14–23.

Danovitch GM. Handbook of Kidney Transplantation. 2d ed. Boston: Little, Brown and Company, 1996.

First MR, Neylan JF, Rocher LL, Tejani A. Hypertension after renal transplantation. J Am Soc Neph 1994; 4(suppl 1):S30–S36.

Fishman JA, Rubin RH. Infection in organ-transplant recipients. N Engl J Med 1998; 338: 1741–1751.

Gaston RS, Julian BA, Curtis JJ. Posttransplant erythrocytosis: an enigma revisited. Am J Kidney Dis 1994; 24:1–11.

Gaya SBM, Rees AJ, Lechler RI, Williams G, Mason PD. Malignant disease in patients with long-term renal transplants. Transplantation 1995; 59:1705–1709.

Lindholm A, Albrechtsen D, Frodin L, Tufveson G, Persson NH, Lundgren G. Ischemic heart disease—major cause of death and graft loss after renal transplantation in Scandinavia. Transplantation 1995; 60:451–457.

Markell MS, Armenti V, Danovitch G, Sumrani N. Hyperlipidemia and glucose intolerance in the post-renal transplant patient. J Am Soc Neph 1994; 4(suppl 1):S37–S47.

Moe SM. The treatment of steroid-induced bone loss in transplantation. Curr Opin Nephrol Hypertens 1997; 6:544–549.

Scandling JD. Renal transplantation: long-term management. In: Jamison RL, Wilkinson R, eds. Nephrology. London: Chapman and Hall, 1997, pp. 1098–1112.

28

Treatment of Acid-Base Disorders

F. John Gennari
University of Vermont, Burlington, Vermont

I. INTRODUCTION

The approach to identifying and diagnosing specific disorders of acid-base equilibrium is reviewed in Chapter 11. The present chapter addresses treatment issues for the four major disorders—metabolic acidosis, metabolic alkalosis, respiratory acidosis, and respiratory alkalosis—and also covers treatment of mixed acid-base disorders.

II. METABOLIC ACIDOSIS

Appropriate management of metabolic acidosis is highly dependent on identifying the cause. In some instances prompt treatment is key for survival, and in others little or no intervention is necessary. When the cause of the metabolic acidosis cannot be promptly reversed, the mainstay of treatment is repletion of alkali stores. The general principles of alkali replacement therapy are presented below, followed by a discussion of the specific recommendations for treatment of the major causes of metabolic acidosis.

A. Bicarbonate/Alkali Therapy: General Principles

Although newly added bicarbonate ions are confined to the extracellular compartment, the increase in pH engendered by the addition of these ions activates cell buffers, which release and add new hydrogen ions to this compartment. When HCO_3^- is given intravenously, 50–60% is rapidly removed from the circulation by combining with this newly generated H^+ to form CO_2 and water. This physiological fact is translated into clinical practice by using a ''space of distribution'' for administered bicarbonate of 50% of body weight.

Using this ''space'' and assuming no loss or gain of body alkali, administration of 100 mEq of HCO_3^- to a 70 kg patient is calculated to increase serum [HCO_3^-] by 100/(0.5 × 70) or approximately 3 mEq/L. The assumption that no alkali is gained or lost, however, is rarely fulfilled in patients with metabolic acidosis. In organic acidoses (see later), treatment leads to the production of endogenous alkali, and with ongoing diarrhea bicarbonate losses continue. Moreover, the ''space of distribution'' varies depending on the pH change engendered by the administered HCO_3^- and is larger when the initial serum [HCO_3^-] is very low. Thus, the clinical calculation is only intended to be a ''ballpark'' estimate. When administering HCO_3^-, one should calculate and administer the dose needed to increase serum [HCO_3^-] by only 3–5 mEq/L and never try to fully correct the deficit. Organic anions, such as lactate, can be administered instead of HCO_3^- (e.g., as in Ringer's lactate) and are equivalent to bicarbonate, assuming they can be appropriately metabolized (see Fig. 1).

In contrast to the acute HCO_3^- therapy described above, much smaller doses of oral sodium bicarbonate can help maintain body alkali stores in the face of impaired renal acid excretion. Daily endogenous acid production is approximately 1 mEq/kg body weight. If, for example, the kidney can excrete only half this amount, then administration of 0.5 mEq/kg body weight of $NaHCO_3$ (or about 30–35 mEq/day) is sufficient to maintain acid-base balance. Each 600 mg $NaHCO_3$ tablet contains 7 mEq of HCO_3^-, and thus as few as four tablets a day may be needed. In certain forms of renal tubular acidosis (see later) in which renal bicarbonate wasting occurs, much larger doses are necessary.

B. Metabolic Acidosis with an Increased Anion Gap

The causes of metabolic acidosis with an increased anion gap include organic acidoses, certain intoxications, and advanced renal insufficiency (see Chapter 11). Treatment guidelines are summarized in Table 1.

1. Organic Acidoses

These disorders are caused by runaway endogenous production of one or more organic acids. The organic acids that are produced are rapidly buffered by HCO_3^-, leaving an organic anion and carbonic acid (the latter removed from the body as exhaled CO_2). If the organic anion is retained, it ''replaces'' HCO_3^- and is responsible for the increase in anion gap (Fig. 1). Because retained organic anions regenerate HCO_3^- when they are metabolized to CO_2 and H_2O (Fig. 1), therapy aimed at stopping the their production and/or promoting their metabolism will

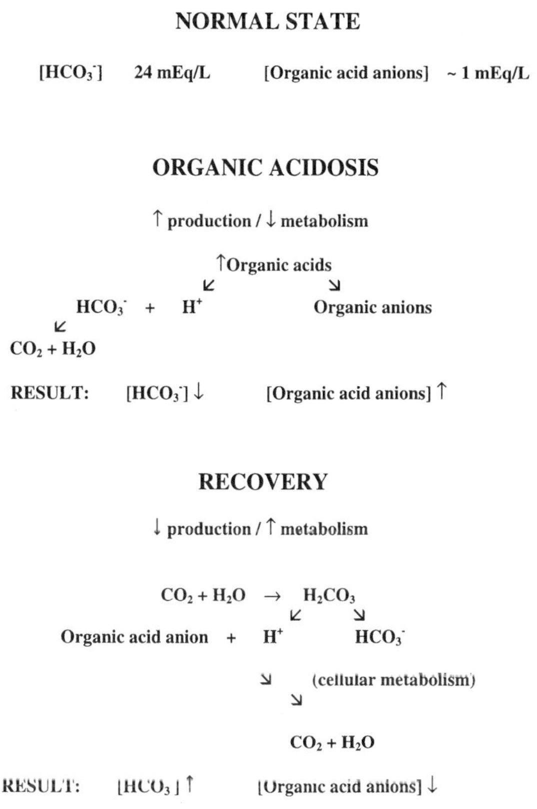

Figure 1 Interactions between organic acids and bicarbonate stores in the body. In the normal state, organic acid production and metabolism is regulated so that the steady-state concentration of organic acid anions (primarily lactate) in the blood is usually only 1 mEq/L. During periods of increased production and/or decreased metabolism of organic acids (e.g., diabetic ketoacidosis), these strong acids are buffered by bicarbonate and organic acid anions "replace" bicarbonate in the blood. In the recovery phase, the circulating organic acid anions remove an H^+ from carbonic acid during their metabolism, regenerating new bicarbonate ions. This process allows for correction of the acidosis without any bicarbonate replacement therapy or any changes in renal acid excretion.

Table 1 General Guidelines for Treatment of Acid-Base Disorders

Disorder	Approach to treatment
Metabolic acidosis	
Diabetic ketoacidosis	Insulin and saline No bicarbonate needed
Alcoholic ketoacidosis	Glucose and saline No bicarbonate needed
Lactic acidosis	Correct underlying problem Bicarbonate rarely needed
Toxin ingestion (methanol, ethylene glycol, salicylates)	Bicarbonate treatment necessary
Advanced renal insufficiency	Oral bicarbonate treatment if serum $[HCO_3^-] < 18$ mEq/L
Diarrhea	Bicarbonate treatment necessary
Renal tubular acidosis	Oral bicarbonate treatment in some instances (see text)
Metabolic alkalosis	
Vomiting, nasogastric drainage	Saline, KCl
Diuretic-induced	KCl or no treatment
Chloride resistant	No treatment—diagnose underlying cause
Respiratory acidosis	Improve ventilation, if possible Bicarbonate not indicated
Respiratory alkalosis	Diagnose underlying cause Rebreathing device in symptomatic patients

rapidly reverse the metabolic acidosis. As a result, administration of bicarbonate is rarely necessary if acid production can be curtailed. Diabetic ketoacidosis, discussed below, illustrates this principle.

(a) Diabetic Ketoacidosis. The cause of diabetic ketoacidosis is overproduction of β-hydroxybutyric acid, due both to insulin deficiency and to insulin resistance. Treatment should be directed at stopping the production of this organic acid and promoting its metabolism by simultaneously reducing insulin resistance and administering insulin. Both goals can be rapidly achieved. Prompt ECF volume repletion with isotonic saline virtually eliminates insulin resistance, and insulin deficiency is addressed by insulin replacement. These therapies are the cornerstones of treatment. As much as 4–6 L of isotonic saline may be necessary to restore ECF volume. Insulin is best administered as a constant infusion at rates of 8–15 units/hr. Because uncontrolled diabetes leads to renal K^+ losses and K^+ deficiency and because insulin promotes K^+ entry into cells, prompt and vigorous K^+ replacement should be undertaken as well (see Chapter 30).

Regardless of the severity of the reduction in serum [HCO_3^-] in patients with diabetic ketoacidosis, there is little evidence that bicarbonate administration speeds recovery or improves outcome. Nonetheless, arterial pH and PCO_2 should always be assessed, and serum [HCO_3^-] calculated, to assure that the ventilatory response is adequate for the reduction in [HCO_3^-] (see chapter 10). If the PCO_2 is inappropriately high, then attention should be paid to the patient's pulmonary status (see Sec. VI).

Treatment with isotonic saline, a critical component of therapy, unfortunately also promotes the excretion of organic anions before they can be metabolized to regenerate HCO_3^-, and this effect can prolong the acidosis (Fig. 2). The rapid excretion of organic anions and their replacement by chloride ions is manifest by the conversion of diabetic ketoacidosis from a high anion gap disorder on presentation to a normal anion gap (hyperchloremic) acidosis after several hours of saline administration. In most instances serum [HCO_3^-] increases by at least several mEq/L during this time interval, ameliorating the acidosis, and no additional treatment is necessary. With correction of the insulin deficiency/resistance, renal mechanisms gradually regenerate the HCO_3^- needed to restore serum [HCO_3^-] to normal levels within 24–48 hours.

(b) Alcoholic Ketoacidosis. This often severe metabolic acidosis is the combined result of starvation and alcohol intoxication, both of which stimulate ketogenesis. In contrast to diabetic ketoacidosis, however, blood sugar levels are

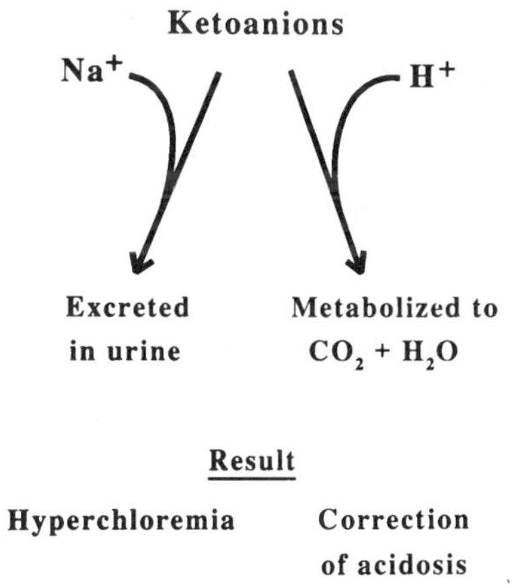

Figure 2 Fate of organic anions during treatment of an organic acidosis. The organic anion (e.g., ketoanion) is either metabolized, generating new bicarbonate ions (see Figure 1), or excreted in the urine, contributing to alkali loss. Administration of saline, necessary for the treatment of most organic acidoses, unfortunately facilitates the latter pathway.

low to normal. The disorder is rapidly reversible by repleting extracellular fluid volume using isotonic saline and by infusing glucose. The infusion of glucose stimulates insulin release, which in turn inhibits ketogenesis and repletes hepatic glycogen stores.

(c) Lactic Acidosis. Lactic acid overproduction is a serious and potentially fatal form of metabolic acidosis. Treatment of this disorder should always be directed primarily at reversing the cause of the lactic acid overproduction. The most common cause of lactic acidosis is inadequate oxygen delivery to tissues (tissue hypoxia), such as occurs in shock, severe congestive heart failure, carbon monoxide poisoning, and severe hypoxemia. Lactic acidosis due to inadequate oxygen delivery is termed type A lactic acidosis. Type B lactic acidosis includes the remaining causes where tissue oxygen delivery appears to be adequate, but another factor interferes with normal mitochondrial metabolism. The causes of type B lactic acidosis include sepsis, hepatic failure, some malignancies, and drugs (Table 2). The oral hypoglycemic agent, metformin, can cause lactic acidosis in patients with renal insufficiency.

Treatment of type A lactic acidosis is straightforward. Maneuvers designed to increase tissue oxygen delivery result in a prompt cessation of lactic acid production and the acidosis is quickly reversed, as circulating lactate ions are metabolized regenerating body alkali stores. Bicarbonate therapy is rarely necessary. Management of type B lactic acidosis should also be directed at reversing the cause, if possible. Treatment of sepsis, or discontinuation of metformin, for example, will promptly reverse the acidosis. When the disorder cannot be rapidly reversed, a variety of interventions have been advocated, all with very limited effi-

Table 2 Causes of Lactic Acidosis

Type A	Type B
Shock	Diabetes mellitus
Severe congestive heart failure	Liver disease
Severe hypoxemia ($PO_2 < 32$ mmHg)	Metformin
Carbon monoxide poisoning	Malignancies
Very severe anemia (Hct < 10% or Hb < 3 g/dL)	acute leukemia
	lymphomas
	Toxins
	cyanide
	ethanol
	methanol
	ethylene glycol
	salicylate intoxication

cacy. Bicarbonate therapy remains the mainstay of treatment, sometimes administered with dialysis therapy to minimize fluid overload. Alternative therapies, including methylene blue, an oxidizing agent that improves NADH oxidation, and dichloroacetate, a promoter of lactate metabolism, have been used to treat type B lactic acidosis without success. These agents are no longer used. At present, the only useful interventions are those that reverse the stimulus for lactic acid production.

2. Intoxications

(a) Salicylate Intoxication. The mainstay of treatment of salicylate intoxication is to speed the removal of this drug from the body. This is accomplished by alkalinizing the urine using intravenous sodium bicarbonate. Ideally the urine pH should be increased to greater than 7.5, if possible. In most instances hemodialysis is not necessary, as the acidosis is not severe or life-threatening.

(b) Methanol/Ethylene Glycol Intoxication. Deliberate or accidental ingestion of either of these organic solvents causes a potentially lethal organic acidosis. The substances themselves are not toxic, but when metabolized they produce large amounts of toxic organic acids (see Chapter 11). Thus, treatment of these disorders is directed at inhibiting the metabolism of these solvents while simultaneously promoting their removal from the body. Until recently, the mainstay of therapy to inhibit metabolism was ethanol. Intravenous ethanol given to maintain the blood alcohol level above 100 mg/dL is sufficient to completely inhibit metabolism of both methanol and ethylene glycol. The problem with this therapy is that ethanol itself is toxic and is also rapidly metabolized and removed by hemodialysis. Therefore maintenance of adequate blood levels is difficult. Fomepizole, an inhibitor of alcohol dehydrogenase, is now available for intravenous use and is a very effective and nontoxic inhibitor of ethylene glycol metabolism. It is given as a loading dose and then redosed every 12 hours, with good maintenance of blood levels even during hemodialysis. Although not yet tested for methanol poisoning in humans, animal studies indicate that it should be an effective inhibitor of methanol metabolism as well. In addition to inhibiting the metabolism of these solvents, hemodialysis should be initiated promptly to speed their removal from the body. Initial therapy should also always include intravenous bicarbonate to improve systemic pH if possible. This maneuver will minimize toxic effects until hemodialysis can be initiated.

3. Advanced Renal Insufficiency

The metabolic acidosis that accompanies advanced renal insufficiency is caused by impaired renal acid excretion. In its milder form (see later), the anions of the strong acids produced are excreted and the anion gap is not increased. As renal insufficiency worsens, these anions (primarily sulfate and phosphate) can no longer be excreted and accumulate, increasing the anion gap. The development of this chronic acidosis is largely dependent on dietary intake and catabolic state. Thus, some patients begin dialysis because of other uremic symptoms with a normal serum [HCO_3^-], whereas some develop a moderately severe acidosis long before other symptoms develop. When present, this form of metabolic acidosis should be treated, because it promotes muscle catabolism, accelerates renal osteodystropy, increases malaise, and reduces appetite. The treatment is oral sodium bicarbonate, 30–50 mEq/day, in divided doses. The limitations of this therapy are Na^+ retention, with worsening hypertension and/or edema. Persistence of a high anion-gap metabolic acidosis, due to intolerance to sodium bicarbonate or lack of effect, is one indication to initiate renal replacement therapy.

C. Metabolic Acidosis with a Normal Anion Gap

1. Diarrhea

The metabolic acidosis induced by diarrhea is the result of HCO_3^- loss in the stool. Patients with diarrhea also lose NaCl and K^+, but, because of the disproportionate loss of HCO_3^-, serum chloride rises and the anion gap remains normal. Treatment should include intravenous NaCl, KCl, and $NaHCO_3$. The exact prescription should be individualized, recognizing that, unless serum [HCO_3^-] is <10 mEq/L, ECF volume and K^+ repletion are more critical than correction of the accompanying metabolic acidosis.

2. Renal Tubular Acidosis

Treatment of renal tubular acidosis (RTA) varies, depending on the type of defect present and on the age of the patient. (See Chapter 11 for diagnosis of the specific types of RTA.)

(a) Type 1 RTA. Type 1 RTA is due to a defect in acid excretion that leads to acid retention, loss of bone calcium, nephrocalcinosis, and renal K^+ wasting. Bicarbonate replacement therapy has been shown to ameliorate these effects and improve outcome, and oral replacement therapy should always be initiated. In adults, a dose of 0.5–1.5 mEq/kg body weight is usually sufficient to correct the acidosis and to prevent the complications of this disease. The bicarbonate is usually given as a mixture of Na^+ and K^+ bicarbonate (or a bicarbonate precursor such as acetate or citrate), in varying amounts, depending on the individual need of the patient. In children with type 1 RTA, the above dosage is insufficient to

correct the associated impairment in growth, and larger amounts of bicarbonate, 2–5 mEq/kg body weight, are recommended.

(b) Type 2 RTA. Type 2 RTA can occur as an isolated defect or in association with the Fanconi syndrome. In either instance the metabolic acidosis is due to impaired renal HCO_3^- reabsorption. As a result correction of the acidosis requires large amounts of HCO_3^-, and replacement therapy leads to flooding the distal nephron with $NaHCO_3$, causing renal K^+ wasting and hypokalemia. In adults with acquired isolated type 2 RTA, no alkali therapy is recommended unless the acidosis is severe (serum $[HCO_3^-] < 16$ mEq/L). In children with type 2 RTA and in all patients with Fanconi syndrome, an attempt should be made to correct the acidosis to prevent complications. Treatment should include Na^+ as well as K^+ bicarbonate (or citrate or acetate), usually in a dosage of 3–6 mEq/kg body weight. In these patients, bicarbonate replacement therapy is sometimes coupled with a thiazide diuretic to limit renal bicarbonate losses. When these two treatment modalities are coupled, close attention should be paid to K^+ replacement as losses of this cation are increased.

(c) Type 4 RTA. Type 4 or hyperkalemic RTA is a common component of chronic renal insufficiency. The acidosis is typically quite mild (serum $[HCO_3^-] = 18$–22 mEq/L), and little attention has been paid to treating it. However, even this mild degree of acidosis can contribute to muscle catabolism and bone disease in patients with renal insufficiency. As a result, oral bicarbonate replacement has been advocated by some experts for all such patients. If the acidosis is more severe, then most agree that bicarbonate supplementation should be initiated. Because it is related to a defect in acid excretion and not in bicarbonate reabsorption, only a small amount of $NaHCO_3$ (0.5–1 mEq/kg body weight) is needed to correct the disorder. The major cost of such therapy is Na^+ retention, exacerbating hypertension and edema.

III. METABOLIC ALKALOSIS

The causes of metabolic alkalosis are subdivided into those that are chloride-responsive and those that are chloride-resistant (see Chapter 11). In either case, the first line of therapy is to attempt to reverse the underlying cause. In contrast to metabolic acidosis, even moderately severe metabolic alkalosis (serum $[HCO_3^-]$ as high as 40 mEq/L) is well tolerated, and correction of the acid-base disorder is almost never an urgent requirement. Treatment guidelines are shown in Table 1. When the serum $[HCO_3^-]$ exceeds 45 mEq/L, more immediate intervention is indicated (see below).

A. Chloride-Sensitive Metabolic Alkalosis

The most common causes of metabolic alkalosis are those due to selective chloride losses from the gastrointestinal tract (vomiting, nasogastric drainage) or kidney (diuretic use).

1. Vomiting/Nasogastric Drainage

In the patient with metabolic alkalosis caused by gastrointestinal losses, ECF volume depletion is always a feature. As discussed in Chapter 11, these patients are also K^+ and chloride depleted. Treatment should be directed at ECF volume and K^+ and chloride repletion, using intravenous isotonic saline and KCl supplementation. There are no guidelines or formulas for the amount of saline needed to replete ECF volume and chloride stores, but one should administer this solution until the disorder begins to correct itself, or until adequate amounts of Na^+ and chloride appear in the urine (concentrations > 20–30 mEq/L). Typically, the K^+ deficit is 200–400 mEq/L, and this should be replaced gradually as part of the treatment. In addition, therapy should be directed at inhibiting emesis if that is the cause or working to discontinue nasogastric drainage. If nasogastric drainage must be continued, the use of an H^+/K^+ ATPase inhibitor such as omeprazole can ameliorate the alkalosis.

2. Diuretics

The most common form of metabolic alkalosis seen in current clinical practice is caused by the use of diuretics that inhibit chloride reabsorption in the loop of Henle or early distal tubule (loop or thiazide diuretics). The alkalosis produced is usually mild (serum $[HCO_3^-] < 35$ mEq/L), and no specific therapy is required from an acid-base perspective. The more pressing problem is the concomitant K^+ deficiency induced by these drugs (see Chapter 30). Potassium repletion should be undertaken using KCl, achieving the dual goal of replacing both K^+ and chloride losses. Providing chloride in this form also serves to minimize the severity of the alkalosis. With ongoing diuretic use, the alkalosis and K^+ depletion are never fully corrected and continuous KCl supplementation is often necessary. The use of K^+-sparing diuretics (amiloride, triamterene) can also minimize K^+ losses and reduce the severity of the alkalosis.

B. Chloride-Resistant Metabolic Alkalosis

The chloride-resistant forms of metabolic alkalosis include a diverse group of disorders caused either by mineralocorticoid excess or by inherited or acquired disorders of renal tubular epithelial transport (see Chapter 11). In all these disorders, the metabolic alkalosis is usually mild and is a diagnostic clue rather than an abnormality requiring specific therapeutic attention. Therapy should be directed at reversing the underlying cause, if possible (see Chapter 11). When the cause cannot be corrected (e.g., in Bartter's or Gitelman's syndromes), management of the alkalosis and associated hypokalemia is difficult and never completely successful.

C. Metabolic Alkalosis—Special Treatment Issues

Patients with severe metabolic alkalosis (serum $[HCO_3^-] > 40$ mEq/L) often have multiple contributing factors causing the disorder. Management should include a careful review of the patient's medications and intravenous therapy to exclude the contribution of alkali or potential alkali administration. Acetate anions, often a component of parenteral nutrition formulas, citrate administration in blood transfusions, Ringers lactate, and $NaHCO_3$ or $CaCO_3$ administration can all contribute to sustaining or exacerbating metabolic alkalosis, particularly in patients with renal insufficiency who are unable to excrete excess alkali.

In patients with severe metabolic alkalosis who cannot tolerate further volume expansion, saline administration is not an option for therapy. If these patients have sufficient renal function, the carbonic anhydrase inhibitor acetazolamide (diamox) can be used both to promote a diuresis and cause bicarbonate loss. When this agent is used, attention should be paid to serum $[K^+]$, as it also promotes renal K^+ losses. In the patient without adequate renal function, severe metabolic alkalosis can be ameliorated by HCl administration, directly titrating body alkali stores. However, HCl must be administered via a large central vein and its concentration should not exceed 100 mEq/L. Thus, the limitation of this therapy is the large amount of fluid that must be administered (>3 L in a 70 kg individual to reduce serum $[HCO_3^-]$ by 10 mEq/L). Arginine monohydrochloride and ammonium chloride have been used in the past to lower serum $[HCO_3^-]$, but their toxicities limit their usefulness and they are now only rarely used. Instead, the technique of continuous venovenous hemofiltration provides a safe means for lowering serum $[HCO_3^-]$. With this technique, as much as 1–1.5 L of bicarbonate-rich fluid can be filtered each hour and replaced with isotonic saline, reducing serum $[HCO_3^-]$.

IV. RESPIRATORY ACIDOSIS

The primary abnormality in respiratory acidosis is hypercapnia, and therefore treatment should be directed at reducing arterial PCO_2, if possible. Attempts to normalize pH by increasing serum $[HCO_3^-]$ should not be undertaken, as this therapy may inhibit ventilatory drive. In addition, acute HCO_3^- administration can exacerbate pulmonary edema and impair pulmonary gas exchange further.

The one exception to this rule is severe acute asthma that is unresponsive to bronchodilators. If hypercapnia and acidosis are present in this setting, acute administration of HCO_3^- can raise pH and relieve the urgent need to lower PCO_2. In addition, the increase in pH can improve the responsiveness of the lung to bronchodilators. In patients with chronic hypercapnia, there is no role for alkali therapy.

V. RESPIRATORY ALKALOSIS

Respiratory alkalosis is a diagnostic finding that should trigger a search for an underlying illness (see Chapter 11). Only in rare instances, such as the anxiety-hyperventilation syndrome, is direct intervention indicated to increase arterial PCO_2. In this disorder, a rebreathing device (e.g., a paper bag over the mouth and nose) will quickly reverse the symptoms of acute respiratory alkalosis. Before initiating such therapy, however, it is critical that one exclude other causes for acute hyperpnea, such as hypoxemia or severe metabolic acidosis.

VI. MIXED DISORDERS

Mixed disorders are defined as the presence of two or more primary acid-base disorders existing at the same time in a patient (see Chapter 11). The importance of identifying more than one disorder is to direct treatment appropriately. Some mixed disorders require no specific attention, whereas for others, treatment issues are vitally important. Examples of mixed disorders and the approach to treatment are discussed below.

A. Respiratory Acidosis and Metabolic Acidosis

Failure to increase ventilatory rate and lower PCO_2 in response to a metabolic acidosis requires swift therapeutic attention, because it will cause severe acidemia. For example, in a patient with a reduction in serum $[HCO_3^-]$ to 10 mEq/L, concomitant impairment in ventilation and failure to reduce PCO_2 below 40 mmHg will cause pH to fall swiftly to 7.00 or lower. In such patients, if metabolic acidosis cannot be quickly reversed, serious consideration should be given to intubation to lower PCO_2 mechanically and improve blood pH.

B. Respiratory Acidosis and Metabolic Alkalosis

This mixed disorder is probably the most common, developing when patient with chronic respiratory acidosis are treated with diuretics. The diuretic-induced increase in serum [HCO_3^-] serves to bring blood pH into the normal range, 7.40–7.45, and usually no treatment is needed. If pH is higher, it may serve to impede ventilatory effort in these patients, and efforts should be made to correct the problem. This goal can be achieved by using acetazolamide rather than a thiazide or loop diuretic. In any case an effort should be made to correct any potassium deficit caused by diuretic therapy.

C. Metabolic Acidosis and Respiratory Alkalosis

This mixed disorder is characteristic of salicylate intoxication, because salicylates stimulate ventilation directly as well as increasing organic acid production. Thus, the disorder is characterized by an arterial PCO_2 that is lower than expected for the reduction in serum [HCO_3^-] (see Chapter 11 for rule of thumb). As a result, arterial pH is often greater than 7.40 in this disorder. Even when arterial blood pH is alkaline, intravenous bicarbonate treatment is recommended because alkalinization of the urine enhances renal excretion of salicylates.

D. Metabolic Acidosis and Alkalosis

This disorder is characteristic in binge drinkers, who develop nausea and vomiting (hence, metabolic alkalosis), and then become volume depleted enough to develop a superimposed lactic acidosis. The disorder is diagnosed by calculating the delta anion gap (see Chapter 11). In brief, the anion gap is typically much larger than would be expected from the reduction in serum [HCO_3^-]. These patients should always be treated with isotonic saline rather than bicarbonate, because restoration of ECF volume will stop the production of organic acids and regenerate more than sufficient new bicarbonate to correct the acid-base disorder. The administered chloride will also correct the deficit in this anion and allow the final serum [HCO_3^-] to return to normal.

E. Triple Disorder: Metabolic Acidosis and Alkalosis Plus Respiratory Alkalosis

This disorder can occur when excessive hyperventilation accompanies a mixed metabolic alkalosis and acidosis, due to any of a wide variety of causes (see Chapter 11). The picture can be confusing, with an alkaline pH and a large anion gap. The treatment is the same, i.e., resuscitation with isotonic saline.

F. Other Mixed Disorders

The above disorders are the most common, but other combined disorders, such as metabolic alkalosis and respiratory alkalosis, are possible. The guidelines provided in Chapter 11 are the tools for identifying these disorders, and, once identified, treatment should be based on the general principle of addressing the most easily reversed or the most life-threatening component of the disorder.

SUGGESTED READINGS

Adrogue HJ, Madias NE. Management of life-threatening acid-base disorders. N Engl J Med 338:26–35 (Part I), 107–111 (Part II), 1998.

Gennari FJ. Respiratory acidosis and alkalosis. In: Narins R, ed. Clinical Disorders of Fluid and Electrolyte Metabolism. 5th ed. New York: McGraw Hill, 1994, pp. 957–990.

Ishihara K, Szerlip HM. Anion gap acidosis. Semin Nephro 18:83–97, 1998.

Rimmer JM, Gennari FJ. Metabolic alkalosis. J Intensive Care Med 2:137–150, 1987.

29
Treatment of Hypertonicity and Hypotonicity

Alan S. Segal
University of Vermont, Burlington, Vermont

I. INTRODUCTION

As discussed in Chapter 12, a net loss of water from the body will produce hypertonicity and a net gain will produce hypotonicity, abnormalities termed here hypoaquaemia and hyperaquaemia to reflect their respective pathophysiology. Symptoms and signs of the dysaquaemias, discussed in Chapter 4, are related to changes in cell volume, the adaptive response of cells to changes in volume, and the cellular response to therapeutic interventions (see Fig. 1). The goal of therapy is to return cell volume towards normal by restoring the ratio of water to solute in the extracellular fluid (ECF) to normal, in a manner that allows cells to adapt to this correction without further damage.

Effective therapy is based on (1) a careful clinical assessment, including a history to ascertain the duration of the dysaquaemia and the presence of any neurological symptoms, (2) a physical examination, with an emphasis on assessment of ECF volume, (3) an evaluation of laboratory tests, including electrolytes and serum creatinine, and (4) calculation of plasma tonicity (see below and Chapter 12). Based on this information, correction of the abnormality can be undertaken at an appropriate rate to alleviate symptoms while treating any underlying primary or co-existing conditions.

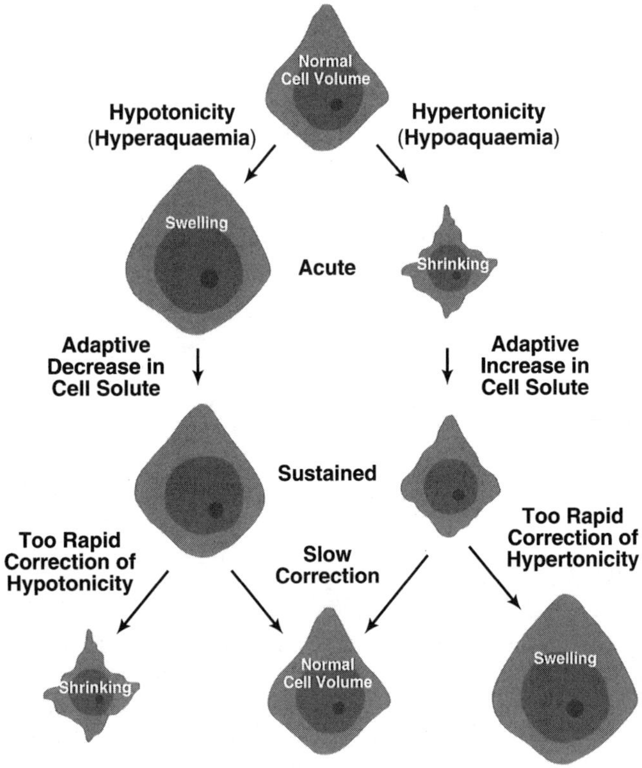

Figure 1 Tonicity-induced changes in (brain) cell volume and the possible sequelae of therapeutic interventions. The left side of the diagram shows the cellular response to hypotonicity (hyperaquaemia). Initial cellular swelling is followed by an adaptive regulatory volume decrease mediated by solute efflux. If the hypotonicity is sustained, cellular solute stores are depleted so that if extracellular tonicity is abruptly increased to ''normal'' levels, water will rush out and dangerous cellular shrinkage may occur. The right side of the diagram shows the cellular response to hypertonicity (hypoaquaemia). Initial cellular shrinkage is followed an adaptive regulatory volume increase mediated by the production of new intracellular solutes. If the hypertonicity is sustained, cellular solute stores are increased so that if extracellular tonicity is abruptly ''normalized,'' water will rush in and dangerous cellular swelling with cerebral edema may occur.

Table 1 Management of Hypertonicity

1. Determine clinical volume status
2. Assess the ability of the patient to signal thirst
   - Able → suggests thirst disorder (hypodipsia)
   - Unable → suggests water access problem
     - unless excessive Na^+ losses, treat with water replacement alone
     - determine underlying cause (e.g., stroke, inadequate water replacement by caregivers)
3. Search for sources of water loss
   - Skin: excessive sweating, burns
   - GI: emesis, diarrhea
   - Renal: osmotic diuresis, diabetes insipidus
4. Check whether hypertonic solutions have been administered
5. Treatment guidelines
   - Replete volume with 0.9% NaCl if hypovolemia co-exists
   - Stop or at least replace any ongoing losses
   - Treat associated problems, since hypertonicity is often associated with significant underlying disease
   - Estimate the water deficit: weight (kg) × [(tonicity/285) − 1] × F, where F = 0.6 for males and 0.5 for females
   - If symptomatic, give d5W with the goal of reducing tonicity by 2–4 mOsm/kg per hour until symptoms resolve, then by 1–2 mOsm/kg per hour (do not exceed 50 mOsm/kg in 24 hours)
   - If acute (<24–48 hours), replace half the deficit over 18–24 hours and aim for a goal of 298 mOsm/kg over the next 36–48 hours
   - If chronic (>48 hours), reduce tonicity by 1–2 mOsm/kg per hour and aim for a goal of 298 mOsm/kg (do not exceed 50 mOsm/kg in 24 hours)
   - Make frequent measurements of plasma tonicity (especially until symptoms resolve) and adjust therapy accordingly

II. TREATMENT OF HYPERTONICITY (HYPOAQUAEMIA)

Guidelines for the approach and treatment of hypertonicity are given in Table 1. The goal of therapy for hypoaquaemia is to curtail further water losses and to replace the existing water deficit. Several formulas have been developed to estimate the magnitude of the water loss in a given patient, but it should be emphasized that these formulas are only intended to be used as estimates:

$$\text{Water deficit (L)} \cong \text{total body water} \times [(\text{tonicity})/285) - 1]$$

For males:

$$\text{Water deficit (L)} \cong 0.6 \times \text{weight (kg)} \times [(\text{tonicity})/285) - 1]$$

For females:

$$\text{Water deficit (L)} \cong 0.5 \times \text{weight (kg)} \times [(\text{tonicity})/285) - 1]$$

Recall from Chapter 12 that tonicity is calculated as 2 × serum [Na^+] + glucose (mg/dL)/18, or as the measured serum osmolality -BUN (mg/dL)/2.8, with a normal value of 285 mOsm/kg H_2O. The above formula for estimating water deficit is based on the assumption that no gain or loss of solute has occurred. In fact, this assumption is almost never correct. In addition, the fraction of water per unit body weight decreases with age in both males and females. For males, the %TBW is about 60% between the ages of 10 and 30, then drops gradually to 50% by age 45, and plateaus. For females, %TBW is 50% between the ages of 16 and 40, then drops to ~40% by age 50, and plateaus. A better estimate of water loss is obtained if the premorbid body weight is known. If it is, the mean of that weight and the current weight may be used.

Finally, it should be emphasized that none of the formulas used to estimate the volume of water needed for correction of hypertonicity take into account urinary output during the correction process. For example, if a patient is excreting 3 L of urine per day, this volume should be added to the water deficit when calculating the amount of fluid needed.

A. Treatment of Associated Volume Depletion

In most instances of hypertonicity, some solute is lost in addition to water. Therefore, most patients present with volume depletion in addition to water depletion. Note that the calculations above underestimate the water deficit in patients who are volume depleted. In patients with significant volume depletion, isotonic saline should always be given first, providing both salt and water to stabilize blood pressure. If the loss included large amounts of bicarbonate (e.g., severe diarrhea), then 5% dextrose in water with 100–150 mEq of sodium bicarbonate added to each liter may be given initially. Once volume deficits are repleted, water deficits should be repaired enterally if possible (oral or nasogastric H_2O) or parenterally.

Rather than beginning therapy with isotonic saline followed by 5% dextrose in water, some authorities recommend using 0.45% (half normal) saline from the outset. Ultimately, the patient probably receives a similar amount of solute and water. However, initial volume repletion with isotonic saline will more rapidly improve renal hypoperfusion and, therefore, the ability of the kidney to conserve free water. Once clinical euvolemia is reestablished, subsequent water administration to achieve a target tonicity is simplified. Therefore, this author prefers the latter approach.

The route of water replacement should include the gastrointestinal tract whenever possible, especially if the hypertonicity is chronic. Enteral replacement helps avoid the glycosuria (and osmotic diuresis) that can potentially occur (especially in diabetics) with rehydration using intravenous 5% dextrose in water. If enteral rehydration is not possible or adequate, parenteral water replacement with either 0.45% saline or 5% dextrose in water is indicated. The former is most useful in cases when some degree of hypovolemia coexists. When 5% dextrose in water is used, plasma glucose level should be followed closely, to assure that an osmotic diuresis is not induced, since hypertonicity is a state of relative insulin resistance.

B. Rate of Tonicity Correction

There are no clear data to indicate the precise rate of correction of hypertonicity needed in a symptomatic hypertonic patient in order to avoid treatment-induced cellular damage. However, the following guidelines are generally recommended (see Table 1). If you know that the hypertonicity developed acutely (<24–48 hours), the deficit can be replaced relatively rapidly. Generally, half of the deficit can be replaced within the first 18–24 hours, regardless of whether symptoms are present. For more chronic hypertonicity (>48 hours), the rate of correction is determined in part by the presence of neurological symptoms. In patients with such symptoms, tonicity should be reduced by 2–4 mOsm/kg H_2O per hour until symptoms improve, and then the rate of correction should be decreased. For asymptomatic patients, the rate of correction should be extremely gradual. As a general rule, it should not exceed 2 mOsm/kg H_2O per hour (Δ [Na^+] < 1 mEq/L per hour) or 50 mOsm/kg per day (Δ [Na^+] < 25 mEq/L per day). Complete correction should never be the aim of initial therapy. Rather the tonicity should only be corrected to 294–298 mOsm/kg H_2O ([Na^+] = 147–149 mEq/L). In states of chronic hypertonicity, decreasing extracellular tonicity to ''normal'' may result in acute cerebral cellular swelling due to the continued presence of intracellular ''idiogenic osmoles'' generated prior to therapeutic interventions (see Chapter 12).

As therapy to replace the water deficit proceeds, the underlying causes of water loss and other co-morbid conditions should be addressed. Careful monitoring of the patient's neurological status, especially during the treatment of chronic hypertonicity, is of paramount importance. Following an initial improvement, any neurological deterioration (e.g., seizures), no matter how slight, may indicate the development of cerebral edema. To avoid further injury, especially catastrophic herniation, water-replacement therapy must be immediately stopped at the first sign of worsening neurological dysfunction.

In the rare instances in which hypertonicity is the result of exogenous solute intake rather than a primary water intake/excretion problem (see Chapter 12), a loop diuretic should be used to facilitate solute excretion during rehydration therapy. Acute renal replacement therapy is indicated if these patients develop pulmonary edema and/or renal failure.

C. Treatment of Chronic Disorders Associated with Hypertonicity

The basic management of central and nephrogenic diabetes insipidus is outlined in Table 2.

1. Central Diabetes Insipidus

The treatment for central diabetes insipidus is hormone replacement. The drug used is 1-desamino-8-D-arginine vasopressin (dDAVP). Unlike AVP (ADH), which binds to both V_1 (pressor) and V_2 (antidiuretic) receptors, dDAVP has essentially no V_1 effect and also has a longer half-life. The usual dose is 10–24 μg intranasally twice a day, but the drug can be given intravenously in acute settings. This dosing schedule is far from the optimal regulation of the native hormonal axis, and additional agents are sometimes used. Chlorpropamide, best known for increasing insulin secretion, can also potentiate the effect of any native ADH that may be released and reduce polyuria by 25–75%. Thiazide diuretics in combination with sodium restriction also decrease the daily urine flow rate by up to 50%. Patients need to be closely monitored for side effects related to the use of these drugs.

2. Nephrogenic Diabetes Insipidus

Hypertonicity should not develop in patients with nephrogenic insipidus (NDI) who have an intact thirst mechanism and adequate access to water. Rather, these patients almost always present with polydipsia and polyuria (see Chapters 1 and 4). Potentially reversible defects in urinary concentration should be addressed by

Table 2 Treatment of Diabetes Insipidus

Central DI
1-Desamino-8-D-arginine vasopressin (dDAVP) as an effective ADH analog
Chlorpropamide to amplify the effect of ADH
Thiazide to induce mild volume depletion
Nephrogenic DI
Restrict solute intake
Diuretic: a thiazide or amiloride in lithium-induced DI
Indomethacin: add if significant polyuria persists

treatment of the underlying disorder (e.g., hypercalcemia). If drug-induced NDI is suspected, the offending agent (e.g., lithium) should be discontinued if possible. Because patients with NDI often have some level of chronic irreversible parenchymal disease, treatment is usually aimed at reducing polyuria. To this end, restriction of solute (sodium) intake and a thiazide diuretic may reduce urine output by up to 50%. Amiloride may be preferable for patients who must take lithium or in whom thiazide-induced hypokalemia develops. Indomethacin may be added to lessen polyuria but should only be used in refractory cases because it acts by decreasing GFR.

III. TREATMENT OF HYPOTONICITY

The optimal management of patients with hypotonicity continues to be an evolving field of study and remains charged with a fair amount of controversy. Although a complete review of this topic is beyond the scope of this chapter, this section will review the presently accepted principles of management and will point out some important misconceptions in the outcome and complications of therapy. General guidelines and therapeutic recommendations are detailed in Table 3.

A. Clinical Approach

When faced with a hyponatremic patient, the most important initial assessment is to determine whether the patient has symptomatic hypotonicity. If so, a medical emergency exists that carries an overall mortality exceeding 20%. The specific management of this situation is discussed in the next section. More often, hypotonic patients are asymptomatic and the goal of therapy is to identify and treat the underlying cause. If at all possible, determine how long the patient has been hypotonic and take measures to correct the hypotonicity at a rate commensurate with the period of time over which the problem developed. A general rule of thumb is, "if it broke quickly it should be fixed quickly; if it broke more slowly, it should be fixed more slowly." For each case, assess the patient's risk factors for the neurological complications associated with hypotonicity. Finally, devise an initial management strategy that incorporates (1) the type, amount and rate of solutions to be infused, (2) the degree of water restriction that should be imposed, (3) additional medications to be given (e.g., furosemide) and (4) the schedule for monitoring, including a contingency plan.

In most cases, the pathogenesis of the hyperaquaemia defines the therapeutic approach. Because a water excretion defect underlies nearly all cases, maneuvers aimed at improving water excretion combined with restricting water intake should form the initial basis of therapy. In turn, specific maneuvers employed

Table 3 Initial Management of Hypotonicity

1. Determine clinical volume status and if the patient is symptomatic
    - Symptomatic and hypovolemic
        - 0.9% NaCl until euvolemic, then reassess
        - Water restriction
    - Symptomatic and hypervolemic
        - Acute hemodialysis until symptoms resolve or [Na] > 125 mEq/L
        - Furosemide intravenously
        - Salt and water restriction
    - Symptomatic and euvolemic
        - 3% hypertonic NaCl to raise [Na] by 1–2 mEq/L per hour until symptoms resolve or [Na] > 125 mEq/L
        - Do not increase [Na] by more than 25 mEq/L over 24 hours
        - Water restriction
2. If asymptomatic, determine how long the patient has been hypotonic
    - Hypovolemic
        - 0.9% NaCl until euvolemic
        - Water restriction
    - Hypervolemic
        - Salt and water restriction
        - Furosemide intravenously
        - Consider hemodialysis if [Na] <120 mEq/L with acute hypotonicity (<24–48 hr)
    - Euvolemic
        - Acute hypotonicity (<24–48 hr) and [Na] < 120 mEq/L
        - 3% hypertonic NaCl to raise [Na] by 1–2 mEq/L per hour until [Na] > 125 mEq/L
        - Consider intravenous furosemide, especially if hypervolemia is developing
        - Water restriction
        - Acute hypotonicity (<24–48 hr) and [Na] > 120 mEq/L
    - Water restriction
        - Chronic hypotonicity (>48 hr) and [Na] < 120 mEq/L
        - 3% hypertonic NaCl to raise [Na] by 1–2 mEq/L per hour until [Na] > 125 mEq/L
        - Consider intravenous furosemide, especially if hypervolemia is developing
        - Water restriction
        - Consider demeclocycline
        - Chronic hypotonicity (>48 hr) and [Na] > 120 mEq/L
        - Water restriction
        - Consider demeclocycline
        - Consider more aggressive therapy, especially for postmenopausal women
3. Discontinue any medications that could possible stimulate ADH release or potentiate its effect
4. Treat the underlying disorder (e.g., a malignancy)

are those that take the underlying condition(s) (e.g., increased ADH effect due to medications and/or CNS, pulmonary or neoplastic processes) and clinical volume status into account. For example, replacement therapy with thyroid or adrenal hormones will correct the hypotonicity associated with endocrinopathies. Maintenance treatment for patients with secondary adrenal insufficiency is hydrocortisone 15–20 mg/m^2 in three divided doses; patients with primary adrenal insufficiency and mineralocorticoid deficiency should also receive fludrocortisone.

B. Symptomatic Hypotonicity: General Treatment Guidelines

The symptoms associated with hypotonicity range from confusion to seizures and coma (see Chapters 4 and 12) and are due do cell swelling in the brain. Regardless of the underlying cause, symptomatic hypotonicity is a medical emergency that requires immediate active intervention. The overall mortality exceeds 20% (>40% if [Na^+] < 120 mEq/L), so it is crucial to identify high-risk patients early. These include perioperative hyponatremia in menstruant women and prepubescent children, and chronic hyponatremia in postmenopausal women and patients with psychogenic polydipsia, SIADH, or those taking thiazide diuretics. It appears that the danger of undertreating these patients (i.e., withholding hypertonic saline) far outweighs the risk of the osmotic demyelination syndrome.

The goals of acute treatment are to ameliorate but not completely correct the hypotonic state. With the exception of the patient with associated hypovolemia, 3% saline is the mainstay of treatment. If present, hypovolemia should be repleted with 0.9% saline. In all other patients, 3% (514 mEq/L) saline should be administered at a rate to increase serum [Na^+] by ~1–2 mEq/L per hour (but never exceeding 25 mEq/L in a 48-hour period). Treatment with hypertonic saline should continue until either (1) the patient becomes asymptomatic, (2) serum [Na^+] increases by 25 mEq/L or (3) serum [Na^+] is greater than 125 mEq/L—whichever occurs first. A loop diuretic may be added in some patients, especially those with SIADH, to promote additional water excretion. If present, hypokalemia should be corrected because it can contribute to hypotonicity. As a rough guideline for the amount of hypertonic saline to give, the following formula can be used:

$$\text{Liters of 3\% saline needed} = \frac{\text{TBW} \times (\text{desired increase in serum } [\text{Na}^+])}{514}$$

For example, a 38-year-old woman weighing 50 kg develops symptomatic postoperative hyponatremia and has a serum [Na^+] of 110 mEq/L. Your goal is to increase serum [Na^+] by 15 mEq/L (to 125 mEq/L) over 48 hours using 3%

saline. Her total body water (TBW) is 25 L (0.5 × body weight in kg), so she requires 25 L × 15 mEq/L or 375 mEq of sodium which, divided by 514, equals 0.73 L of 3% saline. This amount should be administered at 15 mL per hour for 48 hours and her electrolytes checked every 2–3 hours.

As indicated in the example above, electrolytes should be checked frequently because the above equation contains assumptions that may not apply in specific situations. To avoid complications of therapy such as the cerebral demyelinating lesions (see Chapter 4), it is crucial that serum [Na^+] not be increased at a rate exceeding 25 mEq/L in a 48-hour period, or to an absolute level beyond 125–130 mEq/L.

C. Asymptomatic Hypotonicity: General Treatment Guidelines

Most patients with chronic hypotonicity (>48-hour duration) are asymptomatic, especially if serum [Na^+] ≥ 125 mEq/L. Such patients do not usually require emergency intervention, and initial treatment is based on their clinical volume status.

1. Hypovolemic Hyperaquaemia

Treatment of the volume depleted hypotonic patient is usually straightforward, with volume repletion being the cornerstone of therapy. Infusion of isotonic saline (0.9%) will simultaneously replete volume while enhancing renal excretion of free water and decreasing the volume-mediated stimulus for ADH release. Diuretic drugs should be discontinued. Isotonic bicarbonate solution (e.g., a liter of 5% dextrose in water with three 50 mEq ampules of sodium bicarbonate added) may be useful as initial therapy in patients who have suffered excessive bicarbonate loss (e.g., from diarrhea). Volume repletion should continue until the patient is clinically euvolemic, and electrolytes should be monitored to assess tonicity.

In all hypovolemic patients, the possibility of Addison's disease should be considered (see above), as such patients require mineralocorticoid and/or glucocorticoid replacement. Interestingly and ironically, this therapy may result in a rather brisk aquaresis, particularly if cortisone has been given.

Particular attention should be paid to patients with edematous disorders who have become hypotonic and hypovolemic in association with overzealous or inappropriate diuretic use (e.g., prolonged combination therapy with metolazone and furosemide). These patients may develop severe hypotonicity in a short time, and differentiating the effect of the diuresis from that resulting from their underlying pathology can be challenging.

2. Hypervolemic Hyperaquaemia

Edematous hypotonic patients are salt and water overloaded but have retained an additional component of solute-free water. The goals of therapy in these cases are usually much easier to state than they are to achieve—promote natriuresis and aquaresis while working to improve the underlying pathophysiology. The latter goal is the greatest challenge, as these patients often have irreversible heart or liver disease. Hypotonicity is typically an ominous prognostic sign in patients with heart or hepatic failure.

Loop diuretics (thiazides should not be used) combined with salt and water restriction form the basis of therapy for congestive heart failure and cirrhosis with ascites or anasarca. In heart failure, efforts should be made to improve cardiac performance (e.g., inotropic agents), but cardiac transplantation is usually the only definitive treatment. Similarly, liver transplantation is the best hope in patients with end-stage cirrhosis. In either case, the goal of short-term therapy is to temporize until surgery can be performed. Diuretic therapy in these patients is often limited by the lack of "effective circulating volume" in that net water excretion also requires increased distal delivery and suppression of ADH release.

Lithium and demeclocycline, drugs that promote water excretion by interfering with the action of ADH on the kidney, have been used with limited success. Lithium is not recommended because its effects are erratic, it is associated with interstitial nephritis, and there is a risk of acute or chronic intoxication. Demeclocycline (600–1200 mg/day) is preferred and has been shown to be superior to lithium. Several oral V_2 receptor antagonists, so-called aquaretic agents, are currently undergoing clinical trials and may soon be available for treatment as well.

3. Hyperaquaemia with Clinical Euvolemia

Most euvolemic patients with hypotonicity have postoperative hypotonicity or a disorder associated with an increased release or effect of ADH. Strictly speaking, such patients have expansion of all body fluid compartments due to water retention and will have gained several kilograms. However, other than the weight gain they do not show significant clinical signs of volume overload and are therefore assessed as "clinically euvolemic." Tests of thyroid and adrenal function should be performed because hormone replacement therapy will correct hyperaquaemia in patients with hypothyroidism and adrenal insufficiency (see above). Any medications that can stimulate ADH secretion or potentiate its effect on ADH-sensitive nephron segments (see Chapter 12) should be discontinued. A malignancy must be suspected in patients who do not have evidence of pulmonary, CNS, or endocrine disease that can account for the inappropriate ADH secretion.

Water restriction, which takes advantage of insensible water losses, is effective if it is not limited by the patient's ability to comply. In patients with ongoing losses (e.g., vomiting due to chemotherapy), one must be careful not to replace solute and water losses with only water. If fluid restriction cannot control the hypotonicity (due to inability to comply), demeclocycline, (600–1200 mg/day) can be used in combination with more moderate fluid restriction to combat SIADH.

D. Approach to Hypotonicity in Specific Situations

1. Reset Osmostat

Most of these patients have debilitating illness such as tuberculosis, quadriplegia, malnutrition, or cancer. Such patients maintain salt and water balance, but they regulate their water excretion around a level that is clearly hypotonic. Typically the hypotonicity is relative mild (serum $[Na^+] > 125$ mEq/L) and is not associated with symptoms. Because patients with the reset osmostat are able to excrete excess water, no specific treatment is required, and the problem tends to correct if the underlying condition improves. During pregnancy, tonicity regulation is adjusted downward such that serum $[Na^+]$ decreases by ~5 mEq/L during gestation (see Chapter 12). This is a normal component of pregnancy and no specific interventions are necessary.

2. Diuretic-Induced Hypotonicity

As discussed in Chapter 12, mild hypotonicity is a common component of diuretic therapy in many patients. Much more rarely, severe hypotonicity occurs as a complication of treatment with the thiazide diuretics. Although only a small percentage of patients have this complication, diuretic-induced hypotonicity is still relatively common because millions of patients are treated with these agents. The best treatment is prevention. Therefore, electrolytes should be monitored frequently, particularly during the first month of therapy. Patients, especially elderly women, treated with thiazides should not receive any other drugs that might further impair water excretion (e.g., nonsteroidal anti-inflammatory agents) or stimulate thirst and/or ADH (e.g., chlorpropamide). Obviously, in any patient who develops severe hypotonicity (serum $[Na^+] < 125$ mEq/L), the diuretic should be stopped and sodium and potassium deficits should be repleted.

3. Hypotonicity Associated with Inadequate Solute Intake

Individuals consuming primarily beer (''beer potomania'') or ingesting high-water, low-protein diets may have very low solute loads, limiting their ability to excrete free water (see Chapter 12). These patients respond well to treatment with 0.9% saline or, if symptomatic, hypertonic saline (see above). After acute treatment, dietary counseling is recommended.

4. Hypotonicity in the Neurosurgical Patient

The course of patients suffering head injuries, brain tumors, stroke, intracranial infections, and subarachnoid hemorrhage is not infrequently complicated by hypotonicity due either to SIADH or the cerebral salt wasting syndrome (CSWS) (see Chapter 12). CSWS is characterized by volume depletion and hypotonicity resulting from the renal loss of NaCl. Making the differential diagnosis between SIADH and CSWS is important because euvolemic patients with SIADH should be treated with water restriction (or hypertonic saline) and may worsen if given isotonic saline, whereas those with the CSWS should be treated with isotonic saline and may worsen if water is restricted. Therefore, careful assessment of clinical volume status should guide therapy. Administration of isotonic saline tends to correct both the hypovolemia and the hypotonicity in CSWS, whereas water restriction or hypertonic saline is recommended for SIADH (see earlier).

5. Perioperative Hypotonicity

Primary prevention of the development of hypotonicity should be a constant pursuit. Because postoperative patients have multiple reasons for volume depletion and/or stimulation of ADH secretion, defects in free water excretion should be anticipated and solute-free water avoided in order to prevent hyperaquaemia. Although there are few absolutes in the practice of medicine, one can now uncquivocally state that hypotonic solutions should never be given perioperatively unless a patient has developed acute hypertonicity (e.g., from postoperative central diabetes insipidus). Adherence to this principle should greatly reduce the number of complications, although it may not prevent all cases.

As is the case for hypotonicity in general, an optimal approach to therapy of established perioperative hypotonicity (POH) remains elusive. This is due in part to variability among patients and in part because the precise pathogenesis of POH is incompletely understood. In general, postoperative patients who are volume depleted should receive isotonic solutions (or packed red blood cells) at a rate appropriate to achieve and maintain euvolemia and an adequate hemoglobin while avoiding volume overload. Symptomatic patients should be treated with hypertonic saline (see above for specific recommendations) until symptoms resolve. All patients should be in an intensive care unit setting and closely monitored, keeping in mind that the transient abnormalities in AVP release may resolve at any time, necessitating immediate changes in the course of therapy.

SUGGESTED READINGS

Arieff AI. Hyponatremia, convulsions, respiratory arrest, and permanent brain damage after elective surgery in healthy women. N Engl J Med 314:1529–1535, 1986.

Arieff AI. Hyponatremia associated with permanent brain damage. Adv Intern Med 32: 325–344, 1987.

Arieff AI. Management of hyponatraemia. Br Med J 307:305–308, 1993.

Arieff AI, Ayus JC, Fraser CL. Hyponatraemia and death or permanent brain damage in healthy children. Br Med J 304:1218–1222, 1992.

Ayus JC, Arieff AI. Brain damage and postoperative hyponatremia: the role of gender. Neurology 46:323–328, 1996.

Ayus JC, Arieff AI. Chronic hyponatremic encephalopathy in postmenopausal women: association of therapies with morbidity and mortality. JAMA 281:2299–304, 1999.

Ayus JC, Krothapalli RK, Arieff AI. Changing concepts in treatment of severe symptomatic hyponatremia. Rapid correction and possible relation to central pontine myelinolysis. Am J Med 78:897–902, 1985.

Ayus JC, Krothapalli RK, Arieff AI. Treatment of symptomatic hyponatremia and its relation to brain damage. A prospective study. N Engl J Med 317:1190–1195, 1987.

Ayus JC, Wheeler JM, Arieff AI. Postoperative hyponatremic encephalopathy in menstruant women. Ann Intern Med 117:891–897, 1992.

Batlle DC, von Riotte AB, Gaviria M, Grupp M. Amelioration of polyuria by amiloride in patients receiving long-term lithium therapy. N Engl J Med 312:408–414, 1985.

Dzau VJ, Hollenberg NK. Renal response to captopril in severe heart failure: role of furosemide in natriuresis and reversal of hyponatremia. Ann Intern Med 100:777–782, 1984.

Forrest JN Jr, Cox M, Hong C, Morrison G, Bia M, Singer I. Superiority of demeclocycline over lithium in the treatment of chronic syndrome of inappropriate secretion of antidiuretic hormone. N Engl J Med 298:173–177, 1978.

Fraser CL, Arieff AI. Epidemiology, pathophysiology, and management of hyponatremic encephalopathy. Am J Med 102:67–77, 1997.

Lang F, Busch GL, Ritter M, Völkl H, Waldegger S, Gulbins E, Häussinger D. Functional significance of cell volume regulatory mechanisms. Physiol Rev 78:247–306, 1998.

Lauriat SM, Berl T. The hyponatremic patient: practical focus on therapy. J Am Soc Nephrol 8:1599–1607, 1997.

Packer M, Medina N, Yushak M. Correction of dilutional hyponatremia in severe chronic heart failure by converting-enzyme inhibition. Ann Intern Med 100:782–789, 1984.

Sterns RH. Severe symptomatic hyponatremia: treatment and outcome. A study of 64 cases. Ann Intern Med 107:656–664, 1987.

Sterns RH, Riggs JE, Schochet SS, Jr. Osmotic demyelination syndrome following correction of hyponatremia. N Engl J Med 314:1535–1542, 1986.

30
Treatment of Hypokalemia and Hyperkalemia

Geetha Narayan and James A. Strom
St. Elizabeth's Medical Center and Tufts University School of Medicine, Boston, Massachusetts

John T. Harrington
Tufts University School of Medicine, Boston, Massachusetts

I. INTRODUCTION

The causes and clinical presentation of disorders of potassium balance (hypo- and hyperkalemia) are reviewed in Chapter 13. This chapter focuses on the management of these disorders. Hypokalemia is discussed in the first section, which covers the indications, approaches, and risks of potassium replacement therapy. The second half of the chapter discusses the modalities and approaches to the management of acute and sustained hyperkalemia.

II. HYPOKALEMIA

Over 98% of the potassium in the body resides within cells. However, any ingested or administered K^+ must traverse the relatively small extracellular space before it is taken up by the cells. A large oral dose of rapidly absorbed K^+, e.g., 40–60 mEq, can raise serum K^+ concentration ($[K^+]$) by 1–1.5 mEq/L, but this effect is normally very transient because most of the newly absorbed K^+ moves quickly into cells. Nonetheless, rapid or overzealous K^+ administration can lead to dangerous hyperkalemia, a potentially life-threatening complication, particularly in patients with impairment of the normal mechanisms facilitating K^+ entry (see Chapter 13). Hence, in most instances correction of hypokalemia should be approached conservatively and with careful monitoring of the patient.

Although serum $[K^+]$ is not a precise indicator of total body K^+ stores, a predictable and roughly linear relationship exists between the two in the absence of other factors influencing internal K^+ distribution. As discussed in Chapter 13, a decrement in serum $[K^+]$ from 4.0 to 3.0 mEq/L correlates with a loss of approximately 200–400 mEq of K^+. A further decline in serum $[K^+]$ to 2.0 mEq/L is associated with a total deficit of 400–800 mEq. With continued K^+ losses, more severe hypokalemia is generally minimized by the continued release of K^+ from cells. Rare instances of a serum $[K^+]$ of <2.0 mEq/L may reflect profound losses of 1000 mEq or more.

It is important to emphasize that these correlations do not hold when abnormal transcellular potassium shifts occur. For example, in diabetic ketoacidosis where insulin deficiency and hyperosmolality promote K^+ exit from cells, serum $[K^+]$ is often within the normal range or may occasionally even be elevated despite the presence of substantial K^+ deficits. In patients with periodic paralysis, by contrast, severe hypokalemia can occur in the absence of any K^+ deficits. Potassium therapy is not usually required for hypokalemia due entirely to transcellular redistribution, which is a transitory event. Most cases of hypokalemia, however, result from K^+ deficits due to external losses, and replacement is required. Therapy requires a consideration of the magnitude of the deficit, the type of K^+ salt to be administered, and the route and rate of administration.

A. Magnitude of Deficit

Modest levels of K^+ depletion, reflected by a serum $[K^+]$ of 3.0–3.5 mEq/L, are not generally associated with symptoms, except in the setting of acute myocardial infarction or coronary artery ischemia, digitalis treatment, or hepatic failure. Treatment in the asymptomatic patient should consist of oral K^+ replacement in a dose of 40–80 mEq per day and treatment of the underlying disorder, e.g., vomiting, diarrhea. Treatment of mild hypokalemia in diuretic-treated patients is discussed later. More severe deficits are associated with both symptoms and more profound hypokalemia (serum $[K^+] < 3.0$ mEq/L) and may require more aggressive therapy. In selected cases vigorous oral therapy can be successful with careful monitoring and dose adjustment. With life-threatening hypokalemic complications, such as ventricular arrythmias, paralysis, or digoxin toxicity, more rapid intravenous therapy may be appropriate (see below for quantitative details). In such cases, cardiac monitoring in an intensive care unit is necessary.

B. Potassium Preparation

Three types of K^+ salts are available for oral or intravenous use: potassium chloride, potassium phosphate, and potassium bicarbonate or bicarbonate precursors such as citrate or gluconate. The choice of the preparation depends on the accompanying metabolic disorder. Potassium chloride, the most widely used salt, is the drug of choice for hypokalemia associated with metabolic alkalosis because (1) chloride is the optimal anion to correct the chloride deficit and the accompanying metabolic alkalosis, (2) the chloride anion minimizes renal K^+ losses in these circumstances and therefore is most effective in correcting the K^+ deficit, (3) potassium chloride may raise serum [K^+] more rapidly than potassium bicarbonate because the cell is less permeable to chloride than bicarbonate, limiting the initial cellular uptake of K^+, and (4) potassium chloride is an effective way to replete body K^+ stores even when the deficit is not associated with metabolic alkalosis, and the other salts are ineffective when metabolic alkalosis is present.

Dietary supplementation with foods rich in K^+ is generally less effective as a repletion strategy because the K^+ in foods is primarily associated with nonreabsorbable anions such as citrate and phosphate rather than chloride. These salts are not only ineffective in correcting alkalosis but can lead to enhanced K^+ secretion in the distal tubule. In addition, even foods "rich" in K^+ have small amounts of K^+ relative to the patients' large deficits. For example, a banana contains only 1 mEq of K^+ per inch.

Potassium bicarbonate, citrate, or gluconate salts are appropriate for repleting K^+ in patients with K^+ losses associated with metabolic acidosis, e.g., chronic diarrhea, diabetic ketoacidosis, and renal tubular acidosis. Potassium phosphate is most suitable for patients with concomitant phosphate losses. In all these instances, however, potassium chloride is also effective.

C. Route and Rate of Replacement

1. Oral Therapy

Most patients with hypokalemia can be treated successfully with oral K^+ replacement. Oral therapy is the preferred mode and should be used if possible, except in urgent, life-threatening conditions. Oral potassium preparations are available as liquid and slow release tablets or capsules. The liquid form, the least expensive and safest, unfortunately has an unpleasant taste. The current generation of slow-release preparations, while quite safe, on rare occasion can produce ulceration of the gastrointestinal tract. The microencapsulated formulations of KCl probably have a lower risk of GI ulceration and bleeding than wax-matrix formulations. Salt substitutes, which contain KCl in crystalline form, are a surprisingly good form of oral replacement, because they are safe, well tolerated, inexpensive, and provide 50–65 mEq of K^+ per level teaspoon. The typical dose of oral K^+ replacement therapy is 40–120 mEq/day, depending on the degree of deficit, in divided doses, with single doses limited to 20–40 mEq.

2. Intravenous Administration

As described earlier, intravenous K^+ replacement should be undertaken only if hypokalemia is severe and/or producing life-threatening symptoms or if oral therapy is not possible. When intravenous therapy is used in a nonurgent setting, the concentration of K^+ should not exceed 40 mEq/L, and the rate of infusion should not exceed 10 mEq/hr. Potassium concentrations over 60 mEq/L can cause pain and sclerosis of peripheral veins. In life-threatening situations (e.g., ventricular arrhythmias, paralysis), K^+ can be administered more rapidly, up to 20 mEq/hr for short periods of time. In rare instances, even higher rates have been used when treating life-threatening complications. If fluid administration is limited, a higher concentration of K^+, 20 mEq in 100 mL of fluid (i.e., a concentration of 200 mEq/L), can be used provided the solution is infused into a large vein, preferably the femoral vein. Although central venous administration has been used safely, it is less desirable because of the possibility of local increase in $[K^+]$ within the heart and the subsequent risk of arrhythmias.

Because of their inherent danger, all infusions of K^+ must be carried out with extreme caution and, if administered at a rate of greater than 10 mEq/hr, should only be given with cardiac monitoring in an intensive care setting. Although potassium can be administered in either a dextrose or saline solution, the latter is preferred because dextrose infusions promote K^+ entry into cells by stimulating insulin release, blunting the rise in serum $[K^+]$. In some instances serum $[K^+]$ may even fall when K^+ is given in dextrose solutions. Frequent measurement of serum $[K^+]$ and appropriate dose adjustment are the key to safe and successful parenteral K^+ replacement therapy.

D. Additional Therapeutic Measures

Potassium-sparing diuretics are often used as an alternative to supplemental K^+ for prevention, rather than treatment, of hypokalemia. These drugs are particularly valuable in patients with ongoing urinary K^+ losses due to diuretic therapy or primary hyperaldosteronism (see later). Concomitant hypomagnesemia is a feature of these settings, and this deficiency can cause independent urinary potassium wasting (see Chapter 13). Potassium-sparing diuretics are quite effective in maintaining K^+ balance by limiting further urinary losses of both K^+ and magnesium.

Spironolactone acts by inhibiting the binding of aldosterone to the mineralocorticoid receptor in the distal nephron. Maximal inhibition may require doses of 200–400 mg/day. However, doses in excess of 200 mg/day are not desirable because they are associated with gynecomastia, amenorrhea, and decreased libido. Triamterene and amiloride act independently of aldosterone by direct inhibition of epithelial Na^+ channels in the distal nephron. The usual dosage of triamterene is 100 mg/day and the maximum dose is 400 mg/day. Adverse effects include gastrointestinal symptoms and, rarely, radiolucent renal stones and megaloblastic anemia. The usual dosage of amiloride is 5–20 mg/day. Adverse effects include nausea, vomiting, and diarrhea. Amiloride is our preferred drug since it has a lower incidence of adverse effects than the other two drugs. All of these agents have the potential to cause hyperkalemia, particularly when used in combination with K^+ supplements or in patients with renal insufficiency. Such combinations should be avoided or used only with careful monitoring of serum [K^+].

E. Specific Clinical Situations

1. Diuretic Usage

The thiazide and loop diuretics can cause excessive urinary K^+ losses, leading to K^+ depletion and hypokalemia. They also cause chloride and magnesium losses. The resultant metabolic alkalosis and hypomagnesemia can perpetuate the hypokalemia by promoting further renal K^+ wasting. The K^+ deficit in most patients receiving diuretic therapy is relatively modest and is manifested by mild hypokalemia (serum [K^+] = 3.0–3.5 mEq/L). The extent to which supplemental K^+ replacement therapy should be pursued in these patients is controversial. All agree that patients with underlying heart disease or who are receiving digitalis therapy should be treated. In all others with mild hypokalemia, the benefits of K^+ replacement are less clear. Correction of hypokalemia may reduce blood pressure slightly, an effect that may have therapeutic relevance when a thiazide diuretic is used to treat hypertension. Replacement therapy is indicated in all patients receiving diuretic therapy with serum [K^+] less than 3.0 mEq/L.

Either KCl supplements (40–60 mEq per day) or K^+-sparing diuretics can be used to minimize hypokalemia and maintain K^+ balance. As indicated earlier, the chloride salt helps correct the accompanying alkalosis, but not the hypomagnesemia, while K^+-sparing diuretics have the advantage of limiting both K^+ and magnesium wasting. As noted earlier, the use of both K^+ supplements and a K^+-sparing diuretic can cause hyperkalemia and should be avoided.

2. Magnesium Depletion and Hypomagnesemia

The causes of magnesium depletion are described in Chapter 13. Hypomagnesemia-induced hypokalemia requires magnesium as well as K^+ replacement therapy to fully restore serum [K^+] to normal levels; KCl replacement alone will not correct the hypokalemia. Magnesium depletion can be treated with oral tablets of magnesium chloride or magnesium lactate. Both are available in sustained release forms and provide 5–7 mEq of magnesium per tablet. The dose is two to four tablets per day for mild depletion and six to eight tablets for more severe losses. When the hypomagnesemia is due to the chronic use of diuretics that cannot be discontinued, the addition of a K^+-sparing agent such as amiloride limits both K^+ and magnesium losses (see above) and is the recommended treatment.

3. Primary Hyperaldosteronism

The treatment of hypokalemia in patients with primary hyperaldosteronism is determined largely by the underlying pathology (see Chapter 9). The majority of patients have a unilateral adrenal adenoma, and in these individuals surgical removal is the preferred mode of therapy. In patients with an adenoma who are unsuitable for surgery and in all patients with bilateral adrenal hyperplasia, the treatment of choice is a K^+-sparing diuretic. In addition to restoring K^+ balance, these agents help to minimize Na^+ retention and hypertension. Either spironolactone or amiloride is generally used, and higher than usual doses are required for both drugs to achieve adequate blockade of the effects of the heightened aldosterone activity.

The dose of spironolactone usually required is 200–400 mg, but this high dose is frequently associated with endocrine and gastrointestinal effects (see earlier). Amiloride is an alternative agent, in doses of 10–40 mg, because, as mentioned above, it has fewer side effects and is better tolerated. These agents may not fully correct the hypertension in patients with adrenal hyperplasia, however. Other antihypertensive agents such as calcium channel blockers, angiotensin-converting enzyme inhibitors or beta blockers, all of which have a potential for decreasing aldosterone secretion, can be used.

4. Bartters's and Gitelman's Syndromes

These rare hereditary disorders are due to genetic mutations that impair NaCl transport in the loop of Henle (Bartter's) or early distal tubule (Gitelman's) and cause hypokalemia and metabolic alkalosis (see Chapters 11 and 13). Because of the inability to reverse the primary tubular transport defect, treatment of the hypokalemia caused by these disorders remains difficult and is, for the most part, unsatisfactory. Treatment is directed at replacing K^+ and magnesium losses with oral supplements and counteracting the effects of increases in aldosterone and prostaglandin activity induced by salt loss. The latter therapeutic goal is accomplished by using a K^+-sparing diuretic and a prostaglandin inhibitor (NSAID). Angiotensin-converting enzyme inhibitors have been tried with some modest success, but hypotension often limits their use. The best results are obtained when oral K^+ supplements are combined with a K^+-sparing diuretic (spironolactone

100–300 mg or amiloride 10–40 mg) and/or a prostaglandin inhibitor (indomethacin 100–200 mg/day). Even when all three agents are used, the achievement of normal K^+ and magnesium balance remains an elusive goal in some of these patients.

5. Diabetic Ketoacidosis

Potassium depletion is invariably present in diabetic ketoacidosis due to K^+ loss in the urine in uncontrolled diabetes. Despite these losses serum $[K^+]$ is normal in most patients, and about one third actually present with hyperkalemia. The absence of hypokalemia despite potassium depletion is due to the abnormal movement of K^+ out of the cells, induced by the combination of insulin deficiency and hypersomolality. To prevent the sudden development of hypokalemia when insulin therapy is begun, KCl should be added to intravenous replacement fluids at 20–40 mEq/L when the serum $[K^+]$ falls below 4.5 mEq/L.

If hypokalemia is already present prior to insulin therapy, more vigorous K^+ repletion is needed. In such instances, 40–50 mEq of KCl should be added per liter of intravenous fluids, preferably in 0.45% saline to avoid exacerbating the patient's hypersomolality. In the presence of severe hypophosphatemia (<1.5 mmol/L), part of the K^+ may be given as potassium phosphate. Otherwise, intravenous phosphate repletion is not required.

6. Hypokalemic Periodic Paralysis

Hypokalemic periodic paralysis is a rare hereditary condition characterized by episodic sudden shifts of K^+ into cells (see Chapter 13). General measures to prevent such episodes include avoidance of high-carbohydrate meals, high Na^+ intake, or vigorous exercise. Although the hypokalemia is due to redistribution and not K^+ loss, administration of KCl is appropriate for managing acute attacks and can ameliorate paralysis. In the familial form, acetazolamide in doses of 250–750 mg/day appears to be helpful in preventing attacks. Nonselective beta blockers and K^+-sparing diuretics have been tried with limited success. In thyrotoxic patients, treatment is directed at correcting the endocrine disorder. Beta blockers may be especially useful in decreasing the frequency and intensity of attacks in this subgroup.

III. HYPERKALEMIA

Hyperkalemia is a potentially lethal electrolyte abnormality due to its ability to induce catastrophic cardiac and neuromuscular effects, namely, ventricular standstill and paralysis of the respiratory muscles. The speed and intensity of therapy are determined by the severity of the hyperkalemia, the associated electrocardiographic changes, and the underlying clinical condition.

A. Emergency Therapy of Hyperkalemia

In the patient with severe hyperkalemia (serum $[K^+] > 6.5$ mEq/L), the serum value should be rapidly verified and treatment begun. If spurious hyperkalemia is suspected, conditions that predispose to it (e.g., in vitro hemolysis, leukocytosis, and thrombocytosis; see Chapter 13) should be carefully sought and excluded. Once convinced that the hyperkalemia reflects a true increase in ECF $[K^+]$, one should evaluate the patient rapidly for evidence of end-organ dysfunction, particularly in the heart and skeletal muscle. Characteristic electrocardiographic abnormalities start to appear when serum $[K^+]$ exceeds 5.5 mEq/L, but significant signs and symptoms of impaired cardiac and neuromuscular excitability do not usually occur until serum $[K^+]$ exceeds 7–7.5 mEq/L. It is important to emphasize, however, that patients respond with great variability to hyperkalemia. Thus, it is prudent to institute careful monitoring of the EKG (and muscle strength) even with moderate degrees of hyperkalemia (serum $[K^+] = 5.5$–6.5 mEq/L). The presence of any electrocardiographic (EKG) abnormalities warrants immediate attention; mild to moderate EKG changes may abruptly deteriorate into dangerous arrhythmias.

Patients with severe hyperkalemia, but without symptoms or EKG changes, can swiftly develop life-threatening arrhythmias without warning. Therefore, prompt and aggressive treatment is required if serious electrocardiographic changes (i.e., widening of the QRS complex or atrioventricular conduction disturbances) are present, if significant muscle weakness is present, or if the serum $[K^+]$ exceeds 6.5–7.0 mEq/L. A similar aggressive approach is needed even if the initial severity is less than that described above, but the clinical circumstance has the potential for a progressive increase in serum $[K^+]$, e.g., acute renal failure in the presence of rhabdomyolysis and rapid endogenous K^+ release. In such patients, all of the modalities described below and outlined in Table 1 should be instituted simultaneously.

There are three major therapeutic strategies to reverse dangerous hyperkalemia. The first two are temporizing measures that do not alter body K^+ stores. They serve to remove the immediate threat to life posed by severe hyperkalemia and allow time to enable the removal of excessive K^+ from the body through the third strategy. The three strategies are presented below and summarized in Table 1.

1. Stabilize Cardiac Conduction

Intravenous administration of calcium salts directly antagonizes the membrane effects of hyperkalemia, stabilizing cardiac conduction. After an initial increase

Table 1 Therapy of Severe Hyperkalemia

Drug	Dose	Onset	Duration	Comment
Stabilize cardiac conduction				
Calcium gluconate	90 mg elem. calcium (10 mL of 10% solution) IV over 2–5 min; may repeat 1–2 times at 5–10 min intervals	Within min	30–60 min	Cardiac monitoring essential
Movement of K^+ into cells				
Glucose and insulin	Glucose: 50 g (100 mL of 50% solution) IV Insulin: 10 units of regular insulin IV	15–30 min	4–6 hr	Blood glucose monitoring essential
Albuterol				
Nebulized	10–20 mg in 4 mL of isotonic saline over 10 min	15–30 min	2–4 hr	May be ineffective in 40% of end-stage renal disease patients; tachycardia, angina can occur
Intravenous	0.5 mg in 100 mL of 5% dextrose solution over 15 min	15–30 min	2–4 hr	Not available in the United States
Sodium bicarbonate	44 mEq (1 amp. of 7.5%) IV over 5 min; may repeat 1–2 times at 30-min intervals	30–60 min	Hours	Response is delayed; limited effect in end-stage renal disease
Removal				
Diuretics	Furosemide 40–240 mg IV Acetozotamide 250–500 mg IV	Within 60 min	Variable	Effective only with adequate renal function
Kayexalate	Oral 40 g	1–2 hr	4–6 hr	
	Rectal 50–100 g	30–60 min	4–6 hr	Avoid sorbitol
Dialysis	Hemodialysis for 3–4 hr using a low-potassium bath			More efficient than peritoneal dialysis; avoid zero K^+ bath

in membrane excitability, hyperkalemia inactivates Na^+ channels in the cell membrane and thereby depresses excitability, producing the clinical manifestations of impaired cardiac conduction and muscle weakness. Intravenous calcium reverses this effect by a mechanism that is not well understood. Calcium should be given when EKG changes show widening of the QRS complex and/or loss of P waves or if serum $[K^+]$ is >7.0 mEq/L. Calcium can be life saving and is an absolute requirement when it is potentially dangerous to wait the 15–30 minutes for insulin or β_2 agonists to act. Calcium can be given as the gluconate or chloride salt, but gluconate is the preferred form. The usual dose is 10 mL (1 ampule) of a 10% calcium gluconate solution given over 2–5 minutes with constant cardiac monitoring. The dose can be repeated at 5- to 10-minute intervals if life-threatening EKG changes persist. The effect is immediate, often occurring within seconds to minutes, but is relatively short-lived. Calcium cannot be mixed with sodium bicarbonate because it will precipitate (as calcium carbonate), but it can be added to the glucose and insulin infusion. In patients taking digitalis, calcium should be administered more cautiously, as a slow infusion over 30 minutes, because it can induce digitalis toxicity.

2. Promote Movement of K^+ into Cells

(a) Insulin and Glucose. This is a time-honored modality to lower serum $[K^+]$ through insulin-mediated stimulation of cell membrane Na^+/K^+-ATPase activity, which in turn promotes cellular uptake of K^+. Glucose administration alone stimulates endogenous insulin release, but this maneuver produces a lesser effect on serum $[K^+]$ than the combination of glucose and exogenous insulin. In the nondiabetic patient, 10 units of regular insulin, given with 40–50 g of glucose as a 50% solution, reduces serum $[K^+]$ by 0.5–1.5 mEq/L. The onset of action is in 15 minutes, the peak effect is in 60 minutes, and the effect lasts several hours. If one uses less glucose, delayed hypoglycemia can occur in up to 75% of patients. A continuous dextrose infusion after the initial dose and frequent monitoring of serum glucose levels will further protect against hypoglycemia. In the diabetic patient, care should be taken not only to avoid hypoglycemia but, more importantly, to avert hyperglycemia, which can worsen the hyperkalemia by increasing serum osmolality. Optimal therapy in the diabetic patient varies with the initial serum glucose concentration. If the latter is normal or only slightly high, both insulin (10 units of regular insulin) and glucose (25 g given as 50 mL of 50% dextrose solution) are given. If serum glucose is significantly elevated, insulin alone is sufficient.

(b) β_2 Adrenergic Agonists. These agents lower serum $[K^+]$ acutely by transferring K^+ into cells. Although intravenous epinephrine has been used in the past, it is not desirable, both because of its concomitant alpha-adrenergic effects and its arrythmogenic potential. β_2 Agonists such as albuterol and salbuta-

mol are effective when administered intravenously or by inhalation in nebulized form and can lower serum [K^+] by 0.5–1.5 mEq/L. It should be emphasized that up to 40% of patients with end-stage renal disease may be refractory to the hypokalemic action of albuterol. β_2 Agonists may have synergistic action when given in combination with insulin plus glucose. This variable responsiveness has led to conflicting recommendations from experts regarding its use in the treatment of hyperkalemia. We believe that, given the advantages of rapid and easy administration as an inhalant and the absence of significant adverse effects, β_2 Agonists should be used as adjunctive therapy with glucose and insulin in the acute treatment of hyperkalemia. The dose of albuterol is 10–20 mg in 4 mL of saline by nasal inhalation over 10 minutes. The effect starts at 15–30 minutes, peaks at about 90 minutes, and lasts 2–4 hours. Mild tachycardia appears to be the only side effect. However, these drugs can precipitate angina in patients with active coronary disease.

(c) Sodium Bicarbonate. Alkali therapy lowers serum [K^+] by promoting K^+ entry into cells, but the effect is variable and slow in onset. The effect is mediated both through an increase in pH and by a pH-independent effect that is ill-defined. Sodium bicarbonate produces only a trivial reduction in serum [K^+] acutely and has only a modest delayed effect (after a few hours) in patients with end stage renal disease without concomitant metabolic acidosis. Whether it is more effective in individuals with mild to moderate impairment in renal function remains to be determined. The usual dose is 44 mEq (1 ampule of a 7.5% solution) infused slowly over 5 minutes; this dose can be repeated one to two times at 30-minute intervals. The effect may start in 30–60 minutes and may last a few hours. Alkali therapy is effective and appropriate when used in patients with concomitant metabolic acidosis. Caution should be exercised when using sodium salts in patients with significant fluid overload, e.g., patients with heart failure or advanced renal failure.

3. Remove Excess K^+ from the Body

(a) Diuretics. Loop diuretics can induce substantial urinary K^+ losses if renal function is adequate and in some instances may be useful as adjunctive therapy of hyperkalemia. However, the most common cause of hyperkalemia is impaired renal K^+ excretion due to renal insufficiency or failure, and in this setting the kidney is unlikely to respond adequately to diuretic therapy. When renal impairment is mild to moderate (serum creatinine < 4.0 mg/dL), loop diuretics such as furosemide in a dose of 40–120 mg intravenously may be tried. With more advanced renal impairment, provided the GFR is greater than 10–15 mL/min., larger doses (120–240 mg) should be used. An alternative to a loop diuretic is the carbonic anhydrase inhibitor, acetazolamide, which causes bicarbonaturia and a consequent increase in renal K^+ excretion. If used, it should be given in

a dose of 250–500 mg intravenously and requires adequate renal function for its effectiveness.

(b) Cation Exchange Resins. Sodium polystyrene sulfonate (kayexalate), a cation exchange resin available for oral or rectal use, is not absorbed from the gastrointestinal tract. It releases Na^+ and, in exchange, binds to secreted K^+ in the colon, thus causing permanent loss of K^+ from the body. At equilibrium each gram of the resin binds to approximately 1 mEq of K^+. The resin can be given either orally or as a retention enema. When used as an enema, K^+ is removed immediately; when given by mouth there is a greater opportunity for equilibrium to be achieved but the effect may be delayed for 2 or more hours. A reasonable oral dose is 40 g (smaller doses of 20–30 g may be used) dissolved in 20–100 mL of water or other aqueous solution. To avoid the constipating effect of the drug and to promote rapid transit through the gut, it is usually given with sorbitol, either a 20% or a 70% solution depending on the volume desired. The dose should be repeated every 4 hours or so until serum $[K^+]$ reaches the desired range. The rectal dose is 50–100 g of the resin mixed with 200 mL of either water or a 10% glucose solution, given as a retention enema. Using a Foley catheter and balloon inflation, the solution should be retained in the rectum for at least 30–60 minutes. The enema can be repeated every 2–4 hours as needed. With repeated use, either by mouth or as an enema, significant amounts of Na^+, released from the resin, are absorbed from the colon. Thus, one should be alert for symptoms of ECF volume overload in susceptible patients.

Although sorbitol traditionally has been used as a vehicle for kayexelate, use of sorbitol is less desirable than either water or a glucose-containing solution and should not be used in the postoperative period because of the potential for this combination to cause colonic necrosis. This life-threatening complication has been described in postoperative patients receiving kayexalate in sorbitol solutions both as an enema and orally. Animal experiments suggest that sorbitol is the culprit, but we believe that kayexalate, even without sorbitol, should be avoided in this patient population. The use of the resin with correctol (a docusate-phenolphthalein combination) rather than sorbitol is effective in normal individuals and has fewer side effects than sorbitol. However, there are no data regarding its use or effectiveness in patients with renal failure.

(c) Dialysis. Hemodialysis is far superior to peritoneal dialysis with respect to speed and efficiency of K^+ removal. While a single exchange of peritoneal dialysis can remove approximately 10 mEq in one hour, hemodialysis can remove 25–35 mEq per hour using a dialysis bath $[K^+]$ of 1–2 mEq/L. Hemodialysis should be initiated when (1) cation exchange therapy and efforts to move K^+ into cells are unable to control serum $[K^+]$ or are not feasible, or (2) hyperkalemia is severe, in the face of rapid and continuing endogenous release of K^+ due to catabolism and tissue injury, such as rhabdomyolysis or a necrotic or

ischemic extremity. The main limitation of dialysis is the time required to set up the procedure, which sometimes can take a few hours. Additionally, rapid K^+ shifts occur with dialysis, and these changes can provoke cardiac arrhythmias; cardiac monitoring thus is crucial in such cases.

B. Therapy of Chronic Hyperkalemia

Most patients with chronic hyperkalemia or a predisposition for it have chronic renal disease with significant renal functional impairment. Treatment is aimed at preventing or minimizing the hyperkalemia. Several measures can be employed concurrently. The regimen chosen should be tailored to the individual needs of the patient and the clinical situation. The first step should always be to educate the patient to restrict dietary K^+ to <60 mEq per day. Second, severe dietary Na^+ restriction should be avoided as this may impair distal K^+ secretion. Dietary sodium intake should be at least 4 g per day. Most patients with renal insufficiency and hyperkalemia have associated Na^+ retention and may require concomitant diuretic therapy, particularly if Na^+ intake is liberalized. Such a therapeutic strategy, combining the benefits of adequate Na^+ intake and diuretics, can maximize renal K^+ excretion if done carefully. This strategy is not practical or advisable in patients with severe ECF volume overload or in patients with advanced renal failure. Both thiazide and loop diuretics can be used to promote kaliuresis, but recall that the thiazides, used alone, are ineffective in moderate to advanced renal insufficiency.

When the above maneuvers are ineffective, several additional maneuvers should be attempted. Kayexalate (see above) given orally in relatively small doses, 15–20 g per day, is ideal for long-term therapy. Its constipating effect can be countered by the use of a mild laxative such as dulcolax (bisacodyl). Fludrocortisone acetate in doses of 0.1–0.2 mg/day is effective therapy when hyperkalemia is the result of mineralocorticoid deficiency (see below and Chapter 13). The side effects of fludrocortisone, hypertension, and edema are due to Na^+ retention; it is best used with diuretics to avoid volume overload. Finally, drugs that predispose to hyperkalemia should be avoided. These drugs include angiotensin receptor antagonists and converting enzyme inhibitors, nonselective beta blockers, nonsteroidal anti-inflammatory drugs, K^+-sparing diuretics, and trimethoprim in high doses.

C. Specific Clinical Situations

1. End-Stage Renal Disease

Patients with end-stage renal disease are especially at risk for the acute development of severe hyperkalemia. Because they have no capacity to excrete K^+, excess intake resulting from dietary indiscretion or superimposed illnesses that cause K^+ to exit from cells can rapidly lead to life-threatening hyperkalemia. An example is a dialysis patient who sustains a hip fracture and develops hyperkalemia due to the release of K^+ from the hematoma around the fracture. With the exception of diuretics, all the maneuvers described above should be used when appropriate to treat acute hyperkalemia in this population. Kayexalate is effective and can be given while the patient is waiting for dialysis or when the hyperkalemia is less severe. As noted earlier, β_2 agonists may be used, but a significant fraction of patients with end-stage renal disease may not respond.

2. Mineralocorticoid Deficiency

Hyporeninemic hypoaldosteronism (see Chapter 13) can be managed effectively with the same therapeutic measures described above for the treatment of chronic hyperkalemia. Mineralocorticoid replacement is especially appropriate for this problem, in patients who cannot be managed using diet and diuretics. As noted earlier, the limitation of this agent is that it can exacerbate hypertension and ECF volume overload. The dose of fludrocortisone that has been found effective in this disorder, 0.2–1.0 mg per day, is much higher than the physiological replacement dose, suggesting a component of aldosterone resistance. Oral sodium bicarbonate supplements [e.g., liquid bicitra (sodium citrate and citric acid)] in doses of 15–30 mEq per day can help correct the metabolic acidosis and enhance urinary K^+ excretion. In patients with Addison's disease and hyperkalemia, mineralocorticoid replacement is essential. Fludrocortisone should be given in physiological replacement doses, 0.05–0.2 mg per day. These patients also require glucocorticoid replacement in the form of prednisone or dexamethasone.

3. Primary Tubular Defects in K^+ Secretion

Tubular defects in K^+ secretion occur in a variety of renal diseases, including obstructive nephropathy, sickle cell nephropathy, amyloidosis, lupus erythematosis, and renal transplantation. In these patients the primary approach is dietary K^+ restriction. Mineralocorticoid therapy is not effective in these disorders and the response to diuretics generally is poor. Some patients have a kaliuretic response to thiazide diuretics. Alkali therapy may be of benefit if there is associated acidosis.

4. Hyperkalemic Periodic Paralysis

This disorder is caused by rare hereditary defect in the cell membrane Na^+ channel, leading to episodic bouts of hyperkalemia (see Chapter 13). General measures, including avoidance of K^+-rich foods, salt substitutes, or other K^+ supplements and avoidance of exposure to cold, may be of some value. Specific therapy with the β_2 agonist salbutamol, given as two inhalations, seems to be effective for attacks in progress. Acetazolamide also appears to be an effective treatment for this disorder, but its mechanism of action is unknown. The two drugs have been used successfully in combination in some patients.

SUGGESTED READINGS

Allon M. Hyperkalemia in end-stage renal disease: mechanisms and management. J Am Soc Nephrol 1995; 6:1134–42.

Allon M, Copkney C. Albuterol and insulin for treatment of hyperkalemia in hemodialysis patients. Kidney Int 1990; 38:869–872.

Androgue HJ, Lederer ED, Suki WN, Eknoyan G. Determinants of plasma potassium levels in diabetic ketoacidosis. Medicine 1986; 65:163–172.

Berne RM, Levy MN. Cardiovascular Physiology. 4th ed. St. Louis: Mosby, 1981; pp. 7–71.

Blumberg A, Weidmann P, Shaw S, Gnadinger M. Effect of various therapeutic approaches on plasma potassium and major regulating factors in terminal renal failure. Am J Med 1988; 85:507–512.

Blumenfeld JD, Sealey JE, Schlussel Y, et al. Diagnosis and treatment of primary hyperaldosteronism. Ann Intern Med 1994; 121:877–885.

DeFronzo RA. Nephrology forum. Hyperkalemia and hyporeninemic hypoaldosteronism. Kidney Int 1980; 17:118–134.

Griffing GT, Komanicky P, Aurecchia SA, et al. Amiloride in Bartter's syndrome. Clin Pharmacol Ther 1982; 31:713–718.

Griggs RC, Engel WK, Resnick JS. Acetazolamide in the treatment of hypokalemic periodic paralysis. Ann Intern Med 1970; 73:39–48.

Kassirer JP, Harrington JT. Diuretics and potassium metabolism: a reassessment of the need, effectiveness and safety of potassium therapy. Kidney Int 1977; 11:505–515.

Kruse JA, Carlson RW. Rapid correction of hypokalemia using concentrated intravenous potassium chloride infusions. Arch Intern Med 1990; 150:613–617.

Kunis CL, Lowenstein J. The emergency treatment of hyperkalemia. Med Clin North Am 1981; 65:165–176.

Liou HH, Chiang SS, Wu SC, et al. Hypokalemic effects of intravenous infusion or nebulization of salbutamol in patients with chronic renal failure: Comparative study. Am J Kidney Dis 1994; 23:266–271.

Rose BD. Clinical Physiology of Acid-Base and Electrolyte Disorders. 4th ed. New York: McGraw-Hill, 1994.

Rose BD. Treatment of hypokalemia. In: Rose BD, ed. Up to Date. Wellesley, MA, 2000.

Saggar-Malik AK, Cappuccio FP. Potassium supplements and potassium-sparing diuretics: a review and guide to appropriate use. Drugs 1993; 46:986–1008.

Schwartz WB, Van Ypersele de Strihou C, Kassirer JP. Role of anions in metabolic alkalosis and potassium deficiency. N Engl J Med 1968; 279:630–639.

Sopko JA, Freeman RM. Salt substitutes as a source of potassium. JAMA 1977; 238:608–610.

Sterns RH, Fieg PU, Pring M, et al. Disposition of intravenous potassium in anuric man: a kinetic analysis. Kidney Int 1979; 15:651–660.

Tannen RL. Potassium disorders. In: Kokko JP, Tannen RL, eds. Fluids and Electrolytes. 3rd ed. Philadelphia: WB Saunders, 1996, pp. 111–199.

Wang P, Clausen T. Treatment of attacks in hyperkalemic periodic paralysis by inhalation of salbutamol. Lancet 1976; 1:1–7.

Weiner ID, Wingo CS. Hypokalemia: consequences, causes and corrections. J Am Soc Nephrol 1997; 8:1179–1188.

31

Treatment of Calcium, Phosphorus, and Magnesium Disorders

F. John Gennari
University of Vermont, Burlington, Vermont

I. INTRODUCTION

The pathophysiology and diagnosis of disorders of calcium, phosphorus, and magnesium metabolism are discussed in Chapter 14. The present chapter focuses on the treatment of these disorders.

II. CALCIUM

The only abnormalities in serum calcium concentration that require treatment are those associated with abnormalities in ionized calcium concentration ($[Ca^{2+}]$). As discussed in Chapter 14, such abnormalities can be uncovered either by direct measurement of ionized $[Ca^{2+}]$ or by applying a ''correction'' for serum albumin concentration to the routine measurement of serum calcium concentration. One should always be circumspect in interpreting such a ''correction,'' particularly when the serum calcium concentration is only mildly increased or decreased or when the serum albumin concentration is markedly reduced. Whenever there is a question about the diagnosis, direct measurement of serum $[Ca^{2+}]$ should be undertaken.

A. Hypercalcemia

Hypercalcemia is defined as a serum $[Ca] > 10.5$ mg/dL (after an estimated correction for serum albumin concentration), or as an ionized $[Ca^{2+}] > 1.3$ mmol/

L. Mild elevations in serum [Ca] (10.6–12.0 mg/dL) should serve primarily as a focus for further diagnostic evaluation unless the patient is clearly symptomatic (see Chapter 4 and 14). In all instances, exogenous sources of excess calcium (e.g., Tums) and vitamin D should be sought for and discontinued. Serum [Ca] values of >12.0 mg/dL are of more concern, and timely attention should be paid to uncovering the cause. In this group of patients, one should initiate treatment promptly if the patient is symptomatic. When the value is >13.5 mg/dL ($[Ca^{2+}] > 1.65$ mmol/L), treatment should be the first consideration and be undertaken very expeditiously, as higher values can rapidly cause mental status changes and acute renal failure. The approach to treatment is presented below and outlined in Table 1.

1. General Measures

(a) Extracellular Fluid Volume Repletion and Expansion. Patients with hypercalcemia are often volume depleted because of the systemic and renal effects of hypercalcemia. Thus, the first step in treatment is to reexpand the extracellular fluid (ECF) volume with intravenous isotonic saline. Saline treatment should be continued beyond restoring normal ECF volume because ECF volume expansion promotes a saline diuresis, which in turn promotes calcium excretion. In the patient with reasonable cardiac function, isotonic saline should be given at 200–250 mL/hr. Unless signs of fluid overload develop, 2–4 L should be given in the first 24 hours.

(b) Loop Diuretics. Once assured that ECF volume is increased, one should use a loop diuretic to accelerate calcium excretion. Furosemide, bumeta-

Table 1 Treatment of Acute Hypercalcemia

Measures to promote calcium excretion
Replete ECF volume and establish a saline diuresis with intravenous isotonic saline.
When saline diuresis is established, add loop diuretic to enhance calcium excretion.
Measures to inhibit calcium release from bone
Salmon calcitonin intramuscularly or subcutaneously—rapid in onset (1–2 hrs), short duration of action.
Pamidronate intravenously—onset of effect, 1–3 days
Alternatives: Other bisphosphonates—etidronate, clodronate
Plicamycin
Gallium nitrate
Other measures
Prednisone only if hypercalcemia due to excess activity of calcitriol

nide, torsemide, and ethacrynic acid all inhibit calcium reabsorption and will increase calcium excretion dramatically when ECF volume is expanded. The danger of these agents is that they can decrease ECF volume and reverse the salutary effects of saline loading. To avoid this problem, these agents should be administered in low dose and in conjunction with continued saline infusion. Note that thiazide diuretics should not be used to treat hypercalcemia because they reduce calcium excretion.

2. Specific Measures

The above treatments promote calcium excretion but do not address the pathophysiology of the hypercalcemia, which is virtually always due to unregulated calcium release from bone. The rare exception is unregulated calcium absorption from the gut, as occurs with vitamin D intoxication. A variety of agents inhibit the release of calcium from bone. The choice of agent is dependent to some extent on the severity of the hypercalcemia as well as the underlying cause, but in most instances, the combination of calcitonin and a bisphosphonate should be used. These agents are discussed below.

(a) Calcitonin. Subcutaneous injection of calcitonin is a rapid and effective method to decrease serum [Ca^{2+}]. The drug acts primarily by inhibiting osteoclast bone resorption, although it also promotes renal calcium excretion. The preparation available, salmon calcitonin, is generally well tolerated; side effects include occasional nausea, diarrhea, and facial flushing. Calcitonin reduces serum calcium concentration within 1–2 hours, and the reduction lasts for 12–24 hours. Although calcitonin is effective in the short run, its effect is gone within 24 hours, and the response to subsequent injections is reduced. Thus, for a sustained effect one should couple this agent with one of those discussed below.

(b) Bisphosphonates. This group of agents, which includes etidronate, pamidronate, clodronate, and alendronate, inhibits both bone resorption and new bone formation by forming links to calcium (in hydroxyapatite) that are resistant to enzymatic hydrolysis. Of these four drugs, pamidronate is the one recommended for the treatment of acute hypercalcemia. It is the most potent and can be given in a dose that inhibits osteoclast activity without interfering with new bone formation. All of these drugs are very poorly absorbed from the gastrointestinal tract and thus should be given intravenously when treating acute hypercalcemia. Daily intravenous pamidronate (60–90 mg) causes a sustained decrease in serum [Ca^{2+}] that is evident within 1–3 days. In many cases, the treatment can be discontinued after three to four doses, and the effect is sustained for 1–2 weeks. The bisphosphonates are cleared by the kidney, and therefore dosage ad-

justment is necessary in patients with renal insufficiency. In patients with renal failure, a single loading dose is sufficient to produce a sustained effect on serum $[Ca^{2+}]$.

(c) Other Agents. Plicamycin (mithramycin) is an antitumor agent that causes a sustained inhibition of osteoclast function. Prior to the introduction of the bisphosphonates, it was the agent of choice, and it is quite effective, causing a sustained reduction in serum $[Ca^{2+}]$ for up to 1–2 weeks. Inhibition of synthesis of bone marrow elements (particularly platelets) limits its usefulness. Gallium nitrate has also been shown to be effective in causing a sustained reduction in serum $[Ca^{2+}]$, but it has major nephrotoxicity and is no longer used. Glucocorticoids are effective agents only when the cause of the hypercalcemia is excessive calcium absorption from the gut as occurs with vitamin D intoxication or a disease that results in the excessive production of endogenous calcitriol (e.g., sarcoidosis, lymphoma; see Chapter 14). In the absence of specific knowledge about the cause, glucocorticoids should not be used because they are ineffective when the increase in $[Ca^{2+}]$ is due to an abnormal release of calcium from bone.

3. Long-Term Management of Hypercalcemia

Once serum $[Ca^{2+}]$ is controlled by the acute measures outlined above, attention should be directed at reversing the underlying cause if possible. For the patient with primary hyperparathyroidism, the next step is a parathyroidectomy. Antitumor chemotherapy can reverse the hypercalcemia of malignancy. When the cause of the hypercalcemia is not reversible, long-term therapy with either an oral or intravenous bisphosphonate can control the hypercalcemia. In certain cancers, e.g., multiple myeloma, long-term bisphosphonate therapy can also reduce the progression of the tumor in bone.

B. Hypocalcemia

Hypocalcemia is defined as a serum $[Ca] < 9.0$ mg/dL (after an estimated correction for serum albumin concentration) or as an ionized $[Ca^{2+}] < 1.1$ mmol/L. Mild hypocalcemia ([Ca] 8.0–9.0 mg/dL or ionized $[Ca^{2+}]$ 1.0–1.1 mmol/L) is not usually associated with symptoms, and acute treatment is not necessary. Rather the presence of hypocalcemia should serve as a focus for further diagnostic evaluation. More severe hypocalcemia, particularly when acute in onset, can produce symptoms of tetanus, mental status changes, and seizures (see Chapter 4), and acute treatment should be undertaken. Recall that the most common cause of a low total serum [Ca] is a low serum albumin concentration. If the [Ca] is low or even at the low end of normal after adjustment for serum albumin concentration, one should obtain an ionized $[Ca^{2+}]$ in most instances to ascertain whether hypocalcemia is actually present. The main treatments for hypocalcemia, discussed below, are calcium and vitamin D.

1. Acute Treatment

In the acutely symptomatic patient with hypocalcemia, either oral or intravenous calcium should be administered. Oral administration is preferred whenever possible because it is safer and is effective when symptoms are mild (see below under subacute/chronic treatment). Several intravenous preparations are available (see Table 2), but calcium gluconate (10% solution in a 10 mL ampule) is recommended. One ampule delivers 90 mg (2.25 mmol) of elemental calcium. Calcium chloride is also available as a 10% solution in a 10 mL ampule, but this preparation delivers a far larger amount of calcium, 360 mg (9.0 mmol). Even the smaller amount must be given cautiously, as life-threatening cardiac arrhythmias can occur, particularly in the patient receiving digoxin. In some instances (e.g., immediately postparathyroidectomy), a sustained infusion of calcium is necessary to prevent symptomatic hypocalcemia. Whenever possible, one should switch to oral therapy.

2. Subacute/Chronic Treatment

A variety of oral calcium preparations are available (see Table 2). Recall that only a fraction of oral calcium is absorbed from the gut. Absorption of all formulations is best when taken on an empty stomach. Calcium carbonate provides 200 mg of calcium per tablet, is inexpensive, and can be given in as large a dose as tolerated (up to 20 tabs/day as needed). Calcium acetate provides 170 mg of calcium per tablet and may have slightly better absorption characteristics. Calcium citrate is also well tolerated but increases aluminum absorption from the gut and should be avoided in patients with renal insufficiency. The specific dosage

Table 2 Oral and Parenteral Calcium Preparations

	Elemental Calcium
Parenteral	
Calcium gluconate (10% solution)	90 mg/10 mL
Calcium chloride (10% solution)	360 mg/10 mL
Oral	
Calcium carbonate	
500 mg (e.g., Tums)	200 mg/tablet
750 mg (e.g., Xstrength Tums)	300 mg/tablet
1250 mg (e.g., Os-cal)	500 mg/tablet
Calcium acetate, Phos-Lo	169 mg/tablet
Calcium citrate, Citrical	200 mg/tablet

needed is dependent in part on the cause and severity of the hypocalcemia. The starting dose is typically 2–4 tablets/day, but the amount should be increased until the serum [Ca^{2+}] returns to the normal range.

In patients with accompanying vitamin D deficiency (e.g., the patient with renal insufficiency), calcitriol should be given along with oral calcium replacement. When vitamin D is needed it should always be given as calcitriol to assure that adequate amounts of the active form of the vitamin are available. If magnesium depletion is a contributing factor in causing the hypocalcemia (see Chapter 14), magnesium replacement therapy (see below) is necessary for repair of the hypocalcemia.

III. PHOSPHORUS

Phosphorus exists in the body only as inorganic and organic phosphate but is measured in the laboratory as phosphorus. Its normal concentration in serum is 2.5–4.5 mg/dL (0.8–1.5 mmol/L). Both hypophosphatemia and hyperphosphatemia occur as clinical entities and require treatment.

A. Hyperphosphatemia

As discussed in Chapter 14, hyperphosphatemia is virtually always a consequence of impaired renal phosphate excretion, and, with the rare exception of hypoparathyroidism, the decrease in phosphate excretion is always due to a reduction in GFR. In catabolic patients, release of phosphate from cells can worsen the severity of the hyperphosphatemia that occurs in renal failure, and serum phosphorus levels can rise to as high as 20 mg/dL. Treatment is discussed below separately for acute renal failure and chronic renal insufficiency.

1. Acute Renal Failure

Unless severe (serum [P] $>$ 10 mg/dL), hyperphosphatemia in acute renal failure requires no specific treatment. Only when the high serum phosphate level causes a clinically significant reduction in serum [Ca^{2+}] should an intervention be considered. Severe hyperphosphatemia is an indication to initiate dialysis treatment. Although oral phosphate binders (see below) will lower serum [P] even in the patient who is not eating, hemodialysis is a speedier way to correct both the hyperphosphatemia and the hypocalcemia. Only when acute renal failure is prolonged ($>$7–10 days), should one begin the dietary and binder therapy described below.

2. Chronic Renal Insufficiency/Failure

The mainstays of treatment of hyperphosphatemia in patients with chronic renal insufficiency or failure are oral phosphate binders and dietary phosphate restriction. The most potent oral phosphate binder is aluminum hydroxide, which releases its hydroxyl group in the stomach and binds to dietary phosphate, preventing its absorption. Unfortunately the prolonged use of aluminum-containing phosphate binders leads to aluminum accumulation in the body, contributing to bone disease in patients with renal failure. For this reason, aluminum-containing phosphate binders should be avoided. Instead, calcium carbonate or acetate (Table 2), taken with meals, should be used to bind dietary phosphate. To the extent that calcium is absorbed, it will provide additional calcium to the patient. To the extent that it is not absorbed, calcium dissociates from carbonate or acetate in the stomach and combines with phosphate, preventing the absorption of this ion.

Calcium binders are less potent that aluminum binders because a portion of the calcium is absorbed and a portion remains combined with carbonate or acetate. As a result calcium binders often have to be taken in large amounts (4–6 tablets with each meal) to bring serum [P] down to normal or near normal levels. A problem with the ingestion of large amounts of calcium-containing binders is hypercalcemia due to unregulated absorption in the gut. In the past this problem was addressed by using a combination of calcium and aluminum containing binders. Now a new organic phosphate binder, sevelamer hydrochloride (Renagel), is available to bind dietary phosphate without providing either calcium or aluminum to the patient. Although effective, this binder is expensive and has gastrointestinal side effects that limit its tolerability. A far better way to manage this problem is through dietary phosphate restriction. The use of a phosphate binder should always be coupled with dietary education. The patient should be instructed to avoid foods high in phosphate, such as dairy products. A diet limited to 1 g of phosphate a day is ideal, but often difficult to attain.

B. Hypophosphatemia

Hypophosphatemia occurs in a wide variety of settings (see Chapter 14) and, unless very severe (serum [P] < 1.0 mg/dL), does not require specific therapy. Because, in most instances, hypophosphatemia is a reflection of phosphate depletion, the treatment is phosphate replacement. If at all possible, phosphate supplements should be given by mouth. Either sodium or sodium/potassium phosphate mixtures (Neutraphos) are available in 1 g tablets, and two or three tablets a day are adequate for replacement in most instances. The risk of oral phosphate therapy is inducing diarrhea, which can exacerbate the hypophosphatemia. Intravenous phosphate must be used with caution as it can cause acute reductions in serum

$[Ca^{2+}]$. In patients with the familial disorder hypophosphatemic rickets (or vitamin D–resistant rickets), oral phosphate supplements are combined with vitamin D therapy. Calcitriol, the active form of vitamin D, not only increases phosphate absorption in the gut, it also decreases renal phosphate losses by stimulating renal phosphate absorption.

IV. MAGNESIUM

Disorders of magnesium homeostasis are common and often unrecognized. Both hypomagnesemia (virtually always a clinical manifestation of magnesium depletion) and hypermagnesemia are clinical entities (see Chapter 14) that require appropriate treatment.

A. Hypomagnesemia

Hypomagnesemia is defined as a serum level less than 1.5 mEq/L (or 0.75 mmol/L). In all patients with a low serum $[Mg^{2+}]$, the first approach to management is to identify the cause if possible (see Chapter 14) and to attempt to reverse the underlying pathophysiology. The serum magnesium level at which to initiate replacement therapy is a subject of controversy. Some experts advocate aggressive replacement therapy, regardless of the presence of symptoms and even when the level is only mildly reduced. Most advocate that treatment should be initiated even in the asymptomatic patient when serum $[Mg^{2+}]$ is <1.0 mEq/L (0.5 mmol/L). When symptoms of hypomagnesemia (see Chapter 4) or refractory hypocalcemia or hypokalemia are present, treatment should be initiated for any degree of hypomagnesemia.

Intravenous therapy is effective acutely in increasing serum $[Mg^{2+}]$ but is less useful for long-term therapy because the rapid rise in serum concentration promotes renal magnesium excretion and most of the administered magnesium is rapidly lost in the urine. When used, 4–8 mmol should be given as a bolus and then 25 mmol given per day. Magnesium can also be administered intramuscularly in patients who are unable to take oral medications. Whenever possible, however, oral magnesium replacement should be used. Several oral preparations are available, but the best tolerated is magnesium oxide. One 400 mg tablet provides 10 mmol of elemental magnesium, so that in most instances two tablets per day provide adequate supplementation. Other preparations include magnesium gluconate, which provides only 1.2 mmol/tablet, magnesium hydroxide, and magnesium sulfate. The usefulness of the latter two preparations is limited by their laxative effect.

B. Hypermagnesemia

Hypermagnesemia is defined as a serum [Mg^{2+}] > 2.5 mEq/L (1.3 mmol/L) and can be a life-threatening complication when severe ([Mg^{2+}] > 4.0 mEq/L). When cardiac arrhythmias or neurological symptoms are present, emergency treatment with intravenous calcium can be life-saving. In some cases emergency dialysis may be necessary to remove excess magnesium. In most instances, hypermagnesemia is iatrogenic. Medications should be reviewed, and magnesium-containing drugs (e.g., laxatives) should be discontinued.

SUGGESTED READINGS

Berenson JR, Lipton A. Bisphosphonates in the treatment of malignant bone disease. Annual Rev Med 1999; 50:237–248.

Bilezikian JP. Management of acute hypercalcemia. N Engl J Med 1992; 326:1196–1203.

Weisinger JR, Bellorin-Font E. Magnesium and phosphorus. Lancet 1998; 352:391–396.

32
Drug Dosing in Renal Insufficiency

Carl J. Possidente
University of Vermont, Burlington, Vermont

I. INTRODUCTION

Adverse drug reactions occur much more frequently in patients with renal insufficiency than in patients with normal renal function, highlighting the central role of the kidney in the clearance and metabolism of many drugs. Patients with renal insufficiency can have altered pharmacokinetics (i.e., what the body does to the drug) or a modified pharmacodynamic response (i.e., what the drug does to the body) to many drugs, changes that expose them to potential drug toxicities. Perhaps the most common cause of adverse drug reactions in patients with renal insufficiency is the failure to modify drug doses. In one study, 44% of patients were found to be receiving drug doses higher than the manufacturer's recommendations based on an estimated creatinine clearance.

Many drugs are excreted at least partially by the kidney, necessitating drug dosage adjustment in patients with renal insufficiency for safe, efficacious therapy and to minimize toxicity. The proliferation of new drugs has added to the challenge of rational drug therapy in this patient population. This chapter provides information about the changes in drug disposition in patients with renal insufficiency and offers guidelines for designing appropriate dosage regimens.

II. PHARMACOKINETIC CONSIDERATIONS

Although guidelines for drug dosing typically focus on changes in renal excretion, it is important to emphasize that changes in absorption, distribution, and biotransformation also alter drug disposition and influence a patient's response to a drug. Renal disease may influence all these pharmacokinetic factors, and therefore a full understanding of drug absorption and disposition is important for developing an appropriate drug regimen.

A. Bioavailability

Bioavailability is the percentage of the administered drug dose that reaches the systemic circulation. Factors that can influence bioavailability include the dissolution and absorption characteristics of the drug, the drug product formulation, route of administration, stability of the drug in the gastrointestinal (GI) tract, characteristics of the GI mucosa, and extent of drug metabolism before reaching the systemic circulation.

In general, drug bioavailability varies more in patients with renal insufficiency than in patients with normal renal function due to alterations in drug absorption. Gastric pH may be more alkaline due to the conversion of excess urea to ammonia by gastric urease or due to the use of antacids either to treat GI symptoms or to bind dietary phosphate. Antacids can alter the bioavailability for drugs with pH-dependent absorption (e.g., ketoconazole, iron) or reduce absorption secondary to chelation (e.g., fluoroquinolone antibiotics). Nausea, vomiting, and diarrhea are also common conditions that can alter drug absorption. The most common cause of renal insufficiency in the United States is diabetes mellitus, a disease that also is associated with altered gastric motility due to autonomic neuropathy, and this group of patients has a particular susceptibility to alterations in drug absorption.

B. Drug Distribution

After a drug reaches the bloodstream, it distributes throughout the body. The volume of distribution (Vd) is a mathematical concept relating the amount of drug in the body to the serum concentration. Highly lipid-soluble drugs penetrate cells more easily and have a large Vd, while drugs that are highly protein bound or water soluble are limited to the intravascular compartment and have a small Vd. Renal disease may increase or decrease the Vd, in part due to altered plasma protein binding, tissue binding, and changes in total body water or body composition. For example, edema and ascites generally increase the Vd of hydrophilic or highly protein-bound drugs, while volume contraction decreases the Vd.

Hypoalbuminemia is common in patients with renal insufficiency, and this abnormality can increase free or active drug and cause an enhanced pharmacological effect at normal drug concentrations. The clinical action of a drug is determined by the free, unbound fraction, the only portion available for distribution to sites of action, metabolism, and excretion. This change is a clinically relevant issue, as most methods to assess plasma drug concentration measure both free and protein-bound drug and do not distinguish between the two.

The protein binding of acidic drugs (e.g., salicylate, phenytoin, warfarin) is reduced in patients with uremia because of decreased serum albumin concentration, altered albumin binding sites, and accumulation of endogenous inhibitors of protein binding (see Table 1). Binding of organic bases is less affected by uremia. As an example, the protein binding of phenytoin is significantly reduced in patients with renal insufficiency, resulting in an increased fraction of free drug from approximately 10% normally to 20%. The relationship between total plasma drug concentration and efficacy and toxicity changes, shifting the therapeutic range lower as the percentage of free drug increases (see Sec. IV).

C. Biotransformation

1. Liver

Many drugs are metabolized in the liver to water-soluble metabolites that are excreted by the kidney. In patients with renal insufficiency, hepatic clearance of drugs may be decreased (erythromycin), increased (phenytoin), or remain unaffected (metoprolol). Unfortunately there is limited information concerning the effect of renal insufficiency on hepatic drug metabolism. Thus, predicting the effect of renal insufficiency on the hepatic clearance of many drugs is not possible. The dose of a drug with significant hepatic metabolism should be carefully adjusted based on serum levels and clinical effect.

2. Kidneys

The kidneys play an important role in drug metabolism. When standardized to organ mass, the renal cytochrome P450 system may equal the metabolic activity

Table 1 Drugs with Decreased Protein Binding in Renal Insufficiency

Barbiturates
Diazepam
Diflunisal
Furosemide
Morphine
Phenytoin
Salicylates
Sulfamethoxazole
Triamterene
Valproic acid
Warfarin

of the liver. Thus renal insufficiency may alter drug metabolism. For example, impaired conversion of 25-hydroxycholecalciferol in the kidney contributes to renal osteodystrophy and is the reason many dialysis patients require supplementation with the active form of vitamin D (calcitriol). The prolonged hypoglycemic response to insulin in patients with renal insufficiency is due in part to diminished insulin metabolism in the kidneys.

Several drugs are metabolized to pharmacologically active metabolites that are excreted by the kidneys (see Table 2). In patients with impaired renal function, these metabolic products can accumulate resulting in toxicity. For example, meperidine is metabolized to normeperidine, a renally excreted metabolite with central nervous system stimulant activity. This metabolite has little analgesic effect but can produce seizures. Alternatively, a metabolite could have pharmacological activity similar to the parent drug and contribute to increased therapeutic effect. The metabolite of procainamide, *N*-acetylprocainamide (NAPA), is active with different antiarrhythmic properties compared to the parent agent. The metabolite has a long half-life, is predominantly renally excreted, and accumulates in patients with renal insufficiency. Evaluation of both parent and NAPA drug levels is recommended to avoid potential changes in the electrocardiogram in patients with renal insufficiency.

D. Renal Excretion

Most drugs follow elimination by first-order pharmacokinetics, that is, the amount of drug eliminated per unit time is proportional to the amount in the body. For such drugs, the elimination rate constant is inversely proportional to the drug

Table 2 Drugs with Active Metabolites Excreted Primarily by the Kidney

Drug	Active metabolite	Potential clinical effect
Acetaminophen	*N*-Acetyl-*p*-benzo-quinoneimine	Hepatic toxicity
Allopurinol	Oxipurinol	Suppress xanthine oxidase
Azathioprine	Mercaptopurine	Immunosuppressive activity, hematological
Codeine	Morphine-6-glucuronide	Prolonged narcotic effect
Enalapril	Enalaprilat	Active therapeutic agent
Meperidine	Normeperidine	CNS stimulation
Morphine	Morphine-6-glucuronide	Prolonged narcotic effect
Procainamide	*N*-Acetylprocainamide (NAPA)	Antiarrhythmic activity
Propoxyphene	Norpropoxyphene	Cardiac toxicity
Sulfonamides	Acetylated metabolites	Increased toxicity

Source: Frye and Matzke, 1999.

half-life (the time required for the serum drug concentration to be reduced by 50%). Knowledge of the drug's half-life provides important information for modifying a drug regimen. For patients with renal insufficiency, drugs eliminated primarily by the kidney will exhibit a prolonged half-life and a dosage reduction is required to reduce the risk of toxicity. Examples include aminoglycosides, digoxin, lithium, and vancomycin.

III. PRINCIPLES OF DRUG DOSING FOR PATIENTS WITH RENAL INSUFFICIENCY

The primary goal of choosing a specific dosing regimen is to provide efficacious therapy and minimize drug toxicity. Dosage adjustments in patients with renal insufficiency are generally intended to produce serum drug concentrations similar to those obtained in patients with normal renal function. Particular attention must be paid to accurate dosage adjustments for drugs with a narrow therapeutic index, that is, where the difference between therapeutic and toxic serum concentrations is small, because they have a higher potential for serious adverse effects.

Because patients with renal disease may have a variable response to drug therapy, published guidelines and nomograms should be used as general recommendations, not as absolute formulas. Patient as well as drug considerations should be taken into account (see below). For many drugs, specific guidelines for dosing in patients with renal insufficiency are not available. An understanding of the drug characteristics can assist the clinician in deciding whether to modify the dose. The following sections describe important factors to consider and an outline for developing a dosage regimen is provided (see also Tables 3 and 4).

A. Patient Considerations

Before developing a dosage regimen, it is important to review the patient's medical history, physical examination, drug history. Specific factors to consider in-

Table 3 Factors Determining Whether a Drug Will Require Dose Adjustment in Renal Insufficiency

Greater than 40% of a drug or its active/toxic metabolite is excreted by the kidney
The drug or active metabolite has a narrow therapeutic index
The kidney is a major site for metabolism of the drug
There is a significant decrease in the drug plasma protein binding (acidic, highly protein bound, small volume of distribution)

Table 4 Stepwise Approach to Developing a Dosage Regimen in Patients with Renal Insufficiency

Patient considerations
Perform initial patient assessment
Consider the risks and benefits of drug therapy
Calculate accurate estimated creatinine clearance
Determine if renal function is stable
Determine the etiology of renal insufficiency and if the disease is acute or chronic
Determine what patient factors may alter the drug's pharmacokinetic parameters
Drug considerations
Use medications only for specific indications
Determine how much of the drug is eliminated unchanged in the urine
What is the therapeutic index of the drug?
Know the potential toxicity of the drug
Are active or toxic metabolites excreted by the kidney?
Will renal insufficiency effect the ability of the drug to reach its site of action?
Does the elimination of the drug follow first order elimination?
Dosage regimen
If indicated, adjust dose based on the patient's renal function
Consult published guidelines, if available, as to initial dosage
Determine a loading dose, if required
Determine a maintenance dose
Select practical doses and administration schedules
Guide dosing with serum drug levels, if available
Monitor the patient's clinical status and adverse effects
If toxicity occurs, modify therapy

Source: Adapted from Ball, 1983.

clude serum albumin concentration, extracellular fluid volume, and the presence of hepatic or cardiac disease. One should assess whether renal function is stable or changing (as assessed from day-to-day variations in serum creatinine concentration), so that an appropriate estimate of renal function can be calculated (see Chapter 5 for techniques for estimating GFR).

B. Drug Considerations

The route of elimination of the drug should be reviewed. Drugs that are eliminated primarily by renal excretion generally require the greatest dosage modification. (e.g., aminoglycosides, lithium, vancomycin). If a drug has a narrow therapeutic index and is eliminated primarily by the kidney, careful dosage adjustments are required to prevent toxicity. The drug's potential for direct renal injury should also be considered before prescribing to a patient with preexisting renal insufficiency.

C. Dosage Regimen

Steady state, the condition when the rate of drug administration equals drug elimination, is obtained for drugs that follow first-order elimination after four to five drug half-lives. Reduced renal elimination causes the half-life to be prolonged and delays the time to obtain a steady-state serum drug concentration. If a rapid achievement of therapeutic effect is desired, a loading dose may be required. Loading doses are often required if the drug half-life is especially prolonged in a patient with renal insufficiency.

Provided a patient's extracellular fluid volume is normal, a standard loading dose is administered to a patient with renal insufficiency to achieve therapeutic drug levels rapidly. Patients with edema or ascites may require a larger loading dose and conversely volume depleted patients may require a smaller loading dose. An exception to this general principle is digoxin, because the Vd is often lower in patients with advanced renal insufficiency due to decreased tissue binding. The recommended loading dose is generally decreased by 25–50%. If a loading dose is not necessary, a maintenance dose can be utilized to initiate therapy. Three methods are used to adjust maintenance doses:

1. Extending the dosing interval between doses and administering the same dose (interval extension method)
2. Reducing the dose, while maintaining the same dosing interval (dose reduction method)
3. Combination of both methods

Selecting the appropriate method depends on the patient's clinical status, drug characteristics, and also on whether a target peak or trough drug concentration or a constant drug level is needed between dosing intervals. Both the interval extension and dose reduction methods produce similar mean plasma drug concentrations. The interval extension method causes greater fluctuation between peak and trough concentrations and is recommended when a constant serum drug concentration is not required (e.g., aminoglycosides). This method is obviously more convenient, promotes patient compliance with fewer doses, and is less expensive. The dose reduction method is recommended when a more constant serum drug level is desired (e.g., β-lactam antibiotics). Dosage adjustments directed by serum drug levels and clinical response may dictate a combination of both methods.

D. Enhancing Clinical Effectiveness and Drug Safety

Evaluating the need for adjustment of dosage regimens requires assessment of clinical endpoints. If serum drug levels are available and a good relationship exists between drug level and outcomes, monitoring serum drug concentrations is a valuable tool to guide drug dosing and enhance the safety and efficacy of therapy. When measuring serum drug levels, it is important to sample under steady-state conditions (achieved after four to five drug half-lives) and to understand the time of sampling in relation to the time of drug administration. Interpretation of drug levels also requires clinical evaluation of the patient, because considerable overlap can occur between toxicity and efficacy within the "therapeutic range." The antirejection drug cyclosporine is an example of a drug where such overlap is common. Therapeutic drug monitoring is particularly useful in patients with changing renal function, especially when published drug guidelines for patients with renal insufficiency are not available, the drug follows nonlinear or unpredictable pharmacokinetics, or the drug has a narrow therapeutic index.

E. Reference Information

Clinicians are able to gather information for informed therapeutic decisions by reviewing published drug-specific nomograms, dosing guidelines, and pharmacokinetic parameters. Prior to using these references, the clinician should understand their limitations. Most guidelines are based on patients with stable, chronic renal insufficiency, and extrapolation of this information to patients with acute renal failure should be performed cautiously, because pharmacokinetic factors will differ. The data from which the guidelines were developed may be based on a small number of patients or people with characteristics different from those of an individual patient. An important assumption is changes in drug clearance are proportional to reductions in creatinine clearance. Published guidelines often categorize renal insufficiency into mild, moderate, or severe and provide dose recommendations for each group. The limitation of this method is the wide range of renal function within each category. Thus, the recommended drug regimen may not be optimal for all patients within the range.

Secondary references such as the *Physicians Desk Reference* (PDR), American Hospital Formulary Service Drug Information, and the Suggested Readings at the end of this chapter provide drug-specific pharmacokinetic information. Consultation with a pharmacist may assist in the interpretation of published information and the development of appropriate dosing regimens, an important consideration for drugs with a narrow therapeutic index. Dosing recommendations for commonly prescribed drugs are provided in Tables 5 and 6. Table 5 lists the drugs for which a dosing adjustment is necessary in patients with renal insufficiency, and Table 6 lists the drugs for which no dosing adjustment is necessary.

IV. DRUGS WITH SPECIAL CONSIDERATIONS

A. Aminoglycosides

This class of drugs is well known to cause acute renal failure, even when given in the appropriate dose and when serum drug concentrations are followed closely

Table 5 Selected Commonly Prescribed Drugs Requiring a Dosage Adjustment in Renal Insufficiency

Drug	Dosing stategy
Allopurinol	Dose reduction required in relation to degree of renal insufficiency
Aminoglycosides	Increase dosage interval to prevent drug accumulation
Cephalosporins[a]	Dose reduction required in relation to degree of renal insufficiency
Ciprofloxacin	Dose reduction required in relation to degree of renal insufficiency
Digoxin	Dose reduction required in relation to degree of renal insufficiency
Fluconazole	Dose reduction required in relation to degree of renal insufficiency
H-2 antagonists	Dose reduction required in relation to degree of renal insufficiency
Insulin	Lower dosage requirements due to reduced renal metabolism
Meperidine	Use with caution, avoid regular dosing schedule
Morphine	Dose reduction required in relation to degree of renal insufficiency
Procainamide	Dosage reduction required due to renally excreted metabolite
Sulfamethoxazole	Use carefully, not recommended for use if CrCl < 15mL/min
Vancomycin	Dose reduction required in relation to degree of renal insufficiency

[a] Dose reduction not required for cefoperazone or cetriaxone.

(see Chapter 20). As a result, aminoglycosides should only be prescribed to patients with renal insufficiency when clearly indicated and the risks and benefits of therapy have been reviewed. The therapeutic response to aminoglycoside therapy is related to its concentration-dependent antimicrobial activity, and the risk of nephrotoxicity is correlated with elevated trough drug levels. Thus, dosage

Table 6 Selected Commonly Prescribed Drugs That Do Not Require a Dosage Adjustment in Renal Insufficiency

Amlodipine
Amoxicillin
Atorvastatin
Azithromycin
Conjugated estrogens
Diltiazem
Fluoxetine
Levothyroxine
Omperazole
Stertraline
Simvastatin
Warfarin

regimens should be designed to obtain sufficient peak serum aminoglycoside concentrations to achieve efficacy and to allow adequate time between doses to achieve low serum trough concentrations and prevent drug accumulation.

B. Angiotensin-Converting Enzyme Inhibitors

Drugs in this class undergo renal elimination, and the drug half-life is prolonged in patients with renal insufficiency. Initial dosage reduction is recommended to avoid hypotensive effects, with subsequent titration to achieve appropriate blood pressure control. Due to a compensatory increase in fecal elimination, fosinopril is the only angiotensin-converting enzyme (ACE) inhibitor that does not require dosage adjustment in patients with renal insufficiency. ACE inhibitors are recommended therapy for most patients with chronic renal insufficiency (see Chapters 16–18), but they can also cause an abrupt decline in GFR in certain settings (ECF volume depletion, severe congestive heart failure, renal artery stenosis). In addition, by reducing serum aldosterone, they can cause or worsen hyperkalemia. Thus, serum creatinine and potassium levels should be monitored regularly when these drugs are used in patients with renal insufficiency. Because of their unpredictable effects on GFR, these agents should always be avoided or discontinued in any setting in which renal function is changing from day to day (e.g., acute renal failure from any cause or during the first 3–6 months post–kidney transplant).

C. Cisapride*

Cisapride is associated with serious cardiac side effects (prolonged QT intervals, torsades de pointes, cardiac arrest) in patients predisposed to cardiac arrhythmias or when prescribed concurrently with drugs that inhibit its metabolism. Thus, cisapride should not be used in patients receiving drugs that inhibit its primary route of metabolism, the cytochrome P450 enzymes (e.g., erythromycin, clarithromycin, fluconazole, nefazadone). Serious adverse effects have recently been reported in patients with renal insufficiency or end-stage renal disease receiving cisapride without concurrent interacting agents. As a result, cisapride should be avoided in patients with renal failure.

D. Digoxin

Renal excretion accounts for a substantial portion of elimination of digoxin from the body. The drug's half-life increases from 36–48 hours in patients with normal renal function to 4–6 days in anephric patients. Dosage reductions are always necessary in patients with renal insufficiency to achieve and maintain therapeutic

---

* Cisapride was removed from the market in July of 2000.

serum drug concentrations and prevent toxicity. Because of the extended drug half-life in patients with renal insufficiency, the time to achieve a steady-state drug concentration is prolonged, and this will correspondingly delay the time to obtain an appropriate serum drug level (see section on enhancing clinical effectiveness and drug safety). Steady-state dosages as low as 0.125 mg every other day are not uncommon in patients with renal failure.

E. Diuretics

A reduction in glomerular filtration presents a distinct issue for drugs that act in the renal tubules of the kidney. Loop diuretics (e.g., furosemide, bumetanide) and benzothiadiazides (e.g., hydrochlorothiazide) must be filtered by the glomerulus or secreted by the tubules to reach their site of action in the nephron. Renal insufficiency reduces renal blood flow and consequently the amount of drug excreted in the urine, thus reducing the drug's effectiveness. Benzothiadiazides are particularly affected in this regard, and this class of drugs, even when given at the highest recommended dose, is not effective in patients with a creatinine clearance less than 30 mL/min. By contrast, the loop diuretics can overcome this barrier to effectiveness by progressive increases in the dose. In fact, the loop diuretics are unique in that the dosage should be increased in patients with renal insufficiency to achieve the desired therapeutic effect. Because these drugs are relatively nontoxic, dosages as high as 160 mg of furosemide twice daily can be used to achieve an effective diuresis. Potassium-sparing drugs (e.g., amiloride, spironolactone, triamterene) are not recommended for use in patients with renal insufficiency, because serious hyperkalemia can develop.

F. Metformin

Metformin increases blood lactate levels as a result of enhanced lactic acid production. The metabolism of lactic acid is impaired in patients with renal insufficiency, resulting in an increased risk of developing serious lactic acidosis. Metformin is contraindicated in patients with renal insufficiency, defined as a serum creatinine >1.5 mg/dL (males) or 1.4 mg/dL (females), or in patients with abnormal creatinine clearance.

G. Narcotic Analgesics

Despite the fact that narcotic analgesics are largely metabolized in the liver, they have the potential to cause confusion, central nervous system (CNS) stimulation, or respiratory depression in patients with renal insufficiency, even when given in standard doses and time intervals. The commonly prescribed analgesics codeine, morphine, and meperidine are drugs with active metabolites that are excreted primarily by the kidney (see Table 2). The dose of these agents should always be reduced in patients with renal insufficiency to compensate for decreased renal excretion and to limit the possibility of developing adverse effects.

H. Nonsteroidal Anti-inflammatory Drugs

Drugs in this class are well known for their effects on renal blood flow, GFR, and renal sodium reabsorption, as well as for their nephrotoxicity (see Chapter 20). In patients with hypertension, nonsteroidal anti-inflammatory drugs (NSAIDs) can increase blood pressure by promoting renal sodium retention. In any setting in which renal blood flow is reduced, these drugs can cause a clinically significant reduction in GFR and simultaneously increase serum potassium concentration. Thus, these drugs should be used with great caution in patients with renal insufficiency, and their use should be confined to short periods of time to treat acute conditions. When their use is indicated, no dosage adjustment is necessary because they undergo extensive hepatic metabolism. An exception to this rule is ketorolac. Because of reduced plasma clearance, increased drug half-life, and reduced protein binding, dosage reduction is recommended for ketorolac when prescribed for patients with renal insufficiency. Although a single aspirin a day is efficacious and recommended for cardiovascular protection in patients with severe renal impairment, larger doses of this drug should be avoided because of the potential for hemorrhagic complications.

I. Phenytoin

Determining an effective dose of phenytoin in patients with renal insufficiency is problematic due to decreased binding to plasma proteins. In patients with normal renal function, approximately 90% of phenytoin is bound to albumin and about 10% is free to exert pharmacological effects. Serum albumin levels are often reduced and the binding affinity of phenytoin to albumin changes unpredictably in patients with renal insufficiency, causing an increase in the free fraction of drug. The dosage must be adjusted to account for the increased free drug to achieve a therapeutic, nontoxic regimen. Two approaches can be used to achieve this goal. The first is measure serum total phenytoin levels and then use a corrective equation to adjust for the estimated difference in protein binding. The second is to measure free phenytoin directly and to use this level to guide dosage adjustments.

V. OVERVIEW: DIALYSIS THERAPY AND DRUG DOSING

Dosage guidelines for patients receiving hemodialysis or other forms of renal replacement therapy [e.g., peritoneal dialysis, continuous venovenous hemofil-

Table 7 Properties Determining Drug Removal During Hemodialysis

Low volume of distribution
Low protein binding
Small molecular weight
High serum concentration
Water solubility

tration (CVVH)] are beyond the scope of this book, but some general considerations are presented below.

During hemodialysis or peritoneal dialysis, drugs are removed from the blood by both diffusion and convection across the dialysis membrane. Drug removal occurs primarily because of passive diffusion along a concentration gradient between the blood and the dialysis bath and only to a small extent by convection with ultrafiltered water. Thus, this group of patients has special issues that require consideration when developing appropriate drug regimens.

Factors that determine the amount of drug clearance during hemodialysis (see Table 7) include drug properties, the characteristics of the dialysis membrane, and blood and dialysate flow rates. The major drug properties are its molecular weight, water solubility, volume of distribution, and protein binding. In general, drugs with a molecular weight of >500 daltons are not removed well unless dialysis therapy is with a polysulfone membrane (high-flux filter). Water-soluble drugs are removed more easily by the aqueous dialysate than lipophilic agents. Drugs with a large Vd are not removed efficiently because they are predominately bound to tissue (e.g., digoxin). Drugs that are highly bound to plasma proteins (>60–80%) are not removed well during hemodialysis because only free drug (e.g., warfarin) is small enough to pass through the filter membrane. If a drug is extensively removed, supplemental doses after hemodialysis are required to maintain adequate drug levels. Management of drug therapy in patients receiving renal replacement therapy should be undertaken in consultation with a nephrologist and/or a pharmacist with special expertise in dialysis pharmacokinetics.

SUGGESTED READINGS

Aronoff GR, Berns JS, Brier ME, et al. Drug Prescribing in Renal Failure: Dosing Guidelines for Adults. 4th ed. Philadelphia: American College of Physicians, 1999.

Aweeka FT. Dosing of drugs in renal failure. In: Young LY, Koda-Kimble MA, eds. Applied Therapeutics, The Clinical Use of Drugs. 6th ed. Vancouver: Applied Therapeutics, Inc., 1995, pp. 32-1–32-21.

Ball WD. Dosing in renal impairment. In: Knoben JE, Anderson PO, eds. Handbook of Clinical Drug Data. 5th ed. Hamilton, IL: Drug Intelligence Publications, Inc., 1983, pp. 21–28.

Cutler RE, Forland SC, John Hammond PG. Pharmacokinetics of drugs and the effect of renal failure. In: Massry SG, Glassock RJ, eds. Textbook of Nephrology. 3rd ed. Baltimore: Williams and Wilkins, 1995, pp. 1597–1612.

Elston AC, Bayliss MK, Park GR. Effect of renal failure on drug metabolism by the liver. Br J Anaesth 1993; 71:282–290.

Frye RF, Matzke GR. Drug therapy individualization for patients with renal insufficiency. In: DiPiro JT, Talbert RL, Yee GC, et al., eds. Pharmacotherapy, A Pathophysiologic Approach. 4th ed. Stamford, CT: Appleton and Lange, 1999, pp. 872–889.

Gambertoglio JG. Dosing in renal impairment. In: Knoben JE, Anderson PO, eds. Handbook of Clinical Drug Data. 7th ed. Hamilton, IL: Drug Intelligence Publications, Inc., 1993, pp. 161–194.

Gibson TP. Influence of renal disease on pharmacokinetics. In: William EE, Schentag JJ, Jusko JW, eds. Applied Pharmacokinetics: Principles of Therapeutic Drug Monitoring. 2nd ed. Spokane: Applied Therapeutics, Inc., 1986, pp. 83–115.

Gibson TP. Renal disease and drug metabolism: An overview. Am J Kidney Dis 1986; 8:7–17.

Golper TA, Bennett WM. Use of drugs in renal failure. In: Massry SG, Glassock RJ, eds. Textbook of Nephrology. 3rd ed. Baltimore: Williams and Wilkins, 1995, pp. 1612–1625.

Lam YWF, Banerji S, Hatfield C, et al. Principles of drug administration in renal insufficiency. Clin Pharmacokinet 1997; 32:30–57.

Matzke GR, Frye RF. Drug administration in patients with renal insufficiency: Minimising renal and extrarenal toxicity. Drug Safety 1997; 16:205–231.

McCormack JP, Cooper J, Carleton B. Simple approach to dosage adjustment in patients with renal impairment. Am J Health-Syst Pharm 1997; 54:2505–2509.

St Peter WL, Halstenson CE. Pharmacologic approach in patients with renal failure. In: Chernow B, ed. The Pharmacologic Approach to the Critically Ill Patient. Baltimore: William & Wilkins, 1994, pp. 41–79.

Swan SK, Bennett WM. Drug dosing guidelines in patients with renal failure. West J Med 1992; 156:633–638.

Talbert RL. Drug dosing in renal insufficiency. J Clin Pharmacol 1994; 34:99–110.

Turnheim K. Pitfalls of pharmacokinetic dosage guidelines in renal insufficiency. Eur J Clin Pharmacol 1991; 40:87–93.

Index

Abscess, 421, 422
  renal, 421, 422
  urinary tract, 421, 422
ACE inhibitors, 124, 125, 33, 276, 277, 304, 305, 314, 315, 375, 472–474, 584
  in diabetic nephropathy, 314, 315
  dosing in renal insufficiency, 584
  hemodynamic effects of, 375
  hyperkalemia and, 233
  hypertension and, 304, 305
  in nephrotic syndrome, 124, 125
  in pregnancy, 472–474
  in renal insufficiency, 276, 277, 304, 305
  renoprotective effects, 276, 277, 304, 305
Acetazolamide, 32
Acid-base balance, 169–171
  Henderson equation, 169
  Henderson-Hasselbalch equation, 169
  normal regulation of, 171, 172
  normal values, 170
  pH, PCO_2, 170, 171
  Total CO_2, bicarbonate, 170
Acid-base disorders, 169–189, 521–534
  anion gap in, 176, 188
  characterization, 172–174
  delta anion gap calculation, 188
  diagnosis, 172–174
  metabolic acidosis, 176–182, 521–529
  metabolic alkalosis, 182–185, 529–531
  mixed disorders, 187, 188, 532–534
  potassium in, 176
  renal compensation in, 174, 175
  respiratory acidosis, 186, 531, 532
  respiratory alkalosis, 186, 187, 532
  respiratory compensation in, 174, 175
  rules of thumb in, 175
  treatment of, 521–534
  triple disorders, 188, 533
Acidosis, lactic, 178, 526, 527
  causes of 526, 527
  treatment of, 526, 527
  type A, 526
  type B, 526

Acidosis, metabolic, 70, 176–180, 283, 521–529
  bicarbonate treatment, 521, 522
  diabetic ketoacidosis, 177, 178, 524–526
  diarrhea, 179, 180, 528
  ethylene glycol intoxication, 178, 179
  with increased anion gap, 177–179
  lactic acidosis, 178, 526, 527
  methanol intoxication, 178, 179, 527
  with normal anion gap, 179–182
  in renal insufficiency, 283, 284, 527, 528
  renal tubular acidosis, 180–182, 528, 529
  salicylate intoxication, 178
  symptoms in, 70
  treatment of intoxications, 527
  treatment of organic acidoses, 522–527
Acidosis, renal tubular, 180–182, 226, 401, 528, 529
  calcium stones in, 401
  distal RTA, 180, 181, 528
  Fanconi syndrome in, 181
  hyperkalemia in, 182
  hypokalemia in, 181, 226
  proximal RTA, 181, 528
  treatment, 528, 529
  type 1 RTA, 180, 181, 528
  type 2 RTA, 181, 528
  type 3 RTA, 181, 182
  type 4 RTA, 182, 529
Acidosis, respiratory, 71, 72, 186, 531, 532
  symptoms in, 71, 72
  treatment, 531, 532
ACTH secretion, ectopic, 225
Acyclovir, 373
  nephrotoxicity, 373
Addison's disease, 233, 544
  hyperkalemia, 233
  hyponatremia and, 544
Aldosteronism, glucocorticoid-responsive, 225
Alkalosis, metabolic, 72, 182–185, 224–226, 529–531
  alkali administration and, 185
  apparent mineralocorticoid excess and, 184, 185
  Bartter's syndrome, 185
  chloride resistant, 184, 185, 530, 531
  chloride responsive, 182–184, 530
  diuretics and, 183, 184, 530
  Gitelman's syndrome, 185
  HCl treatment, 531
  hypokalemia and, 224–226
  nasogastric suction and, 183, 530
  primary hyperaldosteronism and, 184
  severe, treatment, 531
  symptoms in, 72
  treatment, 529–531
  treatment by hemofiltration, 531
  vomiting and, 183, 530
Alkalosis, respiratory, 72, 86, 187, 467, 532
  causes, 186, 187
  in pregnancy, 467
  salicylates and, 186
  severe illnesses and, 186
  symptoms in, 72
  treatment, 532
Alport's syndrome, 99, 458–460
  clinical findings, 459
  deafness in, 459
  diagnosis, 459, 460
  genetics, 458
  hematuria in, 99
  pathology, 458, 459
  treatment, 460
Aminoglycosides, 370, 371, 415, 582, 584
  dosing in renal insufficiency, 582, 584
  management, 370, 371
  nephrotoxicity of, 370, 371
  pathology, 370
  for pyelonephritis, 415
Amphotericin, 372, 373
  nephrotoxicity, 372, 373

Amyloidosis, 349–351, 389
clinical features, 350
epidemiology, 349, 350
heroin use and, 389
laboratory findings, 350
pathology, 350
treatment, 350, 351
Analgesic nephropathy, 383–385
clinical presentation, 383
epidemiology, 383–385
Analgesics, 383–385
abuse and chronic renal disease, 383–385
ANCA, 356, 357
Anemia, 51, 284–287, 493
in chronic renal disease, 284–287
erythropoietin treatment, 285–287
and left ventricular hypertrophy, 493
Angiotensin receptor blockers, 277, 305, 315, 375
in diabetic nephropathy, 315
hemodynamic effects of, 375
hypertension and, 277, 305
renal insufficiency and, 277, 305
renoprotective effects, 277, 305
Anion gap, 176–179, 188
calculation of delta anion gap, 188
increased, and metabolic acidosis, 177–179
in metabolic acidosis, 177
in mixed disorders, 188
normal, and metabolic acidosis, 179–182
Antibiotics, 369–374, 410–413
allergic interstitial nephritis and, 371
nephrotoxicity of, 369–374
for urinary tract infection, 410–413
Antidiuretic hormone (ADH), 195, 196, 208
hyponatremia and, 208
hypotonicity and, 208
inappropriate secretion of, 208
Antineutrophilic cytoplasmic antibodies (ANCA), 356, 357
Antiphospholipid syndrome, 347, 362, 363
systemic lupus erythematosis and, 347
Anuria, 1–3
cortical necrosis and, 3
definition, 1
pelvic injury and, 3
rapidly progressive glomerulonephritis and, 3
shock wave lithotripsy and, 3
Ascites, 34, 35
Atheroemboli, 262
acute renal failure and, 262
Atrial natriuretic peptide, 21
Azathioprine, 326, 485, 508
in pregnancy, 485
in transplantation, 508
for treatment of glomerular diseases, 326
Azotemia, prerenal, 4
oliguria and, 4

Bacteriuria, 163, 419–421
asymptomatic, 163, 419–421
due to prostatitis, 421
foley catheter-induced, 163
in pregnancy, 419, 420
in surgical patients, 421
Baroreceptors, 21
Bartter's syndrome, 185, 225, 464, 554, 555
hypokalemia in, 225, 554, 555
Beer potomania, 546
Berger's disease (*see* IgA nephropathy), 335, 336
Beta-blockers, 230, 474
hyperkalemia and, 230
in pregnancy , 474
Biopsy, renal, 322, 323
Bisphosphonates, 567, 568
treatment of hypercalcemia, 567, 568
Blood pressure, 301, 467
circadian rhythm, 301
in pregnancy, 467
Blood urea nitrogen (BUN), 89–92
measurement of, 92

Bone disease, 287–289
  adynamic, 288, 289
  in chronic renal insufficiency, 287–289
  osteitis fibrosa, 288, 289
BUN/creatinine ratio, 92

Calciphylaxis, 45
Calcitonin, 567
  side effects, 567
  treatment of hypercalcemia, 567
Calcitriol, 287–289
  in chronic renal insufficiency, 287–289
Calcium, 237–240
  in bone, 237, 238
  bound fraction, 238, 239
  correction for serum albumin, 238
  correction formula, 238
  gut absorption of, 240
  hypercalcemia, 240–246
  interpretation of serum measurement, 238, 239
  ionized, 238, 239
  normal regulation of, 239, 240
  parathyroid hormone and, 240
  units of measurement, 239
  vitamin D and, 240
Calcium channel blockers, 26, 303, 304, 315, 316, 474, 475
  in diabetic nephropathy, 315, 316
  edema and, 26
  in pregnancy, 474, 475
  in renal insufficiency, 303, 304
Cancer, 242
  hypercalcemia and, 242
Cardiovascular disease, 489–497
  in chronic renal insufficiency, 489–497
Cast nephropathy, 351–353
  clinical features, 352
  epidemiology, 351
  Fanconi syndrome in, 352
  pathology, 351, 352
  treatment, 352, 353
Cephalosporins, 371
  allergic interstitial nephritis and, 371
Cirrhosis, 25, 34, 35
  edema in, 25
  treatment of ascites, 34, 35
Clearance, 9, 77–79
  creatinine, 78, 79
  free water, 9
  inulin, 78
  measurement of, 77, 78
  osmolar, 9
  solute, 9
Cockcroft-Gault formula, 84
Congestive heart failure, 22
Contrast media, 374
  nephrotoxicity of, 374
Coronary artery disease, 494–496
  in renal insufficiency, 494–496
Creatinine, 80–88
  in acute renal insufficiency, 87
  in chronic renal insufficiency, 88
  clearance, 82
  excretion, extrarenal, 84
  generation, 83, 84
  measurement, effect of drugs, 86, 87
  measurement errors, 86
  measurement, serum, 84
  monitoring progression of renal insufficiency, 89
  renal handling of, 80–83
  use for drug-dosing, 88
Creatinine serum, 80
Cryoglobulinemia, mixed essential, 342, 359
  hepatitis C and, 342
  membranoproliferative glomerulonephritis and, 342
Cushing's syndrome, 151, 152, 225
  dexamethasone suppression test in, 151, 152
  hypokalemia in, 225
Cyclophosphamide, 98, 324–326
  hematuria, 98
  for treatment of glomerular diseases, 324–326
Cyclosporine, 233, 248, 326, 377–380, 485, 505–510
  acute nephrotoxicity, 378

[Cyclosporine]
chronic nephropathy, 378–380
drug interactions, 509, 510
hemolytic uremic syndrome and, 380
hyperkalemia and, 233
hypomagnesemia and, 248
nephrotoxicity, 377–380
pathology of nephrotoxicity, 378–380
in pregnancy, 485
striped fibrosis in, 379
for transplantation, 506, 507
for treatment of glomerular disease, 326
Cystic disease, medullary, 463
Cystinuria, 463
Cystitis, 161, 416, 417
recurrent, 417
reinfection, 417
relapse, 417
treatment regimen, 416, 417

Demeclocycline, 372
nephrogenic diabetes insipidus and, 372
Dent's disease, 463, 464
Diabetes insipidus, 9, 11, 200–202, 372, 540
central, 9, 201, 540
due to demeclocycline, 372
due to hypercalcemia, 202
due to lithium, 202
familial, 11
nephrogenic, 9, 11, 201–202, 540, 541
nephrogenic, acquired, 201–202
nephrogenic, familial, 201
Diabetes mellitus, 272, 276, 277, 309–320, 514, 524, 525
ACE inhibitors in, 276
blood sugar control in, 277, 316
chronic renal insufficiency and, 272, 273
DCCT trial, 277, 316
diagnosis of, 309
nephropathy in 309–320
[Diabetes mellitus]
post-transplant, 514
prevention of renal failure in, 277, 316, 317
treatment of ketoacidosis, 524, 525
Diabetic nephropathy, 24, 309–320
ACE inhibitors in, 314, 315
blood pressure control, 312–314
blood pressure goals, 313
calcium channel blockers in, 315, 316
diagnosis of, 310
drug therapy of hypertension in, 313, 314
edema in, 24
incidence of, 310
microalbuminuria screening, 310, 311
nephrology referral, 318
nonpharmacological treatment of hypertension in, 313
protein restriction in, 316, 317
smoking and, 317
treatment of, 312–318
treatment of hyperlipidemia, 317
Dialysis, peritoneal, 486
and pregnancy, 486
Diarrhea, 179, 180
hypokalemia in, 179, 180
Digoxin, 584, 585
dosing in renal insufficiency, 584, 585
Diuresis, 12, 442–444
postobstructive, 442–444
solute, 12
Diuretics, 30–33, 183, 184, 207, 248, 281, 474, 530, 544, 546, 552–557, 585
acetazolamide, 32
amiloride, 553, 554
in chronic renal insufficiency, 281
dosing in renal insufficiency, 585
edema mobilization, 32
hypokalemia and, 224, 553
hypomagnesemia and, 248
hyponatremia and, 207, 544, 546

[Diuretics]
hypotonicity and, 207
loop diuretics, 30, 31
metabolic alkalosis and, 183, 184, 530
potassium-sparing, 32, 552, 553
in pregnancy, 474
spironolactone, 552–554
treatment of hypercalcemia, 566, 567
triamterene, 553
Drug dosing, 575–588
ACE inhibitors, 584
active metabolites in renal insufficiency, 578
aminoglycosides, 582–584
bioavailability, 576
and dialysis therapy, 586
digoxin in renal insufficiency, 584, 585
distribution, 576
diuretics in renal insufficiency, 585
effects of hypoalbuminemia, 576
enhancing drug safety, 581, 582
increasing time interval, 581
liver metabolism, 577
metformin in renal insufficiency, 585
narcotic analgesics in renal insufficiency, 585, 586
patient considerations, 579, 580
pharmacokinetic considerations, 575–579
phenytoin in renal insufficiency, 586
protein binding, 577
reference information, 582
renal excretion, 578
in renal insufficiency, 575–588
renal metabolism, 577, 578
therapeutic index, 580
using reduced dosages, 581

ECF volume depletion, 538, 539
treatment in hypertonicity, 538, 539
Edema, 19–38, 121, 125, 134, 206, 280, 281
causes of, 27
in chronic renal insufficiency, 280, 281
chronic venous insufficiency and, 27
cirrhosis and, 25, 34, 35
[Edema]
congestive heart failure and, 22, 23, 34
diabetic nephropathy and, 24
dietary sodium restriction, 33
diuretic therapy, 30–38
diuretic unresponsiveness, 36–38
drug-induced, 25, 26
glomerulonephritis and, 24
hyponatremia in, 206, 207
hypotonicity in, 206, 207
idiopathic, 25
laboratory evaluation of, 29
in nephritic syndrome, 134, 135
nephrotic syndrome, 24, 35, 36, 121
overfill hypothesis, 24, 121
postdiuretic, 25
pregnancy, 26
pulmonary, treatment, 34
refractory, 36–38
renal insufficiency and, 23, 36
treatment of, 30–38, 125, 281
underfill hypothesis, 24, 121
Effective vascular volume, 21
Endocarditis, bacterial, 340
glomerulonephritis in, 340
End-stage renal disease, 269–271, 426
due to obstructive uropathy, 426
Erythropoietin, 285–287
in chronic renal insufficiency, 285–287
dosage, 286
resistance to, 286
Ethylene glycol intoxication, 178, 179, 527
osmolar gap in, 179
treatment, 527
Extracellular fluid (ECF) volume, 4, 20, 28, 206
assessment of by physical examination, 28
depletion, 206
extravascular sequestration and, 4
hyponatremia and hypotonicity, 206
laboratory evaluation, 28

Fanconi syndrome, 181, 352
in multiple myeloma, 352
in type 2 renal tubular acidosis, 181

Fluoroquinolones, 413, 415
  for pyelonephritis, 415
  for urinary tract infections, 413
Foscarnet, 373
  nephrotoxicity, 373, 374
Fractional excretion of sodium (FE_{Na}), 9
Frequency, 1, 7

Genetics, 447–464
  autosomal mutations, 450
  dominant inheritance, 450
  introduction to, 449–450
  Mendelian, 450
  mutations, 449–450
  phenotype, 450
  recessive inheritance, 450
  and renal diseases, 447–464
  X-linked mutations, 450
Gitelman's syndrome, 185, 225, 249, 464, 554, 555
  hypokalemia in, 225, 554, 555
  hypomagnesemia in, 249
Glomerular disease, 321–365
  azathioprine in, 326
  clinical syndromes, 323
  collapsing glomerulopathy, 331
  cryoglobulinemia, mixed essential and, 342, 359
  cyclophosphamide in, 324–326
  cyclosporine in, 326
  due to amyloidosis, 349–351
  due to anti-glomerular basement membrane antibodies, 347–349
  due to antiphospholipid syndrome, 362, 363
  due to bacterial endocarditis, 340
  due to cryoglobulinemia, 359
  due to fibrillary glomerulonephritis, 353
  due to Goodpasture's syndrome, 347–349
  due to Henoch-Schönlein purpura, 359
  due to IgA nephropathy, 335, 336
  due to immunotactoid glomerulopathy, 353
[Glomerular disease]
  due to lupus nephritis, 344–347
  due to membranoproliferative glomerulonephritis, 333, 334
  due to minimal change disease, 328, 329
  due to poststreptococcal glomerulonephritis, 337–339
  due to scleroderma, 363–365
  due to vasculitis, 354–359
  focal and segmental glomerular sclerosis, 329–331
  glucocorticoids in, 324
  hepatitis B and, 340, 341
  hepatitis C and, 341–343
  HIV associated, 343, 344
  infection associated, 337–344
  membranous nephropathy, 331–333
  methotrexate in, 326
  mycophenolate mofetil in, 326
  nephritic syndrome definition, 323
  nephrotic syndrome definition, 323
  nephrotic-range proteinuria, 323
  rapidly progressive glomerulonephritis definition, 323
  treatment, general principles, 323, 324
  vasculitis definition, 323
Glomerular filtration rate (GFR), 75–79, 84, 85, 89, 272
  in chronic renal insufficiency, 272
  estimation of, 79
  estimation of from serum creatinine, 84
  estimation of from serum values, 85
  initiation of dialysis and, 89
  measurement, 77–79
  normal range, 76
  physiology of, 76, 77
Glomerulonephritis (*see also* Glomerular disease), 24, 129–136, 258, 321–365
  acute renal failure and, 258
  clinical features, 340
  crescentic, 323, 357
  edema in, 24
  endocarditis-associated, 340

[Glomerulonephritis]
epidemiology, 340
fibrillary, 353
immunotactoid, 353
laboratory findings, 340
nephritic syndrome and, 129–136
pathology, 340
Glomerulonephritis, membranoproliferative, 333, 334, 341, 342
clinical features, 334
epidemiology, 333
hepatitis B associated, 341
hepatitis C associated, 342
laboratory findings, 334
pathology, 334
treatment, 334
Type I, 333
Type II, 333
Type III, 333
Glomerulonephritis, membranous (*see* Nephropathy, membranous)
Glomerulonephritis, poststreptococcal, 337–339
clinical features, 337–339
epidemiology, 337
laboratory findings, 337–339
pathology, 337
treatment, 339
Glomerulonephritis, rapidly progressive, 323, 347, 348, 356, 357, 389
anti–glomerular basement membrane disease and, 347–348
definition, 323
due to penicillamine, 389
small vessel vasculitis and, 356, 357
Glomerulosclerosis, 329–331
clinical features, 330
collapsing glomerulopathy, 331
epidemiology, 329
focal and segmental, 329–331
laboratory findings, 330
pathology, 330
treatment, 331
Glomerulus, 321, 322
structure and function, 321, 322
Glucocorticoids, 324, 509
for transplantation, 509
for treatment of glomerular diseases, 324
Goodpasture's syndrome, 258, 347, 348
acute renal failure and, 258
clinical features, 348
epidemiology 347, 348
laboratory findings, 348
pathology, 348
treatment, 348, 349

Heart failure, 206
hyponatremia in, 206
hypotonicity in, 206
HELLP syndrome, 468, 469, 478
acute renal failure in, 478
Hematuria, 95–103, 131, 132, 335, 336, 455, 459, 461–463
abnormal, definition of, 96
asymptomatic, 99
CT scanning in, 101
cyclophosphamide and, 98
cystoscopy in, 102
detection of, 96
diagnosis of, 97
drug-induced, 98
due to Alport's syndrome, 459
due to IgA nephropathy, 335, 336
due to medullary sponge kidney, 462, 463
due to polycystic kidney disease, 455
due to sickle cell nephropathy, 461
due to thin glomerular basement membrane disease, 461
dysmorphic red cells, in, 100
exercise and, 98
familial, benign, 99
fever and, 98
glomerular disease and, 99
glomerular vs. nonglomerular source, 99
imaging studies in, 100–102
intravenous pyelography (IVP) in, 101

[Hematuria]
in nephritic syndrome, 131, 132
polycystic kidney disease and, 99
source of, 97
transient vs. persistent, 98
unexplained, 103
urine cytology in, 102
urine dipstick measurement of, 96, 97
Hemodialysis, 486, 560, 561
and pregnancy, 486
treatment of hyperkalemia, 560, 561
Hemolytic uremic syndrome (HUS), 264, 359–362, 380, 479, 480
acute renal failure and, 264
clinical features, 361
due to cyclosporine, 380
epidemiology, 361
laboratory findings, 361, 362
pathology, 361
postpartum, 479, 480
treatment, 362
Henoch-Schönlein purpura, 358, 359
Hepatic failure, 206, 263
hepatorenal syndrome, 263
hyponatremia in, 206
hypotonicity in, 206
Hepatitis B, 340, 341
glomerular disease in, 340, 341
membranoproliferative glomerulonephritis and, 340, 341
membranous nephropathy and, 340
polyarteritis nodosa and, 340, 341
Hepatitis C, 341–343
cryoglobulinemia, mixed essential and, 342
glomerular disease and, 341–343
Hepatorenal syndrome, 263, 264
acute renal failure in, 263, 264
HIV infection, 343, 344
glomerular disease and, 343, 344
Homocysteine, 495, 496
Hydronephrosis, 426, 466
definition, 426
in pregnancy, 466
Hyperaldosteronism, glucocorticoid-responsive, 225
Hyperaldosteronism, primary, 147–149, 184, 224, 299
adrenal venography in, 149
aldosterone level in, 148, 149
aldosterone/renin ratio in, 148, 149
CT scanning in, 149
hyperkalemia in, 224
hypokalemia in, 148
laboratory evaluation in, 148
metabolic alkalosis in, 184
MR scanning in, 149
renin level in, 148, 149
sodium loading test in, 149
Hyperaquaemia (*see also* Hypotonicity and Hyponatremia), 193, 541–546
treatment, 541–546
Hypercalcemia, 65–67, 202, 240–246, 248, 288, 400, 565–568
bisphosphonates for, 567
calcitonin treatment, 567
and calcium stones, 400
in chronic renal insufficiency, 288
drug-induced, 243
due to granulomatous diseases, 242
due to malignancy, 242
due to primary hyperparathyroidism, 241, 242
due to vitamin D intoxication, 242, 243
ectopic calcitriol and, 242
familial hypocalciuric, 243
gallium nitrate in, 568
glucocorticoids for, 568
hypomagnesemia and, 248
loop diuretics for, 566, 567
mithramycin treatment, 568
nephrogenic diabetes insipidus and, 202
osteoclast activating cytokines and, 242
pamidronate for, 567
parathyroidectomy for, 568
plicamycin treatment, 568
PTH-related peptide and, 242
in renal failure, 243
saline administration in, 566
symptoms in, 66, 67
treatment, 565–568

Hyperglycemia, 204, 205
hyponatremia and, 204, 205
Hyperkalemia, 64, 228–236, 282, 382, 511, 555–563
ACE inhibitors and, 233
β_2 adrenergic agonists in, 558, 559
calcium salts and, 556–558
cardiac effects, 64
cation exchange resins, 560
chronic treatment, 561
cyclosporine and, 233
diagnosis of cause of, 234, 235
dietary potassium restriction in, 561
drug-induced, 233
due to Addison's disease, 233
due to aldosterone deficiency, 231–233
due to β-blockers, 230
due to exercise, 230
due to hemolysis, 228
due to high potassium intake, 228
due to high white cell count, 228
due to hypertonicity, 229, 230
due to hyporeninemic hypoaldosteronism, 231–233
due to impaired potassium excretion, 231
due to insulin deficiency, 229, 230
due to mineral acids, 230
due to periodic paralysis, 230
due to thrombocytosis, 228
due to transcellular shifts, 229–231
EKG changes in, 64
emergency treatment, 556–561
in end-stage renal disease, 561, 562
fludrocortisone treatment, 561
hemodialysis, 560, 561
heparin and, 233
insulin and glucose in, 558
kayexelate treatment, 560, 561
loop diuretics for, 559, 561
mineralocorticoid deficiency, 562
muscle paralysis in, 64, 562, 563
nonsteroidal anti-inflammatory drugs and, 233, 382
periodic paralysis and, 562, 563
peritoneal dialysis, 560, 561
[Hyperkalemia]
potassium-sparing diuretics and, 234
in renal insufficiency, 282
in renal transplantation, 511
sodium bicarbonate treatment, 559
spurious, 228
symptoms in, 64
tacrolimus and, 233
transtubular potassium gradient (TTKG) in, 234
treatment, 555–563
trimethoprim and, 234
tubular defects in potassium secretion, 562
tubulointerstitial disease and, 234
type 4 RTA and, 232
Hyperlipidemia, 122, 126, 279, 494, 495, 513, 514
LDL in chronic renal insufficiency, 494, 495
LP(a) in chronic renal insufficiency, 494, 495
in nephrotic syndrome, 122
in renal insufficiency, 279, 494, 495
in renal transplantation, 513, 514
treatment, 126, 495
Hypermagnesemia, 69, 249, 250, 573
in preeclampsia, 250
symptoms in, 69
treatment, 573
Hypernatremia, 60, 61, 200–203, 537–541
coma in, 61
diabetes insipidus, 200–202
due to hypertonic solutions, 203
due to increased water losses, 200
osmotic diuresis and, 200
symptoms in, 61
treatment, 537–541
Hyperoxaluria, 401, 402
calcium stones and, 402
primary, 402
secondary, 402
Hyperparathyroidism, 40–42, 241, 242, 493
and left ventricular hypertrophy, 493
hypercalcemia in, 241
primary, 241, 242

Hyperphosphatemia, 68, 246, 288, 570, 571
in acute renal failure, 570, 571
aluminum hydroxide, treatment, 571
calcium acetate, treatment, 571
calcium carbonate, treatment, 571
in chronic renal insufficiency, 288
dietary phosphate restriction for, 571
due to hypoparathyroidism, 246
due to pseudohypoparathyroidism, 246
due to renal failure, 246
oral phosphate binders in, 570, 571
sevelamer (Renagel), 571
symptoms in, 68
Hypertension, 46, 134, 137–155, 227, 273, 289, 290, 293–307, 382, 444, 456, 465–477, 491, 492, 504, 512, 513
ACE inhibitors, 304, 305
alcohol and, 153, 154
α–blockers in renal insufficiency, 303
angiotensin receptor blockers, 304, 305
β-blockers in renal insufficiency, 303
calcium-channel blockers in renal insufficiency, 303, 304
causing renal failure, 273
circadian rhythm of blood pressure in, 301
diuretics in renal insufficiency, 303
drug-induced, 152–154
due to cocaine in pregnancy, 476
due to Cushing's syndrome, 151, 152
due to hyperaldosteronism, 147–149
due to immunosuppressive drugs, 512, 513
due to known cause (secondary), 137–155
due to Liddle's syndrome, 299
due to pheochromocytoma, 149–151
due to polycystic kidney disease, 456
[Hypertension]
due to primary hyperaldosteronism, 299
due to renal artery stenosis, 144–147
due to renal disease, 141–144, 293–300
due to renovascular disease, 144–147
essential, in pregnancy, 471, 472
hydronephrosis and, 444
hyperaldosteronism in pregnancy, 476
hypokalemia in, 227
left ventricular hypertrophy in, 492
in nephritic syndrome, 134
nonsteroidal anti-inflammatory drugs and, 154, 382
obstructive uropathy and, 295
oral contraceptives and, 154
pathophysiology of in renal disease, 295–300
pheochromocytoma in pregnancy, 476
in pregnancy, 465–477
in pregnancy, classification, 468
in pregnancy, epidemiology, 468
in pregnancy, treatment, 472–476
in renal transplantation, 504, 512, 513
risk of preeclampsia, 475,476
risk of renal damage, 302
symptoms of, 46
treatment in chronic renal insufficiency, 289, 290, 302–305
treatment in renal transplantation, 513
unilateral renal injury, 293–294
Hypertonicity, 61, 192, 200–203, 537–541
calculation of water deficit, 537, 538
diabetes insipidus, 200–202
due to hypertonic solutions, 203
due to impaired assess to water, 202
due to increased water losses, 200
osmotic diuresis and, 200
rate of correction, 539, 540
symptoms in, 61
treatment, 537–541

Hypervolemia, 192
Hypoaldosteronism, 231–233
  drug-induced, 233
  heparin-induced, 233
  hyperkalemia and, 231–233
Hypoaquaemia (*see also* Hypertonicity and Hypernatremia), 193, 537–541
  treatment, 537–541
Hypocalcemia, 65, 243–245, 249, 568–570
  calcium salts for, 569
  due to citrate, 245
  due to hypomagnesemia, 249, 570
  due to hypoparathyroidism, 243, 244
  due to pseudohypoparathyroidism, 244
  due to PTH unresponsiveness, 244
  familial, 244
  intravenous therapy for, 569
  oral therapy, 569, 570
  seizures in, 65
  symptoms in, 65
  treatment, 568–570
  vitamin D deficiency and, 244, 245, 570
Hypodipsia, 198
Hypokalemia, 62–64, 148, 180, 219–227, 549–555
  alcoholism and, 222
  amiloride for, 554
  cardiac effects, 62
  daily dosage of potassium salts, 551, 552
  diabetic ketoacidosis and, 226
  diagnosis of causes of, 227
  distal RTA and, 226
  diuretic-induced 224, 553
  due to alkalemia, 221
  due to apparent mineralocorticoid excess, 225, 226
  due to Bartter's syndrome, 225, 554, 555
  due to catecholamines, 221
  due to chloride depletion, 224
  due to Cushing's syndrome, 225
[Hypokalemia]
  due to diarrhea, 180, 222
  due to ectopic ACTH production, 225
  due to Gitelman's syndrome, 225, 554, 555
  due to glucocorticoid-responsive hyperaldosteronism, 225
  due to inadequate intake, 219–221
  due to insulin, 221
  due to magnesium depletion, 227
  due to nasogastric suction, 224
  due to renal artery stenosis, 227
  due to renal potassium losses, 223–227
  due to sweating, 222
  due to transcellular shifts, 221
  due to vomiting, 224
  eating disorders and, 222
  ECG changes in, 62
  hypomagnesemia and, 553, 554
  independent of chloride depletion, 224–226
  intravenous therapy, 552
  in malignant hypertension, 227
  metabolic acidosis and, 226–227
  muscle paralysis in, 62
  oral therapy, 551, 552
  in periodic paralysis, 221, 222
  potassium deficit and, 550
  potassium salts, 551
  potassium-sparing diuretics for, 552, 553
  in primary hyperaldosteronism, 148, 554
  proximal RTA and, 226
  spironolactone for, 554
  symptoms in, 62–64
  treatment, 549–555
Hypomagnesemia, 69, 248, 249, 553, 554, 572
  cyclosporine and, 248
  diagnosis of, 249
  diarrhea and, 248
  drug-induced, 248
  Gitelman's syndrome and, 249

[Hypomagnesemia]
hyperaldosteronism and, 248
hypercalcemia and, 248
hypocalcemia and, 249
hypokalemia and, 553, 554
intravenous therapy, 572
laxative abuse and, 248
magnesium oxide for, 572
malabsorption and, 248
oral therapy, 572
poor dietary intake and, 248
symptoms in, 69
tacrolimus and, 248
thiazide diuretics and, 248
Hyponatremia (*see also* Hypotonicity), 58–60, 203–214, 284, 382, 541–547
calculation of solute required, 543, 544
caused by transcellular water shifts, 204, 205
central nervous system disorders and, 208
central pontine myelinolysis and, 60
cerebral salt-wasting and, 208, 213, 547
in chronic renal insufficiency, 207
clinical approach to, 213
drug-induced, 210, 211
due to diuretics, 207, 546
due to ECF volume depletion, 206, 543, 544
due to ectopic ADH secretion, 211
due to endocrine disorders, 208
due to inadequate solute intake, 212, 546
due to inappropriate ADH secretion (SIADH), 208
due to pulmonary disease, 208
due to reset osmostat, 212, 546
due to tumors, 211
due to water-excreting defect, 205–211
in edema, 206, 545
head injuries and, 547
in hepatic failure, 206
[Hyponatremia]
hyperglycemia, 204, 205
in nephrotic syndrome, 207
nonsteroidal anti-inflammatory drugs and, 382
perioperative, 211, 547
pseudohyponatremia, 204
in renal insufficiency, 284
sports and exercise induced, 213
subarachnoid hemorrhage and, 547
symptoms in, 58–60
treatment, 541–546
in asymptomatic patients, 543, 544
in euvolemic patients, 543–545
in symptomatic patients, 543–545
in volume depleted patients, 543, 544
water restriction in, 545, 546
Hypoparathyroidism, 243, 244
hypocalcemia in, 243, 244
Hypophosphatemia, 67, 68, 246, 247, 571, 572
alcoholism and, 247
due to hyperparathyroidism, 247
Fanconi syndrome and, 247
hyperventilation and, 247
kidney transplantation and, 247
phosphate depletion and, 247
sodium/potassium phosphate therapy, 571, 572
symptoms in, 67, 68
vitamin D–resistant rickets, 572
Hyporeninemic hypoaldosteronism, 231–233
hyperkalemia and, 231–233
Hypotonicity (*see also* Hyponatremia), 192, 203–214, 541–547
calculation of solute required, 543, 544
cerebral salt-wasting and, 208, 213, 547
in chronic renal insufficiency, 207
clinical approach to, 213
in congestive heart failure, 206
diuretic-induced, 207, 546
drug-induced, 210, 211

[Hypotonicity]
due to ECF volume depletion, 206
due to ectopic ADH secretion, 211
due to inadequate solute intake, 212, 213, 546
due to reset osmostat, 212, 546
due to tumors, 211
due to water-excreting defect, 205–211
in edema, 206, 545
head injuries and, 547
in hepatic failure, 206
in nephrotic syndrome, 207
perioperative, 211, 547
sports and exercise induced, 213
subarachnoid hemorrhage and, 547
treatment, 541–546
in asymptomatic patients, 543, 544
in euvolemic patients, 543–545
in symptomatic patients, 543–545
in volume depleted patients, 543, 544
water restriction in, 545, 546
Hypovolemia, 20, 192

IgA nephropathy, 99, 335, 336
clinical features, 335
epidemiology, 335
hematuria in, 99
laboratory findings, 335
pathology, 335
secondary causes, 336
treatment, 336
Immunosuppressive drugs, 485, 501, 505–509, 512–514
azathioprine, 508
basiliximab, 506
cardiovascular disease and, 512
causing diabetes mellitus, 514
corticosteroids, 509
cyclosporine, 506, 507
daclizumab, 506
FK506, 507, 508
hypertension and, 512, 513
long-term effects, 512
mycophenolate mofetil, 508
[Immunosuppressive drugs]
nephrotoxicity, 501
OKT3, 506
and pregnancy, 485
sirolimus, 509
tacrolimus, 507, 508

Ketoacidosis, alcoholic, 525, 526
Ketoacidosis, diabetic, 177, 178, 226, 524, 525, 555
hypokalemia in, 226, 555
treatment of 524, 525

Lead, 386, 387
clinical presentation, 387
diagnosis, 386
nephrotoxicity, 386, 387
pathogenesis, 386, 387
treatment, 387
Liddle's syndrome, 226, 299, 464
Lithium, 202, 243
hypercalcemia and, 243
nephrogenic diabetes insipidus and, 202
Loop diuretics, 30, 31
Lupus nephritis, 344–347, 482, 483
clinical features, 344–346
effect on fetal survival, 483
epidemiology, 344
laboratory findings, 344–346
pathology, 344
in pregnancy, 482, 483
treatment, 346–347
Lymphoma, 242
hypercalcemia and, 242

Magnesium, 248, 249
hypermagnesemia, 249, 250
hypokalemia and magnesium depletion, 227
hypomagnesemia, 248, 249
normal regulation of, 248
normal values, 248
Malnutrition, 496
in chronic renal insufficiency, 496
Medullary sponge kidney, 462, 463

Medullary washout, 12
Methanol intoxication, 178, 179, 527
  osmolar gap in, 179
  treatment, 527
Methyldopa, 474
Microalbuminuria, 107, 310, 311
  measurement of 310, 311
  screening for, 310, 311
Minimal change disease, 328, 329
  clinical features, 328
  laboratory findings, 328
  pathology, 328
  secondary causes, 329
  treatment of, 329
Mycophenolate mofetil, 326, 508
  for kidney transplantation, 508
  for treatment of glomerular disease, 326
Myeloma, multiple, 351–353
  renal disease in, 351–353

Narcotics, 585, 586
  dosing in renal insufficiency, 585, 586
Nephritic syndrome, 129–136, 337
  clinical presentation, 130
  due to poststreptococcal glomerulonephritis, 337
  edema in, 134, 135
  hematuria in, 131, 132
  history of, 129
  hypertension in, 134
  laboratory evaluation in, 135, 136
  pathophysiology, 130
  proteinuria in, 132
  red cell casts in, 132
  renal abnormalities in, 133
  renal insufficiency in, 133
Nephritis, interstitial, 234, 260, 371, 381, 382, 389
  acute renal failure and, 260
  allergic, due to cephalosporins, 371
  allergic, due to penicillin, 371
  due to nonsteroidal anti-inflammatory drugs, 260, 381, 382
  due to penicillamine, 389
  hyperkalemia in, 234
Nephronophthisis, juvenile, 463
Nephropathy, 343, 351, 383
  due to analgesics, 383
  due to cast nephropathy, 351–353
  due to multiple myeloma, 351–353
  HIV associated, 343, 344
Nephropathy, membranous, 331–333, 340
  clinical features, 332
  epidemiology, 332
  hepatitis B associated, 340
  laboratory findings, 332
  pathology, 332
  secondary causes, 333
  treatment, 332, 333
Nephropathy, obstructive, 425–444
  fibrosis due to, 436
  GFR in, 437
  hypertension and, 444
  pathophysiology, 433–438
  ureteral pressures in, 434, 435
  vasoconstriction in, 435, 436
Nephrotic syndrome, 24, 35, 36, 113–128, 323, 328–333, 381, 382, 388–390
  ACE inhibitors in, 124
  acute renal failure in, 127
  associated diseases, 119
  complications of, 120–127
  diagnosis, 116, 117
  dietary protein in, 126
  drugs associated with, 120
  due to cocaine, 388
  due to focal and segmental glomerulosclerosis, 329–331
  due to gold, 389, 390
  due to membranous nephropathy, 331–333
  due to mercury exposure, 390
  due to minimal change disease, 328, 329
  due to penicillamine, 389
  edema in, 24, 35, 36, 121, 125
  endocrine abnormalities in, 123
  history in, 117
  hypercoagulability in, 122, 123, 126, 127

[Nephrotic syndrome]
hyperlipidemia in, 122, 125
hyponatremia in, 207
infection in, 123
laboratory evaluation in, 118
lymphoma and, 120
malignancy and, 119, 120
measurement of protein excretion in, 117
nephrotic-range proteinuria, 323
nonsteroidal anti-inflammatory drugs and, 120, 381, 382
overfill hypothesis, 24
pathophysiology, 113–116
physical examination in, 117
renal biopsy in, 118, 119
renal vein thrombosis in, 123
severe hypoalbuminemia in, 125
treatment of, 124
underfill hypothesis, 24
Nephrotoxicity, 367–391
aminoglycosides, 370, 371
management, 370, 371
pathology, 370
drug-induced, 369–385
due to ACE inhibitors, 375
due to acyclovir, 373
due to amphotericin, 372, 373
due to analgesics, 383–385
due to angiotensin receptor blockers, 375
due to cadmium, 387, 388
due to cyclosporine, 377–380
due to foscarnet, 373
due to gold, 389, 389
due to heavy metal exposure, 390, 391
due to illicit drug use, 388, 389
due to lead exposure, 386, 387
due to mercuric chloride, 390
due to methotrexate, 377
due to mithramycin, 377
due to nitrosoureas, 376
due to nonsteroidal anti-inflammatory drugs, 380–382
due to penicillamine, 389
due to pentamidine, 373
[Nephrotoxicity]
due to platinum, 376
due to radiocontrast media, 374
due to rifampin, 372
due to streptozotocin, 376
due to sulfonamides, 372
due to tacrolimus, 380
due to tetracyclines, 372
due to vancomycin, 372
pathophysiology, 368, 369
toxin-induced, 386–391
Neuropathy, 47–49
Nitric oxide, 21
Nitrofurantoin, 411, 413
Nocturia, 1, 7, 50
Nonsteroidal anti-inflammatory drugs, 120, 154, 233, 260, 380–382, 586
acute renal failure and, 260, 381
anaphylactic reactions, 382
hyperkalemia and, 233, 382
hypertension and, 154, 382
interstitial nephritis and, 260, 381, 382
nephrotic syndrome and, 120, 381, 382
nephrotoxicity of, 380–382
papillary necrosis and, 381
sodium retention and, 382
use in renal insufficiency, 586
water retention and, 382

Obstructive uropathy, 256–258, 295
hypertension and, 295
management of, 258
radiological evaluation, 257
ultrasound in, 257
Oliguria, 1, 3–6
acute interstitial nephritis and, 5
acute renal failure and, 3
acute tubular necrosis and, 5
aminoglycoside antibiotics and, 5
amphotericin and, 5
angiotensin converting enzyme (ACE) inhibitors and, 4
congestive heart failure and, 4

[Oliguria]
definition, 1
fractional excretion of sodium (FE_{Na}) in, 4, 5
glomerular disease and, 5
hepatorenal syndrome and, 4
myoglobinuria and, 5
nonsteroidal anti-inflammatory drugs and, 4
obstruction and, 6
in pregnancy, 474
prerenal azotemia and, 4
radiocontrast dye and, 5
sepsis and, 4
urine sediment and, 5
urine sodium concentration and, 5
Oral contraceptives, 154
hypertension and, 154
Osmolality, 197, 198
calculation of, 197, 198
measurement of, 197
Osmolar gap, 179
Osteodystrophy, renal, 287–289

Paralysis, periodic, 221, 222, 230, 555, 562
hyperkalemic, 230, 562
hypokalemic, 221, 222, 555
Parathyroid hormone (PTH), 287–289
in chronic renal insufficiency, 287–289
Penicillin, 371
allergic interstitial nephritis and, 371
Pentamidine, 373
nephrotoxicity, 373
Pericarditis, 45, 46
Phenytoin, 586
dosing in renal insufficiency, 586
Pheochromocytoma, 149–151, 476
CT scan in, 151
history in, 150
laboratory evaluation in, 150
magnetic resonance imaging in, 151
metanephrines in, 150
physical examination in, 150
in pregnancy, 476
Phosphorus, 245–247, 288
hyperphosphatemia, 246, 288
hypophosphatemia, 246, 247
normal regulation of, 245, 246
Polyarteritis nodosa, 340, 341
hepatitis B associated, 340, 341
Polycystic kidney disease, 454–458, 462
autosomal dominant, 454–458
autosomal recessive, 462
bleeding, 456
cerebral aneurysms in, 455, 457
clinical manifestations, 455
colonic diverticuli, 457
complications, 456, 457
diagnosis, 455, 456
genetics, 454
hypertension, 456
infection, 457
liver cysts, 457
management, 458
mitral valve prolapse, 457
pain, 456
pathology, 454, 455
stones, 457
Polydipsia, 11, 199
Polyuria, 1, 6, 8, 11, 14–16, 50, 431, 442–444
causes of, 8
definition, 1
diagnosis, 14
due to postobstructive diuresis, 442–444
in obstructive nephropathy, 431
pregnancy and, 11
solute diuresis and, 8
treatment, 16
water diuresis and, 8
water restriction test, 15
Potassium, 176, 217–236
in acid-base disorders, 176
hyperkalemia, 228–236
hypokalemia, 219–227
intracellular stores, 218
normal intake and balance, 217–219
renal excretion of 218, 219

Potassium salts, 551, 552
intravenous administration, 552
potassium bicarbonate, 551
potassium chloride, 551
potassium citrate, 551
salt substitutes, 551
wax-matrix preparations, 551
Preeclampsia, 465–486
acute fatty liver, 478, 479
acute renal failure in, 477–479
cortical necrosis in, 479
differentiation from primary renal disease, 477
drug treatment of hypertension, 472–476
effect on preexisting renal disease, 481, 482
HELLP syndrome, 468, 469, 476
pathophysiology, 469, 470
prognosis, 476
seizure prophylaxis, 471
treatment, 470, 471
Pregnancy, 465–486
acid-base changes, 467
azathioprine in, 485
changes in renal function, 466, 467
cyclosporine in, 485
in dialysis patients, 486
HELLP syndrome, 468, 469, 476
hemodynamic changes, 467
hemolytic uremic syndrome and, 479
hydronephrosis in, 466
hypertensive emergencies, 475
kidney and ureters, anatomical changes, 465, 466
lupus nephritis and, 482, 483
normal blood pressure, 467
prednisone therapy in, 485
prognosis with preeclampsia, 476
proteinuria in, 480–482
pyelonephritis in, 484
in renal transplant patients, 484–486
salt and water regulation, 467
urinary tract infections in, 483, 484
Prostatitis, 162, 421
Proteinuria, 104–110, 117, 310, 311, 389, 390, 480, 481
due to gold, 389, 390
due to penicillamine, 389
evaluation, 107,108
glomerular, 105
laboratory evaluation, 109
measurement of, 106, 107, 117
microalbuminuria, 107, 310, 311
orthostatic, 108, 109
overflow, 105
pathophysiology, 105
persistent, 109
in pregnancy, 480
in pregnancy, effect on fetal survival, 481
prognosis, 109, 110
protein/creatinine ratio, 108, 117
quantitation, 108
renal biopsy for, 109
transient, 108
tubular, 105
ultrasound in, 109
Pruritus, 40–42
calcium-phosphorus product and, 40
due to hyperparathyroidism, 40–42
Pseudohyponatremia, 204
Pseudohypoparathyroidism, 244
hypocalcemia in, 244
Pyelonephritis, 162, 413–415, 418, 484
aminoglycosides, 415
ampicillin treatment, 415
antibiotic treatment, 413–415
aztreonam treatment, 414
ceftazidime treatment, 414
ceftriaxone treatment, 414
fluoroquinolones, 415
piperacillin treatment, 414, 415
in pregnancy, 484
treatment recommendations, 418
trimethoprim/sulfamethoxazole treatment, 415
Pyuria, urinary infection and, 164, 165

Radiocontrast dyes, nephrotoxicity of, 374

Renal artery stenosis, 144–147
aortography in, 147
doppler ultrasound, 146, 147
evaluation for, 144–147
indications for invasive studies, 146
prevalence, 144
rationale for evaluation, 144, 145
renogram, 146
screening tests, 146, 147
Renal disease, inherited, 447–464
Alport's syndrome, 458–460
Bartter's syndrome, 464
clinical manifestations, 453
cystinuria, 463
Dent's disease, 463, 464
family history, 452
genetic counseling, 454
Gitelman's syndrome, 464
Liddle's syndrome, 464
management, 453, 454
medullary cystic disease, 463
medullary sponge kidney, 462, 463
Mendelian inheritance, 452, 453
polycystic kidney disease, 454–458, 463
sick cell nephropathy, 461
thin glomerular basement membrane disease, 460, 461
Renal failure, acute, 2, 3, 4, 6, 127, 251–268, 381, 388, 389, 477–479, 503
anuria and, 2,3
assessment of renal function in, 252
BUN/creatinine ratio in, 256
conservative support in, 265, 266
CT scan in, 257
definition of, 251
diagnosis of 252–254
due to acute tubular necrosis (ATN), 260–262
due to atheroemboli, 262
due to cyclosporine, 503
due to glomerular disease, 258–260
due to hepatorenal syndrome, 263, 264
due to illicit drug use, 388, 389
[Renal failure]
due to nonsteroidal anti-inflammatory drugs, 381
due to obstructive uropathy, 256–258
due to postrenal causes, 256–258
due to prerenal azotemia, 255, 256
due to thrombotic microangiopathy, 264
epidemiology of, 251
fractional excretion of sodium (FE_{Na}) in, 4, 6, 256, 261
Goodpasture's syndrome and, 258
hemolytic uremic syndrome and, 264
in hospitalized patients, 252
hyperphosphatemia, treatment, 570
nephrotic syndrome and, 127
nutritional treatment, 266, 267
obstruction and, 6
obstruction, management of, 258
oliguria in, 3
physical examination in, 254
pigment nephropathy, 262, 263
postrenal, definition, 254
in pregnancy, 264, 477–479
prerenal, definition, 254
prevention of, 268
radiological evaluation, 257
radionucleotide scan in, 257
in renal transplant patients, 503
rhabdomyolysis and, 262, 263
thrombotic thrombocytopenic purpura (TTP) and, 264
treatment of, 264–268
treatment of hyperkalemia in, 266
ultrasound in, 257
urine sodium excretion in, 256
use of loop diuretics in, 267
use of mannitol in, 267
vasculitis and, 258
Wegener's granulomatosis and, 258
Renal failure, chronic (*see* Renal insufficiency), 269–291
Renal function, Cockcroft-Gault formula, 272

Renal insufficiency, 36, 133, 207, 231, 269–291, 294, 295, 299, 301, 302, 305, 455, 459, 461, 462, 463, 482, 489, 490, 491, 494, 495, 496, 527, 528, 571, 575–588
ACE inhibitors in, 276
acute vs. chronic 253, 254
anemia in 284–287
antinuclear antibodies (ANA) in, 274
blood pressure control in, 275–277
bone disease in, 287–289
calcitriol treatment, 287–289
cardiovascular complications, 489–497
causes, 272
circadian rhythm of blood pressure in, 301
complement levels in, 274
coronary artery disease in, 490, 491, 494, 496
definition, 269
diabetes mellitus and, 272, 273, 277, 278
dietary phosphate restriction in, 288, 571
drug dosing in, 575–588
due to Alport's syndrome, 459
due to autosomal recessive polycystic kidney disease, 462
due to hypertension, 273
due to IgA nephropathy, 273
due to medullary cystic disease, 463
due to polycystic kidney disease, 455
due to renovascular disease, 275
due to sickle cell disease, 461
ECF volume regulation in, 295–300
edema in, 36, 280, 281
effect on fetal survival, 482
epidemiology, 269, 270
history in, 273, 274
homocysteine in, 495, 496
hypercalcemia in, 288
hyperkalemia in, 231
[Renal insufficiency]
hyperlipidemia, control of, 279, 494, 495
hyperphosphatemia in, 288, 571
hypertension in, 289, 290, 294, 295, 302–305, 491, 492
hyponatremia in, 207, 284
left ventricular hypertrophy in, 490, 491
malnutrition in, 496
maneuvers to slow progression, 275–280
metabolic acidosis and, 283, 284, 527, 528
nephrology referral, 290, 291
in nephrotic syndrome, 133
obstructive nephropathy in, 274
osteodystrophy, 287–289
oxidant stress in, 495
pathophysiology of hypertension in, 295
phosphate binders in, 288, 571
physical findings in, 274
pressure natriuresis and, 296–298
protein restriction in, 278
PTH in, 287–289
renal biopsy in, 274
smoking and, 279
sodium restriction in, 281
target blood pressure in, 305
urinalysis in, 274
vascular resistance in, 299, 300
Renal tubular acidosis (RTA), 180–182, 528, 529
distal RTA, 180, 181
Fanconi syndrome in, 181
proximal RTA, 181
type 1 RTA, 180, 181, 528, 529
type 2 RTA, 181, 529
type 3 RTA, 181, 182
type 4 RTA, 182, 529
Renovascular disease, 144–147
aortography in, 147
doppler ultrasound, 146, 147
evaluation for, 144–147
indications for invasive studies, 146

[Renovascular disease]
prevalence, 144
rationale for evaluation, 144, 145
renogram, 146
screening tests, 146, 147
Rhabdomyolysis, acute renal failure and, 262, 263
Rifampin, nephrotoxicity, 372

Salicylates, intoxication, 178, 527
Salt-wasting, cerebral, 208, 213, 547
Scleroderma, 363–365
clinical features, 364
epidemiology, 364
laboratory features, 364
pathology, 364
renal crisis in, 364
treatment, 364, 365
Sclerosis, systemic (*see* Scleroderma), 363–365
Sickle cell disease, 461
chronic renal insufficiency, 461
hematuria in, 461
Sodium, restriction of in renal insufficiency, 281
Solute diuresis, 12
Starling forces, 21
Stones, 393–407, 457, 463
24 hour urine measurements, 398, 399
calcium excretion and, 399
calcium intake and, 398
citrate excretion and, 399
clinical presentation, 394
CT scan for diagnosis, 394
due to cystinuria, 463
due to Dent's disease, 463, 464
epidemiology, 393, 394
evaluation of, 395–399
history, features, 397
intravenous pyelography, 394
laboratory evaluation, 397
lithotripsy treatment, 406
management of, general measures, 398
management, acute, 394, 395
[Stones]
multiple episodes, 398, 399
oxalate excretion and, 399
in polycystic kidney disease, 457
protein intake and, 398
renal ultrasound in, 398
single episode, 395–398
sodium restriction and, 398
surgical treatment, 406
uric acid excretion and, 399
urinalysis in, 397
urine pH and, 399
Stones, calcium, 399–403
due to hyperoxaluria, 401–402
due to hyperuricosuria, 402, 403
due to hypocitraturia, 401
hypercalcemia and, 400
hypercalciuria and, 399, 400
idiopathic, 403
primary hyperparathyroidism and, 400
in type 1 renal tubular acidosis, 401
Stones, cystine, 405, 406
Stones, struvite, 404, 405
and infection, 404
urease inhibitors and, 404
Stones, uric acid, 403, 404
dietary purines and, 403, 404
urine pH and, 403
Sulfonamides, nephrotoxicity, 372
Syndrome of inappropriate ADH secretion (SIADH), 208–211
adrenal insufficiency and, 210
central nervous system disease and, 208
diagnosis of, 211
drug-induced, 210, 211
ectopic ADH secretion and, 211
hyponatremia in, 208
hypothyroidism and, 208
hypotonicity in, 208
pulmonary disease and, 208
tumors and, 211
Systemic lupus erythematosis, 344–347, 482, 483
nephritis and, 344–347
nephritis in pregnancy, 482, 483

Tacrolimus, 233, 248, 380, 507–510
  drug interactions, 509, 510
  hyperkalemia and, 233
  hypomagnesemia and, 248
  nephrotoxicity, 380
Tetracyclines, nephrotoxicity, 372
Thiazides, 31
  hypokalemia and, 31
  metabolic alkalosis and, 31
Thirst disorders, 198, 199
  hypodipsia, 198
  polydipsia, 199
Thrombocytopenia, 359–362
  due to hemolytic uremic syndrome, 359–362
  thrombotic (TTP), 359–362
Thrombocytopenia, thrombotic, 264, 359–362
  acute renal failure and, 264
  clinical features, 361, 362
  epidemiology, 361
  pathology, 361
  treatment, 362
Tonicity disorders, 191–215, 535–548
  treatment, 535–548
Tonicity, normal regulation of, 191–197
Transplantation, renal, 499–520
  acute renal failure in, 502, 523
  annual rate, 500
  bone disease in, 518
  causing diabetes mellitus, 514
  cervical cancer in, 517
  chronic rejection in, 502, 504
  erythrocytosis in, 519
  factors influencing graft survival, 500, 501
  gout and, 518
  graft dysfunction, 502, 503
  graft survival, 500
  hyperlipidemia in, 513, 514
  hypertension in, 504, 513
  immunosuppressive drugs, 501, 505–509
  infection in, 515, 516
  Kaposi's sarcoma in, 517
[Transplantation]
  long-term care, 500
  lymphoma in, 517
  malignancy in, 516–518
  management of chronic rejection, 504
  and pregnancy, 484–486
  reproductive function in, 519
  serum creatinine in, 502, 503
  skin cancer in, 516, 517
  treatment of hypertension in, 513
  urinalysis in, 503
  weight gain in 514, 515
Trimethoprim/sulfamethoxazole, 411, 415
  for pyelonephritis, 415
  for urinary tract infections, 411
Tubular necrosis, acute, 260–262
  fractional excretion of sodium (FE_{Na}) in, 261
  physical examination in, 261
  renal failure in, 260–262
  sodium excretion in, 261
  urinalysis in, 261

Urea, 90, 92
  measurement of, 92
  metabolism, 90
  renal handling of, 90
Uremia, 39–54
  acute vs. chronic renal failure, 52, 53
  anorexia in, 49
  arthritis in, 45
  bleeding diathesis in, 51
  bone disease in, 43, 44
  calciphylaxis in, 45
  cardiomyopathy in, 46
  central nervous system symptoms in, 47
  convulsions in, 47
  diarrhea in, 50
  effect of dialysis on, 53, 54
  mental status changes in, 47
  myopathy in, 42, 43
  nausea and vomiting in, 49, 50
  pericarditis in, 45, 46

[Uremia]
peripheral neuropathy in, 47–49
psychiatric symptoms in, 47
red eye syndrome in, 45
restless leg syndrome in, 48
tendon rupture in, 44
time course of symptoms, 52
vascular disease in, 45
white blood cell function in, 51, 52
Urethritis, 162
Urinalysis, 164, 165, 503
pyuria, 164, 165
in renal transplantation, 503
Urinary tract infection, 157–168, 409–423, 457, 483, 484
abscess, 162, 163, 421, 422
antibiotic therapy, 410–413
asymptomatic, 163
bacterial characteristics, 159, 160
blood culture in, 166
catheter associated, 422
cephalosporins, 413
ciprofloxacin, 413
complicated, 418, 419
cystitis, 161
definition of, 158
diagnosis of, 164
epidemiology of, 157, 158
fluoroquinolones, 413
fungal, 422
inflammatory response to, 160
laboratory evaluation of, 164
microbiology of, 160
nitrofurantoin, 411–413
normal host defenses, 159
pathogenesis, 158–160
in polycystic kidney disease, 457
in pregnancy, 483, 484
prophylaxis, 409, 410
prostatitis, 162, 421
pyelonephritis, 162
pyuria, 164, 165
radiology evaluation in, 166, 167
recurrent, 417
reinfection, 417
relapse, 417
[Urinary tract infection]
renal ultrasound in, 166, 167
treatment, 409–423
trimethoprim, 411
trimethoprim/sulfamethoxazole, 411
urethritis, 162
urinalysis in, 164, 165
urine culture in, 165
Urinary tract obstruction, 3, 425–444
causes, 427–429
clinical findings, 431
complicated by infection, 433
CT scanning, 440
cystography, 440
diagnosis, 438–442
diuretic renogram in, 440, 441
polyuria in, 431
post-obstructive diuresis, 442–444
radioisotope renogram in, 440, 441
resistive index in, 440
symptoms, 429–431
treatment, 442
ultrasonography in, 438–440
Whitaker test, 441, 442
Urine concentration and dilution, 7, 8
antidiuretic hormone in, 8
Urine solute excretion, 13
electrolytes, 13
nonelectrolytes, 13
Urine volume, 1
normal, 1
Uropathy, obstructive (*see* Urinary tract obstruction), 425–444
causes, 427–429
causing end-stage renal disease, 426
congenital abnormalities and, 426
incidence, 426

Vancomycin, nephrotoxicity, 372
Vasculitis, 258, 354–359, 388
acute renal failure and, 258
due to cryoglobulinemia, 359
due to heroin, 388
due to methamphetamines, 388
due to microscopic polyangiitis, 356–358

[Vasculitis]
  due to polyarteritis nodosa, 354–356
  due to Wegener's granulomatosis, 356–358
  pauci-immune, 356–358
  small vessel, 356–359
Vasopressin, 195, 196
Ventricular hypertrophy, 492, 493
  anemia and, 493
  and control of hypertension, 492, 493
  hyperparathyroidism and, 493
Vitamin D, in chronic renal insufficiency, 287–289
Water balance, 1, 193–197
  antidiuretic hormone and, 195, 196
  aquaporin 2 and, 196
  cell volume regulation and, 197
  kidney and, 194, 195
  normal, 193, 194
  serum osmolality and, 197, 198
  tonicity and, 197, 198
  vasopressin and, 195, 196
Water diuresis, 10
Wegener's granulomatosis, 258, 356–358
  acute renal failure and, 258
  clinical features, 357
  laboratory findings, 357, 358
  treatment, 358

About the Editor

F. JOHN GENNARI is the Robert F. and Genevieve B. Patrick Professor of Medicine and Director of the Nephrology Division, University of Vermont College of Medicine, Burlington. The author or coauthor of over 90 articles, book chapters, and books, Dr. Gennari is a Fellow of the American College of Physicians and a member of the American Society of Nephrology, the International Society of Nephrology, and the American Society of Clinical Investigation. He received the B.S. degree (1959) from Yale University, New Haven, Connecticut, and the M.D. degree (1963) from Yale University School of Medicine, New Haven, Connecticut.